PRACTICAL CONTACT DERMATITIS

NOTICE

PRACTICAL CONTACT DERMATITIS

A Handbook for the Practitioner

EDITOR

JERE D. GUIN, M.D.

Professor and Chairman
Department of Dermatology
University of Arkansas for Medical Sciences
Little Rock, Arkansas

McGraw-Hill, Inc.
HEALTH PROFESSIONS DIVISION

New York • St. Louis • San Francisco • Auckland • Bogotá • Caracas
Lisbon • London • Madrid • Mexico City • Milan • Montreal • New Delhi • San Juan
Singapore • Sydney • Tokyo • Toronto

1234567890   DOCDOC   98765

ISBN 0-07-025169-X

This book was set in Times Roman by Monotype Composition Company, Inc.
The editors were Michael Houston and Muza Navrozov;
the production supervisor was Clare B. Stanley;
the cover was designed by Marsha Cohen/Parallelogram;
the index was prepared by Alexandra Nickerson.
R. R. Donnelley & Sons Company was printer and binder.
This book was printed on acid-free paper.

Library of Congress Cataloging-in-Publication Data

Practical contact dermatitis: a handbook for the practitioner /
   editor, Jere D. Guin.
       p.   cm.
   Includes bibliographical references and index.
   ISBN 0-07-025169-X :
   1. Contact dermatitis—Handbooks, manuals, etc.   I. Guin, Jere D.
RL244.H36   1995
   616.5'1—dc20   94-7880

CONTENTS

PART II
STANDARD PATCH-TEST ANTIGENS

PART III
SPECIAL CATEGORIES
IN CONTACT DERMATITIS
AND ECZEMA

PART IV
PRACTICAL MANAGEMENT, METHODS,
AND SOURCES OF MATERIALS

Color Plates appear between pages 430 and 431.

CONTRIBUTORS*

Robert M. Adams, M.D. [43]
Clinical Professor of Dermatology
Stanford University School of Medicine
Stanford, California

Michael H. Beck, M.D. [49]
University Department of Dermatology
The Skin Hospital
Salford, Lancs, United Kingdom

Donald V. Belsito, M.D. [34]
University of Kansas Medical Center
Division of Dermatology
Kansas City, Kansas

Derk P. Bruynzeel, M.D. [7]
Professor
Free University Academic Hospital
Amsterdam, The Netherlands

Magnus Bruze, M.D., Ph.D. [5]
Department of Occupational Dermatology
University Hospital
Malmö, Sweden

Jyoti B. Burruss, M.D. [37]
Indianapolis, Indiana

Jose G. Camarasa, M.D. [39]
Professor and Chairman, Department
of Dermatology
Universitat Autonoma de Barcelona
Unitat Docent, Hospital Del Mar
de Barcelona
Barcelona, Spain

Ponciano D. Cruz, Jr., M.D. [1]
Department of Dermatology
University of Texas Southwestern
Medical Center
Dallas, Texas

Arthur D. Daily, M.D. [52]
Associate Clinical Professor of Medicine
Brown University
Fall River, Massachusetts

Vincent A. DeLeo, M.D. [8, 9]
Associate Professor of Dermatology
Columbia University
Chief of Dermatology Service (Interim)
St. Luke's–Roosevelt Hospital Center
New York, New York 10019

**An Dooms-Goossens, R. Pharm.,
Ph.D.** [6]
Associate Professor
Department of Dermatology
University Hospital
Catholic University of Leuven
Leuven, Belgium

**Tuula Estlander, M.D.,
Ph.D.** [30, 35]
Section of Dermatology
Finnish Institute of Occupational Health
Helsinki, Finland

Susan E. Feinman, Ph.D. [20]
Immunotoxicologist
Potomac, Maryland

* The numbers in brackets following the contributor name refer to chapter(s) authored or co-authored by
the contributor.

xi

Torkel Fischer, M.D.   [33]
Professor of Dermatology
Departments of Dermatology
  and Occupational Dermatology
Karolinska Hospital
  and National Institute
  of Occupational Health
Solna, Sweden

Lars Förström, M.D., Ph.D.   [42]
Department of Dermatology
Helsinki University Central Hospital
Helsinki, Finland

Joseph F. Fowler, M.D.   [37]
Associate Professor of Dermatology
University of Louisville
Louisville, Kentucky

Anthony F. Fransway, M.D.
                              [14, 23, 40]
Associates in Dermatology
Fort Myers, Florida
Assistant Professor of Dermatology
University of South Florida
Tampa, Florida

**C. L. Goh, M.D., F.R.C.P.
  (Edin.)**   [3]
Clinical Associate Professor
Medical Director
National Skin Centre
Singapore

**Anton C. de Groot, M.D.,
  Ph.D.**   [32]
Carolus-Liduina Hospital
's-Hertogenbosch, The Netherlands

Jere D. Guin, M.D. [10, 11, 12, 13,
  15, 16, 17, 18, 19, 21, 22, 24, 25,
  26, 27, 28, 29, 36A, 36B, 38, 45,
    48, 50, Appendixes B and C]
Professor and Chairman
Department of Dermatology
University of Arkansas for Medical Sciences
Little Rock, Arkansas

Jeff D. Harvell, M.D.   [2]
Department of Dermatology
University of California,
  San Francisco
San Francisco, California

Riitta Jolanki, D. Tech.   [30, 35]
Section of Dermatology
Finnish Institute of Occupational Health
Helsinki, Finland

**Lasse Kanerva, M.D.,
  Ph.D.**   [30, 35]
Section of Dermatology
Finnish Institute of Occupational Health
Helsinki, Finland

Kaija H. Lammintausta, M.D.   [2]
Department of Dermatology
Turku University Central Hospital
Turku, Finland

**Antti I. Lauerma, M.D.,
  Ph.D.**   [42]
Department of Dermatology
Helsinki University Central Hospital
Helsinki, Finland

Howard I. Maibach, M.D.   [2, 7]
Professor
Department of Dermatology
University of California Medical School
San Francisco, California

**Deborah F. Mac Farlane,
  M.D.**   [8, 9]
Department of Dermatology
College of Physicians and Surgeons
Columbia University
New York, New York

Susan B. Mallory, M.D.   [44]
Associate Professore of Medicine
Department of Dermatology and Pediatrics
Washington University School of Medicine
  and St. Louis Children's Hospital
St. Louis, Missouri

Hideo Nakayama, M.D.   [46, 47]
Saiseikai Central Hospital
Tokyo, Japan

Bo J. Niklasson, B.Sc.
[51, Appendix A]
Department of Occupational Dermatology
University Hospital
Malmö, Sweden

Deborah K. Phillips, M.D.   [18]
Longview, Texas

Patricia Podmore, F.R.C.P.   [31]
Anderson House
Altnagelvin Area Hospital
Londonderry, North Ireland

Sakari Reitamo, M.D.   [42]
Department of Dermatology
Helsinki University Central Hospital
Helsinki, Finland

Elizabeth Sherertz, M.D.   [41]
Professor and Vice Chairman
Department of Dermatology
Bowman Gray School of Medicine
Wake Forest University
Winston-Salem, North Carolina

James S. Taylor, M.D.   [4]
Head, Section of Industrial Dermatology
The Cleveland Clinic Foundation
Cleveland, Ohio

William J. Work, Ph.D. [36A, 36B]
Corporate Exploratory Research
Rohm and Haas Company
Bristol, Pennsylvania

PREFACE

When clinicians are confronted with a difficult and recalcitrant eczema, both patients and physicians ask themselves what is wrong and why the problem is unresponsive. The reason patients with eczema fail to get well is certainly not a lack of potent topical medications. The pharmaceutical industry has not been slack in providing a procession of powerful therapeutic agents. Patients with eczema frequently fail to respond to effective pharmacologic agents because the cause has not been removed, and that cause is often contact dermatitis, either irritant or allergic. Why then is the subject not more emphasized in training programs and why do dermatologists not do more testing for contact allergy? For a period of time the test materials were not available commercially in the United States. Now the answer most often heard is that despite so much scholarly information published, it is difficult to know what to tell people because even when positive tests are found there is relatively little information in the patient's language which will clearly explain how to recognize and avoid the causative agent.

Now why publish another book on contact dermatitis? There are several scholarly publications in the field, with more than one published in the last three years. There are also two journals concerned with contact reactions and other occupational and general dermatology journals which publish manuscripts on contact dermatitis. Computerized data bases are available to aid in finding the material, but it takes time and with today's emphasis on efficiency, uncovering the information for individual patients becomes overwhelming. Therefore there is a need then for an immediate source of information for patients known to be allergic to standard (and indeed nonstandard) contact allergens. Patients expect their doctors not only to provide an understanding of their problems, but also to furnish sources of both exposure and products which can be safely substituted. Currently such expectations seem unrealistic, but unless we as physicians can provide it, the remainder of the treatment program will also be in jeopardy. Therefore, we have written this book to try to furnish busy practitioners with practical, usable information which can easily be transferred to their patients.

The major asset of this book is the handouts, designed specifically for patients. Because no source can cover everything about a subject, patients should be told that handouts are furnished as an aid to understanding.

The intent of each author is to provide practical information to the physician and through the physician to the patient. We have attempted to help in the area of contact dermatitis by furnishing information both on individual antigens used in testing and on special sources of contact such as medications, clothing, plants, cosmetics, sunlight, fragrances, etc. In addition, we have included methodology for testing to standard test agents as well as testing to materials not in the standard kit, and we have attempted to describe to the readers our approach to recognition and management of patients with contact dermatitis.

Recently, during my illness my patients were tested by other physicians, many of whom were still in training. To my delight, on returning I found the patients to be improving nicely as they were surprisingly well informed about their conditions. They had received their information mostly through handouts, the same ones published in the book, especially those in the chapters on standard antigens. The compelling reason for the book then is to provide a source of practical information, much of which can easily be copied and handed to the patient. Hopefully, not only will furnishing this information to patients improve the quality of their care, but it will also allow many physicians who might not have undertaken patch testing and prick testing to add this methodology to their practices.

I would like to thank Dr. Sigfrid Fregert, Dr. Magnus Bruze, Dr. Riitta Jolanki, and Dr. Ann-Therese Karlberg for their help in reviewing some of the material.

PRACTICAL CONTACT DERMATITIS

I

CONTACT DERMATITIS
AND PATCH TESTING

1

BASIC MECHANISMS UNDERLYING CONTACT ALLERGY

Ponciano D. Cruz, Jr.

The skin is an integral part of the immune system; as such, it can be involved in a variety of disorders as the initiator, regulator, or target organ of immune responses. The immunologic function of skin is perhaps best exemplified by allergic contact dermatitis, a disorder that was considered even early on as a model of the cellular or delayed type of hypersensitivity (Table 1-1). Recent advances indicate that allergic contact dermatitis is a T-cell-mediated disorder that develops in genetically susceptible individuals following epicutaneous contact with particular chemical substances.

Most contact allergens are haptens—that is, simple chemicals that bind to proteins to form a complete antigen. Key to understanding the pathogenesis of contact allergy is an appreciation of the discriminate nature in which chemicals can serve as antigens. Clearly, not all chemicals act as allergens. In fact, experimental data implicate three sequential criteria necessary for a chemical to serve as a contact allergen (Fig. 1-1). First, the chemical must be able to penetrate the principal barrier in skin, namely the stratum corneum, and thereby reach living cells of the epidermis. Although many chemicals can accomplish this, not all produce contact allergy. Because only molecules with molecular mass less than 500 Da are capable of penetrating the stratum corneum, it is generally accepted that most contact allergens share the common characteristic of being low-molecular-weight compounds. Another property that promotes transit through the stratum corneum is lipophilicity, or lipid-solubility. Thus, most (if not all) contact allergens are small, lipophilic molecules.[1]

Within the epidermis, chemicals can bind to different cell-associated and cell-free proteins. The hapten-protein conjugates that form are potentially antigenic. The second criterion that governs whether a hapten can become an allergen is its appropriate presentation by antigen presenting cells (APCs) to T lymphocytes. During the primary sensitization process, the actual presentation of the antigen to T cells is thought to occur within draining lymph nodes. In this scenario, antigen is taken up and processed in skin by APCs, which migrate to regional lymph nodes to interact with T cells.

Langerhans cells, which are the principal APCs within epidermis, appear to be responsible in great part for presentation of contact allergens. Recent laboratory studies

3

**TABLE 1–1. Gell and Coombs'
Classification of Immune-
Mediated Reactions**

Humoral	
Type I	Anaphylactic
Type II	Cytotoxic
Type III	Immune complex
Cellular	
Type IV	Delayed hypersensitivity

indicate that haptens (unlike irritants) cause Langerhans cells to (1) acquire more endocytic organelles,[2] (2) upregulate expression of major histocompatibility complex (MHC) molecules on their surfaces[3] and of particular cytokines such as interleukin-1β (IL-1β), (3) migrate in greater numbers to draining lymph nodes,[4] and (4) exhibit augmented APC function.[5] These data, however, do not exclude the possibility that other cells in skin, especially in the dermis, may serve as APCs for contact allergens, including Langerhans cell precursors, other dendritic cells, and macrophages.[6]

In general, protein antigens are processed within APCs into relatively short oligopeptides that are recognized by T cells. Such antigen processing may encompass a series of biochemical events that includes internalization of proteins within APCs, degradation into peptide fragments within acidic intracellular vacuolar compartments such as endosomes and lysosomes, linkage of peptide fragments with MHC molecules, and finally expression of the peptide-MHC complexes on the APC surface.[6] In the case of haptens, it is not certain whether similar processing is required or whether mere binding of the chemical to MHC molecules (already present on the APC surface) will suffice. In either case, APCs bearing antigen-MHC complexes are capable of interacting with responder T cells via their T-cell receptor complexes.

The third determinant of whether or not a chemical can act as an allergen is the potential to activate T cells and cause their proliferation in a clonal fashion. Activation results in the induction of transmembrane signals within T cells that trigger responses manifested ultimately as expression of new T-cell surface molecules, secretion of a host of lymphokines, and proliferation and differentiation of the T cells.[6] Clonal proliferation, which assumes the presence of precursor T cells that specifically recognize the contact allergen, may account for variable genetic susceptibility to different allergens. Thus, individuals lacking precursor T cells for the antigenic form of urushiol may never be sensitized to poison ivy.

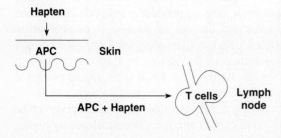

FIG. 1–1. For a chemical to serve as a hapten for contact allergy, it must (1) be able to penetrate the stratum corneum, thereby reaching living epidermal cells; (2) interact with and activate antigen presenting cells in skin, and (3) be capable of stimulating proliferation of T cells in an antigen-specific (or clonal) manner.

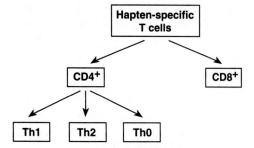

FIG. 1–2. The spectrum of T cells that may be activated in contact allergy includes CD4+ and CD8+ T cells as well as Th1, Th2, and Th0 subsets within the CD4-bearing population.

Different types of T cells possess disparate phenotypic and functional properties. For example, T cells are categorized into those bearing CD4 or CD8 molecules on their surfaces (Fig. 1-2). In addition, CD4+ T cells are now classified into Th1 and Th2 subsets, based on the lymphokines they secrete (Fig. 1-2). Th1 cells produce IL-2 and interferon γ (IFNγ), both of which are proinflammatory cytokines believed to be the soluble mediators of delayed hypersensitivity reactions. By contrast, Th2 cells produce IL-4, IL-5, and IL-6, which are responsible for helping B cells produce antigen-specific antibodies. These two T-cell subsets are capable of counterregulating each other, since IFNγ secreted by Th1 cells can inhibit proliferation of Th2 cells, whereas IL-10, an additional cytokine secreted by Th2 cells, can inhibit proliferation of Th1 cells.[6]

The disparate (even opposing) functions of T-cell subsets may explain the observation that effector and suppressor mechanisms are set in motion simultaneously during the induction of contact allergy. Although yet unproven, the proinflammatory Th1 cells may indeed be the mediators of the effector response, whereas the Th2 cells may mediate the suppressor response. Both CD4+ and CD8+ T cells are activated during the induction of contact allergy in mice.[7] In similar studies, a spectrum of CD4+ T cells were activated, including populations with Th1, Th2, and even overlapping Th1/Th2 (or Th0) characteristics (unpublished observations).

Following initial sensitization, there would then exist an expanded population of antigen-specific T cells capable of reacting to subsequent antigenic exposures. The clinical outcome of each confrontation or challenge with antigen depends upon several factors. First and foremost is the integrity of the stratum corneum. Obviously, an injured or diseased stratum corneum that allows greater penetrance of exogenous substances will increase the chances for a chemical to activate APCs in skin. A second factor is the viability of Langerhans cells or other APCs in skin, since these cells need to seek and bind appropriate responder T cells. Third is the presence or absence of extracellular factors, including cytokines produced by keratinocytes, that can promote or hinder APC–T-cell engagement. For example, IL-1 and granulocyte-macrophage colony stimulating factor (GM-CSF) produced by keratinocytes can potentiate the APC function of Langerhans cells. The final factor is the preexisting mix of T-cell subtypes specific for the antigen. A higher frequency of cells of an effector subtype increases the likelihood that a dermatitis will result, whereas a higher frequency of cells of a suppressor subtype may dampen or prevent the dermatitis.

Knowledge of the different factors that govern the development of allergic contact dermatitis provides a useful framework for potential diagnostic and therapeutic interventions. In the future, it may be possible to predict those chemicals that can serve as haptens based on their physicochemical characteristics (which enable them to penetrate the stratum corneum and to activate APC). Genetic predisposition toward specific allergens may be identified based on the precursor frequency of effector and suppressor T cells. Finally, established sensitivities may be prevented or alleviated by manipulating the interaction between APC and haptens or between APC and T cells.

REFERENCES

1. Baer RL: The mechanism of allergic contact hypersensitivity, in Fisher AA (ed): *Contact Dermatitis.* Philadelphia, Lea & Febiger, 1986, pp 1–8.
2. Kolde G, Knop J: Different cellular reaction patterns of epidermal Langerhans cells after application of contact sensitizing, toxic, and tolerogenic compounds: A comparative ultrastructural and morphometric time-course analysis. *J Invest Dermatol* 89:19–23, 1987.
3. Aiba S, Katz S: Phenotypic and functional characteristics of in vivo–activated Langerhans cells. *J Immunol* 145:2791–2796, 1990.
4. Enk A, Katz S: Early molecular events in the induction phase of contact sensitivity. *Proc Natl Acad Sci USA* 89:1398–1402, 1992.
5. Kripke ML, Munn CG, Jeevan A, Bucana C: Evidence that cutaneous antigen presenting cells migrate to regional lymph nodes during contact sensitization. *J Immunol* 145:2833–2838, 1990.
6. Cruz PD, Bergstresser PR: Antigen processing and presentation by epidermal Langerhans cells, in Sauder DN (ed): Dermatologic Clin 8:633–647, 1990.
7. Gocinski BL, Tigelaar RE: Roles of CD4[+] and CD8[+] T cells in murine contact sensitivity revealed by in vivo monoclonal antibody depletion. *J Immunol* 144:4121–4127, 1990.

2

IRRITANT CONTACT DERMATITIS

Jeff D. Harvell
Kaija Lammintausta
Howard I. Maibach

Contact dermatitis is *dermatitis invoked as a result of exposure to an exogenous agent.* In occupational settings, contact dermatitis accounts for approximately 90 percent of skin disease.[1] Contact dermatitis is divided into two types, based on differences in mechanism—irritant contact dermatitis, the subject of this chapter, and allergic contact dermatitis. Irritant dermatitis accounts for approximately 70 percent of occupationally induced contact dermatitis and allergic contact dermatitis for 30 percent.[1] In both irritant and allergic types, *contact* with an exogenous substance is key in pathogenesis. The difference between the two is largely mechanistic. In the case of allergic contact dermatitis, the substance is an allergen and the mechanism is that of a delayed (type IV) hypersensitivity reaction, mediated by T cells and requiring prior sensitization. In contrast, irritant reactions encompass mechanisms which do not require previous sensitization and do not proceed via type IV pathways. This distinction may be simplistic, but it reflects the fact that less is known regarding the mechanisms of irritant contact dermatitis. In this chapter, the term *irritant contact dermatitis* is used in an all-encompassing way to describe lesions that probably arise through diverse mechanisms, including histiocytic proliferation (giving rise to granulomas), direct effects on melanocytes (giving rise to hyper- or hypopigmentation), and effects on the pilosebaceous unit (giving rise to pustular and acneiform reactions).

The main distinction to be made in clinical practice, however, is as to whether the dermatitis is allergic or irritant. This is not an easy task, as the morphology of irritant and allergic contact dermatitis reactions can be virtually identical. General clinical differences have been noted. Allergic contact dermatitis reactions are more likely to exhibit a delayed onset of symptoms, to produce symptoms of itch over sting and burn, to produce vesicles, and to occasionally generalize (e.g., into erythroderma).[2] Despite these clues, a definitive diagnosis of irritant contact dermatitis is made based on a history of contact with a known irritant and negative patch tests to relevant allergens (i.e., one must exclude allergic contact dermatitis).

Of course, allergic contact dermatitis is not the only dermatologic condition which exists in the differential diagnosis, and, based on the site of the reaction, the differential can sometimes be extensive. In the case of hand dermatitis, for example, the differential diagnosis includes psoriasis, atopic dermatitis, fungal infection, and allergic contact dermatitis. The first two can usually be distinguished from irritant contact dermatitis based on the characteristic lesions at other sites; fungal infection is excluded by potassium hydroxide preparation; and allergic contact dermatitis can be ruled out through proper patch testing. Biopsy is of less value, especially when one is attempting to distinguish between irritant and allergic contact dermatitis, as the histopathology may be virtually identical.

Further complicating the issue is the fact that in many instances, irritant and allergic contact dermatitis coexist. In other words, irritant contact dermatitis predisposes to the development of allergic contact dermatitis (and vice versa), as irritant contact dermatitis disrupts properties of the cutaneous barrier, allowing the ingress of allergens.[3-7] Therefore, allergic contact dermatitis may in some cases represent the primary disease process, while in others it may be superimposed upon an irritant contact dermatitis.

TYPES OF IRRITANT CONTACT DERMATITIS

Differences in the clinical presentation of irritant contact dermatitis has generated a classification scheme as seen in Table 2-1. Irritant contact dermatitis is classified into acute irritant dermatitis (primary irritation), irritant reaction, delayed acute irritant contact dermatitis, cumulative irritant dermatitis, pustular and acneiform irritant dermatitis, mechanically induced dermatitis, and subjective irritation. This classification is meant to draw attention both to the varied morphology and mode of onset of irritant contact dermatitis; however, it is recognized that the terminology may cause confusion.

The "classic" classification of contact dermatitis (both irritant and allergic) is one based mainly on morphology (i.e., *acute*—erythema, vesicles, weeping, crusting, edema; *subacute*—erythema, dryness, scale, fissuring; and *chronic*—lichenification, dryness, scale, fissuring, hyperpigmentation). The latter scheme is especially useful for describing treatment options, so it is used in the treatment section of this chapter.

Acute Irritant Dermatitis (Primary Irritant Dermatitis)

Acute irritant dermatitis results from contact with a primary irritant of high potency. Exposure is often industrial and accidental. The classic symptoms of "acute" dermatitis (erythema, edema, vesicles and/or bullae, and weeping) develop at the exposed site. This type usually heals soon after exposure, but in rare cases it may persist for a longer period of time.

Irritant Reaction

This type of irritant contact dermatitis is most frequently seen among individuals who are newly engaged in "wet work" (i.e., neophyte hairdressers, bartenders, food preparers, waiters/waitresses, nurses, surgeons etc.). The dermatitis consists of erythema and chapping, which develop soon after wet work is initiated. Typically, the dermatitis subsides after the skin adapts to the new environmental exposure through as yet unknown mechanisms.[8-10]

TABLE 2-1. Types of Irritation in Humans

Type	Onset	Characteristics
Acute irritant dermatitis	Acute	Vesicles/bullae, erythema, edema
Irritant reaction	Acute	Erythema, papules, dryness
Delayed acute irritant contact dermatitis	Delayed (8 to 24 h)	Vesicles/bullae, papules, erythema
Cumulative irritant contact dermatitis	Slow (weeks to years)	Erythema, papules, dryness scale, fissuring
Pustular and acneiform contact dermatitis	Moderately slow (weeks to months)	Papules, pustules, comedones
Mechanically induced irritant contact dermatitis	Moderately slow (weeks to months)	Lichenification, callus, bullae (blisters), hyperpigmentation
Subjective irritation	Immediate (within 1 h)	No visible changes

Source: Adapted with permission from Lammintausta and Maibach.[34]

Delayed Acute Irritant Contact Dermatitis

Some contactants can induce an acute irritant dermatitis picture, as described above, only after a lag period of 8 to 24 h or more after exposure. Examples include anthralin, *bis* (2-chloroethyl) sulfide, butanedioldiacrylate, dichlor (2-chlorovinyl) arsine, epichlorhydrin, ethylene oxide, hydrofluoric acid, hexanedioldiacrylate, hydroxypropylacrylate, podophyllin, and propane sulfone.[11-12]

Cumulative Irritant Dermatitis

This type of contact dermatitis is the most frequently encountered in clinical practice. It is due to substances which are capable of inducing a visible reaction only after repeated exposures, sometimes occurring over a period of days, weeks, or years. With each repeated exposure, the threshold for visible irritation is decreased until, finally, an episode of minor damage produces a visible dermatitis. The classic morphology of this type consists of erythema and dryness, followed by scaling and fissuring.[11,13-15]

Pustular and Acneiform Irritant Dermatitis

Pustules, papules, and comedones are often produced by contact with metals,[16-18] cutting oils, greases, tar, asphalt, chlorinated naphthalenes, and polyhalogenated naphthalenes.[19] Similar acneiform lesions can result from the combined effects of occlusion, pressure, and friction, as described by Mills and Kligman[20] (acne mechanica). These are evident on the shoulders of football players due to shoulder pads, on the backs of truck drivers due to pressure in the seated position, and on the necks of violinists and violists ("fiddler's neck").[21]

Mechanically Induced Irritant Contact Dermatitis

Mechanical processes of friction and pressure can induce varied reaction patterns which include lichenification, fissuring, calluses, bullae (blisters), and hyperpigmentation.[22-24]

Calluses and blisters are frequently seen at characteristic sites, depending upon a person's occupation (i.e., occupational stigmata).[25] The pustules and papules of acne mechanica (described above) are also forms of mechanically induced irritant contact dermatitis.[20] It should be emphasized that repeated microtrauma may, by itself, produce irritant contact dermatitis; however, often physical trauma and exposure to irritants are seen together in industrial processes, one exacerbating the other.

Subjective Irritation

In this form of reaction, no visible dermatitis is seen. Rather, the patient, frequently labeled as having "sensitive skin," reports subjective symptoms of burning, stinging, and itching after contact with certain substances. Symptoms usually develop within 1 h of exposure. Since the reaction is "immediate," these reaction patterns may represent a form of contact urticaria. Compounds which have been shown to cause such reactions include benzoic acid, sorbic acid, and sodium benzoate (found in many cosmetics as preservatives) and cinnamic aldehyde (found in mouthwash as a flavoring agent), among others. Several thorough reviews of contact urticaria are available.[26-28]

MORPHOLOGY

The morphology of irritant contact dermatitis reactions is wide and in some cases agent-specific (Table 2-2). The morphology of irritant contact dermatitis comprises a spectrum which includes acute dermatitis reactions with erythema, edema, vesicles as well as weeping to chronic dermatitis reactions with lichenification, fissuring, dryness, and scale. In addition, pustular reactions, granulomas, hyper- and hypopigmentation, and miliaria can also be manifestations of irritant contact dermatitis (Table 2-2). Follicular pustules, especially on the extensor surfaces of the forearms, are frequent in industrial processes in which the worker is exposed to cutting fluids and oils.[19] Granulomas arise from a foreign body reaction to inorganic materials such as silica, berrylium, and talc.[29] Hyperpigmentation is often seen as a late manifestation of a healing irritant reaction or, on the other hand, can be caused by substances which have a direct effect on melanocytes, such as coal tar, pitch, asphalt, creosote, and other coal derivatives.[30] Hypopigmentation is often the result of direct damage to melanocytes by phenolic or benzyl organics (Table 2-2).[31] The papules and vesicles of miliaria (commonly known as heat rash) are produced as a result of sweat duct occlusion and are frequently seen among hospitalized, bedridden patients. Occlusive exogenous materials such as clothing and tapes in combination with overheating are probably involved in the pathogenesis of this eruption.

LOCALIZATION

In general, irritant dermatitis is localized to the site of contact. In some cases, localization of the dermatitis can provide valuable clues as to causative agents. Dermatitis localized to exposed areas (face, arms, hands) is often a clue to airborne irritant gases and vapors.[32] Exposure to solid airborne particles such as dust or fibers often causes dermatitis on

TABLE 2–2. Clinical Features That May Suggest the Etiology of Irritant Contact Dermatitis

Ulcerations
  Strong acids, especially chromic, hydrofluoric, nitric, hydrochloric, sulfuric
  Strong alkalis, especially calcium oxide, sodium hydroxide, ammonium hydroxide, calcium hydroxide,
    sodium metasilicate, sodium silicate, potassium cyanide, trisodium phosphate
  Salts, especially arsenic trioxide, dichromates
  Solvents, especially acrylonitrile, carbon bisulfide
  Gases, especially ethylene oxide, acrylonitrile
Folliculitis and acneiform lesions
  Arsenic trioxide
  Glass fibers
  Oils and greases
  Tar
  Asphalt
  Chlorinated naphthalenes
  Polyhalogenated biphenyls
  Mechanical processes
  Metals
Miliaria
  Occlusive clothing and dressing
  Adhesive tape
  Ultraviolet
  Infrared
  Aluminum chloride
Pigmentary alterations
  Hyperpigmentation
    Any irritant (healing phase)
    Metals, such as inorganic arsenic (systemically), silver, gold, bismuth, mercury
    Radiation: ultraviolet, infrared, ionizing
  Hypopigmentation
    p-tert-Amylphenol
    p-tert-Butylphenol
    Hydroquinone
    Monobenzyl ether of hydroquinone
    Monomethyl ether of hydroquinone
    p-Cresol
    3-Hydroxyanisole
    Butylated hydroxyanisole
    1-*tert*-Butyl-3,4-catechol
    1-Isopropyl-3,4-catechol
    4-Hydroxypropiophenone
Granulomas
  Keratin, silica, beryllium, talc, cotton fibers

Source: Adapted with permission from Lammintausta and Maibach.[34]

covered parts of the body (i.e., beneath belts or collars).[33] Clothing dermatitis typically involves the anterior thighs, upper back, periaxillary areas, and feet.[34]

EXTERNAL FACTORS

Such factors as the nature of the irritant and the exposure conditions also affect the degree of reactivity seen in the skin. The type of irritation produced depends upon physicochemical properties of the substance, such as molecular size, ionization, polarization, and solubility. Also, exposure conditions such as concentration, volume, application time, and duration on and in the skin can determine the degree of irritation seen. Usually, long exposure time and large volume increase cutaneous penetration and lead to an acute response. Occlusion also enhances penetration and thus increases irritation.[35] Gloves and clothing, while normally providing protection from potentially irritating substances, can enhance irritancy if they become soaked or if the irritant becomes trapped beneath the garment. Also, sweating beneath the glove causes moisture to accumulate, which itself can be irritating. Frequent changes of these articles are recommended, especially when they become contaminated. Finally, the effect of simultaneous exposure may produce irritant contact dermatitis by even the most innocuous of substances. Even though each substance alone would elicit only a minor reaction or none at all, the additive effect of many such chemicals can lead to increased reactions.[36]

ENDOGENOUS FACTORS

Various endogenous factors which influence one's propensity to develop irritant contact dermatitis or the severity of symptoms include regional anatomic differences, age, race, sex, and previous or preexisting skin disease.

Regional Anatomic Differences

Great regional differences in normal skin architecture probably account for the skin's site-to-site differences in reactivity. For example, the upper back has been found to be the most reactive site for both irritant and allergic patch testing,[37] while the thin skin of the eyelids and scrotum is more reactive than thicker skin elsewhere. Additionally, the threshold for irritation is low on the vulva, which may be of importance in cases of vulvodynia.[38-40]

Age

The threshold for skin irritation is decreased in babies and children below the age of 8,[41-44] so they can react to substances which will not produce dermatitis in adults. The ability to generate an inflammatory response to an exogenous substance is, in general, decreased in the elderly. The elderly exhibit decreased responses to primary irritants both in terms of total numbers of individuals responding and the overall intensity of the responses.[40,45-48]

Race

Experimental data concerning differences in irritant contact dermatitis among the races has not yet reached a consensus. A number of studies have demonstrated a decreased irritation response among black subjects as compared to whites.[49,50] On the other hand, some experimental studies have demonstrated that black skin is more irritated by surfactants, as evidenced by higher transepidermal water loss and blood flow values.[51] The differences may relate to the fact that erythema is more difficult to visualize in black individuals. Alternatively, there may be true differences in the way in which the skin of black individuals reacts to irritants. For instance, Morrison et al.[52] concluded that, unlike Caucasians, African-Americans do not experience much erythema when exposed to surfactant-containing products. Rather, the irritation manifested as dryness and hyperpigmentation.

Sex

Females may be more prone to develop irritant contact dermatitis than males. The incidence of irritant contact dermatitis, mostly of the hands, is higher in females,[15,53,54] but most experimental studies addressing a possible constitutional susceptibility to irritant contact dermatitis have not found a difference in cutaneous reactivity between male and female skin.[55,56] The concept that females develop irritant contact dermatitis more easily than males may simply be a reflection of a greater degree of exposure to wet work and irritants.

Previous and Preexisting Skin Disease

Patients with atopic dermatitis appear to have an increased susceptibility to irritant contact dermatitis.[57,58] In wet work, for example, in which exposure to water, detergents, or other chemicals is commonplace, subjects with a history of atopic dermatitis develop hand dermatitis more often than those without such a history.[59–60] Atopic dermatitis patients demonstrate a decreased baseline skin barrier function, as evidenced by a high transepidermal water loss and a reduced stratum corneum water binding capacity.[62–65] As indicated earlier, any process which damages the skin barrier function allows for easier access by exogenous chemicals. This concept is especially important in cases of hand dermatitis, where many endogenous processes, such as psoriasis, may increase one's susceptibility to irritation by exogenous substances.[66]

TREATMENT

Treatment depends upon the stage of the dermatitis and, as indicated earlier, the terms *acute, subacute,* and *chronic* will be used to describe morphologically the stage of dermatitis and its appropriate treatment. Key to the successful treatment of all types of irritant contact dermatitis is prevention. Therefore, patients should be instructed in proper skin care, especially the avoidance of harsh soaps and too frequent washings, and in the use of protective garments, such as gloves and aprons when necessary (Table 3-3—patient guide).

TABLE 2–3. Patient Guide

What is irritant contact dermatitis?
There are two types of contact dermatitis: irritant contact dermatitis and allergic contact dermatitis. Both are caused by environmental substances which contact the skin during everyday activity. Allergic contact dermatitis is caused by allergens through allergic mechanisms. This is sometimes called "delayed hypersensitivity" and may take a day or two to break out after exposure. In contrast, irritant contact dermatitis is nonallergic and it occurs more rapidly. While these two conditions have very different causes, their appearances can be quite similar. To differentiate between the two, a physician may have to perform a patch test.

How does one develop irritant contact dermatitis?
One can develop irritant contact dermatitis reactions to many different substances commonly encountered in the workplace, at home, or while pursuing hobbies. Even normal, everyday hygiene can cause irritant contact dermatitis. It is important not to overbathe your skin, as this can damage its natural protective barrier.

How is irritant contact dermatitis best treated?
Depending upon the stage of dermatitis, your physician may prescribe or recommend one or all of the following:
Prevention. To prevent future episodes of irritant contact dermatitis, it is necessary to identify and subsequently avoid those substances likely to cause a reaction. Your physician can help you with this. Furthermore, you must avoid the frequent use of harsh soaps. These tend to dry your skin, making it more vulnerable to contact dermatitis. If your work makes contact with potentially irritating substances unavoidable, make sure that you use protective garments such as gloves and an apron.
Compresses. Soak a clean cotton cloth in plain water or the solution recommended by your doctor and apply it to the affected area. Do not wring it dry. Leave the cloth in place for 20 to 30 minutes and then remove it. Repeat this procedure two to six times a day. Once the blisters have resolved, discontinue the compress and begin applying the topical corticosteroid prescribed by your doctor.
Oral medication. Your physician may prescribe one or all of the following: an oral corticosteroid (such as prednisone), which will help to decrease inflammation; an antihistamine, which will help to relieve itching and enhance sleep; an oral antibiotic if there is any infection. As with all medications, take the proper dosage as indicated by your physician and pharmacist.
Topical corticosteroids. Topical corticosteroids are commonly used for many types of irritant contact dermatitis. They should be applied evenly over the affected area. In some cases, your physician may recommend that you occlude the area with a plastic wrap or vinyl glove after application of the topical steroid. Occlusion enhances the ability of the medication to penetrate the skin. Remember, these topical medications are potent and can cause side effects if they are not used properly. Therefore you should use these medications *only* under the supervision of a physician.
Lubrication. Frequent lubrication (three to four times a day) of the affected area with a lotion or ointment recommended by your physician helps to minimize drying. Lotions or ointments are best used immediately after bathing and toweling, while the skin is still moist. If your physician has also prescribed a topical corticosteroid, it is best to apply the lotion or ointment 2 to 3 hours *after* the topical corticosteroid, In other words, alternate the application of topical corticosteroid and lubricant lotion throughout the day.

Acute Dermatitis

Treatment for acute dermatitis includes (1) cold compresses of Burow's solution or plain water left on the affected area for 20 to 30 min and repeated 2 to 6 times per day; (2) oral corticosteroid therapy—prednisone, 40 to 60 mg/day in divided doses for 14 to 21 days with gradual taper; and (3) antihistamines as a sedative and antipruritic. When the vesicles resolve, one may institute a topical corticosteroid and discontinue wet compresses.

Subacute Dermatitis

Treatment for subacute dermatitis includes (1) a medium-potency (group III–V) topical corticoid cream (with or without occlusion) or ointment (an ointment is preferred for drier lesions) and (2) lubrication with lotions or ointments. The patient should be instructed to apply emollients 2 to 3 h after topical corticoids and informed that emollients are most efficacious when applied while the skin is still moist (i.e., after bathing and toweling).

Chronic Dermatitis

Treatment for chronic dermatitis consists of (1) group II–V topical corticoids with vinyl glove or plastic wrap occlusion (overnight or for a few hours a day) or group I topical corticoids without occlusion and (2) lubrication, as described above. Intralesional corticoids may be efficacious for recalcitrant lesions.

It is important always to be aware of the possibility of bacterial superinfection. Such infections are not uncommon in irritant contact dermatitis and should be suspected especially in those cases which are unresponsive to appropriate therapy. Appropriate antibiotics are those active against *Staphylococcus aureus*.

Some forms of irritant contact dermatitis require special treatment. Only brief mention is made of their diagnosis and treatment in the following paragraphs. The reader is referred to textbooks on occupational dermatology for more complete descriptions.

Dermatitis due to fiberglass is a pruritic dermatitis *with or without* visible lesions. when lesions are present, they are often follicular papules. The dermatitis mainly involves exposed areas such as the arms, face, and neck, but it can localize beneath clothing and footwear (i.e., airborne dermatitis). It is diagnosed definitively by stripping an area of affected skin with Scotch tape and examining the tape under a microscope for the presence of glass fibers.[67] Often, however, the fibrous strands cannot be seen and the diagnosis rests on the history and clinical appearance. Treatment for fiberglass dermatitis consists of removing the entrapped fibers from the skin. This can be accomplished with the use of adhesive tape, such as plumber's duct tape, applied directly to the affected skin. Often the skin of workers so afflicted becomes "hardened,"[68–70] so that the initial symptoms disappear within 1 to 4 weeks.

Hydrofluoric acid burns are seen among workers in the electronics and semiconductor industries. These burns are frequently localized to the fingers and hands and have a delayed onset of hours to eventually produce a deep, throbbing, excruciating pain, and, in the most advanced stage, extensive tissue necrosis. The damage is due to the free fluoride ion, and the goal of treatment is to complex the ion by administering a 10% calcium gluconate solution directly into the affected tissue with a small 30-gauge needle. Close follow-up of these patients is important for two reasons. First, patients may require repeated calcium gluconate infusions and, second, these patients should be monitored for the possibility of fluoride poisoning due to systemic absorption.[71]

REFERENCES

1. Goh CL, Soh SD: Occupational dermatoses in Singapore. *Contact Dermatitis* 11:288–293, 1984.
2. Rietschel R: Diagnosing irritant contact dermatitis, in Jackson EM, Goldman R (eds): *Irritant Contact Dermatitis*. New York, Dekker, 1990, pp 167–174.

3. Van Ketel WG: Clinical factors promoting the development of allergic contact dermatitis. *Derm Beruf Umwelt* 25:78, 1977.

4. Bjornberg A: Skin reactions to primary irritants in patients with hand eczema (thesis). Gothenburg, Sweden, Oscar Isacsons Tryckeri AB, 1968.

5. Mitchell JC: Angry back syndrome. *Contact Dermatitis* 7:359–360, 1981.

6. Bruynzeel DP, van Ketel WG, Scheper RJ: Angry back of the excited skin syndrome: A prospective study. *J Am Acad Dermatol* 8:392–397, 1983.

7. Bruynzeel DP, Maibach HI: Excited skin syndrome (angry back). *Arch Dermatol* 122:323–328, 1986.

8. Fregert SF: Irritant contact dermatitis, in Fregert SF (ed): *Manual of Contact Dermatitis,* 2d ed. Copenhagen, Munksgaard, 1981, pp 55–62.

9. Griffiths WAD, Wilkinson DS: Primary irritants and solvents, in Griffiths WAD, Wilkinson DS (eds): *Essentials of Industrial Dermatology,* Oxford, Blackwell, 1985, pp 58–72.

10. Hjorth N, Avnstorp C: Rehabilitation in hand eczema. *Derm Beruf Umwelt* 34:74–76, 1986.

11. Malten KE, den Arend J, Wiggers RE: Delayed irritation: Hexanediol diacrylate and butanediol diacrylate. *Contact Dermatitis* 5:178–184, 1979.

12. Lovell CR, Rycroft RCG, Williams DMJ, Hamlin JW: Contact dermatitis from the irritancy (immediate and delayed) and allergenicity of hydroxy acrylate. *Contact Dermatitis* 12:117–118, 1985.

13. Malten KE, den Arend J: Topical toxicity of various concentrations of DMSO recorded with impedance measurements and water vapor loss measurements. *Contact Dermatitis* 4:80–92, 1978.

14. von Hagerman G: Uber das "traumiterative" (Toxische) Ekzem. *Dermatologica* 115:525–529, 1957.

15. Agrup G: Hand eczema and other dermatoses in South Sweden (Thesis). *Acta Derm Venereol (Stockh)* 49(suppl 161):1969.

16. Cronin E: Metals, in Cronin E (ed): *Contact Dermatitis.* New York, Churchill Livingstone, 1980, pp 279–390.

17. Fisher AA: Dermatitis and discolorations from metals, in Fisher AA (ed): *Contact Dermatitis,* 3d ed. Philadelphia, Lea & Febiger, 1986, pp 710–744.

18. Fischer T, Rystedt I: False positive, follicular and irritant patch test reactions to metal salts. *Contact Dermatitis* 12:93–98, 1985.

19. Wahlberg JE, Maibach HI: Identification of contact pustulogens, in Marzulli FN, Maibach HI (eds): *Dermatotoxicology,* 2d ed. Washington DC, Hemisphere Publishing, 1982, pp 627–635.

20. Mills OH, Kligman A: Acne mechanica. *Arch Dermatol* 111:481–483, 1975.

21. Harvell J, Maibach HI: Skin disease among musicians. *Medical Problems of Performing Artists* 7:114–120, 1992.

22. Samitz MH: Repeated mechanical trauma to the skin: Occupational aspects. *Am J Ind Med* 8:265–271, 1985.

23. Menne T: Frictional dermatitis in post office workers. *Contact Dermatitis* 9:172–173, 1983.

24. Susten AS: The chronic effects of mechanical trauma to the skin: A review of the literature. *Am J Ind Med* 8:281–288, 1985.

25. Ronchese F: *Occupational Marks and Other Physical Signs: A Guide to Personal Identification.* New York, Grune & Stratton, 1948.

26. Frosch PJ, Kligman AM: Rapid blister formation in human skin with ammonium hydroxide. *Br J Dermatol* 96:461–473, 1977.

27. Lammintausta, Maibach HI, Wilson D: Mechanisms of subjective (sensory) irritation propensity to nonimmunologic contact urticaria and objective irritation in stingers. *Derm Beruf Umwelt* 36:45–49, 1988.

28. Harvell J, Bason M, Maibach HI: Contact urticaria (immediate reaction syndrome). *Clin Rev Allergy* 10:303–324, 1992.

29. Kresbach H, Karl H, Wawschink O: Cutaneous mercury granuloma. *Berufsdermatosen* 18:173–186, 1971.

30. Gellin GA: Contact dermatitis due to irritation: pigmentary changes, in Adams RM (ed): *Occupational Skin Disease,* 2d ed. Philadelphia, Saunders, 1990, pp 21–25.

31. Gellin GA: Occupational disorders of pigmentation, in Maibach HI (ed): *Occupational and Industrial Dermatology,* 2d ed. Chicago, Year Book, 1987, pp 134–141.

32. Lachapelle JM: Industrial airborne irritant or allergic contact dermatitis. *Contact Dermatitis* 14:137–145, 1986.

33. Lammintausta KH, Maibach HI: Irritant dermatitis syndrome. *Immunol Allergy Clin North Am* 9:435–446, 1989.

34. Lammintausta KH, Maibach HI: Contact dermatitis due to irritation, in Adams RM (ed): *Occupational Skin Disease,* 2d ed. Philadelphia, Saunders, 1990, pp 1–15.

35. Wester RC, Maibach HI: Dermatopharmacokinetics, in Maibach HI, Bronaugh RL (eds): *Percutaneous Absorption*. New York, Dekker, 1985, pp 525–530.
36. Malten KE: Thoughts on irritant contact dermatitis. *Contact Dermatitis* 7:238–247, 1981.
37. Magnusson B, Hersle K: Patch test methods: II. Regional variation of patch test responses. *Acta Derm Venereol (Stockh)* 45:257–261, 1965.
38. Britz MB, Maibach HI: Human cutaneous vulvar reactivity to irritants. *Contact Dermatitis* 5:375–377, 1979.
39. McKay M: Vulvodynia: A multifactorial clinical problem. *Arch Dermatol* 125:256–262, 1989.
40. Elsner P, Wilhelm D, Maibach HI: Sodium lauryl sulfate-induced irritant contact dermatitis in vulvar and forearm skin of premenopausal and postmenopausal women. *J Am Acad Dermatol* 23:648–652, 1990.
41. Jordon WE, Blaney TL: Factors influencing infant diaper dermatitis, in Maibach HI, Boisits EK (eds): *Neonatal Skin*. New York, Dekker, 1982, pp 205–221.
42. Mobly SL, Mansman HC: Current status of skin testing in children with contact dermatitis. *Cutis* 13:995–1000, 1974.
43. Epstein E: Contact dermatitis in children. *Pediatr Clin North Am* 18:839–852, 1971.
44. Fisher AA: Childhood allergic contact dermatitis. *Cutis* 15:635–645, 1975.
45. Grove GL, Duncan S, Kligman AM: Effect of ageing on the blistering of human skin with ammonium hydroxide. *Br J Dermatol* 107:393–400, 1982.
46. Grove GL, Lavker RM, Hoelzle E, Kligman AM: Use of nonintrusive tests to monitor age-associated changes in human skin. *J Soc Cosmet Chem* 32:15–26, 1981.
47. Coenraads PJ, Bleumink E, Nater JP: Susceptibility to primary irritants: Age dependence and relation to contact allergic reactions. *Contact Dermatitis* 1:377–381, 1975.
48. Cua AB, Wilhelm KP, and Maibach HI: Cutaneous sodium lauryl sulphate irritation potential: Age and regional variability. *Br J Dermatol* 123:607–613, 1990.
49. Weigand DA, Gaylor JR: Irritant reaction in Negro and Caucasian skin. *South Med J* 67:548–551, 1974.
50. Andersen KE, Maibach HI: Black and white human skin differences. *J Am Acad Dermatol* 1:276–282, 1979.
51. Berardesca E, Maibach HI: Racial differences in sodium lauryl sulphate induced cutaneous irritation: Black and white. *Contact Dermatitis* 18:65–70, 1988.
52. Morrison BM, Babulak SW, Scala DD, et al: Evaluation of the response of African-American skin to facial cleansing products using a modified soap chamber test (poster). American Academy of Dermatology, 51st Annual Meeting, December 5–10, 1992.
53. Rystedt I: Factors influencing the occurrence of hand eczema in adults with a history of atopic dermatitis in childhood. *Contact Dermatitis* 12:247–254, 1985.
54. Lantinga H, Nater JP, Coenraads PJ: Prevalence, incidence and course of eczema on the hand and forearm in a sample of the general population. *Contact Dermatitis* 10:135–149, 1984.
55. Bjornberg A: Skin reactions to primary irritants in men and women. *Acta Derm Venereol (Stockh)* 55:191–194, 1975.
56. Lammintausta K, Maibach HI, Wilson D: Irritant reactivity in males and females. *Contact Dermatitis* 17:276–280, 1987.
57. Rystedt I: Work related hand eczema in atopics. *Contact Dermatitis* 12:164–171, 1985.
58. Hanifin JM, Rajka G: Diagnostic features of atopic dermatitis. *Acta Derm Venereol (Stockh)* 92(suppl):44–47, 1980.
59. Lammintausta K, Kalimo K: Atopy and hand dermatitis in hospital wet work. *Contact Dermatitis* 7:301–308, 1981.
60. Nilsson E, Mikaelsson B, Andersson S: Atopy, occupation, and domestic work as risk factors for hand eczema in hospital workers. *Contact Dermatitis* 13:216–223, 1985.
61. van der Walk PGM, Nater JP, Bleumink E: Vulnerability of the skin to surfactants in different groups of eczema patients and controls as measured by water vapour loss. *Clin Exp Dermatol* 10:98–103, 1985.
62. Rajka G: The aetiology of atopic dermatitis, in Rajka G (ed): *Atopic Dermatitis*. London, Saunders, 1975, pp 46–104.
63. Finlay AY, Nocholls S, King CS, et al: The "dry" noneczematous skin associated with atopic eczema. *Br J Dermatol* 102:249–256, 1980.
64. Al Jaberi H, Marks R: Studies of the clinically uninvolved skin in patients with dermatitis. *Br J Dermatol* 111:437–443, 1984.
65. Werner Y, Lindberg M, Forslind B: The water binding capacity of stratum corneum in dry non-eczematous skin of atopic eczema. *Acta Derma Venereol (Stockh)* 62:334–336, 1982.

66. Epstein E: Hand dermatitis: Practical management and current concepts. *J Am Acad Dermatol* 10:395–424, 1984.
67. Bjornberg A: Glass fiber dermatitis. *Am J Ind Med* 8:395–400, 1985.
68. Lim J, Balzer JL, Wolf CR, Milby TH: Fiber glass: Reinforced plastics. *Arch Environ Health* 20:540–544, 1970.
69. Possick PA, Gellin GA, Key MM: Fibrous glass dermatitis. *Am J Ind Hyg Assoc J* 31:12–15, 1970.
70. Sulzberger MB, Baer BL: The effects of fiberglass on animal and human skin. *Ind Med* 11:482–484, 1942.
71. Vance MV: Contact dermatitis due to irritation: Hydrofluoric acid (HF) burns, in Adams RM (ed): *Occupational Skin Disease,* 2d ed. Philadelphia, Saunders, 1990, pp 18–21.

3

ALLERGIC CONTACT DERMATITIS

C. L. Goh

DEFINITION AND CLASSIFICATION OF DERMATITIS/ECZEMA

The term *eczema* is often confusing because it is used in more than one way, and multiple names not infrequently apply to the same condition. In many countries the terms *dermatitis* and *eczema* are used interchangably, and this will be the usage here. The word *eczema*—from Greek *ekzema*—means to erupt or boil out, and indeed this looks somewhat like what is happening. Eczema is recognized clinically by its tendency to show redness, weeping, oozing, crusting, scaling, and—for chronic forms—thickening, hyperkeratosis, and lichenification. Some divide eczema into endogenous and exogenous types, with allergic contact dermatitis (e.g., poison ivy dermatitis) being an example of the exogenous type and an id reaction causing pompholyx representing an endogenous eczema.[1] Sometimes an endogenous cause can precipitate an external type of lesion (e.g., in systemic contact dermatitis).[2] Another way to look at these two entities is to consider contact dermatitis as dermatitis caused by an external/environmental factor (contactants) and endogenous dermatitis to be due to "constitutional" factors.

Contact dermatitis can be subdivided into *irritant, allergic, phototoxic,* and *photoallergic* types. Endogenous eczema is classified according to morphology and presentation, e.g., atopic or seborrheic dermatitis or hand or foot dermatitis (Table 3-1).

The exact incidence of allergic and irritant contact dermatitis is unknown and may be dependent upon the population in question, but it is common, estimated to be more than 10 percent of patients attending any skin clinic.[1,3] Although allergic contact dermatitis is caused by a cell-mediated mechanism and irritant contact dermatitis arises from physical damage to the skin, separating these two entities is not always easy. In many clinical situations, they may overlap. The clinical appearance of irritant and allergic contact dermatitis can be almost identical, and even the histology may not always be separable. However, knowing the cause is important, as avoidance of the agent is necessary in managing the dermatitis. Furthermore, both prognosis and management depend upon an accurate diagnosis.

Contact dermatitis is classified into (1) *allergic contact dermatitis* (a cell-mediated hypersensitivity reaction), (2) *irritant contact dermatitis,* (3) *contact urticaria syndrome* (allergic and nonimmunologic), (4) *phototoxic dermatitis,* and (5) *photoallergic dermatitis.*

TABLE 3-1. Classification of Dermatitis

Endogenous Dermatitis	Exogenous Dermatitis
Atopic dermatitis	Allergic contact dermatitis
Seborrheic dermatitis	Irritant contact dermatitis
Discoid dermatitis	Photoallergic dermatitis
Hand/foot dermatitis	Phototoxic dermatitis
Lichen simplex chronicus	Dermatitis secondary to
Varicose/stasis dermatitis	contact urticaria
Asteatotic dermatitis	
Unclassifiable dermatitis	

ALLERGIC CONTACT DERMATITIS

Allergic contact dermatitis has been found to account for about 31 percent of all cases of dermatitis, 24 percent of all hand dermatitis, and 24 percent of occupational and dermatitis seen at the Contact and Occupational Dermatoses Clinic in Singapore.[3,4]

The immunologic mechanism is a type IV hypersensitivity reaction, frequently known as a cell-mediated hypersensitivity reaction. In contrast, the inflammatory response in irritant contact dermatitis is caused by direct cell damage from a contact irritant. Allergic contact dermatitis, unlike endogenous dermatitis and other types of exogenous dermatitis, can often be diagnosed objectively with a positive patch-test reaction. However the ability to make an accurate diagnosis will also depend on the experience and skill of the investigating dermatologist.

The contactant causing allergic contact dermatitis is called an *allergen* or *antigen*. The list of such agents is incredibly long, with some contactants being strong sensitizers and some individuals susceptible to developing allergy to contactants. Fortunately, most individuals do not become allergic to the more moderate sensitizers. However, the potent sensitizers (e.g., dinitrochlorobenzene) cause allergy in 90 percent of normal individuals who are adequately exposed to that allergen.[5] Some contactants become allergenic only after exposure to ultraviolet light. Such contactants are known as *photocontact allergens.*

Sensitization is the process whereby an individual becomes allergic to an allergen. Contact allergy is always acquired, with the time taken by a person to manifest allergic contact dermatitis after repeated exposure to an allergen called the *latent period.* The latent period is not constant, but there is a minimal time required to initiate sensitization.

The *sensitizing index* of an allergen is the relative capacity of an allergen to induce contact allergy in the population. This may be influenced by the exposure, and that, in turn, partly depends upon how the specific antigen is used. For example, if a cosmetic company were to use a more highly sensitizing ingredient or an injudicious concentration of mildly sensitizing preservative or fragrance in a popular product, this would very likely cause a higher incidence of sensitivity in the general population. Those who were sensitized would now break out to the lower levels found in many other products. The sensitizing index can often be predicted by animal and human studies, and industry spends a generous amount of money to try to minimize risk.

Cross-sensitivity may be a "true" or a "false" cross-reaction.[6] The first is a reaction to a chemical different from but structurally similar to the original sensitizer. In such instances, allergy to the primary allergen is probably due to allergy to a part of its structure that is common to both chemicals. False cross-sensitivity is a reaction to the same chemical contained in different sources, such as weeds or fragrance materials. In that case, a person with contact dermatitis to *Parthenium hysterophorus* might break out when patch tested to ragweed, as both plants contain ambrosin.[7] This is a shared antigen, and while it seems to cause allergies, it really evokes a reaction to the same chemical in two patch test materials.

CLINICAL FEATURES

Morphology

Allergic contact dermatitis may present with acute, subacute, or chronic dermatitis, but it is the pattern more than anything else that causes one to look for a contactant. Furthermore, many experienced clinicians will patch test patients with classic pictures of other eczemas and will uncover causative or aggravating sensitivities. Perhaps the principal diagnostic feature of contact dermatitis is the appearance of an eczematous process in an unnatural distribution, suggesting an association with the causative contactant. For example, someone who has recently become sensitized to the posts in pierced earrings will likely have a weeping, oozing, crusting, and perhaps scaling eruption located where the earrings are worn in the earlobes and especially around the earrings.

The same person will eventually be exposed to other sources and will possibly develop more chronic forms of dermatitis, which may show lichenification and scratch papules from rubbing a pruritic site (e.g., where the bare midriff contacts metal snaps in blue jeans). Both the initial and chronic eruptions are caused by nickel sensitivity and both are forms of allergic contact dermatitis.

Another artificial pattern occurs with strong allergens as finger marks occur where poison ivy or oak is transferred by the contaminated hands and fingers. This produces a linear pattern from the finger spread.

The morphologic features of acute contact dermatitis include redness, itching, weeping, oozing, crusting, scaling, and fissuring. A biopsy at this time would show prominent spongiosis in most cases. In more severe cases, frank bullae may be seen. Again, the pattern will depend upon the nature of the antigen, the exposure, and the level of sensitivity, among other things.

In subacute dermatitis, a milder reaction with mild erythema, papules, and occasional vesiculation is seen. The features of chronic dermatitis include thickening, scaling (hyperkeratosis), and lichenification comprising scratch papules, sometimes with pigmentary changes and with dryness and/or fissuring.

The symptoms and signs of allergic contact dermatitis may appear hours to days after an exposure to an allergen. The dermatitis may persist from several days to several weeks after cessation of contact with the allergen.

Although allergic contact dermatitis is usually eczematous, it may manifest itself as lesions which morphologically might not seem to be eczematous.[8,9] A classic example might be dermal contact dermatitis, which is sometimes seen in nickel-allergic persons. These lesions include erythema multiforme–like eruptions (urticarial, papular, and

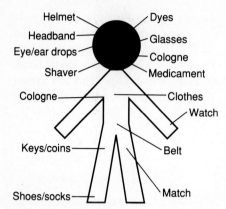

FIG. 3-1. Male: common contact allergens by site (*front*).

plaque eruptions), purpuric eruptions, lichen planus–like eruptions, pigmented reactions, and granulomatous reactions. Another unusual type of contact dermatitis simulates parapsoriasis. Such reactions are often seen with a specific antigen, as with lichenoid dermatitis from color film developers and parapsoriasis-like eruptions with cyanoacrylate sensitivity. Why these antigens cause such unusual morphologic pictures is not clear.

Lesion Sites

The contact site in allergic contact dermatitis often gives a clue to the diagnosis and to the possible contact allergen. The following are some common contact allergens with characteristic localization and morphology (Figs. 3-1 through 3-4).

HANDS AND ARMS. Hand dermatitis may be due to contact allergy such as from nickel (e.g., in keys and coins) or foodstuffs (among chefs and housewives). Chronic dermatitis on the hands and wrists with clear cutoff lines are suggestive of contact allergy to gloves (e.g., rubber chemicals). Hand dermatitis is often a manifestation of occupational allergic contact dermatitis[2,3,10,11] (e.g., contact allergy to chromates in cement or to epoxies, acrylates, and isocyanates, which are resins used in the electronics industry). An eczema of the tips of the thumb, index, and middle fingers suggests contact with

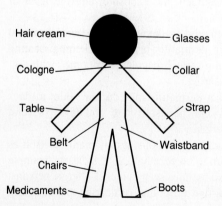

FIG. 3-2. Male: common allergens by site (*back*).

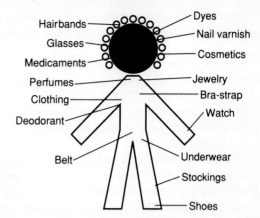

FIG. 3-3. Female: common allergens by site (*front*).

an object or substance gripped, and involvement of the finger webs suggest contact with irritants or allergy to lotions, etc.

Chronic or subacute dermatitis around the wrists is suggestive of contact allergy to nickel from watch straps and nickel-plated costume jewelry or to *p*-tertiary butyl phenolformaldehyde resins from leather watch straps.

AXILLAE. Dermatitis in the axillae is suggestive of contact allergy to fragrances and preservatives in deodorants, antiperspirants, and medicaments. When the axillae are spared but the surrounding area is involved, one might suspect clothing.

FACE. Dermatitis of the face and lips is suggestive of allergy to cosmetics. The common contact allergens in cosmetics include fragrances and preservatives. Lip dermatitis may also result from contact allergy to flavors in toothpastes. Earlobe dermatitis is suggestive of nickel allergy to nickel in costume jewelry. Gold allergy from jewelry, although rare, does occur. Acute or subacute dermatitis on the scalp, hairline, and eyelids is suggestive of contact allergy to *p*-phenylenediamine in hair dye or to glyceryl monothioglycolate in permanent-wave solution. Eyelid dermatitis may be caused by

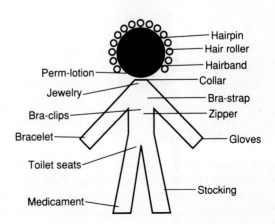

FIG. 3-4. Female: common allergens by site (*back*).

contact allergy to preservatives, dyes, fragrances, and other ingredients in eye makeups, medications (eyedrops), or contact lens solution.

NECK. Nickel contact allergy from costume jewelry and fragrance allergy from cologne are common causes of contact allergy around the neck.

TRUNK. Contact allergy to clothing dyes and resins may cause dermatitis on the trunk. Such dermatitis tends to be most intense on skin folds and flexures.

FEET AND LOWER LIMBS. Dermatitis on the feet is suggestive of contact allergy to footwear. Common allergens here include p-tertiary butyl-phenolformaldehyde resins, which are glues used on rubber and leather shoes; chromates in chrome-tanned leather; and rubber chemicals in rubber shoes and sandals. Allergic contact dermatitis from footwear is often characterized by the presence of well-defined cutoff lines around the ankles or lower legs. Contact allergy to topical medicaments, lanolin, and preservatives is not uncommon in patients with stasis dermatitis and ulcers. In fact, it is wise to suspect almost anything that has been used to treat stasis dermatitis, including corticosteroids.

Presentation and Lesion Morphology

The pattern of the dermatitis sometimes gives a clue to the diagnosis and the causative allergen. Streaks of acute eczematous lesions on limbs are suggestive of poison ivy/ oak dermatitis. Discoid dermatitis may be associated with allergic contact eczema to metals (e.g., nickel and chromate).[12] Rectangular patch dermatitis bearing a plaster outline is suggestive of colophony allergy from sticky plaster. Scaly, fissuring finger-pulp eczema is suggestive of contact allergy to a foodstuff (e.g., garlic), proteinaceous substances, or resins (e.g., epoxies).

A dermatitis affecting exposed parts of the face but sparing the shaded areas— eyelids, the submental area, and the postauricular areas—is suggestive of *photoallergic contact dermatitis*. Such an eruption also tends to involve the V of the chest, the back of the neck, and exposed parts of limbs (e.g., the dorsal forearms) while sparing the ventral forearms. The common photocontact allergens nowadays include sunscreens, musk ambrette and its derivatives (fixatives and fragrances in cologne), phenothiazines, and phenyl-propionic acid derivatives used as nonsteroidal anti-inflammatory drugs.

Lichen planus–like eruptions on the limbs can be caused by contact allergy to color photographic developers. Lichen planus–like eruptions on the *buccal mucosa* may suggest contact allergy to mercury in (amalgam) dental restorations. Histologically, granulomatous eruptions on the earlobes can be caused by contact allergy to gold and gold salts.

Secondary Spread

In contact allergy, dermatitis tends to be most intense on the primary contact sites. However, the dermatitis may spread from the primary contact site to distant parts of the body that are not in direct contact with the allergen. This phenomenon is referred to as *secondary spread*. The exact mechanism of secondary spread is unknown. Passive transfer of allergens from primary to distant sites is one explanation. Systemic absorption and systemic spread of allergen from primary sites could be another explanation. Some allergens (e.g., medications and metals) may cause such secondary spread.

Airborne Contact Dermatitis

Light-particle allergens may be carried in the air and cause an *airborne contact dermatitis*. The typical picture in airborne contact dermatitis is an eczematous eruption on exposed parts of the body, (i.e., the face, neck, and exposed parts of the limbs), with mild secondary spread to covered parts. It may mimic photodermatitis except that, in typical cases, the protected areas (e.g., eyelids, postauricular and submental areas) are not spared, as in photodermatitis. There are exceptions to this rule for both contact and photocontact in such cases. Examples of airborne allergens include fragrance from cologne sprays, insecticides from insecticide sprays, chromate from cement dust, plant resins, plant pollens, and wood dust. Dust-borne allergens may cause allergic contact dermatitis on truck and skin folds. It may mimic atopic dermatitis.

Diagnosis

Perhaps the first principle of diagnosing allergic contact dermatitis is to be suspicious that it may be present. This becomes especially important when one realizes the time required to establish relationships and to decide upon a course of testing to look for underlying causes. The diagnosis of allergic contact dermatitis is based on an accurate, detailed history and a thorough physical examination. To help with this, a questionnaire is included in Appendix B. This could be given to the patient before the examination and, in referral practices, it may be mailed to the patient when the appointment is made.

In the history, the *age, race, sex, occupation, and hobbies* of patients should be sought, as they may give clues to the causative allergen and its source.

The *primary site* of the dermatitis and the evolution and *progress* of a dermatitis may give a clue to the diagnosis and type of allergen.

In a patient suspected of having occupational allergic contact dermatitis, the occurrence of a similar morphology and distribution of dermatitis among coworkers and the effect of the dermatitis on *weekends, vacations, and off days* may give a clue as to the occupational source of the allergen. Material safety data sheets are also important parts of the history for this group.

A patient with suspected allergic contact dermatitis should also be questioned on his or her past or recent history of over-the-counter or prescribed *medication*. Many cases of allergic contact dermatitis are due to topical medicaments. Perhaps the most important part of the history is the items (including medications) which have been applied. Sometimes, after a printed history has been completed and an oral history taken, important new items are brought out by directed questions. Another practical way to find unsuspected sources of exposure is to have the patient bring in *all* the lotions, cosmetics, and medications used in the recent and even distant past. Some, (e.g., soaps, shampoo, etc.) are too irritating to use as is, but knowing what is used helps in correcting the routine until the workup is completed.

The *physical examination* should be carried out in a well-lit room. The morphology and location of any dermatitis should be carefully noted, as these are clues to the cause of the allergic contact dermatitis. A general examination of the rest of the body apart from the primary dermatitis site may help exclude endogenous or noneczematous disorders.

Treatment

Treatment of allergic contact dermatitis is covered in Chap. 51. Basically it requires removal from the offending irritants and allergens, but the basic treatment of the dermatitis is the same as for any other dermatitis.

For acute dermatitis, wet compresses (e.g., normal saline, Burow's solution, or potassium permanganate in a 1:10,000 dilution) can be used. For subacute and chronic dermatitis, a moderately potent topical steroid (e.g., betamethasone valerate cream or fluocinolone acetonide cream) should be used. The use of potentially sensitizing antibiotics such as neomycin should be avoided, as this can promote sensitization to the antibiotic.

Oral antihistamines may be prescribed for itching. Systemic antibiotic therapy is indicated when secondary bacterial infection is present, but this is not always easy to know.

A short course of oral steroids (e.g., prednisolone) may be indicated when dermatitis *of known cause* is acute, widespread, or located on the face. However, any secondary infection must be treated before administering systemic steroids. The effectiveness of systemic glucocorticoids sometimes causes the patient to be less careful, and flares commonly occur on withdrawal.

Identifying the Cause

Allergic contact dermatitis can often be suspected by the appearance and—for some strong allergens such as the toxicodendrons—the diagnosis can be presumed, although one can be fooled even there. For most allergens, patch testing is required for confirmation, and it helps in many cases where the allergen might not have been otherwise suspected. Patch testing is an extremely important tool in understanding what probably happened. For optimum success, it helps for the dermatologist to be sufficiently experienced and skilled to select the right allergens at the right concentration. The details of patch-testing procedure are discussed in Chap. 5.

Education and Rehabilitation

Once the cause of allergic contact dermatitis has been identified, the patient should be taught how to avoid the allergen. This includes providing material on sources of the allergen and how to avoid them. Handouts on each standard allergen are included in the respective chapters of Part II. One classic approach is avoidance. Another is allergen substitution, which allows the patient to live normally using products that serve the same purpose but which do not contain the allergen.

In patients with occupational allergic contact dermatitis, information on protection from allergens can often be obtained from material safety data sheets present in the

ALLERGIC CONTACT DERMATITIS—PATIENT HANDOUT

WHAT IS ALLERGIC CONTACT DERMATITIS?

Contact allergy is an allergic reaction of the skin developed by some people after contact with substances that are generally harmless to the nonallergic. These substances, often called *antigens* or *allergens,* can penetrate the skin, causing a rash where they are applied. We are not born allergic but must learn to react to chemicals that are foreign to our bodies. This is a protective mechanism the body uses to defend itself against harmful agents such as ringworm, viruses, and tumor cells. Some causes, such as poison ivy, are common; others such as Vaseline, rarely cause a problem.

HOW DOES ONE RECOGNIZE CONTACT DERMATITIS?

The picture of contact dermatitis is that of an itching (eczematous) eruption localized to the spot where the "antigen" comes in contact with the skin. This produces what can sometimes be recognized as an artificial pattern and sometimes an eruption indistinguishable from other eczemas.

A typical case might be an eczema of the earlobes, which suggests a metal used in earrings as a cause. A rash outlining a beltlike pattern around the waist is produced by allergy to rubber chemicals in the elastic in underclothing. Very strong allergens (e.g., poison ivy or poison oak) tend to cause severe reactions in streaks, where the fingers spread the allergen to other areas. In looking for the source, you should have a better idea about what comes into contact with that area than anyone else.

WHAT ARE THE MOST COMMON CONTACT ALLERGENS?

The most prevalent contact allergy in the United States is sensitivity to poison ivy and poison oak. About 85 percent of the population is either allergic to poison ivy or will become so after adequate exposure. Other common sources of contact sensitivity include costume jewelry (nickel), cosmetics (fragrances, preservatives), dyes (colorants, mordants, etc.), perfumes, metal, industrial chemicals, and rubber products. Medications are a very large problem and the practice of treating every rash with a topical medication has caused many cases of contact dermatitis to the medication. In fact, people sometimes become allergic to things which seem impossible, such as the "cortisone" in a topical medication prescribed to treat a rash. Most such reactions to an object or to whole products are actually allergies to one or more ingredients rather than to the whole product.

This information is provided to help persons with contact dermatitis in the understanding of their problem. The contents are subject to change as more information becomes available and are not intended as a substitute for medical treatment.

ALLERGIC CONTACT DERMATITIS—PATIENT HANDOUT

(Continued)

IS THERE A CURE FOR CONTACT ALLERGY?

In many cases, removing the cause of the allergy should sooner or later cause the problem to subside, but how can this be done? First, one must know all of the ingredients to which he or she is allergic and must avoid all of them. To do this, it is necessary to know where the allergen is found, i.e., what contains it. Third, it helps to have available substitutes for the problem product which do not contain that antigen.

Let's look at some examples. If one is allergic to earrings, the substance in the earrings causing allergy is probably nickel. There is a test you can do at home which will detect nickel in metals, so you can tell which earrings will and will not cause the condition. Therefore you can wear earrings and not break out provided that only those free of the "allergen" are purchased and worn.

Another patient who is allergic to formaldehyde tries to avoid this allergen, but still breaks out on the hands and ears to a shampoo containing formaldehyde. A list of formaldehyde-free shampoos is available, and using a shampoo free of formaldehyde allows that patient to live normally without breaking out (at least to shampoos).

With a practical understanding of the problem—knowing where one is likely to be exposed and what can be used as a safe substitute—most patients suffering from allergic contact dermatitis can live normal lives. However, they must still use this knowledge and apply the self-discipline necessary to avoid the causative agent.

ONCE ALLERGIC, HOW LONG DOES ONE STAY ALLERGIC?

Contact allergy in some cases seems to disappear, but it may not. In any event, it will probably last a very long time, so the allergic patient would do well to learn how to tell what is and what is not safe. Success depends upon early diagnosis and cooperation between doctor and patient. Medications can help reduce your symptoms, but they are no substitute for finding and eliminating the cause. In fact, treating the condition without eliminating the cause may result in the development of an allergy to medications used to treat the condition.

HOW IS AN ALLERGEN IDENTIFIED?

Proof of contact sensitivity usually depends upon patch testing. This involves applying "patches" of standard dilutions of "antigens" to the skin of the upper back. The patches are usually removed after two days and read twice after this. When a patient or doctor suspects an allergy, a case history will be taken which will include information on home and work, living habits, and time of year that the symptoms occur. The doctor will help in deciding from this what patch tests are necessary, and the results of these tests, together with the case history, will help him or her decide what should be avoided and what treatment is needed.

workplace. These documents should also provide the telephone number of a toxicologist familiar with the specific chemical and product. It is often possible to work with the plant safety officer of larger employers to provide protection or to institute a job change to protect the patient.

REFERENCES

1. Burton JL: Eczema, lichenification, prurigo and erythroderma, in Champion RH, Burton JL, Ebling FJG (eds): *Textbook of Dermatology,* 5th ed. Oxford, Blackwell, 1993.
2. Guin JD, Phillips D: Erythroderma from systemic contact dermatitis: A complication of systemic gentamicin in a patient with contact allergy to neomycin. *Cutis* 43:564, 1989.
3. Fregert S (ed): *Manual of Contact Dermatitis,* 2nd ed. Copenhagen, Munksgaard, 1981.
4. Goh CL: An epidemiological comparison between occupational and non-occupational hand eczema. *Br J Dermatol* 120:77, 1989.
5. Ahmed AR, Blose DA: Delayed-type hypersensitivity skin testing: A review. *Arch Dermatol* 119:934, 1983.
6. Benezra C, Maibach H: True cross-sensitization, false cross-sensitization, and otherwise. *Contact Dermatitis* 11:65, 1984.
7. Mitchell JC, Dupuis G: Allergic contact dermatitis from sesquiterpenoids of the *Compositae* family of plants. *Br J Dermatol* 84:139, 1971.
8. Goh CL: Urticarial papular and plaque eruptions: A noneczematous manifestation of allergic contact dermatitis. *Int J Dermatol* 28:172, 1989.
9. Goh CL: Non-eczematous contact reactions, in Rycroft RJG, Menne T, Frosch P, Benezra C (eds): *Textbook of Contact Dermatitis.* Berlin, Springer-Verlag, 1992.
10. Goh CL: An epidemiological comparison between hand eczema and non-hand eczema. *Br J Dermatol* 118:797, 1988.
11. Goh CL: An epidemiological comparison between occupational and non-occupational hand eczema. *Br J Dermatol* 120:77, 1989.
12. Fregert S, Hjorth N, Magnusson B, et al: Epidemiology of contact dermatitis. *Trans St Johns Hosp Dermatol Soc* 55:17, 1969.

4

RECOGNIZING ALLERGIC CONTACT DERMATITIS

James S. Taylor

Allergic contact dermatitis (ACD) has been recognized since ancient times in written descriptions of cutaneous reactions to common allergens.[1] It occurs as either a single event, as intermittent or recurrent episodes, or as a persistent, chronic disease. ACD is a common disorder in medical and dermatologic practice; it may also result in significant occupational and avocational impairment. Fortunately, with the development of patch testing almost 100 years ago,[1] along with the subsequent standardization and refinement of this procedure, ACD today can be scientifically and reliably diagnosed. However, the clinician must know how to recognize potential cases of allergic contact dermatitis, who should be patch tested, and to what. This chapter discusses those important parts of the history and physical examination which offer important clues to the recognition of ACD.

HISTORY

The patient history is an integral part of the diagnosis of ACD, especially in cases of chronic dermatitis and putative occupational contact dermatitis. According to Fischer et al.,[2] in attempting to recognize allergic contact dermatitis on the basis of history alone, a clinician may be only 50 percent right, on average, ranging from 80 percent correct for nickel to 50 percent for moderately common allergens, to about 10 percent for less common allergens. Even with obvious causes, the specific allergen may not be known, and ACD to other chemicals may be associated. Considerable skill is also required to differentiate ACD from a past history of contact urticaria and irritant dermatitis. The yield from the history may also be related to the memories and observational skills of the patient. Published history forms are available which may be utilized by physicians or their assistants or adapted for self-administration by patients.[3,4] One such form can also be found in Appendix B. An initial examination of the area of chief complaint often helps direct the questioning. This is especially true in patients with hand, foot, stasis, and facial dermatitis. In the broadest sense, contact dermatitis should be considered in the differential diagnosis of any patient with eczema. However, patients with generalized, disseminated dermatitis (e.g., quaternium-15 allergy), including exfoliative erythroderma, those with chronic actinic dermatitis (e.g., corticosteroid or photoallergic contact dermatitis), stasis dermatitis (topical medicament allergy), and other forms of eczema should also be questioned and patch tested.[5,6] ACD should also be considered as a secondary diagnosis in patients with other skin disorders.

Taking the history is easier when there is a chief complaint of dermatitis or allergy to a specific substance. In less obvious cases, the patient's own detailed, chronological description of the reaction is especially important. A picture of vesicles with itching, erythema, and edema is typical. These findings may be harder to elicit on a background of chronic lichenified dermatitis and other dermatoses such as psoriasis. Direct questioning may elicit further clues. The cause of abrupt-onset contact dermatitis may be established by taking a careful history of all contactants used during the days immediately preceding the eruption. This includes those personal care, therapeutic, and occupational substances with direct contact as well as sources of indirect exposure such as airborne, connubial (consort), or photocontact dermatitis.[5]

The timing of the reaction is important. Onset of symptoms within minutes or an hour or two points more to contact urticaria[7] or irritant dermatitis.[8] Onset after 1 to 2 days or as long as 1 week suggests contact allergy, especially in first-time cases of dermatitis or in recurrent, intermittent acute dermatitis. This distinction is often blurred in chronic cases. It is also important to remember that irritation, contact urticaria, and contact allergy may coexist. Irritation or chemical burns may predispose one to the development of ACD from the same or other chemicals. A number of contact allergens are also skin irritants. Contact urticaria with onset delayed up to several hours has also been reported.[9] Timing on a longer basis would include seasonal variations in exposure, which may be present with plants and fragrance.

We typically try to elicit a history of overt contact allergy to one or more of the major contact allergens, such as nickel, rubber, topical medicaments, cosmetics (fragrances, preservatives, and dyes), and obvious occupational or avocational exposures which are known potential contact allergens (such as chrome, epoxy, acrylics, gloves, clothing, first aid creams, preservatives, plants, and other chemicals). A history of prior contact allergy may point to inadvertent contact dermatitis in an otherwise unexplained eruption. Patients with stasis dermatitis frequently have allergy to medicaments and over-the-counter products. While most cosmetic reactions are irritant, allergic reactions to cosmetics are most often caused by fragrances.[9]

Other clues in the general medical and dermatologic history may come from a review of past and present therapy, both prescription and over-the-counter, and from a detailed review of personal care products.[3] A complete history of recent drug intake may point to a diagnosis of systemic contact dermatitis. Contact allergy to a medicament may result in generalized eczema with accentuation on the buttocks (baboon syndrome), trunk, and body folds, dyshidrosis, flares at sites of existing or previous eczema, or flares of prior positive patch tests when the same drug or a chemically related drug is administered.[10]

A detailed work history is important in order to evaluate occupational factors. This includes review of job descriptions, lists of work contactants, material safety data sheets, protective equipment, barrier creams, first aid treatment, methods used to clean the skin, previous jobs, second jobs, previous worker's compensation claims, and predisposing factors, including atopic dermatitis, other skin disorders, elevated or decreased temperature and humidity, and personal hygiene.[3] Establishing occupational causation of contact dermatitis is often a challenge to the practicing physician. Criteria listed by Mathias[11] include the following: (1) Is the clinical appearance consistent with contact dermatitis? (2) Are there workplace exposures to potential cutaneous irritants or allergens? (3) Is the anatomic distribution of dermatitis consistent with cutaneous exposure from workplace substances? When the answer to questions 2 and 3 is yes, determining the type of exposure is important. Was there contact with chemicals in a container, as, for example, following an accidental spill? With contaminated surfaces, tools, or rags? With aerosol mist or soluble powders, spray droplets, or permeation through protective clothing?[12] (4) Is the temporal relationship between exposure and onset consistent with contact dermatitis? (5) Are nonoccupational exposures excluded as probable causes? (6) Does dermatitis improve away from work exposures to the suspected irritants or allergens? (7) Do patch or provocation tests identify a probable causal agent? A yes answer to four of the seven criteria is probably adequate for establishing causation in worker's compensation claims.

As Marks and DeLeo[4] illustrate, both patients and physicians often have a number of misconceptions about ACD. These fallacies, along with the correct concepts, include the following:

1. "Allergy only develops to new substances." In fact, allergy can develop years after contact. The statement of William P. Jordan, Jr., M.D., often made at medical meetings, that "life is one big induction period" illustrates this concept.
2. "Allergy is dose-dependent." Allergy is not, within a wide range, dose-dependent. Occasional contact with an object should not exclude it as an allergen. Examples include eyelash curlers, steering wheels, and cosmetic applicators.
3. "If change in medications or cosmetics does not lead to clearing of the rash, those products are not the cause." Many products contain the same or cross-reacting antigens. Also, the composition of a product may be altered without a change in trade name of the product.
4. "Contact allergy occurs only at the site of exposure to the offending agent." Contact allergy can spread by direct or indirect contact, airborne exposure, or connubial contact. Stasis dermatitis with autoeczematization, with or without allergic contact dermatitis on the legs, is a classic example of spread of dermatitis beyond the site of contact.
5. "Expensive products are not allergenic." In fact, allergy is cost-independent.
6. "Negative allergy, prick, or RAST tests exclude contact allergy." Only patch testing is diagnostic of allergic contact dermatitis.

PHYSICAL EXAMINATION

MORPHOLOGY

Allergic contact dermatitis usually appears as either an acute or chronic eczematous dermatitis. Acute contact allergy presenting with vesicles, erythema, and edema may appear anywhere but is best visualized on the palms, sides of the fingers, periungual areas, and soles of the feet. Frequently occurring or persistent episodes of acute contact dermatitis often become chronic with an erythematous, scaling, crusted, and later lichenified eruption. Vesicles may be noted at the periphery of involved skin. Acute dermatitis is more likely to be caused by recent exposure, and accordingly the cause is more obvious. On the other hand, the onset of allergic contact dermatitis is often more subtle. A low-grade subacute to chronic eczema may appear as primarily a scaly or chapped eruption, especially on the face or on the dorsa of the hands.[5,13]

DISTRIBUTION

The distribution of the dermatitis is often the single most important clue to the diagnosis of contact allergy. The area of most intense dermatitis usually corresponds to the site of most intense contact with the allergen. In contact allergy from solid objects, such as tape or dressings, the pattern corresponds to the shape of the causative agent. Liquid allergens may run, leaving a trail or streaks. Both acute and chronic dermatitis may be bilaterally symmetrical, but both are often asymmetrical or unilateral. Dermatitis may be uniform and confluent or involve discrete, patchy areas. Exceptions to the rule occur, however, and the site of greatest exposure is not always the site of greatest involvement. The example most often cited is nail polish allergy, which typically occurs on ectopic sites, especially the eyelids, face, and neck. Onycholysis, nail dystrophy, and periungual dermatitis may also occur, especially with acrylic nail preparations. In addition to the transfer of allergens to distant sites, volatile airborne chemicals may cause dermatitis on exposed body areas.[4]

Regional differences in susceptibility to contact allergens also exist. The thinner eyelid and genital skin is more susceptible to both allergic and irritant contact dermatitis. Maibach and Prystowsky[14] showed that on the soles of six glutaraldehyde-sensitive persons, the application of 25 percent glutaraldehyde produced no reaction, whereas on the arms a concentration of 2.5 percent as a "use test" showed definite reactions. Scalp hair is often protective, with allergic reactions to hair cosmetics involving the upper face, eyelids, postauricular area, and neck. Other areas have higher or lower exposures to allergens which are not always clear and which are reflected in unusual distributions of dermatitis. Allergens in lotions and creams applied all over the body sometimes produce reactions in skin folds and intertriginous areas, where the chemicals tend to concentrate. Attempting to recognize ACD on the basis of the physical examination alone is risky, as the diagnosis may be only partially accurate. Linear vesicular streaks are commonly seen in poison ivy, oak, and sumac allergy, but contact with other plants may give a similar picture. Dermatitis caused by furocoumarins in *Umbelliferae* is typically phototoxic and may be followed by marked hyperpigmentation. Contact with other liquids may also produce linear vesicles. Failure to examine the entire skin may result in misdiagnosis. An eczematous eruption of the trunk and arms may in fact represent autoeczematization from contact or stasis dermatitis of the legs.[4,5,13]

REGIONAL CONTACT DERMATITIS

There are significant regional variations in contact dermatitis, and a knowledge of substances which cause dermatitis of specific body sites will facilitate the diagnosis.

In cases of diagnostic dilemmas, in which the standard patch-test tray is negative, we will sometimes review the texts by Waldbott[15] and Fisher,[5] the atlas by Larsen et al.,[16] and the recent chapter by Veien.[13] We have compiled lists of regional contactants from these sources for patient review.

Hand Eczema

Hand eczema is a significant cause of both occupational and consumer impairment. Allergic contact dermatitis should be considered as the sole or contributing cause in anyone with hand eczema, and patch testing may be the only way to distinguish between irritant and allergic contact dermatitis. Although Cronin[17] believes there are few correlations between clinical patterns of hand eczema and their cause, characteristic patterns of contact allergy do occur. Clues that hand eczema is likely to be allergic include fingertip eczema and change in the pattern of dermatitis from the palm to the dorsum of the hand. Causes of allergic fingertip eczema are glyceryl thioglycolate and paraphenylenediamine in hairdressers; acrylic allergy in dentists; primula, tulip, and *Alstromeria* in florists; and garlic in food handlers. Vesicular finger dermatitis may be associated with nickel, cobalt, and neomycin. Foods—especially fish, meat, poultry, and spices—cause protein contact dermatitis (contact urticaria) with vesicles along the fingers, itching, and contact urticaria. While glove dermatitis may present as bilateral finger and dorsal hand dermatitis with a sharp cutoff at the wrist, it is often patchy with a nonspecific pattern. Anyone with hand eczema who wears gloves, especially rubber or latex gloves, should be evaluated for allergic contact dermatitis and contact urticaria from gloves.[9]

Scalp Dermatitis

According to Fisher,[5] the scalp is resistant to contact dermatitis, and substances applied to this area produce dermatitis of the eyelids, neck, ears, and hands, sparing the scalp. While this is often true, close examination often reveals some scalp dermatitis, especially in cases of hair dye and conditioner allergy. Contact dermatitis has infrequently been reported from wash-off products. Items with occasional contact should not be overlooked, such as hair clips, straps, and caps.

Facial Dermatitis

The differential diagnosis of facial dermatitis is long and cosmetic allergy is the paradigm of allergy from directly applied agents. The face is one of the most common sites of cosmetic allergy. In many cases, the diagnosis is not suspected by the patient or physician, and patch testing is needed to determine the cause. These facts were shown in an American study in which the most common cosmetic allergens were fragrances, preservatives, hair colors, and permanent waves.[18] Cosmetic dermatitis is usually bilateral; the exception is nail polish allergy, which may be unilateral. Nail polish allergy is the paradigm of ectopic contact dermatitis, often affecting the eyelids. In our experience, other areas of the face are typically involved, especially the forehead, cheeks, and neck; the external ear and perineum are occasionally involved. Photocontact dermatitis typically involves exposed areas of the body—the face, neck, and dorsa of the hands—sparing the submental and retroauricular areas in early disease. Fragrances and sunscreens are the most common causes of photoallergic contact dermatitis. Airborne contact dermatitis is often difficult to differentiate from photosensitivity, and these patients should be patch tested with an oleoresin screening tray of selected Compositae as well as pieces of the patient's house and office plants. Other causes of facial dermatitis are allergens with occasional contact (e.g., a pillow), autoeczematization to the face, connubial (consort) contact dermatitis, and systemic contact dermatitis. Atopic dermatitis and seborrheic dermatitis are probably the two most common endogenous dermatoses affecting the face.[19]

Eyelid Dermatitis

The causes of eyelid dermatitis are similar to those affecting the face. Specific substances to consider are nail polish, eye cosmetics and their applicators, eyelash curlers, paper (perfume, formaldehyde), plants, and matches. Many cases of eyelid dermatitis sent for patch testing are negative, especially in those without accompanying erythema and edema.[4,5,13,15,16]

Ear and Earlobe Dermatitis

Nickel allergy from ear piercing is the most common cause of earlobe contact dermatitis. A number of these patients are also cobalt-sensitive, and a few are gold-allergic. Ear canal dermatitis may be caused by objects put into the ear, such as paper clips, matches, and hearing aids as well as by ingredients in topical otic preparations, such as neomycin, propylene glycol, and hydrocortisone.[4,5,13,15,16]

Trunk Dermatitis

According to Veien,[13] the principal sensitizers causing dermatitis of the trunk are nickel in clothing straps; zippers and buttons; rubber in elastic undergarments; fragrances used in soaps, skin-care products, and detergents; and formaldehyde, formaldehyde-containing textile resins, and dyes. Clothing dermatitis is usually most pronounced in places where clothing fits most snugly and at sweat-retention sites—anterior and posterior axillary folds, the sides of the neck, the inner aspects of the thighs, and the gluteal folds. Formaldehyde resin allergy is usually chronic, whereas dye allergy tends to be acute and rapid in onset. An example of contact dermatitis of the waistband area which may be overlooked is the bleached-underwear-elastic syndrome, in which dermatitis is produced only by wearing bleached elastic. Patch testing with a piece of bleached elastic is also positive. The allergen is *n, n*-dibenzyl carbamyl chloride, but its parent chemical, zinc dibenzyl dithiocarbamate, as well as the carba mix on the standard tray, are patch-test negative.[20] Nonbleached elastic causes no clinical dermatitis and is patch-test negative. Antiperspirant and deodorant dermatitis involves the axillae but in some cases may spare the axillary vaults because the allergen is washed out by perspiration.[4,5,13,15,16]

Anogenital Dermatitis

Anogenital dermatitis may be caused by devices and substances used in sexual intercourse or personal hygiene, cosmetics and topical medicaments, clothing, plants such as poison ivy, and a number of other substances with which the patient comes into direct or indirect contact. In a recent study of vulvar dermatoses and contact allergy, the following chemicals were considered relevant: neomycin, quinolone mix, ethylenediamine, imidazoles, topical corticosteroids, fragrance, quaternium-15, diazolidinyl urea, formaldehyde, lanolin, and parabens. Relevant allergens in perianal dermatitis included balsam of Peru, lanolin, neomycin, preservatives, and mercurials. In this area, contact urticaria from condoms and gloves should not be forgotten.[4,5,13,15,16]

Dermatitis of the Thighs, Legs, and Feet

Dermatitis of the thighs may be due to objects inside pockets, such as coins, keys, and matches. Patients with chronic stasis dermatitis and ulceration, like those with anogenital dermatitis, have a high incidence of contact allergy to a number of contactants, especially active ingredients and vehicles in topical medicaments—neomycin, lanolin, parabens, fragrances, etc. Additional allergens include stocking dyes, rubber in support hose, and shoe constituents. Nylon stocking dye dermatitis usually affects the areas of most intense contact—the dorsa of the feet and toes, the backs of the knees, and the inner aspects of the upper thigh. Shoe dermatitis is initiated when the heels and soles of the feet are affected. Shoe dermatitis may involve any part of the foot, often corresponding to the site of the shoe allergen and sparing the arch, except in cases of sport-shoe dermatitis. With chronic dermatitis and sweating, shoe allergens bleed, affecting other parts of the feet.[4,5,13,16,21]

CONNUBIAL CONTACT DERMATITIS

Clues to connubial or consort contact dermatitis are an intermittent eruption resulting from sharing or changing topical products by the spouse or significant other. The onset of symptoms is often related to sexual intercourse or close personal contact. The eruption is usually eczematous or urticarial, especially involving the face, neck, hands, or genitals. Products to suspect are cosmetic hair dyes and fragrances, topical medicaments, contact lens solutions, transdermal patches, intercourse devices, and the handling or mixing of medications for others.[5,22]

SYSTEMIC CONTACT DERMATITIS

When patients with allergic contact dermatitis are subsequently exposed to the same or a related allergen by systemic ingestion, injection, inhalation, or absorption, several different reaction patterns may occur. These include flare of eczema, a flare of patch-test reaction sites, dyshidrosis, or a diffuse erythema (baboon syndrome). The baboon syndrome appears with diffuse or erythema involving the buttocks, upper inner thighs, and axillae and has been caused by ampicillin, nickel, hair dyes, mercury, and disulfiram (Antabuse). Fixed drug eruption and a keratotic eruption of the elbows have also been described in cases of systemic contact dermatitis.[5,10]

NONECZEMATOUS CONTACT DERMATITIS

Contact allergy may have other clinical presentations. Erythema multiforme has been produced by tropical woods and plants, topical medications, certain laboratory chemicals, and other substances.[5] However, most patients with erythema multiforme do not have allergic contact dermatitis. Purpuric contact dermatitis has been reported from rubber or elastic garments or devices, especially those containing the rubber antioxidant *n*-isopropyl-*n*-phenyl-paraphenylenediamine.[5] Pigmented contact dermatitis has been reported from optical whitening agents formerly present in laundry powders in Europe and from azo dyes in textiles and formerly present in some Japanese cosmetics.[5] Lichenoid contact dermatitis in the United States and elsewhere has been reported from contact with color film developers, and lichen planus–like oral eruptions have been reported from certain dental metals, copper, nickel, and mercury.[5] Pustular allergic contact dermatitis from nitrofurazone cream was reported by Burkhart,[23] and allergic granulomas have been seen from zirconium, beryllium, and chromium.[5]

ECZEMATOUS CONTACT DERMATITIS IN OTHER SKIN DISORDERS

Contact dermatitis may appear as a secondary eruption in seborrheic dermatitis,[24] psoriasis,[25] Hailey-Hailey disease,[26] prurigo nodularis,[27] palmar-plantar pustulosis,[24] lichen planus,[5] and probably a number of other disorders. One of our patients with morphea involving her leg was allergic to topical corticoids. Aggravation or unexplained persistence of any dermatosis should raise the question of an associated contact dermatitis.

CHEMICAL LEUKODERMA

Chemical leukoderma, indistinguishable from vitiligo, may occasionally be a sign of allergic contact dermatitis. A careful history may reveal that little or no dermatitis preceded the leukoderma. Patch testing with the putative agent may result in a negative reaction, followed by depigmentation at the test site within 1 to several weeks. Other cases of chemical leukoderma may be preceded by dermatitis. The diagnosis of chemical leukoderma is more readily made in cases that are clustered in a factory and when there is exposure to a known depigmenting chemical, such as monobenzyl ether of hydroquinone or one of the alkyl phenols and catechols. Histologic differentiation from vitiligo is often impossible.[5,28] Zelickson[29] has reported ultrastructural changes associated with 4-isopropylcatechol depigmentation which he can distinguish from vitiligo. Chemical leukoderma usually occurs from direct contact with the offending agent, but inhalation or ingestion has been suggested in some factories.[5,29] Differentiation from postinflammatory hypopigmentation, Koebner-induced depigmentation in vitiligo, and numerous other genetic and metabolic causes of leukoderma is required.

CONCLUSION

Allergic contact dermatitis may occur as an acute event, once or intermittently, or may cause or contribute to chronic eczematous dermatoses. It may be a "background factor" in atopic, seborrheic, irritant contact, and stasis dermatitis as well as in dyshidrosis, contributing to acute or chronic flares of these dermatoses. It may also occur as a secondary factor in a number of other dermatoses. Both the history and physical examination yield important clues in recognizing the presence of ACD. This, in turn, sets the stage for the sound and reliable use of patch testing in accurately diagnosing ACD and providing appropriate allergen avoidance and substitution.

REFERENCES

1. Lachapelle JM: Historical aspects, in Rycroft RJG, Menne T, Frosch P, Benezra C (eds): *Contact Dermatitis.* Berlin, Springer-Verlag, 1992, pp 1–5.
2. Fischer TI, Hansen J, Breilgard B, Maibach HI: The science of patch test standardization in urticaria and the exogenous dermatoses. *Immunol Allerg Clin North Am* 9:417–434, 1989.
3. Freeman S: Diagnosis and differential diagnosis, in Adams RM (ed): *Occupational Skin Disease,* 2nd ed. Philadelphia, Saunders, 1990, pp 194–214.
4. Marks JG Jr, DeLeo VA: *Contact and Occupational Dermatology.* St. Louis, Mosby Yearbook, 1992.
5. Fisher AA: *Contact Dermatitis.* Philadelphia, Lea & Febiger, 1986.
6. Wilkinson SM, English JSC: Hydrocortisone sensitivity: Clinical features of fifty-nine cases. *J Am Acad Dermatol* 27:683–687, 1992.
7. Lahti A, Maibach HI: Immediate contact reactions, in Marzrilli FN, Maibach HI (eds): *Dermatotoxicology,* 4th ed.: New York, Hemisphere, 1991, pp 473–495.
8. Rietschel RL: Diagnosing irritant contact dermatitis, in Jackson EM, Goldner R (eds): *Irritant Contact Dermatitis.* New York, Dekker, 1990, pp 167–171.
9. Taylor JS: Latex allergy. *Am J Contact Dermatitis* 4:114–117, 1993.
10. Menne T, Maibach HI: Systemic contact-type dermatitis, in Marzulli FN, Maibach HI (eds): *Dermatoxicology.* New York, Hemisphere, 1991, pp 453–472.
11. Mathias CGT: Contact dermatitis and worker's compensation: Criteria for establishing occupational causation and aggravation. *J Am Acad Dermatol* 20:842–848, 1989.
12. Cohen BS, Popendorf W: A method for monitoring dermal exposure to volatile chemicals. *Am Indus Hyg Assoc J* 50:216–223, 1989.
13. Veien NK: Clinical features, in Rycroft RJG, Menne T, Frosch PJ, Benezra C (eds): *Contact Dermatitis.* Berlin, Springer-Verlag, 1992, pp 151–204.
14. Maibach HI, Prystowsky SD: Glutaraldehyde (pentanedial) allergic contact dermatitis. *Arch Dermatol* 113:170, 1977.
15. Waldbott GL: *Contact Dermatitis.* Springfield, Ill, Charles C Thomas, 1953, pp 218.
16. Larsen WG, Adams RM, Maibach HI: *Color Atlas of Contact Dermatitis.* Philadelphia, Saunders, 1992.
17. Cronin E: Hand eczema, in Rycroft RJG, Menne T, Frosch PJ, Benezra C (eds): *Contact Dermatitis.* Berlin, Springer-Verlag, 1992, pp 205–218.
18. Adams RM, Maibach HI: A five year study of cosmetic reactions. *J Am Acad Dermatol* 13:1062–1069, 1985.
19. Dooms-Goosens AE, Debusschere KM, Gevers DM, et al: Contact dermatitis caused by airborne agents. *J Am Acad Dermatol* 15:1–10, 1986.
20. Jordan WP Jr, Bourlas MC: Allergic contact dermatitis to underwear elastic. *Arch Dermatol* 111:593–595, 1975.
21. Podmore P: Shoes, in Rycroft RJG, Menne T, Frosch PJ, Benezra C (eds): *Contact Dermatitis.* Berlin, Springer-Verlag, 1992, pp 515–526.
22. Williford PM, Scherertz EF: Connubial contact dermatitis due to thimerosal. *Am J Contact Dermatitis* 3:92–94, 1992.
23. Burkhart CG: Pustular allergic contact dermatitis: A distinct clinical and pathological entity. *Cutis* 27:630–636, 638, 1981.
24. Sherertz EF: Contact dermatitis as a factor in other skin disorders. Syllabus, Ohio Dermatological Association Meeting. Columbus, Ohio, September 18, 1993.

25. Heidenheim M, Jemec GBE: Concomitant psoriasis and allergic contact dermatitis; co-existent inter-related clinical entities. *Am J Contact Dermatitis* 2:175–180, 1991.
26. Retaimo S, Remitz A, Lauerma AI, Forstrom L: Contact allergies in patients with Hailey-Hailey disease. *J Am Acad Dermatol* 21:508–510, 1989.
27. Zelickson BD, McEvoy MT, Fransway AF: Patch testing in prurigo nodularis. *Contact Dermatitis* 20:321–325, 1989.
28. Stevenson CJ: Occupational vitiligo: Clinical and epidemiological aspects. *Br J Dermatol* 105(suppl 20):51, 1981.
29. Zelickson A: *The Clinical Use of Electron Microscopy in Dermatology,* 4th ed. Minneapolis, Bolger Publications, 1985, p 38.

5

PATCH TESTING

Magnus Bruze

Dermatitis accounts for perhaps 25 percent of patients seen in many dermatologists' offices; half of these patients suffer from contact dermatitis.[1] Contact dermatitis comprises irritant contact dermatitis, allergic contact dermatitis, phototoxic contact dermatitis, and photoallergic contact dermatitis. Most of these exogenous cases are either irritant or allergic contact dermatitis. The diagnosis of allergic contact dermatitis is a two-step process: (1) the establishment of delayed hypersensitivity and subsequently (2) the demonstration that the patient is exposed to the sensitizer and that the hypersensitivity and exposure explain the dermatitis under investigation. To make a diagnosis of irritant contact dermatitis, clinically relevant hypersensitivities have to be excluded.

There are two major ways to establish delayed hypersensitivity: by patch testing and by performing laboratory (in vitro) tests. Presently, there is no in vitro technique available which can replace patch testing as a method for establishing contact allergy, although some things supplement it. Patch testing has the advantage over in vitro techniques of being carried out on the skin, the target organ for allergic contact dermatitis. In the skin, metabolism of a compound and/or binding to a certain biologic molecule may be necessary for the hypersensitivity reaction; these can occur with (in vivo) patch tests, but not as yet with in vitro tests. Furthermore, patch testing is not only a bioassay for delayed hypersensitivity but also a provocation test.

HISTORY

Individual intolerance to wood (e.g., toxicodendrons) and other products has been known since antiquity.[2] Idiosyncratic reactions to various substances were recognized during the early nineteenth century, and a method using a strip of blotting paper was described in 1847 for testing for this. However, it was Jadassohn in 1895 who introduced the method of application, which is accepted as the beginning of modern patch testing.[1-3]

INDICATIONS

The major indication for patch testing is a suspicion of allergic contact dermatitis. However, even in cases of endogenous dermatitis, patch testing can be indicated, as that condition can have allergic dermatitis superimposed on it, or it can be provoked by exposing a hypersensitive person to a sensitizer. While contact dermatitis may be of minor significance for endogenous dermatitis, the exposure to the sensitizer may be the only factor that can be altered and that thus can permanently change the severity of the eczema. Occasionally, contact allergy can more closely resemble diseases other than eczemas.[4] In these "noneczematous" cases, patch testing can be indicated, particularly when the skin disease does not fit within the traditional diagnostic framework.

THE PATCH-TEST PROCEDURE

The present patch-test technique is the result of an ongoing process in development and improvement since its first application in the late nineteenth century. Still, there is no ideal patch test,[1] and further improvements will be expected. The overall goal of patch testing is establishing contact allergy rather than diagnosing allergic contact dermatitis, although it is an important contribution to the diagnosis. A perfect patch test should give no false-positive and no false-negative reactions. A test with high specificity would not have false negatives. Furthermore, the ideal patch test should cause as few adverse reactions as possible, particularly active sensitization. False positives, false negatives, and adverse reactions are all dose-dependent. With a sufficiently low concentration of the sensitizers, there will be no false-positive reactions or other adverse effects. In fact, a false-positive reaction is an irritant reaction with the same morphology as, and thus indistinguishable from, an allergic patch-test reaction. However, with a low test concentration, there will be false-negative reactions. Finding the ideal test concentration is complicated, and the current recommended concentrations have been determined taking all of the important factors into account.

In addition to the concentration, the elicitation of a positive patch-test result in a given individual depends upon (1) the dose—that is, the number of molecules of the sensitizer applied, (2) the patch test technique—meaning the vehicle used and the type of occlusion, and (3) the occlusion time.[5-8] The dose is determined by the concentration and volume/amount of the test preparation applied. Thus, if the same amount/volume of a test preparation is applied all the time with the same test technique, it is appropriate to use concentration as a parameter for the dose.

METHODS

Some standard methods of patch testing are included in Table 5-1. All methods except the TRUE test and the Epiquick ready test must be supplemented with test materials from one or more other sources to be complete.

AL-TEST

For years the Al-test was the standard method of applying antigens. The Al-test consists of filter paper disks with a diameter of 1 cm attached to polyethylene-coated aluminum foil.[9] The Al-test has the advantage that the test preparations come into contact mainly

TABLE 5–1. Suppliers of Patch-Test Devices Including Test Allergens

Patch Test Device	Supplier	
A1-test	Hollister-Stier Laboratories P.O. Box 3145 Spokane, WA 99220 Phone 509-489-5656 FAX 509-484-4320	
Finn chambers	Hermal Pharmaceutical Laboratories, Inc. 163 Delaware Ave. Delmar, NY 12054 Phone 1-800-Hermal-1 FAX 518-475-0180	Hermal Kurt Herrmann D 21462 Reinbek/Hamburg Scholtzstrasse 3A Federal Republic of Germany
Van der Bend chambers	Van der Bend B. V. Postbus 73, NL-3230 AB Brielle The Netherlands Phone 31 1810-18055 FAX 31 1810-17450	
TRUE test	Glaxo Dermatology Glaxo Inc. 5 Moore Drive Research Triangle Park, NC 27709 FAX 919-941-3012	
Patch test allergens	Hermal Pharmaceutical Laboratories, Inc. 163 Delaware Ave. Delmar, NY 12054 Phone 1-800-Hermal-1 FAX 518-475-0180	Hermal Kurt Herrmann D 21462 Reinbek/Hamburg Scholtzstrasse 3A Federal Republic of Germany
	Dormer Pharmaceuticals 91 Kellfield Street Unit 5 Rexdale, Ontario M9W 5A3, Canada Phone 416-242-6167 FAX 416-242-9487	Chemotechnique Diagnostics P.O. Box 80, 230 42 Tygelsjö Malmö, Sweden Phone 46-40-160236 FAX 46-40-158640

with inert materials and solutions are easily applied to the attached filter paper disks. The major disadvantage of the Al-test is the size of the patch, as relatively few tests can be applied at the same time.

PATCH TEST

Most other tests consist of aluminum or polypropylene plastic chambers and cups.[10–12] Today the Finn chamber test is probably the most common method used (Figs. 5-1 to 5-10). It has the same accuracy as the Al-test but uses a smaller test area, making it possible to apply numerous tests when they are needed.[13–15] A disadvantage with aluminum is that it is not an inert material but can react with metals such as mercury, cobalt, and nickel.[16–19] It can also increase the rate of acrylate polymerization, probably by acting as a catalyst.[20] Such interactions are probably not a practical problem when the allergens are mixed in petrolatum.

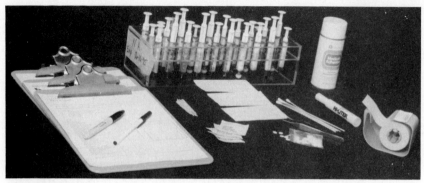

FIG. 5–1. Materials used for patch testing are usually placed in a convenient arrangement close to where the procedure is to be done.

READY-TO-USE SYSTEMS

Recently, some new ready-to-use patch-test systems have been introduced. Pharmacia in Sweden developed the TRUE (thin-layer rapid-use epicutaneous) test, which is a ready-to-use test strip of tape in which a measured amount of allergen is placed in a thin hydrophilic gel film printed on a polyester patch measuring 9 by 9 mm.[4,21] The patch contains different sensitizers mounted on strips of acrylic tape protected by sheets of plastic and packaged in airtight envelopes. For testing, the thin sheet of plastic is removed and the strips are placed on the skin. The dry film dissolves into the gel and the allergen is released onto the skin when the strips come into contact with it. The TRUE test has been compared with the Finn chamber test in multicenter studies and found to have the same accuracy as the Finn chamber test.[22,23]

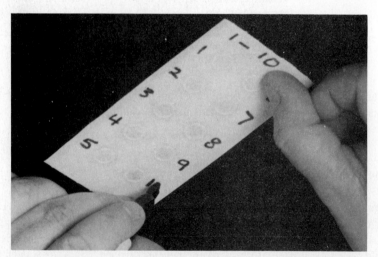

FIG. 5–2. The tape is marked before the protective paper is removed. The reason for this is that the left and right rows are reversed when the chambers are turned over to be loaded. The numbers should be bold enough to be legible through the tape. Inclusive numbers (e.g., 1–10, 11–20, etc.) are placed at the top of the tape strips. These can be left in place when the chambers are removed.

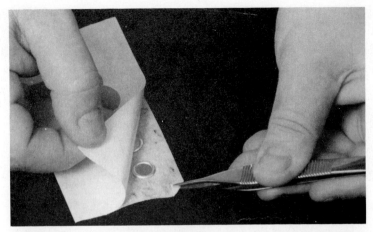

FIG. 5–3. A small corner can be folded over at one edge of the tape strip so that the tape can be handled without sticking. This can be clipped off later with a pair of scissors.

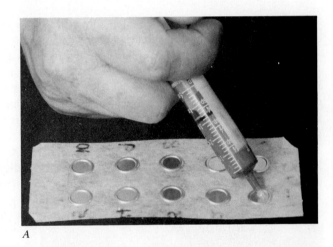

A

FIG. 5–4. *A.* The chambers are loaded with the inclusive numbers placed on the left, so that the order of filling is always the same and in numerical progression. *B.* About 12 to 15 μL of semisolids are added (less than 9 μL will cause false-negative results), which is 50 to 60 percent of the chamber's capacity. Excessive semisolid can be conveniently removed with a toothpick.

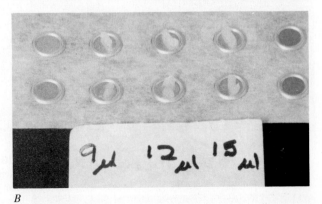

B

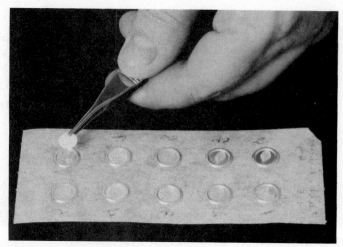

FIG. 5–5. Liquids are added last to prevent unnecessary evaporation. A small dab of petrolatum will hold the cellulose pads used for the liquids (these pads are not used with semisolids). Cellulose pads can easily be mounted to Finn chambers using thumb forceps without teeth.

A condition rarely acknowledged for its significance is the variation in skin absorption of sensitizers with different patch-test systems.[24,25]

Hermal in Germany has developed another new ready-to-use patch test system called Epiquick. Sensitizers of the European standard series are incorporated in petrolatum and applied at a constant volume of 18 μL to Finn chambers on Scanpor tape.[3] The chambers are kept in a special airtight polypropylene aluminum packing until used. Epiquick has been compared not only with other methods but also with itself, with good reproducibility.[26–28]

Recently, a similar ready-to-use patch-test device called *Accupatch* was introduced.[29] It has the antigen incorporated into the nonsensitizing medical-grade acrylic adhesive of the patch.[29] The only antigen that so far seems to have been incorporated is paraphenylenediamine.

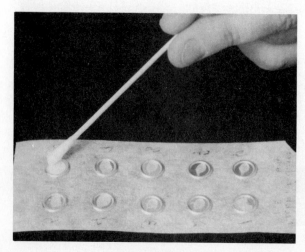

FIG. 5–6. Liquids are added to slight excess; then any excess can be removed with the quick touch of a clean, cotton-tipped applicator.

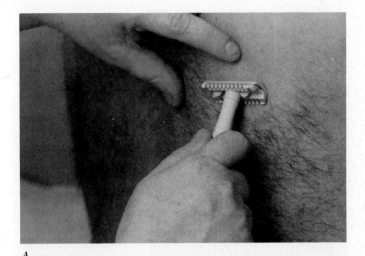

A

B

FIG. 5–7. *A.* Application is made to the skin without cleaning. Alcohol can be used to remove excess oil provided the skin is allowed to dry. Excessively hairy skin may require shaving. Hollister adhesive can be used outside the chamber location where additional adhesive quality may be needed (e.g., in children). *B.* With the patient sitting and leaning a bit forward, the chambers are applied from below upward, smoothing the tape with the palm of the hand and pressing each Finn chamber into position to make sure that good adhesion is present. The skin site chosen should be free of inflammation, ointments, and sebum. The patient should avoid showers and vigorous physical activities for a number of hours after the chambers are applied.

ALLERGENS

Patch testing should be performed when a detailed history and careful clinical examination of a patient's skin disease suggests the presence of an allergic contact dermatitis.

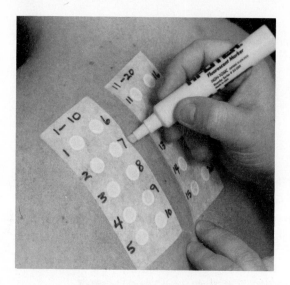

FIG. 5–8. The skin is marked with some type of marking material meeting the criteria outlined in the text. In the United States, many use a fluorescent highlighter which can be detected under a Woods lamp (black light). The tape strips are outlined at the border and rows are then marked in the railroad track pattern both horizontally and vertically.

Occasionally also, endogenous dermatitis and other skin diseases may justify patch testing, which is discussed under the subtitle "Indications," above. Hopefully, the history and the examination will also provide clues to suspected sensitizers. Unfortunately, it is not sufficient to patch test with only primarily suspected sensitizers; unsuspected reagents used in patch testing frequently turn out to be the real cause of the dermatitis.[30] Ideally, one might like to include all known sensitizers, but as there are approximately 3000 currently known allergens,[31] this is impossible. Fortunately, a small number of compounds accounts for the majority of delayed hypersensitivity. Therefore, generally 20 to 25 test preparations consisting of chemically defined compounds and mixes of allergens as well as natural and synthetic compound products are grouped into a standard test series. All over the world, different national and international groups of patch-test specialists recommend use of a standard series, with minor differences in contrast due to differences in culture, industrialization, and use in the various countries. Such series are often revised to adapt to changes in exposure, introduction of new allergens into

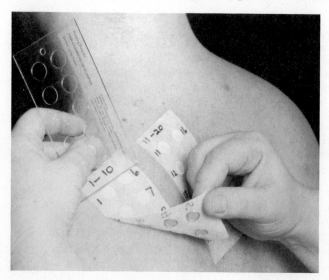

FIG. 5–9. If the chambers are removed in the office, the serrated edge of the template is placed just below the inclusive numbers and the tape strips are cut to remove the Finn chambers but leave the inclusive number firmly fixed to the skin.

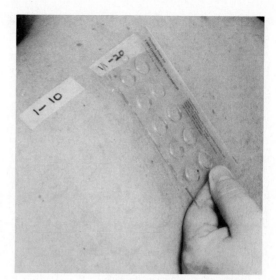

FIG. 5–10. Positive reactions on the back can be identified by the skin marking located under a Woods lamp or with some marking material in room light. A template placed inside the outlined border of the tape strip will help to identify the location of positive reaction.

the market, and experience and information gained on irritant and sensitizing (active sensitization) properties as well as necessary alteration in the test materials themselves.[32–34] The American and European standard series are shown in Tables 5-2 and 5-3. Manufacturers of test preparations are given in Table 5-1. The allergens selected for inclusion are generally those with contact allergy prevalence of 1 percent in routinely patch tested patients with a suspected allergic contact dermatitis. Testing with the test preparations in a standard series is said to detect 70 to 80 percent of all contact allergy,[35–43] but in a study by members of the European Contact Dermatitis Research Group,[43] the sensitivities detected by the standard series alone ranged from 37 to 73 percent of contact allergy, depending upon the testing institution.

The wide variation may partly be due to differences in exposure in the referral areas of participating patch-test clinics, but another possible explanation is differences in patch testing with regard to the number of substances and products tested. The absolute frequency of contact allergy in the general population or in any contact dermatitis population will never be known, but the more test compounds and products that are used in each patient, the more contact allergy will be found. Logically, it follows that a decreasing proportion will be detected by the allergens in the standard series. There is overwhelming evidence for the value of testing to potential sensitizers that are not part of the standard series.[35–43]

Test series for special purposes are commercially available, including series for airborne allergens, coolants, plastics, preservatives, sunscreens, rubber compounds, textile dyes, topical steroids, cosmetics, fragrances, and shoe chemicals. There are also series for allergens present in certain occupations such as hairdressing, bakery work, and dentistry.[1,44–48] Not infrequently, additional patch testing with patient-supplied products has to be performed. Both patch testing with test series other than the standard series and testing with patient-supplied products are discussed in other chapters in this book.

The test preparations in the standard series, except for the ready-to-use tests, are delivered as petrolatum preparations in plastic syringes or water solutions in bottles

TABLE 5–2. The American Standard Patch-Test Series

Test Preparation	Vehicle	Concentration, %
Benzocaine	Pet.	5
Mercaptobenzothiazole	Pet.	1
Colophony	Pet.	20
p-Phenylenediamine	Pet.	1
Imidazolidinyl urea (Germall 115)	Water	2
Cinnamic aldehyde	Pet.	1
Lanolin alcohol (wool wax alcohols)	Pet.	30
Carba mix (carba rubber mix)	Pet.	3
1,3-Diphenylguanidine		1
Zinc diethyldithiocarbamate		1
Zinc dibutyldithiocarbamate		1
Neomycin sulfate	Pet.	20
Thiuram mix (thiuram rubber mix)	Pet.	1
Tetraethylthiuram disulfide		0.25
Tetramethylthiuram monosulfide		0.25
Tetramethylthiuram disulfide		0.25
Dipentamethylenethiuram disulfide		0.25
Formaldehyde (contains methanol)	Water	1
Ethylenediamine dihydrochloride	Pet.	1
Epoxy resin	Pet.	1
Quaternium-15 [N-(3-chloroallyl)-hexaminium chloride]	Pet.	2
p-tert-Butylphenol formaldehyde resin	Pet.	1
Mercapto mix (mercapto rubber mix)	Pet.	1
N-Cyclohexyl-2-benzothiazole-sulfenamide		0.333
2,2-Benzothiazyl disulfide		0.333
Morpholinylmercaptobenzothiazole		0.333
Black rubber (p-phenylenediamine) (P.P.D.) mix	Pet.	0.6
N-Phenyl-N'-cyclohexyl-p-phenylenediamine		0.25
N-Isopropyl-N'phenyl-p-phenylenediamine		0.10
N,N'-Diphenyl-p-phenylenediamine		0.25
Potassium dichromate	Pet.	0.25
Balsam of Peru	Pet.	25
Nickel sulfate (anhydrous)	Pet.	2.5

made from inert polypropylene (Figs. 5-1 and 5-4A). When not used, the test preparations should be kept refrigerated to minimize degradation. To assure accurate test preparations with the labeled sensitizer at the labeled concentration, the preparations should not be used beyond the dates given by the manufacturer. Paraphenylenediamine degrades rapidly, as shown by its color change, but its allergenic properties are not significantly altered.[3] Also, photoallergens stored in sunlight deteriorate rapidly.[49] The antigenicity of fragrances diminishes substantially on aging.[50] On the other hand, some antigens increase in potency with storage (e.g., limonene, which is oxidized to a potent sensitizer).[51]

MIXES

Patch testing with mixes of closely related allergens saves time and space. However, the use of mixes involves problems of concentration, interference, stability, and formula-

TABLE 5–3. The European Standard Patch-Test Series

Test Preparation	Vehicle	Concentration, %
Potassium dichromate	Pet.	0.5
4-Phenylenediamine base	Pet.	1.0
Thiuram mix	Pet.	1.0
tetramethylthiuram monosulfide (TMTM)		0.25
tetraethylthiuram disulfide (TMTD)		0.25
tetraethylthiuram disulfide (TETD)		0.25
dipentamethylenethiuram disulfide (PTD)		0.25
Neomycin sulfate	Pet.	20.0
Cobalt chloride	Pet.	1.0
Benzocaine	Pet.	5.0
Nickel sulfate	Pet.	5.0
Quinoline mix	Pet.	6.0
cliquinol		3.0
chlorquinaldol		3.0
Colophony	Pet.	20.0
Parabens	Pet.	15.0
methyl-4-hydroxybenzoate		3.0
ethyl-4-hydroxybenzoate		3.0
propyl-4-hydroxybenzoate		3.0
butyl-4-hydroxybenzoate		3.0
benzyl-4-hydroxybenzoate		3.0
Black rubber mix	Pet.	0.6
N-isopropyl-N'-phenyl-4-phenylenediamine		0.1
N-cyclohexyl-N'-phenyl-4-phenylenediamine		0.25
N,N'-diphenyl-4-phenylenediamine		0.25
Wool alchols	Pet.	30.0
Mercapto mix	Pet.	2.0
N-cyclohexylbenzothiazyl sulfenamide		0.5
mercaptobenzothiazole		0.5
dibenzothiazyl disulfide		0.5
morpholinylmercaptobenzothiazole		0.5
epoxy resin	Pet.	1.0
Balsam of Peru	Pet.	25.0
4-tert-Butylphenol formaldehyde resin	Pet.	1.0
Mercaptoenzothiazole (MBT)	Pet.	2.0
Formaldehyde	Water	1.0
Fragrance mix	Pet.	8.0
cinnamic alcohol		1.0
cinnamic aldehyde		1.0
hydroxycitronellal		1.0
amylcinnammaldehyde		1.0
geraniol		1.0
eugenol		1.0
isoeugenol		1.0
oakmoss absolute		1.0
Sesquiterpene lactone mix	Pet.	0.
alantolactone		0.033
dihydrocostus lactone + costunolide		0.067
Quaternium 15 (Dowicil 200)	Pet.	1.0
Primin	Pet.	0.01
Cl + Me-isothiazolinone (Kathon CG, 100 ppm)	Water	0.67

tion.[3] Most mixes can induce irritant patch-test reactions. To avoid this, the allergens are incorporated at suboptimal concentrations, sometimes resulting in weak or negative reactions even though a contact allergy is present. Both in cases of morphologically allergic responses and probable irritant responses, it is best to patch test with separate ingredients of the mix.[3,52] The thiuram mix consisting of three thiuram disulfides and one monosulfide represents an interesting example of interference, as the three disulfides change to an equilibrium of six different thiuram disulfides while the monosulfide remains stable.[1] At present, the North American Contact Dermatitis Group recommends mixes of parabens, "caine" anesthetics, and four sets of rubber compounds,[3] while the European Standard contains one more mix (Tables 5-2 and 5-3).

The dose (concentration and volume) of applied sensitizer on a defined area has a decisive effect on a positive patch-test reaction. With petrolatum preparations, it is impossible to apply the same amount/volume of the test preparation every time, but an experienced and trained person can keep the variation within a limited range (Fig. 5-4A and B).[53] The test preparation should cover the test area completely, but it should not spread beyond its limits, as that might cause loosening of the adhesive. The same problems exist with solutions, but it is easier to apply a defined volume of a solution to the filter paper disk. For a Finn chamber with a filter paper disk, the recommended volume is 15 μL, and the corresponding volume for the Al test is 25 μL.

VEHICLES

There are some general demands on a vehicle used for an allergen for patch testing. The vehicle itself should be nonirritating, nonsensitizing, and chemically inert; i.e., it should not react with the allergen. Examples of vehicles that can be used are water, ethanol, acetone, methyl ethyl ketone, olive oil, and petrolatum.[9] The allergens in the standard series are either incorporated into petrolatum or, for a few, dissolved in water. The earlier use of lanolin as a vehicle has been abandoned because of its sensitizing properties. Softisan is a hydrophilic lanolin substitute which has been suggested as a vehicle for patch-test allergens.[54] Control tests are in order, as even petrolatum, olive oil, or acetone may rarely sensitize.[55-59]

The major advantage of the liquid vehicles is the relative ease of applying a fixed volume of the test preparation to the patch. The major disadvantages are problems with stability regarding both the allergens[49] and the solvent. The opposite conditions are true for petrolatum. It is stable and seems to prevent degradation of the incorporated allergen.[49] With petrolatum as the vehicle, it is impossible to apply a determined volume/ amount from time to time (Fig. 5-4A and B). For screening purposes (of detection of contact allergy) this variation is of minor significance, but for most scientific purposes, a vehicle that permits the repeated application of a determined volume should be used.[60]

In the Epiquick test system, the vehicle is petrolatum. The vehicle in the TRUE test contains hydroxypropylcellulose and polyvinylpyrolidone.[3]

ADHESIVE

The tape used to attach the patches to the skin should give good adhesiveness for sufficient occlusion, with a minimal chance of an adverse reaction. Many types of tape can provide proper attachment to the skin but can cause such tight occlusion that miliaria and irritant reactions occur, making the reading of the test impossible. Older adhesive tape consists of a cotton fabric covered with a sticky mass which most often consisted of crepe rubber, rosin, zinc oxide, lanolin, antioxidants, and preservatives.[1] Many of these materials were potential sensitizers, often resulting in tape allergy.[61–63]

Most tapes used today are made of nonwoven textile material and an acrylate adhesive.[1] Still, rosin derivatives are sometimes contained in the adhesive, which can be a source of allergic reactions.[64] Allergic reactions to adhesive acrylates are rare and only occasionally reported.[65] Contact allergy to formaldehyde[66] and diphenylthiourea[67] in tapes has also been reported.

Because of the occlusive property of any tape, mildly irritant, acneiform, and miliarial reactions are relatively common.[68] Scanpor is a finely meshed paper tape with a polyacrylate adhesive[3] used for Finn chambers but commonly for other purposes as well (Fig. 5-3). Miliaria and other adverse effects are seldom induced by Scanpor and similar tapes because of the large number of perforations per square centimeter in the fabric.

Any tape may not adhere well enough when the skin is greasy or when there is excessive sweating. To improve adhesion, oily skin can be washed with ethanol, but the back must be permitted to dry completely before the patches are applied. Also, a hairy back may reduce adhesion of the tape, so sometimes the test site must be shaved before the patches are applied (Fig. 5-7A).

To assure uniform adhesion of the tape strips holding the patches, the patient should be sitting and leaning slightly forward. The tape strips are then applied from below, with firm pressure to remove air bubbles (Fig. 5-7B).[3]

MARKING THE TEST AREA

The location of the various patches applied must be marked in some way to assure the identification of patch-test reactions. Some mark the top edge of each tape strip, leaving this in place when the chambers are removed. Others mark the skin with some marking material, which must remain on the skin up to the time of the first reading (48 to 96 h) (Fig. 5-8). This must neither irritate[69,70] nor sensitize the skin, and it should not discolor clothing.[3] Either fluorescent[71] or colored inks may be used. Coloring substances used for marking include methylrosaniline (chloride), silver nitrate, gentian violet dihydroxyacetone, pyrogallol, and ferric chloride.[1,3,9] Many in the United States use an inexpensive fluorescent highlighter which leaves marks detectable by Woods lamp (black light) examination.

OCCLUSION TIME

When the tape strips with patches are attached to the skin, a process starts whereby the sensitizers migrate from the patches into the epidermis. The rate of this process is governed by a complicated interaction between factors including the patches, the test substance, its vehicle, and the skin. Physical-chemical properties of these factors will determine the nature and rate of the process. The patch-test procedure is standardized with an occlusion time of 48 h. However, this occlusion time does not mean that all the sensitizer is discharged from the patch.[24,60,72-74] As most sensitizers will not leave the patches entirely (in fact, this will never happen for any sensitizer), differences in test technique (for example, different test methods and adhesive tapes) will influence the number of molecules of the sensitizer entering the skin and consequently the outcome of the test.[24,25] Moreover, a change in occlusion time can be expected to affect the patch-test result; that is, a shorter occlusion time with the same test preparation and the same method will therefore result in fewer persons reacting positively.[73]

Three major factors are decisive for the patch test result: (1) the allergen dose, (2) patch-test technique (including vehicle, test method, and adhesive tape), and (3) occlusion time. No one of these factors can therefore be changed without affecting the outcome. However, a decrease in occlusion time can be compensated by a higher dose of the sensitizer. Thus, patch testing with nickel sulphate at 30% under occlusion for 5 h gave a similar patch-test result as for nickel sulfate at 5% under occlusion for 48 h.[75] However, the patch-test procedure has been standardized with an occlusion time of 48 h, so any possible change must be preceded by extensive scientific investigations.

READING THE TEST RESULT

The time for reading is not as standardized as the occlusion time. At some patch-test clinics, the reading is done after 48 h. The test strips are removed at the clinic and the test is read after a half hour (Figs. 5-9 and 5-10).[76] Sometimes this is the only reading, but it is insufficient, as many contact allergies show up first after 48 h. In many countries, the patients themselves, friends, or relatives remove the strips after 48 h and the reading is then made after another 24 h. However, contact allergies may also appear on the back after 72 h.[76-83] A single reading on day 2 (48 h) means that approximately 30 percent of the contact allergies detected by a standard test series are missed, as compared with the number of allergies found when the tests are read frequently during the period of 2 days to 1 week after the application.[79-83] However, the time when the sensitizers appear macroscopically positive varies with the allergen. Neomycin and paraphenylenediamine are among those showing up late.[81,83] With primin, present in the European standard series but not the North American series, all contact allergy seems to be detected with the reading on day 2.[82] However, with regard to all sensitizers in the standard series, no single reading detects all contact allergy. If only one reading is feasible, it should be performed on day 3 or 4.[77,79,81,82] The policy of reading only once and only on day 2 (48 h) may well give inaccurate conclusions and is therefore no longer recommended.[82] Some dermatologists have gone so far as to suggest challenging medicolegal use of results of only a single patch-test reading on day 2 (48 h).[82]

The contact-allergic response in the skin after applying a sensitizer is a dose-response phenomenon characterized by skin inflammation. An erythema precedes infiltration, followed by papules and vesicles, which may coalesce to bullae. These various inflammatory responses can be seen at the same time when reading patch tests with serial dilutions of a sensitizer in a hypersensitive person. The largest dose may produce coalescing vesicles, a lower dose may lead to only erythematous infiltration with a few papules, and an even lower dose may result in a negative reaction. With some variation, patch-test reactions are usually graded according to the evaluation model in Table 5-4.[1,9,84]

If a patch-test reaction is to be considered truly allergic, certain morphologic features

TABLE 5–4. Patch-Test Interpretation Gradings

–	Negative reaction
?	Doubtful reaction; macular erythema only
+	Weak reaction—nonvesicular; erythema, infiltration, papules
+ +	Strong reaction—edematous or vesicular
+ + +	Extreme reaction—ulcerative or bullous
IR	Irritant reaction
NT	Not tested

must be present, ranging from an erythematous infiltration to erythema with coalescing vesicles. Unfortunately, there is no biological response which will, with certainty, guarantee or exclude allergy. The present limit (with at least an erythematous infiltration for a reaction to be considered allergic) has been chosen arbitrarily. The major reason is that most reactions of this intensity or greater represent true allergic responses, while reactions which are only erythematous often turn out to be irritant or nonspecific. Therefore, when there is only erythema without infiltration where standard test sensitizers have been applied, the cause could be either a weak allergic response or an irritant reaction. To establish or rule out contact allergy, patch testing should be repeated. Because of biological and technical reasons, there might be a variation in the test response to the same sensitizer from time to time. Thus, the repeat test reading may be positive, negative, or questionable. If negative, it is likely that the first erythematous reaction represented an irritant reaction, but it is not possible to totally rule out allergy. However, even if the original weak test result were contact-allergic, it is so very weak that it is unlikely to be clinically relevant. To further investigate the possibility of contact allergy, additional testing with in vitro and intradermal tests can be carried out.[84–86]

Irritant reactions may occur to sensitizers in the standard series. Test preparations commonly causing such irritant reactions are formaldehyde, potassium dichromate, fragrance mixes, and carba mix. Irritant reactions present many different morphological types, from homogeneous erythema without infiltration to weak erythema with wrinkling (silk-paper structure), petechiae, pustules, bullae, and necrosis.[1,9,87,88]

CLINICAL RELEVANCE

Often, the patient is found to be allergic to one or more tests. In such instances, we still have not proved that the allergy is relevant (i.e., that it caused or contributed to the presenting problem). To establish relevance, we look for evidence of recent exposure to that sensitizer and then evaluate the likelihood that such exposure would explain what we see clinically, including the type of dermatitis, its localization, and its course. Here, a knowledge of where a person is likely to be exposed to that antigen is invaluable. Much of that information can be found in Part II, on standard patch-test antigens.

PATIENT INSTRUCTIONS

The patient should be told the purpose of patch testing, how it is done, the various symptoms that may occur, and the factors that may influence the outcome of the test.

During the occlusion period, the patient should not shower or bathe or participate in strenuous activities, as the patches may come loose. After removal of the patches, a short shower is permitted provided that the marking tolerates water. All activities causing considerable sweating should be avoided, as this tends to cause the tape to come loose. Should that happen, the patient can reaffix the tape and make a note what part has been loose. If the patient experiences severe symptoms, (most likely itching), he or she should contact the dermatologist and, if necessary, return earlier than the scheduled time for reading the patch tests. At the clinic, the part of the tape covering the skin with the symptoms can be removed. If there is an intense reaction, the test result is recorded and a topical steroid can be used for symptomatic treatment.

Preferably, the patient should get written information on the patch-test procedure and necessary instructions (Table 5-5). Most of our patients want some information on the sensitizers tested, so, at our department, a written information sheet on the sensitizers (Table 5-6) is also given to the patient on the day of patch-test application.

CAUSES OF FALSE-POSITIVE REACTIONS

A false-positive patch-test reaction, by definition, is morphologically indistinguishable from a true allergic reaction, but it is mediated by a mechanism other than contact allergy. Thus, patch-test reactions with an obvious irritant morphology are never examples of false-positive reactions. However, it is sometimes difficult or even impossible to differentiate between allergic and irritant reactions, and an irritant reaction can thus be read as an allergic reaction—a false-positive reaction.

As the reading requires skill and particularly experience, the risk of false-positive reactions is higher when inexperienced dermatologists read the tests. Although the recommended test concentrations for the sensitizers in the standard series are the result of extensive international experience of testing, some of the concentrations (e.g., for chromate and formaldehyde) have been chosen close to the irritancy threshold to diminish the risk of getting false-negative reactions. The frequency of irritant reactions is higher at 48 h as compared with later readings.[79] Atopics are particularly prone to nonspecific (erythematous) reactions, irritant reactions both from the test materials themselves and from the sensitizers.

TABLE 5–5. Instructions for the Patient on the Patch-Test Procedure

To investigate whether or not you are contact-allergic to certain chemicals which may cause allergic contact dermatitis, patch-test strips with potential sensitizers have been applied to your back. These strips should remain on the back for 2 days. During and after these 2 days, redness and itching may appear on one or a few small areas that have been exposed to the sensitizers. Such a skin reaction usually indicates contact allergy.

To increase the reliability of the test, you should observe the following instructions:

1. When you bathe or shower, the test panels must not get wet, as this might cause loosening of the panels.
2. Avoid exercising or other activities that may cause you to sweat, as this might also cause the test panels to loosen.
3. Avoid scratching the test area, as the skin may become irritated and therefore make it difficult for your dermatologist to read the test.
4. If an area of the test strip becomes loose, you should immediately reattach it with adhesive tape and make a note of what part was loose.

TABLE 5–6. Information on the Sensitizers in the Standard Patch-Test Series

Metals	Nickel can be present in costume jewelry, zip fasteners, bra clips, jeans buttons, etc. Chrome can exist as chromate and can be found in cement, anticorrosion agents, matches, etc.
Rubber additives	Black rubber *p*-phenylenedehyde mix, thiuram mix, carba mix, mercapto mix, and mercaptobenzothiazole contain substances used in rubber products to prevent degradation and improve the properties of the material. These additives can be present in gloves, hoses, elastic bands, handles, tires, packings, cables, etc.
Perfumes, balsams	Cinnamic aldehyde and balsam of Peru can be present in cosmetics, cleansers, and toiletries as well as taste-enhancing additives in ice cream, soft drinks, etc.
Resins	Rosin or colophony is a natural resin used in adhesives, tapes, mascara, wart remedies, soldering fluxes, etc.
	Epoxy resin can be present in glues, paints, surface coatings, etc.
	p-tert-Butylphenol formaldehyde resin is used in glues for rubber and leather.
Preservatives	Imidazolidinyl urea, formaldehyde, and quaternium-15 can be found in cosmetics, toiletries, cleansers, coolants, and other industrial products requiring preservation. Formaldehyde can also be present in glues and textiles.
Lanolin	Lanolin or wool alcohols are used in cosmetics, toiletries, medications, etc.
Ethylenediamine	Ethylenediamine can be used as a stabilizing agent in creams and medicines.
p-Phenylenediamine	Paraphenylenediamine is a dye which can be used in textiles, leather objects, cosmetics, etc.
Medicines	Neomycin is a germicidal substance which can be used in topical remedies but also systemically.

Also, irritant reactions which might be misinterpreted as true-positive reactions are dose dependent. Thus, if there is a great variation in the amount/volume of a test preparation applied on the patch, the risk of false-positive reactions is increased. Many sensitizers are also irritant, so an injudiciously high concentration increases the risk of a false-positive reaction.

The "angry back" or "excited skin syndrome" implies that there are many patch test reactions, of which some are false positive.[89–92] However, a patient can have multiple contact allergies, so the presence of some or many morphologically allergic test reactions on the back must never be automatically interpreted as a sign of angry back or excited skin syndrome. In my experience,[60] very few if any morphologically allergic reactions to sensitizers in the standard series represent false positive reactions if they appear on skin with normal skin separating that test from other positive tests. However, sometimes there is a widespread eruption over much of the back, with nonspecific erythematous reactions more or less covering the whole test area. Test reactions appearing where the skin is so affected should be looked upon with skepticism, as they can represent false-positive reactions. This type of reactivity is increased when there is a widespread active dermatitis, so patch testing should be postponed until the dermatitis is more quiescent. In case there are any patch-test reactions believed to be due to an angry back, testing with these preparations must be repeated.

CAUSES OF FALSE-NEGATIVE REACTIONS

To elicit a positive patch-test reaction in a hypersensitive person, the migration of a certain number of molecules of the sensitizer into the skin is required. There are three major factors that determine the number of molecules entering the skin at patch testing:

(1) the dose applied on the patch, (2) the type of occlusion (vehicle used and patch test system), and (3) the occlusion time. If any one of these factors is changed, there is a risk of false-negative reactions. The dose can be low due to a low concentration of the sensitizer in the test preparation and/or a low amount/volume of the test preparation applied on the patch. If the patches come loose during the test procedure, the risk of false-negative reactions increases. The major reason for loosening patches and adhesives is moisture around the test area. This may come from bathing or showering and from sweating from, for example, outdoor summer heat or physically strenuous activities. Scratching the test area may also cause the panel to loosen. Removing the panels before 48 h may increase the risk of false-negative reactions. Reading only once at 48 h also means that there will be many false-negative reactions.

Potent topical corticosteroids applied to the test site for several days before testing may diminish the skin reactivity, with false-negative reactions as a consequence.[3] Also, systemic steroids influence the patch-test results. With daily prednisolone in doses of 15 to 20 mg or less, the risk of false-negative reactions is considered negligible.[92] Other circumstances that may affect a person's skin reactivity are ultraviolet radiation and female sex hormones. In Sweden and Denmark but not in Belgium, a seasonal influence with more positive routine test reactions during the winter has been found.[93-95] In women, the skin reactivity to allergens is increased premenstrually.[96] Another cause of false-negative reactions is the failure to test for photosensitivity, as in this instance light is also necessary to elicit a response.

ADVERSE REACTIONS

Apart from nonspecific reactions to test materials and weak irritant reactions to test preparations in the routine series, adverse reactions are rare.

ACTIVE SENSITIZATION

Induction of contact allergy due to the patch-test procedure (active sensitization) is considered to be an extremely infrequent complication of patch testing.[3] The induction of sensitization is dose dependent, so a proper test technique with use of standardized test preparations, with the sensitizer at the intended concentration and the application of an intended amount/volume of the test preparation, diminishes substantially the risk of active sensitization. By definition, active sensitization is seen by a flareup reaction on the back, with an earliest appearance after 7 to 10 days.[97] Patch testing again with suspected test preparations then gives a positive reaction to one preparation already on the ordinary reading day (3 to 4 days after test application). However, induction of hypersensitivity may also be silent, which would require some special investigations to demonstrate it.[97,98]

REACTION TO THE TEST DEVICE (TEST MATERIALS OTHER THAN THE ANTIGEN)

Apart from a nonspecific erythematous reaction (most often due to the occlusion), adverse reactions to the test device are uncommon. However, colophony and formalde-hyde in the test device can occasionally cause an allergic contact dermatitis.[64,66]

ALTERATION OF PIGMENTATION

Inflammatory reactions in the skin may result in transient alteration of pigmentation, both hypo- and hyperpigmentation. Testing with chemicals known to be potential depigmenting agents may induce depigmentation at the test site. In the present standard test panels (Table 5-2 and 5-3), *p*-tert phenol-formaldehyde resin is a potential depigmenting chemical.

PERSISTENCE OF REACTION

Usually a positive patch test reaction disappears within some weeks. However, occasionally positive reactions may last significantly longer. This refers particularly to gold compounds,[3] but persistent reactions to a Compositae plant[99] and textile dyes[100] have also been reported.

MISCELLANEOUS

Occasionally a flare of dermatitis elsewhere on the skin may occur at the highest intensity level of a positive test reaction. Rarely, psoriasis may appear following irritant or allergic patch-test reactions in psoriatic patients. Other extremely uncommon adverse reactions may occur with substances outside the routine test series, including scarring after extensive irritant reactions and anaphylactoid reactions when potent urticaria-producing substances are tested.

SUMMARY

Many of the patients seen in dermatologists' offices suffer from contact dermatitis. The bulk of contact dermatitis comprises irritant and allergic contact dermatitis. The first step in establishing a diagnosis of allergic contact dermatitis is the establishing of contact allergy. Although patch testing has been used for almost 100 years, no other method for establishing contact allergy has so far been able to replace it. There are various patch-test methods available which in principle can be divided into two major groups. The old methods comprise two separate units: the patch units to which the test preparations are applied from a container. The new methods deliver the test preparations already contained in each patch. The present test concentrations are chosen to minimize the risks of false-negative and false-positive reactions as well as active sensitization. The patch-test procedure is standardized with an occlusion time of 48 h, while the reading usually is performed once 2 to 4 days after the application. However, if the test is read after 2 days, the reading must be repeated at least once more *after that*.

REFERENCES

1. Fischer T, Maibach HI: Improved, but not perfect, patch testing. *Am J Contact Dermatitis* 1:73, 1990.
2. Foussereau J: History of epicutaneous testing: The blotting paper and other methods. *Contact Dermatitis* 11:219, 1984.

3. Adams RM, Fischer T: Diagnostic patch testing, in Adams RM (ed): *Occupational Skin Disease,* 2nd ed. Philadelphia, Saunders, 1990, pp 223–253.

4. Goh CL: Noneczematous contact reactions, in Rycroft RJG, Menne T, Frosch PJ, Benezra C (eds): *Textbook of Contact Dermatitis.* Berlin, Springer-Verlag, 1992, pp 219–236.

5. Upadhye MR, Maibach HI: Influence of area of application of allergen on sensitization in contact dermatitis. *Contact Dermatitis* 27:281, 1992.

6. Webster RC, Maibach HI: Percutaneous absorption relative to occupational dermatology, in Maibach HI (ed): *Occupational and Industrial Dermatology,* 2nd ed. Chicago, Yearbook, 1987, pp 241–257.

7. Bruze M: Patch testing with nickel sulphate under occlusion for five hours. *Acta Derm Venereol* 68:361, 1988.

8. Friedmann PS, Moss C, Shuster S, Simpson JM: Quantitative relationships between sensitizing dose of DNCB and reactivity in normal subjects. *Clin Exp Immunol* 53:709, 1983.

9. Fregert S: *Manual of Contact Dermatitis.* Copenhagen, Munksgaard, 1981.

10. Pirilfi W: Chamber test versus patch test for epicutaneous testing. *Contact Dermatitis* 1:48, 1975.

11. Forsch PJ, Kligman AM: The Duhring chamber: An improved technique for epicutaneous testing of irritant and allergic reactions. *Contact Dermatitis* 5:73, 1979.

12. Dooms-Goossens A: Van der Bend Chamber Test. *Nieuwsbrief Contactdermatologie,* December 1984.

13. Cronin E: Comparison of Al-test and Finn chamber. *Contact Dermatitis* 4:301, 1978.

14. Hammershoy O: Contradictory results following patch testing with Finn chambers. *Contact Dermatitis* 6:216, 1980.

15. Peltonen L: Comparison of Al-test and Finn chamber test. *Contact Dermatitis* 7:192, 1981.

16. Kalveram K-J, Rapp-Frick C, Sorck G: Misleading patch test results with aluminum Finn chambers and mercury salts. *Contact Dermatitis* 6:507, 1980.

17. Lachapelle JM, Douka M-A: An evaluation of the compatibility between aluminum Finn chambers and various mercurials dissolved in water or dispensed in petrolatum. *Dermatosen* 33:12, 1985.

18. Lindemayer H, Berecano ST: Interaction of mercury compounds and aluminium. *Contact Dermatitis* 13:274, 1985.

19. Fischer T, Maibach HI: Aluminum in Finn chambers reacts with cobalt and nickel salts in patch test materials. *Contact Dermatitis* 12:200, 1985.

20. Bjorkner B, Niklasson B: Influence of the vehicle on the elicitation of contact allergic reactions to acrylic compounds in guinea pig. *Contact Dermatitis* 11:268, 1984.

21. Fischer T, Maibach HI: The thin layer rapid use epicutaneous test (TRUE test): A new patch test method with high accuracy. *Br J Dermatol* 112:63, 1985.

22. Lachapelle JM, Bruynzeel DP, Ducombs G, et al: European multicenter study of the TRUE Test. *Contact Dermatitis* 19:91, 1988.

23. Stenberg B, Billberg K, Fischer T, et al: Swedish multicenter study with True test panel 2. in Frosch PJ, Dooms-Goossens A, Lachapelle J-M, et al (eds): *Topics in Contact Dermatitis.* Heidelberg, Springer-Verlag, 1989, pp 518–523.

24. Bruze M: Patch testing with a mixture of phenol-formaldehyde resins. *Contact Dermatitis* 19:116, 1988.

25. Kim HG, Wester RC, McMaster JA, et al: Skin absorption from patch test systems. *Contact Dermatitis* 17:178, 1987.

26. Hornstein M: Anvendung eines neuen Fertigpflasters in der Praxis (Epiquick). *Z Hautkrank* 62:1719, 1987.

27. Lachapelle J-M: Left versus right side comparative study of Epiquick patch test results in 100 consecutive patients. *Contact Dermatitis* 20:51, 1989.

28. Lachapelle J-M, Antoine J-L: Problems raised by the simultaneous reproducibility of positive patch test reactions in man. *J Am Acad Dermatol* 21:850, 1989.

29. Marks JG: The Accupatch: A new patch testing device. *Am J Contact Dermatitis* 2:98, 1991.

30. Adams RM: Patch testing—A recapitulation. *J Am Acad Dermatol* 5:629, 1981.

31. de Groot AC: *Patch Testing: Test Concentrations and Vehicles for 2800 Allergens.* Amsterdam, Elsevier, 1986.

32. Revised European standard series. *Contact Dermatitis* 19:391, 1988.

33. Logan RA, White IR: Carbamix is redundant in the patch test series. *Contact Dermatitis* 18:303, 1985.

34. Bruze M, Gruvberger B, Bjorkner B: Kathon CG—An unusual sensitizer, in Menne T, Maibach HI (eds): *Exogenous Dermatoses.* Boca Raton, FL, CRC Press, 1991, pp 283–289.

35. Hammershoy O: Standard patch test results in 3225 consecutive Danish patients from 1973 to 1977. *Contact Dermatitis* 6:263, 1980.

36. Hirano S, Yoshikawa K: Patch testing with European and American standard allergens in Japanese patients. *Contact Dermatitis* 8:48, 1982.
37. Hjorth N: Routine patch tests. *Trans St John's Hosp Dermatol Soc* 49:99, 1963.
38. Lepine EM: Results of routine office patch testing. *Contact Dermatitis* 2:89, 1976.
39. Gailhofer G, Ludvan M: Zur Anderungen der Allergenspectrums bei Kontaktekzemen in der Jahren 1975–1984. *Dermatosen* 35:12, 1987.
40. Magnusson B, Blohm S-G, Fregert S, et al: Routine patch testing: III. Frequency of contact allergy at six Scandinavian clinics. *Acta Derm Venereol* 46:396, 1966.
41. Young E, Honwing RH: Patch test results with standard allergens over a decade. *Contact Dermatitis* 17:104, 1987.
42. Nethercott JR, Holness DL, Adams RM, et al: Patch testing with a routine screening tray in North America, 1985–1989: I. Frequency of response. *Am J Contact Dermatitis* 2:122, 1991.
43. Menne T, Dooms-Goossens A, Wahlberg JE, et al: How large a proportion of contact sensitivities are diagnosed with the European Standard Series? *Contact Dermatitis* 26:201, 1992.
44. Foussereau J, Benezra C, Maibach HI: *Occupational Contact Dermatitis: Clinical and Chemical Aspects.* Copenhagen, Munksgaard, 1982.
45. *The Trolab Guide for Patch Testing.* Reinbek, Germany, Hermal, Kurt Herrmann, 1992.
46. *Patch Test Allergens: Product Catalogue.* Malmö, Sweden, Chemotechnique Diagnostics AB, 1992.
47. Lachapelle J-M: Industrial airborne irritant or allergic contact dermatitis. *Contact Dermatitis* 14:137, 1986.
48. Dooms-Goossens A, Debusschere KM, Gevers DM, et al: Contact dermatitis caused by airborne agents. *J Am Acad Dermatol* 15:1, 1986.
49. Bruze M, Fregert S: Studies on purity and stability of photopatch test substances. *Contact Dermatitis* 9:33, 1983.
50. Fisher AA, Dooms-Goossens A: The effect of perfume "aging" on the allergenicity of individual perfume ingredients. *Contact Dermatitis* 2:155, 1976.
51. Karlberg A-T, Magnusson K, Nilsson U. Airoxidation of d-limonene (the citrus solvents) creates potent allergens. *Contact Dermatitis* 26:332, 1992.
52. Mitchell JC: Patch testing with mixes: Note on mercaptobenzothiazole mix. *Contact Dermatitis* 7:98, 1981.
53. Fischer T, Maibach HI: Finn chamber patch test technique. *Contact Dermatitis* 11:137, 1984.
54. Vaananen A, Hannuksela M: Softisan—A new vehicle for patch testing. *Contact Dermatitis* 14:215, 1986.
55. Dooms-Goossens A, Degreef H: Contact allergy to petrolatums: I. Sensitizing capacity of different brands of yellow and white petrolatums. *Contact Dermatitis* 9:175, 1983.
56. Dooms-Goossens A, Degreef H: Contact allergy to petrolatums: II. Attempts to identify the nature of the allergens. *Contact Dermatitis* 9:247, 1983.
57. Dooms-Goossens A, Degreef H: Contact allergy to petrolatums: III. Allergenicity prediction and pharamacopoeial requirements. *Contact Dermatitis* 9:352, 1983.
58. Malmkvist Padoan S, Pettersson A, Svensson A: Olive oil as a cause of contact allergy in patients with venous eczema, and occupationally. *Contact Dermatitis* 23:73, 1990.
59. Tosti A, Bardazzi F, Ghetti P: Unusual complication of sensitizing therapy for alopecia areata. *Contact Dermatitis* 18:322, 1988.
60. Bruze M: Contact sensitizers in resins based on phenol and formaldehyde. *Acta Derm Venereol Suppl* 119:1, 1985.
61. Calnan CD: Diethyldithiocarbamate in adhesive tape. *Contact Dermatitis* 4:61, 1978.
62. Cronin E, Calnan CD: Allergy to hydroabietic alcohol in adhesive tape. *Contact Dermatitis* 4:57, 1978.
63. Rasmussen JE, Fischer AA: Allergic contact dermatitis to a salicylic acid plaster. *Contact Dermatitis* 2:237, 1976.
64. Sjoborg S, Fregert S: Allergic contact dermatitis from a colophony derivative in a tape skin closure. *Contact Dermatitis* 10:114, 1984.
65. Jordan WP: Cross-sensitization pattern in acrylate allergies. *Contact Dermatitis* 1:13, 1975.
66. Andersen KE, Hjorth N, Bundgaard H, et al: Formaldehyde in a hypoallergenic non-woven textile acrylate tape. *Contact Dermatitis* 9:228, 1983.
67. Fregert S, Trulsson L, Zimerson E: Contact allergic reactions to diphenylthiourea and phenylisothiocyanate in PVC adhesive tape. *Contact Dermatitis* 8:38, 1982.

68. Marks JG, Rainey MA: Cutaneous reactions to surgical preparations and dressings. *Contact Dermatitis* 10:1, 1984.

69. Bjornberg A: Toxic reactions to a patch test skin marker containing fuchsin-silver nitrate. *Contact Dermatitis* 3:101, 1977.

70. Dooms-Goossens A: Toxic reactions to skin markers. *Contact Dermatitis* 3:280, 1977.

71. Jordan WP: Fluorescent marking ink for patch test site identification. *Contact Dermatitis Newsletter* 10:229, 1971.

72. Fischer T, Maibach HI: Recovery of nickel sulphate from a standard patch test. *Contact Dermatitis* 11:134, 1984.

73. Kalimo K, Lammintausta K, Maki J, et al: Nickel penetration in allergic individuals: Bioavailability versus x-ray microanalysis detection. *Contact Dermatitis* 12:255, 1985.

74. Kalimo K, Lammintausta K: 24 and 48 h allergen exposure in patch testing: Comparative study with 11 common contact allergens and NIC12. *Contact Dermatitis* 10:25, 1984.

75. Bruze M: Patch testing with nickel sulphate under occlusion for 5 hours. *Acta Derm Venereol* 68:361, 1988.

76. Rietschel RL: Contact dermatitis and diagnostic techniques. *Allergy Proc* 10:403, 1989.

77. Mathias TCG, Maibach HI: When to read the patch test. *J Invest Dermatol* 18:127, 1979.

78. Mitchell JC: Day 7 patch test reading—Valuable or not? *Contact Dermatitis* 4:139, 1978.

79. Rietschel RL, Adams RM, Maibach HI, et al: The case for patch test reading beyond day 2. *J Am Acad Dermatol* 18:42, 1988.

80. Paramsothy Y, Collins M, Smith AG: Contact dermatitis in patients with leg ulcers. *Contact Dermatitis* 18:30, 1988.

81. Macfarlane AW, Curley RK, Graham RM, et al: Delayed patch test reactions at days 7 and 9. *Contact Dermatitis* 20:127–132, 1989.

82. Shehade SA, Beck MH, Hillier VF: Epidemiological survey of standard series patch test results and observations on day 2 and 4 readings. *Contact Dermatitis* 24:119–122, 1991.

83. Nethercott JR, Holness DL, Adams RM, et al: Results of first and second readings with standard screening tray in North America 1985–1989. *Am J Contact Dermatitis* 2:255, 1991.

84. Moller H: Intradermal testing in doubtful cases of contact allergy to metals. *Contact Dermatitis* 20:120, 1989.

85. Meneghini C, Angelini G: Intradermal test in contact allergy to metals. *Acta Derm Venereol* 59:123, 1979.

86. Christensen O, Wall L: Open, closed, and intradermal testing in nickel allergy. *Contact Dermatitis* 16:21, 1987.

87. Schmidt H, Schultz-Larsen F, Olholm Larsen P, et al: Petechial reaction following patch testing with cobalt. *Contact Dermatitis* 6:91, 1980.

88. Wahlberg JE, Maibach HI: Sterile cutaneous pustules: A manifestation of primary irritancy? Identification of contact pustulogens. *J Invest Dermatol* 76:381, 1981.

89. Mitchell JC: The angry back syndrome: Eczema creates eczema. *Contact Dermatitis* 1:193, 1975.

90. Mitchell JC: Multiple concomitant positive patch test reactions. *Contact Dermatitis* 3:315, 1977.

91. Bruynzell DP, Maibach HI: The excited skin syndrome (angry back). *Arch Dermatol* 122:323, 1986.

92. Condie MW, Adams RM: Influence of oral prednisone on patch test reactions to *rhus* antigen. *Arch Dermatol* 107:540, 1973.

93. Bruze M: Seasonal influence of routine patch test results. *Contact Dermatitis* 14:184, 1986.

94. Dooms-Goossens A, Lessafre E, Heidbuchel M, et al: UV sunlight and patch test reactions in humans. *Contact Dermatitis* 19:36, 1988.

95. Veien NK, Hattel T, Laurberg G: Is patch testing a less accurate tool during the summer months? *Am J Contact Dermatitis* 3:35, 1992.

96. Alexander S: Patch testing and menstruation (letter). *Lancet* 2:751, 1988.

97. Cronin E: *Contact Dermatitis*. New York, Churchill Livingstone, 1980.

98. Bruze M: Simultaneous patch test sensitization to 4 chemically unrelated compounds in a standard test series. *Contact Dermatitis* 11:48, 1984.

99. Guin JD, Baker GF, Mitchell JC: Persistent open patch test reaction. *Contact Dermatitis* 18:181, 1988.

100. Patrizi A, Lanzarini M, Tosti A: Persistent patch test reactions to textile dyes. *Contact Dermatitis* 23:60, 1990.

6

PATCH TESTING WITHOUT A KIT

An Dooms-Goossens

The main problem in contact allergy is that one can only find what one is looking for. In other words, one can only identify an ingredient as an allergen if it is tested.

Testing with a standard series containing all possible allergens is ideal; it is also impossible. In practice, testing can detect only the most common environmental allergens. In order to estimate the proportion of the allergens detected by testing with an internationally applied standard series, the results obtained by members of the European Contact Dermatitis Research Group were compared.[1] The proportion of positive tests obtained with the "standard series only" varied from 37 to 73 percent. The proportion obtained with "other products only" varied from 5 to 23 percent. How large a proportion of contact sensitivities are detected by testing with the internationally applied standard series depends entirely on the opportunity of the investigator to go deeper into the allergological problem.

Obviously, it is very important to test with allergens other than those in the standard series. These other allergens may be represented in what are called *focused* series, compiled according to various factors:

- Professions, such as a hairdresser's and a baker's series
- Lesion location, such as a lower leg and a face series
- Exposure, such as a textile and a shoe series
- Topical products, such as a cosmetics and a pharmaceuticals series. However, the source of the allergen may also be a product that the patient has used and can supply. This is the subject discussed in this chapter.

REASONS FOR TESTING PATIENT-SUPPLIED PRODUCTS

The reasons for testing patient-supplied products and substances are as follows:

- A standard kit of allergens for testing can never contain all possible allergens.
- Rapid changes in some areas can give rise to the abrupt appearance or disappearance of new allergens.

- In general, one has little information on the composition of most of the products with which the patient has come in contact (cosmetics—at least in Europe—and industrial, household, and other kinds of products). Hence, one cannot identify the potentially allergenic ingredients to be tested.
- The biopharmaceutical characteristics of the substances at the origin of the allergic reaction are not necessarily identical to those of the allergens available or on the market (diluted in petrolatum, water, alcohol, and so on).
- A sensitization to a given product is not always detected when the ingredients are tested separately[2]; Indeed, the allergy can be due to contaminants or intermediary products. Moreover, some substances, like emulsifiers and keratolytic agents, can enhance penetration and thus influence the bioavailability of the allergens. Finally, a new allergen might be formed during storage, which is then known as a *compound allergen*.

GUIDELINES FOR TESTING PATIENT-SUPPLIED PRODUCTS

The way in which skin tests with patient-supplied products are conducted is not based on scientific research but derived from the everyday, pragmatic approach used by clinicians. This accounts for the rather personal approach of this chapter. Nevertheless, there are a number of classic works that treat this subject.[3-8]

Before proceeding to the test, one must always check to see if the container (if labeled) does indeed contain the original product. Thus, one should check the label and all the information accompanying the product carefully. Standardized stickers have been developed to identify dangerous products. If the product is not labeled properly, one should always identify it before testing. Moreover, litmus paper should be kept at hand to check the product's pH: excessive acidity or alkalinity can be harmful to the skin.

Three methods are generally used to test patient-supplied products: patch tests, open tests, and usage tests (repeated open-application tests, or ROATs).[9,10] The choice of the kind of test depends, of course, on the nature of the product. In the last few years, we have been increasingly using "semi-open" tests, that is, the application with a cotton swab of a minute amount (about 1 to 2 µL) of a liquid (solution or suspension of the substance) on about 1 cm² (0.15 sq in.) of the skin (Fig. 6-1). We allow the liquid to dry completely on the skin (the excess liquid may be removed with paper toweling or a cotton swab) and, when it is dry, cover the area with acrylate tape. The site is examined after a few minutes up to about an hour to check for contact urticaria (if suspected), after day 2 (when the adhesive tape is removed), and on day 4 for contact eczema. We perform prick or scratch (chamber) tests if we suspect protein contact dermatitis. On the basis of our experience, we have developed a few general rules for testing with patient-supplied products. Depending upon its nature, one can test with the product as such, with dilutions, or with extracts, the last being particularly suitable for plants and solids like plastics and paper.

When a skin reaction to a given product is obtained, the results may be confirmed by testing with a more diluted solution of the product, but the allergen can be identified only by testing with the individual components of the product.

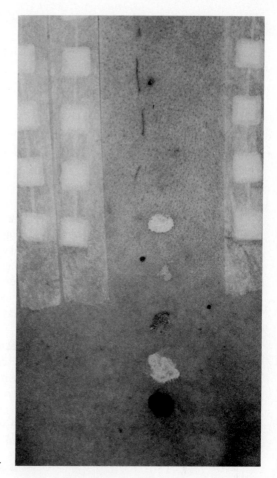

FIG. 6–1. Semi-open tests with paints.

CHEMICAL SUBSTANCES

When a patient brings in chemical substances (in powder or liquid form), one must first read the labels and make every attempt to confirm their identity. The books by Fisher[6] and de Groot[11] provide useful information on the concentrations and vehicles to be used. If the exact nature of the substance is not known, one must at least try to determine the group to which it belongs or the purpose for which it is used. One may then proceed with the testing as recommended for that particular group of materials. It is best to be extremely careful in testing reactive chemicals used as intermediates in the synthesis of raw materials for various industries, like the pharmaceutical industry, as they may sensitize during the testing procedure itself. The literature gives several examples of such occurrences, sensitization by trichloropyridazine being a typical example.[12] To determine whether sensitivity to such a particular component is present is sometimes crucial in cases of occupation-related dermatoses. Therefore, concentrations greater than 0.01% to 0.1% in petrolatum should never be exceeded for testing individuals suspected of being allergic to such substances. Moreover, caution is required with control subjects.

TOPICAL PHARMACEUTICAL PRODUCTS

In most cases, tests can be done in function of the galenical form and of the composition of the products. The product may or may not have to be diluted.

- *Patch tests* (under occlusion) may be used for most creams, ointments, gels, and so on except for products containing substances that could be irritating; for example, some mercury-based antiseptics like phenylmercuriborate (Merfen), quaternary ammonium salts like benzalkonium chloride, or cetrimide (Cetaflex/Cetavlon), and products containing solvents, such as high concentrations of propylene glycol. For such products, open, semi-open, or even usage testing with the undiluted products can be useful. Even creams containing emulsifiers like sodium lauryl sulfate can provoke slight irritant reactions under occlusive dressings.
- *Usage tests,* or ROATs, are administered if the suspected product continues to patch test negatively. This may occur particularly if corticosteroids are present in the preparation, as their anti-inflammatory effect may mask the product's sensitizing properties.
- *Semi-open tests.* This is the case for products that may contain irritants such as tinctures like iodine alcohol and solutions based on antiseptics like iodine, chlorhexidine, and hexamidine, which also contain emulsifiers like nonoxynol. These are also allergens,[13] and, if tested under occlusion, may indeed also be irritants.

   If the toxic or irritative capability of a pharmaceutical ingredient is in doubt, one can always ask the manufacturer or consult books like *Martindale's Extra Pharmacopoeia,*[14] which is an excellent source of such information.

COSMETIC PRODUCTS

As for cosmetics, the testing methods are virtually the same as for pharmaceuticals.

- *Patch tests* (under occlusion) can be done with the skin-care preparations like creams, lotions, and milks; makeup (foundation creams, lipstick, powders, rouge); toilet waters; deodorants; and so on.
- *Usage tests* are generally very helpful when the skin tests with the suspected products remain negative with patch testing.
- *Semi-open tests* are useful if certain emulsifiers, solvents, or other irritant substances are present. This is the way to test mascaras, hair dyes, nail varnish, beauty masks, and so on. Even products like shampoos, liquid soaps, and permanent-wave solutions (Fig. 6-2) can be tested this way if the reactions are interpreted prudently (there can be a soap and shampoo effect). One should take care, however, to apply minute amounts and to allow them to dry completely on the skin.

   Information concerning the composition of cosmetic products by category can be obtained from works such as the book by de Groot.[15]

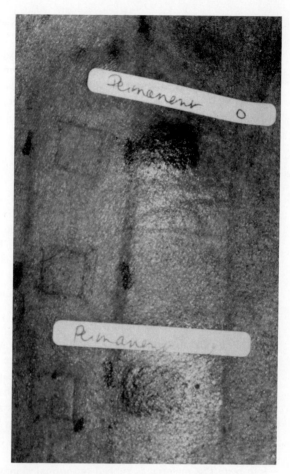

FIG. 6–2. Results of semi-open tests with permanent-wave solutions in a patient allergic to glycerylmonothioglycolate.

WOODS, PLANTS, AND FOODS

Most often, the fresh plant can be tested as such: the flower, stem, fruit, or root. Wood dust can also be tested as such. Nevertheless, some woods and plants can cause irritation reactions and can even induce sensitization when tested in this way. This is the case for primula,[16] which is why its allergen, primin, was reintroduced into the standard battery, although false-negative reactions may be encountered.[17] Primula dermatitis can be very tricky; thus the standard tested primin gives a false sense of security in detecting it. However, patch testing with plant materials as such may also give false-negative reactions. These difficulties can easily be resolved by using extracts made with water, alcohol, acetone, etc. Several books deal with this subject and are useful to the clinician.[16,18–20] The ideal way to detect plant sensitivity, of course, is to test with the causal allergens present in them. The introduction into the standard series of a sesquiterpene lactone mix containing allergens responsible for most cases of Compositae, or Asteraceae, dermatitis is very useful. A positive reaction to this mix might, in some cases, even be a clue to chronic actinic dermatitis, as has been reported.[21]

PROTEINS

Proteins or proteinlike high-molecular-weight substances present in "natural" substances (fruits, vegetables, grains, animals, fish, enzymes, latex, etc.) may be responsible for a combination of an immediate skin reaction presenting as contact urticaria as well as delayed skin reactions presenting as contact eczema or at least an aggravation of an already existing eczematous skin condition. This is called a *protein contact dermatitis*.[22–24]

Such reactions are most often occupation-related and occur particularly in patients with an atopic skin condition and/or with a preexisting dermatitis on the hands (presenting a damaged skin barrier). In some instances, the skin lesions may be accompanied by extracutaneous symptoms such as conjunctivitis, rhinitis, orolaryngeal symptoms, dyspnea, asthma, or even anaphylactic shock.

Patch testing on normal skin and test readings taken after 2 to 4 days are generally inappropriate for revealing the nature of the allergens. In fact, macromolecular allergens are generally not able to penetrate healthy, intact skin; moreover, the test readings have to be performed shortly after application (5 to 20 min).

To detect immediate-type reactions, several test methods[25] may be considered (test readings are done within minutes after application):

- *Open test.* The material is placed on normal skin and fixed with acrylic tape. This test method is preferred when severe reactions are to be expected in, for example, patients who have had severe asthma or even anaphylactic reactions after contact with the offending substance. For example, we have observed a strong urticarial reaction in an open test to chestnut 2 min after its application in an individual who had presented with an anaphylactic condition after having swallowed a small piece of it. If the test is negative, an open application can be performed on previously undamaged skin.
- *Rub test.* The material is rubbed on normal skin. If this test is negative, an open application can be done on damaged skin.
- *Patch test.* On normal skin and, if negative, on damaged skin.
- *Prick test.* A drop of an allergen extract is put on and introduced into the skin with an ultrafine needle. Such testing is performed to detect latex allergy,[26] for example, and is less likely to cause severe reactions than the following methods.
- *Scratch test.* The test area of the skin is scarified and fresh material (e.g., food) is applied and fixed with acrylic tape.
- *Scratch-chamber test.* This seems to be the most appropriate method for diagnosing a protein contact dermatitis to fresh materials—such as fruit, vegetables, and so on—as it prevents desiccation of the material and also provides better fixation: the test material is placed on scarified skin and fixed with a chamber (Finn or Vander Bend chambers). Test readings are made immediately but can also be performed after 24 h. The material should be removed after 24 h because of the danger of deterioration.
- *Intradermal test.* A small quantity of an allergenic extract is injected intradermally with a tuberculin syringe. Unfortunately, only very few allergen extracts are commercially available.

For intradermal, prick, scratch, and scratch-chamber testing, physiologic saline and a histamine solution can be used as the negative or, respectively, the positive control.

One must be extremely cautious with these techniques, particularly in patients with a history of severe immediate reactions, since anaphylactic reactions may occur.[27] They should be performed only in an hospital environment, where the equipment to cope with anaphylactic reactions is available.

Even for protein contact dermatitis, delayed test readings are generally negative. Theoretically, however, delayed responses to proteins can be detected by the following tests:

- *ROATs.* The material is applied twice a day to the inner forearm and the reaction evaluated after several days.
- *Patch tests.* Because fresh test material degenerates quickly, the readings should be made after 1 day.
- *Scratch-chamber tests.* See above.

Remarks

Testing for protein contact dermatitis may, of course, give rise to particular problems: false-positive as well as false-negative reactions may occur. The former may be due to dermographism, irritant reactions, the release of histamine or other vasoactive substances by the material, or the presence of an additive, and so on. The latter may be due to denaturation of the material, too low a concentration of the allergen in the material tested, diminished skin reactivity (which occurs with atopic patients), and—perhaps the most obvious reason to consider—the intake of antihistamines. The administration of β-sympathomimetics a few hours before the test procedure may also influence the test reactivity. Hence, both positive as well as negative controls have to be carried out.

HOUSEHOLD AND INDUSTRIAL PRODUCTS

Because of their diversity and our occasional ignorance of their nature, household and industrial products are more complicated to test than cosmetics or pharmaceuticals. Products like strong detergents, paint strippers, abrasive powders, and strong acids or alkalis must never be tested because they can cause strong irritation reactions (blisters, necrosis, eschars). However, these products may contain perfumes, preservatives, dyes, contaminants, degradation products, and the like, and these can be sensitizers. The dilution of a product to a degree that it does not provoke an irritant reaction in a normal person might yield a false-negative result,[28] since the concentration of the allergen might be too low to cause an allergic reaction. Bruze[29] suggests using buffer solutions for the dilution of acidic or alkaline solutions. In his article, he gives several examples. Buffering allows one to increase the concentration of both acid and alkaline products 300 to 3000 times. Dilutions with buffer solutions alone, of course, will not be sufficient to avoid irritant reactions if the irritation is due to properties other than acidity or alkalinity. For this reason, hydrofluoric acid, for example, should never be tested. Moreover, a product that is labeled to be dangerous to the skin may never be tested without precautions. In such a case, poison-control centers or the manufacturers themselves may be able to supply critical information. Generally, if household or industrial products are suspected as the source of sensitization, the individual ingredients must be tested separately in an appropriately diluted form.

The open or semi-open test is recommended for testing an "unknown" product (after its pH is tested to determine if buffering is called for, since products with a pH below 3 or above 10 should not be tested as such). This is the case for products with solvents or emulsifiers such as paints, resins, varnishes, glues, waxes, cooling oils, and thinners. Minute amounts of the products are applied to the skin, allowed to dry completely, and then covered with acrylic tape. We have rarely seen very strong reactions with this technique. Obviously, all the reactions must be verified should the test be positive.

Solids, from which one can, if necessary, remove scrapings, can be tested as they are (Figs. 6-3 and 6-4). Nevertheless, tests with such materials often turn out to be falsely negative. To get around this problem, the material can be extracted with certain solvents. For example, plastic, rubber,[30] and even paper[31] can be extracted with acetone.

The book by Gosselin and colleagues[32] is an excellent source of information, since it includes the general composition of most household and industrial products. In the clinic, information on the products must be available to those who conduct the tests. It can often be obtained from the occupational physician and from safety data sheets.

CLOTHING, SHOES, AND GLOVES

Gloves can be tested directly with thin strips cut from the gloves to prevent occlusion and pressure effects, which, in general, only disturb the first patch-test reading. The

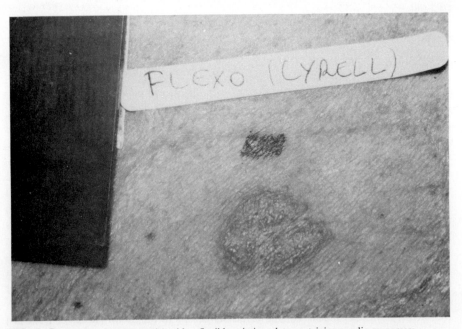

FIG. 6–3. Results of testing (as is) with a flexible printing plate containing acrylic monomers.

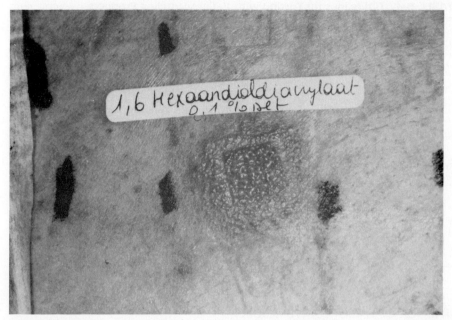

FIG. 6–4. Positive patch-test result to 1,6-hexanediol diacrylate (0.1% petrolatum) in the same patient.

same applies for shoes: one must test pieces removed from the area that matches the site of the contact eczema. If topical pharmaceutical products have been used, they may have contaminated the gloves or the shoes and might be the true source of sensitization.

As regards textiles and shoes, one can easily test small fragments, which should be moistened with water or physiologic saline before they are applied to the skin. Ultrasonic bath extracts can also be made.[30,33]

PROBLEMS

There are a number of problems with tests of patient-supplied products. These are outlined below.

THE PRECISE COMPOSITION OF THESE PRODUCTS IS MOST OFTEN UNKNOWN

The best way to resolve this problem is to contact the manufacturer, but this is not always possible in practice. In our experience, product distributors are not a good source of information, as they are often not aware of the composition of the products they deal with. The time involved in making such inquiries is often prohibitive and, indeed, at the initial stage of the investigation, the product may only be suspected.

TABLE 6–1. Guidelines for Testing with Patient-Supplied Products

1. Check to see that the container (if labeled) contains the original product.
2. Identify the nature of the product to be tested.
3. Check with litmus paper for acidity or alkalinity: products with a pH lower than 3 or higher than 10 should not be tested as such.
4. Perform patch, open, or semi-open tests depending on the nature of the product. Be extremely careful with reactive chemical intermediates.
5. Usage tests or repeated open application tests (ROAT) are useful when the suspected (nonirritant) products give a negative reaction on patch, open, or semi-open testing.
6. When a positive reaction occurs to a given patient-supplied product, test the individual ingredients with the appropriate test concentration and vehicle in order to identify the exact allergen.
7. When a product is strongly suspected but fails to react with the methods suggested above, repeat the investigation, as a small detail in the anamnesis might provide a clue for the detection of the allergen. Test the ingredients separately when the particular product continues to be suspected, as the results with the product itself might have been falsely negative. If solid materials are suspected, testing with extracts might be useful.
8. To diagnose a contact urticaria and/or protein contact dermatitis to high-molecular-weight substances, one usually has to damage the skin barrier (prick, scratch, scratch chamber). These tests should be carried out with emergency equipment at hand.

THE RISK OF FALSE-POSITIVE RESULTS

False positive results are most often irritant reactions. An irritant reaction can sometimes be recognized as such, although considerable experience in reading test results is required to do so. The testing of control subjects can be helpful (testing about 20 individuals is generally recommended).

If the response to the product is positive but negative to the individual ingredients, then one may conclude that the reaction was an irritant reaction. However, a new allergen may have been formed in the final product that is not present when the ingredients are taken individually (compound allergy), or there may be ingredients present that enhance the penetration of the causal allergen, thus increasing its bioavailability. One of the best worked-up examples of a compound allergy was the case reported by Smeenk et al.,[34] who identified the allergen which had been formed by the interaction of thymol and hexahydro-1,3,5-tris(2-hydroxy-ethyl)-triazine (Grotan BK) present in Hirudoid cream.

THE RISK OF FALSE-NEGATIVE RESULTS

If the test results with a product are negative, it still cannot be definitively rejected as a potential source of the responsible allergen. Indeed, it is possible that the concentration of the allergen in the product is too low to cause a positive response with the testing method used. Moreover, the allergen may not be liberated in sufficient quantity or the occlusion may be insufficient, so that other testing methods might be required. In certain cases, repeated open application tests (ROATs) can be very useful. If a product is under serious suspicion, the different ingredients should be tested individually.

The airborne contact allergic reaction to triglycidylisocyanurate is a typical example.[35] Although the sensitized patient reacted to the polyester pigment powders when they were present in the air, patch testing with the powder remained completely negative. It was only when the ingredients of the powder were tested separately that contact sensitivity to a hardener in the product could be confirmed.

THE RISK OF ACTIVE SENSITIZATION

The composition of topical pharmaceutical products and cosmetics makes it unlikely that they will cause active sensitization. The materials with which one has to be careful in this regard are reactive chemical intermediates, plants and woods (see above), and industrial products such as acrylic resins,[36] which may sensitize when patch tested.

RELEVANCE

As with all test results, a patch-test result—positive or negative—is only the beginning.

If the test results remain negative in a patient in whom the signs strongly suggest an allergic contact dermatitis, the investigation must be repeated, with special attention to all the details. The patient may be instructed to keep a diary, in hopes of finding the connection between exposure to a substance and the skin problems.

If a positive patch test is obtained, the patient should be carefully informed about the causes of the contact dermatitis, which usually means a detailed investigation. Bruze[37] advises that one be hesitant with the assessment of "no relevance." Indeed, such a judgment is generally the result of ignorance on the part of the investigator.

CONCLUSION

As Lachapelle argues,[38] skin tests with finished products must be conducted with technical subtlety and interpreted with intellectual flexibility. In addition, the person administering the tests must have access to the critical product information.

Even when these precautions are taken, slight irritant reactions are still possible, but they are certainly preferable to false-negative reactions to an overdiluted product that rules it out from further consideration. There is then the danger that the allergen will not be recognized.

REFERENCES

1. Menné T, Dooms-Goossens A, Wahlberg JE, et al: How large a proportion of contact sensitivities are diagnosed with the European Standard Series? *Contact Dermatitis* 26:201–202, 1992.
2. Dooms-Goossens A: *Allergic Contact Dermatitis to Ingredients Used in Topically Applied Pharmaceutical Products and Cosmetics.* Leuven, Leuven University Press, 1983.
3. Adams R: *Occupational Skin Disease,* 2nd ed. Philadelphia, Saunders, 1990.
4. Cronin E: *Contact Dermatitis.* Edinburgh, Churchill Livingstone, 1980.
5. Ducombs G, Chabeau G: *Dermato-Allergologie de Contact,* 2nd ed. Paris, Masson, 1988.
6. Fisher AA: *Contact Dermatitis,* 3rd ed. Philadelphia, Lea & Febiger, 1986.
7. Foussereau J, Benezra C, Maibach H: *Occupational Contact Dermatitis. Clinical and Chemical Aspects.* Copenhagen, Munksgaard, 1982.

8. Foussereau J: *Les Eczémas Allergiques, Cosmétologiques, Thérapeutiques et Vestimentaires.* Paris, Masson, 1987.
9. Epstein WL: The use test for contact hypersensitivity. *Arch Dermatol Res* 272:279–281, 1982.
10. Hannuksela M, Salo H: The repeated open application test (ROAT). *Contact Dermatitis* 14:221–227, 1986.
11. de Groot AC: *Patch Testing Concentrations and Vehicles for 2800 Allergens.* Amsterdam, Elsevier, 1986.
12. Dooms-Goossens A, De Boulle K, Snauwaert J, Degreef H: Sensitization to 3,4,6-trichloropyridazine. *Contact Dermatitis* 14:64, 1986.
13. Dooms-Goossens A, De Veylder H, Gidi de Alam A, et al: Contact sensitivity to nonoxynols as a cause of intolerance to antiseptic preparations. *J Am Acad Dermatol* 21:723–727, 1989.
14. Reynolds JF (ed): *Martindale: The Extra Pharmacopoeia,* 29th ed. London, Pharmaceutical Press, 1989.
15. de Groot, AC: Adverse Reactions to Cosmetics (thesis). State University of Groningen, 1988.
16. Mitchell J: *Botanical Dermatology: Plants and Plant Products Injurious to the Skin.* Vancouver, Greengrass, 1979.
17. Dooms-Goossens A, Biesemans G, Vandaele M, Degreef H: Primula dermatitis: More than one allergen? *Contact Dermatitis* 21:122–124, 1989.
18. Benezra C, Ducombs G, Sell Y, Foussereau J: *Plant Contact Dermatitis.* Toronto, Dekker, 1985.
19. Hausen B: *Allergiepflanzen, Pflanzenallergene. Handbuch und Atlas der Allergie-induzierenden Wild- und Kulturpflanzen.* Munich, Ecomed, 1988.
20. Guin JD, Beaman JH (eds): Plant dermatitis. *Clin Dermatology:* 4(2), 1986.
21. White I, Norris PG, Hawk JLM: Sesquiterpene lactone sensitivity and chronic actinic dermatitis. *Contact Dermatitis* 23:260, 1990.
22. Hjorth N, Roed-Pedersen J: Occupational protein contact dermatitis in food handlers. *Contact Dermatitis* 2:28–42, 1976.
23. Krook G: Occupational dermatitis from lactuca sativa (lettuce) and chicorum (endive): Simultaneous occurrence of immediate and delayed allergy as a cause of contact dermatitis. *Contact Dermatitis* 3:27–36, 1977.
24. Hannuksela M, Lahti A: Immediate reactions to fruits and vegetables. *Contact Dermatitis* 3:79–84, 1977.
25. von Krogh G, Maibach HI: The contact urticaria syndrome, an updated review. *J Am Acad Dermatol* 5:328–342, 1981.
26. Turjanmaa K, Reunala T, Räsänen L: Comparison of diagnostic methods in latex surgical glove contact urticaria. *Contact Dermatitis* 19:241–247, 1988.
27. Temesvari E, Albonczy E, Somlai B: Kontakturtikaria durch Ei. *Dermatosen* 17(3):69–71, 1979.
28. Malten KE, Nater JP, Van Ketel WG: *Patch Testing Guidelines.* Nijmegen, Dekker and Van de Vegt, 1976, pp 10–25.
29. Bruze M: Use of buffer solutions for patch testing. *Contact Dermatitis* 10:267–269, 1984.
30. Bruze M, Trulsson L, Bendsöe N: Patch testing with ultrasonic bath extracts. *Am J Contact Dermatitis* 3:1–5, 1992.
31. Karlberg A-T, Lidén C: Colophony (resin) in newspapers may contribute to hand eczema. *Br J Dermatol* 126:161–165, 1992.
32. Gosselin R, Hodge M, Smith R, Gleason M: *Clinical Toxicity of Commercially Available Products.* Baltimore, Williams & Wilkins, 1984.
33. Brandão FM, Altermatt C, Pecegueiro M, et al: Contact dermatitis to disperse blue 106. *Contact Dermatitis* 13:80–84, 1985.
34. Smeenk G, Kerckhoffs H, Schreurs P: Contact allergy to a reaction product in Hirudoid cream: An example of compound allergy. *Br J Dermatol* 116:223–231, 1987.
35. Dooms-Goossens A, Bedert R, Vandaele M, Degreef H: Airborne contact dermatitis due to tryglycidyliso-cyanurate. *Contact Dermatitis* 21:202–203, 1989.
36. Kanerva L, Estlander T, Jolanki R: Double active sensitization caused by acrylics. *Am J Contact Dermatitis* 3:23–26, 1992.
37. Bruze, M: What is a relevant contact allergy? *Contact Dermatitis* 23:224–225, 1990.
38. Lachapelle J-M: *Dermatologie profesionnelle.* Paris, Masson, 1984.

7

"ANGRY BACK," OR THE EXCITED SKIN SYNDROME

Derk P. Bruynzeel
Howard I. Maibach

> The routine patch test tends to create a false sense of security
> in the mind of the dermatologist.
> —N. Hjorth, 1963

HISTORY

The concept of a state of skin hyperreactivity has been recognized since Jadassohn introduced the diagnostic patch test at the end of the last century.[1–7] Patients with active eczema are especially prone to show this. Von Zumbusch called it "reflektorisches Ekzem," and since then it has been described frequently, often under different names (Table 7-1[8–18]). The 1968 thesis of Bjornberg[19] is even today an excellent seminal review on hyperreactivity of the skin and reactivity to irritants.

TERMINOLOGY

Enhanced skin reactivity can be seen in patients with active dermatitis as well as strong positive patch-test reactions. Mitchell,[15] emphasizing the problem of false-positive patch reactions, called the phenomenon the "angry back syndrome." However, since hyperreactivity is not restricted to the back and can involve the skin anywhere, "excited skin syndrome" (ESS) may be a better term.[18,20] Patch tests performed where the skin is hyperreactive may produce positive reactions to compounds that are marginal irritants or may enhance subclinical or weak allergic reactions. Retesting done after the skin hyperirritability has disappeared is commonly negative. However, retesting does not completely rule out false-positive reactions, and some very weak true-positive allergic reactions may be lost. Therefore, test results in such patients have to be carefully evaluated. Consequently, the ESS is a phenomenon which occurs in patients presenting with multiple concomitant positive patch-test reactions for allergic contact dermatitis, or with dermatitis elsewhere, in whom the test results are not reproducible with a single

TABLE 7–1. Different Expressions Used to Denote Skin Hyperreactivity, 1921–1981

Reflektorisches Ekzem	1921
Crazy back	1979
Metallergic and parallergic reactions	1939
Status eczematicus	1959
Skin fatigue	1967
Multiple nonspecific reactions	1970
Conditioned hyperirritability	1975
Angry back syndrome	1975
Spillover	1977
Rogue positive reactions	1980
Excited skin syndrome	1981

Source: From Refs. 8 through 18.

repeated challenge. When the ESS complicates patch testing, the expression "angry back" is commonly used.

INCIDENCE OF THE ANGRY BACK

Although the concept of skin hyperreactivity has been widely known for a long time, the incidence and importance of ESS remain controversial. Several studies have been published on this subject since Mitchell's article in 1975. The number of nonreproducible patch-test reactions has been reported to be in the range of 8 to 60 percent. In his first paper on the angry back, Mitchell observed, in 35 patients, that of the 90 one-plus (1+) reactions, 38 (42 percent) were negative or "lost" on repeated testing.[15] A 1+ reaction is defined as redness, induration, and/or papules. Later reports showed figures on the same order.[16,21–23] However, Bandmann and Agathos[24] found far fewer "lost" reactions in their series of 40 patients: 8.6 percent. Differences in the test protocols makes comparison between these studies difficult. The outcome of retesting can be influenced by patient selection and other criteria—such as when (at what moment) and whether it is redone and whether relevant allergens or only those which seem irrelevant are included. Recently, Gollhausen et al.[25] showed again that the reproducibility of weak patch-test reactions is low. Twenty-four patients, who a week previously had shown a positive reaction to one or several allergens of the standard series, were retested on a previously unused side of the back. Of the 70 total reactions, 40 percent were positive on only one of the two occasions. In another group, they performed patch tests in duplicate on the back: 52 percent of the reactions were positive on only one side. Weak positive reactions were far more often not reproducible than strong reactions. Studies on reproducibility, comparing ready-to-use test material (TRUE Test) and the conventional technique, showed results comparable with those of the previous study. In these investigations, in which the test series were applied on the left and right sides of the back, the overall concordance was 67 percent. Half of the weak reactions were disconcordant.[26] Putting this together, we do not know exactly how many weak reactions are not reproducible on retesting, but clearly we may expect that nearly 50 percent might be "lost." In many cases, hyperirritability (ESS) will be responsible for this disturbing phenomenon. The interpretation of a weak positive reaction is usually difficult, especially if we consider that nonreproducibility does not always mean that such a reaction was a false-positive one. The skin reactivity apparently is not constant but fluctuates slightly, so it is also possible that we will miss weak allergic reactions, which is just as troublesome.

DERMATITIS AND PATCH-TEST REACTIVITY

Björnberg proved in human experiments that patients with hand eczema had enhanced skin reactivity to some irritants, so apparently even a limited dermatitis can enhance skin reactivity. Similarly, Magnusson and Hellgren[27] noticed significantly more positive patch-test reactions to a number of allergens and irritants in patients with adhesive-tape dermatitis than in patients without a tape reaction. In patients without dermatitis, but with several strong positive patch-test reactions, lost reactions are frequently seen, suggesting that strong patch-test reactions are capable of inducing skin hyperirritability. Thus, small areas of active dermatitis (e.g., hand eczema), an adhesive-tape dermatitis, and even a strong positive patch-test reaction may induce skin hyperirritability or an angry back. Therefore, patch-test results in patients with even a minor dermatitis should be interpreted very carefully.

LOCALIZATION

In a patient with ESS, we can expect to find false-positive reactions scattered all over the test area. Such responses are not limited to the back. This syndrome involves the entire skin, and other sites such as the arms also can be hyperreactive. A strong reaction on one arm can even elicit a nonspecific response on the other.[18] This points to a systemic effect, but more localized effects are possible as well. This is illustrated by the influence of the tape dermatitis on the outcome of patch testing and the observation that false-positive reactions are often found close to strong patch-test reactions.[22]

This suggests the existence of a "runover" or "spillover" effect (Fig. 7-1). Spillover can be demonstrated experimentally by inducing a strong positive (allergic) patch-test reaction and at the same time eliciting a weak positive skin reaction (? + or 1 +) by means of a marginal irritant like sodium laurylsulfate. If the weak reaction is close to the stronger one, the weak reaction usually will be enhanced compared with a control test performed far away from the others.[28]

While more or less comparable experiments performed by others[29,30] did not demonstrate a spillover effect, experiments by Hamani and Marks[31] support the phenomenon of enhanced skin reactivity adjacent to strong test reactions. They observed an increased skin temperature and blood flow 2 cm from the allergic patch-test reaction compared to control sites. The histology of "normal skin" 1 cm away showed spongiosis and/or increased inflammatory cells.[31] These findings indicate that normal-appearing skin near foci of inflamed skin can have an abnormal blood flow and histology. Therefore humoral mediators of inflammation probably play an important role in ESS and in spillover in particular. Furthermore, previously inflamed skin reportedly has a lower threshold to irritants near areas with eczema.[32] These clinical observations and the results of these experiments support the existence of the spillover reactions and help to explain them.

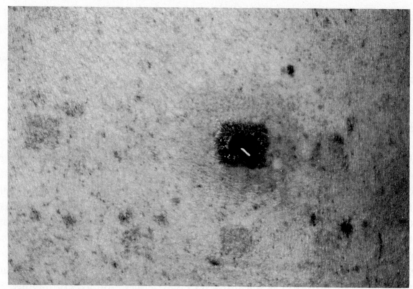

FIG. 7–1. Angry back (spillover phenomenon). A strong positive allergic reaction is surrounded by several (weaker) false-positive reactions. (See color Plate 1.)

Another potential cause of localized skin reactivity is the numerous inflammatory cells present in the dermis weeks after a dermatitis has healed clinically. The increased numbers of Langerhans cells and T lymphocytes are likely to result in an earlier and stronger reaction to an inflammatory stimulus, producing what we see clinically as enhanced skin reactivity and which can result in false-positive patch-test reactions.[33–35] Thus, there are several plausible explanations for how normal-looking skin can react to irritants more prominently than expected and how such phenomena could play a role in spillover and ESS.

REGIONAL SKIN VARIATION

Patch testing is performed with allergens in concentrations that have been adjusted to be nonirritating in practically all patients but that are still high enough to elicit an allergic reaction. The margin between a nonirritating level and one which effectively evokes an allergic reaction is sometimes small. When, instead of the back, a different area is chosen for testing, the possibility exists that the standard concentration will be too high. Magnusson and Hersle[36] observed not only that 5% benzalkonium chloride caused irritant reactions twice as often on the upper back as on the lower back but also that they were stronger. Therefore regional difference in skin sensitivity may contribute to false-positive reactions when marginal irritants are applied to more sensitive skin in areas other than the back.

SERIAL DILUTIONS

The spillover effect is important when dermatotoxicologic assays for contact sensitization or irritancy are performed. The skin of the test subject is challenged with decreasing concentrations to determine the lowest point at which it reacts. Such tests are usually performed, for convenience, with several dilutions at a time. Additional challenges with one dilution at a time will show that several subjects no longer react to the lowest concentration that was positive in the earlier tests.[37] This phenomenon can also occur with open tests. Thus, the end point may be incorrect if one does not consider the influence of spillover.

Patch testing with chemical allergens in a marginal irritant concentration is likely to give nonspecific skin reactions when the threshold for irritation is lowered, as in the case of ESS. This is frequently seen with formaldehyde solution, fragrance mixture, metal salts, rubber chemicals, "para" substances, paraben mixture, and wool wax alcohol.[18,22] The standard test concentrations for formaldehyde and the fragrance mixture have been lowered because of this. However false-positive responses can be seen even with allergens of low irritance. Obviously, one must be extremely circumspect when interpreting reactions to relatively unknown compounds.

In summary, the factors leading to the nonreproducible results are the degree of irritancy of the various compounds, the number of positive reactions observed, the strength of the concomitant reactions, the proximity of the reaction sites, and the existence of a dermatitis elsewhere.

MECHANISMS

The mechanism responsible for the fluctuations in skin reactivity in ESS is not clear, but, from animal experiments, clinical observations, and recent advances in understanding the pathological mechanisms of skin inflammation, humoral factors are probably very important.[38,39] Hypothetically, the irritability state could depend on the balance between mediators of inflammation, like cytokines, that promote and depress inflammation. Depending on this balance, a marginal irritant test substance may elicit a positive reaction or no reaction at all. Fluctuations in immune reactivity do occur.[38] Distribution or compartmentalization of lymphocytes probably plays a role in immune skin reactivity, as do other factors such as the influence of infectious diseases, stress, and circadian rhythm (cortisol levels). Such fluctuations might allow allergens that induced a weak sensitization to evoke either a weak positive reaction or no reaction at all (a false negative). There is no reason to assume that both hypotheses are working independently. A combination of both is more likely.

Interestingly, the opposite of ESS also exists. Extensive and severe dermatitis in guinea pigs resulted in a short period of depressed skin reactivity.[40] The skin reactivity can run a biphasic course, with depression of reactivity in the early phase of a severe acute inflammation followed by enhancement later on. The same phenomenon can also be seen in humans with an acute dermatitis.[41]

RETESTING

When there is possible ESS, patients or volunteers who have been patch tested in toxicologic assays should probably be retested. To prove allergic contact dermatitis, the patient is retested to each patch-test reagent that yielded a positive reaction, one at a time, after a suitable rest period. The length of this rest period has not been defined, but in practice 6 weeks after the skin in the test area is clinically healed, the same test region can be used again for testing. A dermatitis in any other region preferably should be healed or at least in a quiet phase. Unfortunately, false-negative reactions sometimes occur on retesting.

PRACTICAL IMPLICATIONS

How can one avoid mistaking nonreproducible reactions for true positives? Hyperirritability occurs often during patch testing, so how does one deal with patients who have multiple positive patch-test reactions in battery testing? A practical strategy for doing this without unnecessary effort and without sacrificing accuracy can be found in Table 7-2.

When the patient has more than one positive patch-test reaction, we retake the clinical history to examine the relevance of each test result. This procedure often suffices to solve the problem.

It is not always necessary to retest every compound that yielded a positive reaction. For instance, if the material is a chemical that is easily avoided because it is rarely encountered in the patient's surroundings, it is easier to suggest this, question him or her about the previous reactions, and leave it at that. If no relationship is found between the patient's history and the test result, there is no practical need to do further testing, at least not for the time being.

The physician loses credibility when the patient is told that he or she is allergic to something that he or she *knows* does not cause difficulty. When a positive test is related to a ubiquitous substance, however, it becomes very important to retest the patient. When the compound is something like a preservative (the parabens, Cl − + Me-isothiazolinone), a vehicle (wool wax alcohol or lanolin), a medicament (neomycin), a fragrance, rubber chemicals, or formalin, this takes on great importance. The avoidance of these materials requires so much effort that such advice, based on a false-positive reaction, is a needless waste of time and causes loss of confidence in the physician.

TABLE 7–2. How to Deal with a Possible Excited Skin Syndrome in Battery Testing

---

1. When more than one positive reaction is noted, retake the clinical history
2. It may not be necessary to retest positive reactions individually if
   • The material is readily avoided
   • The history strongly negates the positive patch-test results
3. Positive reactions should be retested individually when the material is ubiquitous (e.g., preservative, vehicle, medicament, fragrance, rubber chemical, or formaldehyde)
4. Retest positive reactions in important situations
5. Consider using the provocative use test (repeated open application test) in such an evaluation
6. Special attention to relevance should be made in cases of
   • Possible job change
   • Medical/legal situation
   • Regulatory situation
   • Public health issues
7. Mixtures: testing the individual components is often helpful

---

THE PROVOCATIVE USE TEST

The patch test is still too primitive a bioassay to serve as the only proof of allergic contact sensitization. It assumes that there are appropriate controls, that proper patch-test techniques have been used, and that no irritation is present. In difficult cases, the provocative test is invaluable. The advantage of this open test is that it is far less likely than closed testing to give an irritant response. A single open application, however, results in many false-negative responses, so repeated applications are used. We can call this technique the "repeated open application test" (ROAT) or provocative use test.

We ordinarily apply the material twice daily for approximately a week, although the testing can be stopped if a reaction is noted before the end of the 7-day period. The usual test site is either near the antecubital fossa, on the cheek, or on the neck near the ear. The material is spread over an area 3 cm in diameter. Appropriate controls should be obtained because irritation can occur even with use tests, although this occurs much less often than with occlusive patch testing. Overall, the use test is a simple but often effective way to evaluate patch-test results in patients with a possible ESS.

JOB CHANGE AND MEDICOLEGAL CONSIDERATIONS

Whenever a job change is considered as a way of solving a clinical problem of allergic contact dermatitis, the reliability of the patch-test reaction becomes critical. A patient should not be too lightly advised to change his or her job, as this often involves not only a change in work status but also a change in socioeconomic status and lifestyle. Such a recommendation should be made only on firm evidence. This means that the patch-test reaction should be confirmed and then, after the significant possibility of a false-positive response (e.g., due to ESS) has been ruled out, a recommendation can be made. Incorrect advice given to a patient regarding his or her potential for future employment can have devastating consequences. In some cases, despite all of its complexity, judgment of a legal claim rests almost solely on the patch-test result. The individual, the employer, and the courts are entitled to the most reliable information possible; therefore it is not unreasonable to perform patch testing more than once. This also holds for cases which could result in a government regulatory change. Changing regulations on the basis of several patients with allergic contact dermatitis is a difficult matter, and it is even more troublesome if the data turn out to be nonreproducible.

REFERENCES

1. Jaeger H: De la nature de l'eczema: Recherches expérimentales: Hypersensibilite, idiosyncrasie et anaphylaxie cutanées chez les eczémateux. *Ann Dermatol* 6:109, 1923.
2. Geiger R: Unspezifische Desensibilisierungsversuche an Ekzematikern mit Terpentinöl auf percutanem Wege. *Arch Dermatol* 158:76, 1929.
3. Rostenberg A Jr, Sulzberger MB: Some results of patch tests. *Arch Dermatol* 35:433, 1937.
4. Beek CH: The sensibility of the skin against soap among patients with eczema. *Dermatologica* 93:167, 1946.
5. Grolnick M: Studies in contact dermatitis: The response of healed specific sites to stimulation with another contactant. *J Allergy Clin Immunol* 19:298, 1948.
6. Wilson HTH: Standard patch tests in eczema and dermatitis. *Br J Dermatol* 67:291, 1955.
7. Bettley FR: Non-specific irritant reactions in eczematous subjects. *Br J Dermatol* 76:116, 1964.
8. Von Zumbusch L: Ueber die Behandlung des Ekzems. *Münch Med Wochenschr* 68:401, 1921.

9. Jessner M, quoted by Fisher AA: Occupational, industrial and plant dermatology symposium, San Francisco. *Cutis* 24:143, 1979.

10. Shelmire B: Contact dermatitis from weeds: Patch testing with their oleoresins. *JAMA* 113:1085, 1939.

11. Rostenberg A: Predictive procedures for eczematous hypersensitivity. *Arch Indust Health* 20:181, 1959.

12. Fischer AA: *Contact Dermatitis*. Philadelphia, Lea & Febiger, 1967, p 18.

13. Wilkinson DS, Fregert S, Magnusson B, et al: Terminology of contact dermatitis. *Acta Derm Venereol* 50:287, 1970.

14. Kligman AM, Epstein W: Updating the maximization test for identifying contact allergens. *Contact Dermatitis* 1:231, 1975.

15. Mitchell JC: The angry back syndrome: Eczema creates eczema. *Contact Dermatitis* 1:193, 1975.

16. Mitchell JC: Multiple concomitant positive patch test reactions. *Contact Dermatitis* 3:315, 1977.

17. Fisher AA, quoted by Cronin E: *Contact Dermatitis*. New York, Churchill Livingstone, 1980, p 12.

18. Maibach HI: The ESS: Excited skin syndrome, in Ring J, Burg G (eds): *New Trends in Allergy*. New York, Springer-Verlag, 1981, p 208.

19. Björnberg A: *Skin Reactions to Primary Irritants in Patients with Hand Eczema*. Goteborg, Sweden, Oscar Isacsons Tryckeri AB, 1968.

20. Mitchell JC, Maibach HI: The angry back syndrome: The excited skin syndrome. *Semin Dermatol* 1:9, 1982.

21. Maibach HI, Fregert S, Magnusson B, et al: Quantification of the excited skin syndrome (the "angry back"): Retesting one patch at a time. *Contact Dermatitis* 8:78, 1982.

22. Bruynzeel DP, Van Ketel WG, Scheper RJ, et al: Angry back or the excited skin syndrome: A prospective study. *J Am Acad Dermatol* 8:392, 1983.

23. Von Luderschmidt C, Heilgemeir R, Ring J, Burg G: Polyvalente Kontaktallergie versus "Angry Back": Zur Problematik falsch positiver Epikutantestreaktionen. *Allergie* 5:262, 1982.

24. Bandmann H-J, Agathos M: New results and some remarks to the "angry back syndrome." *Contact Dermatitis* 7:23, 1981.

25. Gollhausen R, Przybilla B, Ring J: Reproducibility of patch testing, in abstracts of the 17th World Congress of Dermatology, part II. G. Braun Druckerei und Verlage Karlsruhe, 1987, p 59.

26. Lachapelle J-M, Bruynzeel DP, Ducombs G, et al: European multicentre study of the True Test. *Contact Dermatitis* 19:91, 1988.

27. Magnusson B, Hellgren L: Skin-irritating and adhesive characteristics of some different tapes. *Acta Derm Venereol* 42:463, 1962.

28. Bruynzeel DP, Nieboer C, Boorsma DM, et al: Allergic reactions, "spillover" reactions and T-cell subsets. *Arch Dermatol Res* 275:80, 1983.

29. Bandmann H-J, Agathos M: Das "Angry Back Syndrome": Untersuchungsergebnisse mit Sequenztestungen, Wiederholungstestungen und dem Cocarden-(Target-) Test. *Hautarzt* 32 Suppl 5:97, 1981.

30. Kligman A, Gollhausen R: The "angry back": A new concept or old confusion? *Br J Dermatol* 115 Suppl 31:93, 1986.

31. Hamani I, Marks R: Abnormalities in clinically normal skin—A possible explanation of the "angry back syndrome." *Clin Exp Dermatol* 13:328, 1988.

32. Roper SS, Jones HE: A new look at conditioned hyperirritability. *J Am Acad Dermatol* 7:643, 1982.

33. Sjöborg S, Andersson A, Christensen OB: The Langerhans cells in healed patch test reactions before and after oral administration of nickel. *Acta Derm Venereol Suppl* 111, 1984.

34. Kanerva L, Estlander T, Jolanki R: Immunohistochemistry of lymphocytes and Langerhans cells in longlasting allergic patch tests. *Acta Derm Venereol* 68:116, 1988.

35. Scheper RJ, Von Blomberg-Van der Flier BME, Boerrigter GH, et al: Induction of immunological memory in the skin: Role of local T cell retention. *Clin Exp Immunol* 51:141, 1983.

36. Magnusson B, Hersle K: Patch test methods: II. Regional variation of patch test responses. *Acta Derm Venereol* 45:257, 1965.

37. Bruynzeel DP, Maibach HI: Excited skin syndrome (angry back). *Arch Dermatol* 122:323, 1986.

38. Bruynzeel DP, Maibach HI: Excited skin syndrome and the hyporeactive state: Current status, In Menne T, Maibach HI (eds): *Exogenous Dermatoses: Environmental Dermatitis*. Boca Raton, FL, CRC Press, 1990, p 142.

39. Pasche-Koo F, Hauser C: How to better understand the angry back syndrome. *Dermatology* 184:237, 1992.

40. Bruynzeel DP, Von Blomberg-Van der Flier BME, Van Ketel WG, et al: Depression or enhancement of skin reactivity by inflammatory processes in the guinea pig. *Int Arch Allerg Appl Immunol* 72:67, 1983.

41. Kligman AM: Poison ivy (Rhus) dermatitis. *Arch Dermatol* 77:149, 1958.

8

PHOTOTOXIC AND PHOTOALLERGIC DERMATITIS

Deborah F. Mac Farlane
Vincent A. DeLeo

The term *photocontact dermatitis* is used to describe a photosensitized reaction in skin caused by a topically applied chemical. This is distinguished from *systemic photosensitivity,* where the chemical is systemically administered. This chapter will deal with the responses to topically applied chemicals, or photoallergic contact dermatitis (PACD) and phototoxic or photoirritant contact dermatitis (PICD).

In both PACD and PICD, chemicals and light are necessary for a response to occur. The chemicals involved in these reactions have structures able to absorb radiation in the solar spectrum typically in the UVA (320 to 400 nm) or visible (400 to 800 nm) ranges. The absorption of radiation by these chemicals results in the conversion of absorbed energy into chemical change. This photochemical reaction, in turn, results in a biologic response. PICD occurs when the response directly damages skin cells. In PACD, the photochemical reaction produces an antigenic molecule—a photoallergen and an immune response of the delayed cellular type. These different mechanisms explain the clinical differences between PACD and PICD.

DIFFERENCES BETWEEN PICD AND PACD

Only sensitized individuals react positively when photopatch tested to a chemical producing PACD. Unsensitized individuals and the population in general do not react. In contrast, a majority of the population react positively when phototested to a phototoxic agent (PICD). In addition, while a reaction occurs in PICD at the first exposure of the chemical agent and light, a sensitization delay is necessary for PACD. As PACD is an allergic dermatitis, timing of the response following testing will be delayed. In contrast, with PICD, timing of the response is dependent on the chemical involved. While tars produce an immediate positive reaction in skin following exposure to radiation, psoralens produce a response 48 to 72 h following light exposure. Clinically, PACD presents as an eczematous response, while PICD causes erythema, edema, and

TABLE 8–1. Differences between Photoallergic and Phototoxic Reactions

	Photoallergy (PACD)	Phototoxicity (PICD)
Incidence	Low	High
Occurrence on first exposure	No	Yes
Onset after UV exposure	24–48 h	Minutes to days
Dose dependence		
Chemical	Not crucial	Important
Radiation	Not crucial	Important
Clinical morphology	Eczematous (erythroderma)	Erythema and edema, bullous; hyperpigmentation; psoriasiform
Histology	Eczema	Necrotic keratinocytes
Action spectrum	UVA	UVA
Diagnosis	Photopatch test	Clinical

bullous lesions and, histologically, keratinocyte necrosis. The dose of chemical and radiation required to produce the response is more critical with respect to PICD than PACD. Often, it may be difficult to distinguish between PACD and PICD clinically. Table 8-1 lists the characteristics that aid in differentiating photoallergic and phototoxic reactions.

PHOTOTOXIC DERMATITIS (PICD)

CLINICAL REACTION

The reaction of PICD occurs in all individuals under appropriate conditions, that is, where there is sufficient light intensity and quantity of photosensitizing chemicals. The type of agent involved determines whether the reaction will occur immediately or be delayed. Tar photosensitization, for instance, occurs quickly, with affected individuals reporting "tar smarting" or burning and stinging during exposure to the sun or an artificial light source. In contrast, with furocoumarins or psoralens, the response is delayed, occurring 2 to 3 days following exposure to chemical and light. Clinically, the involved skin in PICD becomes erythematous, with edema and possible bullae formation, hence the term *exaggerated sunburn*. Following exposure to low-level photoirritants, the inflammatory response may be subclinical, with only hyperpigmentation involved. This is seen with "berloque dermatitis" due to furocoumarins in perfumes, where hyperpigmented macules are visible in "pendant" or "berloque" shapes on the neck.

HISTOLOGY

Histologically, an early lesion of PICD may reveal epidermal inter- and intracellular edema with keratinocyte necrosis and subepidermal blister formation in severe cases.

MECHANISM

The actual pathways involved in PICD vary in an agent-specific manner. Furocoumarins, for example, react with UV radiation to induce monoadducts and DNA cross-linking. Porphyrins, dyes, and probably tars induce cellular damage through the production of excited oxygen species.

DIAGNOSIS

The diagnosis of PICD is made by history and morphology. As these agents are photoirritants and will produce positive reactions in everyone independent of previous exposure, photopatch testing should not be done. Treatment consists of acute local care and instruction to the patient to avoid the agent and UV exposure in future.

AGENTS CAUSING PHOTOTOXIC DERMATITIS (See Table 8-2)

Coal Tar Derivatives

THERAPEUTIC USE. Tars can gain exposure to skin in a therapeutic and in an occupational context. The known photosensitizers in tar include acridine, anthracene, phenanthrene, and pyridene. Tars are used extensively in the treatment of skin disease and are available in prescription and over-the-counter preparations such as shampoos, bar soaps, bath oils, scalp and skin solutions, lotions, creams, and ointments. The action spectrum for tar photosensitization is in the UVA range. Patients may experience a PICD response following tar use and subsequent exposure to radiation filtered through window glass. Patients should be warned not to expose themselves to long periods of sun following the use of a tar preparation.

INDUSTRIAL USE. Products such as creosote and pitch are used to coat roofs and treat lumber (e.g., for telephone poles and railroad ties). It is apparent that exposure to these agents in the outdoor workplace can easily lead to PICD. Interestingly, direct contact with pitch or creosote is unnecessary for photosensitivity to occur, as volatile fumes produced from these products can, in the presence of sunlight, produce a photodermatitis.

Drugs

The phenothiazines and sulfonamides may cause PICD or PACD in health care workers who have skin contact with these agents.

Dyes

Certain dyes such as eosin photosensitize in the visible light region.

TABLE 8–2. Agents Inducing Photocontact Dermatitis

Phototoxicity	Photoallergy
Coal tar derivatives	**Sunscreens**
Acridine	PABA, PABA esters
Anthracene	Benzophenones
Phenanthrene	Cinnamates
	Dibenzoylmethanes
Drugs	**Fragrances**
Phenothiazines	Musk ambrette
Sulfonamides	6-Methylcoumarin
	Sandalwood oil
Dyes	**Antibacterial agents**
Anthraquinone	Sulfanilamide
Eosin	Tribromosalicylanilide
Methylene Blue	Tetrachlorosalicylanilide
Rose Bengal	Triclosan
Dispense Blue 35	Dichlorophene
	Bithionol
Furocoumarins	Fenticlor
Therapeutic	Hexachlorophene
Psoralen	Chlorhexidine
8-Methoxypsoralen	**Therapeutic agents**
4,5,8-Trimethylpsoralen	Diphenhydramine
Fragrance materials[a]	Psoralens
Plants[b]:	Thiazides
Lime, lemon	Sulfonylureas
Celery	Chlorpromazine
Parsley	Promethazine
Parsnip	**Miscellaneous**
Fig	Thiourea
Angelica	Primula

[a] Berloque dermatitis.
[b] Phytophotodermatitis (not all-inclusive).

Furocoumarins

THERAPEUTIC. This group of chemicals constitutes probably the most frequent cause of PICD in the United States. Produced naturally in various plant products and also synthesized for use as therapeutic and fragrance ingredients, these agents include 8-methoxypsoralen (8-MOP), 5-methoxypsoralen (5-MOP), and trimethypsoralen (TMP). 8-MOP and TMP are widely used by dermatologists in the treatment of a variety of skin diseases when combined with UVA radiation for psoralen + UVA (PUVA) photochemotherapy.

PLANTS. When psoralens from certain plants, vegetables, or fruits are accidentally applied to the skin followed by radiation, a form of PICD called *phytophotodermatitis* results. When a patient squeezes limes for beverages and then undergoes exposure to the sun, PICD occurs. The response may present clinically with erythema, edema, and vesicles or bullae formation 48 to 72 h following exposure. The reaction usually resolves with hyperpigmentation but may present with bizarre streaking and whirling patterns and can occur on any body site. Patients may also have noninflammatory blisters on the lateral surfaces of the fingers with no resultant hyperpigmentation. The photosensitizer in limes is present in the colored part of the fruit's skin, not in the juice, and is lipid-soluble, penetrating into the epidermis with ease. High humidity further increases percutaneous absorption of the psoralens and accentuates their phototoxic action. Celery is also frequently reported to induce PICD. Initially only fungus-infected celery was noted to contain enough 8-MOP to induce the response. Recently, however, uninfected celery has been reported to induce PICD, usually in the workplace. This celery is typically grown on the West Coast and bred to be especially hardy and long-lasting—characteristics associated with the natural anti-infective capacity of the plant psoralens. A psoriasiform dermatitis has also been reported, as has systemic photosensitization, following the ingestion of a large quantity of celery root. Other commonly encountered causes of PICD include members of the Umbelliferae family of plants: figs, parsnips, wild carrots, fennel, caraway, anise, coriander, angelica, and parsley.

PHOTOALLERGIC DERMATITIS (PACD)

CLINICAL AND HISTOLOGIC REACTION

The clinical and histologic response in PACD is eczematous, does not vary appreciably among agents, and usually occurs in a delayed fashion 24 to 48 h following exposure.

INCIDENCE

While approximately 20 percent of photosensitivity patients suffer from PACD, the incidence in the population at large is unknown.

MECHANISM

PACD is an immune-mediated response where the chromophore enters the body via the skin, absorbs radiation, and is converted into a complete photoantigen by a poorly defined mechanism which probably involves processing by macrophages and complexing to proteins, possibly the HLA-DR molecule. PACD is a T-cell-mediated, Gell and Coombs type IV reaction which will occur only in a predisposed part of the population and, as sensitization is necessary, not on first exposure. The action spectrum of photosensitivity to the photoantigen, both clinically and in photopatch testing, is in the UVA range. Once the diagnosis of PACD is made and the antigen exposure stopped, the reaction ceases in most cases. Such reactions are called *transient light reactions*. Rarely, the photosensitivity persists long after the exposure to antigen is stopped. In such cases the patient is said to have a "persistent light reaction." In most patients this photosensitivity involves the entire skin surface, even sites not previously exposed to antigen, and the spectrum of photosensitivity becomes altered so that the patient responds not only to antigen and UVA but also to UVB alone. Therefore, in addition to the clinical difference of persistence after antigen avoidance between transient and persistent reactors, the groups will differ with respect to phototesting results. While both will have positive photopatch tests (antigen and UVA), transient reactors will have normal minimum erythema doses (MEDs) to UVB and UVA. Persistent reactors will have abnormal or lowered MEDs in the UVB and possibly UVA range. These responses will usually persist and be eczematous histologically and even clinically. The persistent reaction has been reported with certain salicylanilides and musk ambrette. These patients are classed under the diagnosis of chronic actinic dermatitis.

DIAGNOSIS AND TREATMENT

It is difficult to distinguish clinically between PACD and idiopathic photosensitivity like polymorphous light eruption. And PACD, especially to sunscreens, can complicate the clinical course in patients with other types of photosensitivity. PACD is diagnosed by photopatch testing. As in allergic contact dermatitis, treatment consists of avoidance of contact with the allergen. For most patients, the photosensitivity disappears once this is achieved.

AGENTS CAUSING PHOTOTOXIC DERMATITIS (See Table 8-2)

SUNSCREENS

Increased public awareness of the dangers of ultraviolet radiation has led to a greater use of sunscreens and a consequent increase in exposure to the active ingredients in these products. While the incidence of PACD among sunscreen users is probably very low, the incidence of reactions in groups of patients referred for testing because of photosensitivity is high.

PABA. An excellent UVB absorber, PABA was the first chemical sunscreen in the 1960s. The perception that PABA was highly sensitizing resulted in the production of "PABA-free" sunscreens. Consequently PABA is now an infrequent ingredient of marketed sunscreens. It should be noted that PABA may also be present in moisturizers, emollients, lipsticks, lip balms, shampoos, and hair-care products.

PABA ESTERS. The PABA esters, octyl-dimethyl PABA (padimate O), amyl-dimethyl PABA (padimate A), and glycerol PABA have replaced PABA. Padimate A use was associated with an immediate photoirritancy. Glycerol PABA, once thought to be a high-level photoirritant, has recently become more popular as a sunscreen. Padimate O is currently the most frequently used chemical in the PABA group and is capable of inducing PACD. Cross-reactivity between PABA and its esters has been noted.

BENZOPHENONES. UV-absorbing agents with absorbance in the UVA range, benzophenones were originally used to protect industrial materials from discoloration. Sulisobenzone (benzophenone 4) was the first agent in the benzophenone class to be used in PABA-free sunscreens and is a low-level sensitizer. Oxybenzone (benzophenone 3) is currently the most commonly used active ingredient in U.S.-marketed sunscreens. Reports of PACD to this agent are increasing as its usage in turn increases. Dioxybenzone (benzophenone 8) is similarly used in sunscreens, and 2,2′,4′,4′-tetrahydroxy-benzophenone (benzophenone 2) is a preservative in personal care products.

CINNAMATES. Cinoxate (2-methoxy ethyl-p-methoxycinnamate) is an infrequently used sunscreen in the United States and has been reported to cause PACD in Europe.

DIBENZOYLMETHANES. Butyl methoxydibenzoylmethane (Avobenzone, PARSOL 1789) is a recent addition to U.S.-marketed sunscreens and an excellent UVA absorber. This agent has been reported to cause PACD in Europe and is likely to do the same with increasing usage in this country. Table 8-3 provides a list of products to be avoided by patients with PACD to possible sunscreens and suggests products which may be safely substituted.

Fragrances

Various fragrance ingredients have been associated with PACD. The most commonly implicated include musk ambrette, 6-methylcoumarin, and sandalwood oil.

MUSK AMBRETTE. Musk ambrette is a synthetic fragrance fixative used primarily in men's aftershave and cologne. In the 1970s and '80s, concentrations as high as 15% were used in these products. By the 1980s, musk ambrette was the most frequently reported cause of PACD and many of the men who became sensitized developed persistent

TABLE 8–3. Sunscreen Substitutions

Allergen	Products to Avoid	Substitute
Sunscreens PABA or PABA derivatives	PABA and PABA derivatives-padimate A, padimate O, glyceryl PABA. You may react to thiazide diuretics, sulfonylurea antidiabetic agents, p-aminosalicylic acid, procainamide, benzocaine and p-phenylenediamine in permanent hair dyes. PABA may also be found in moisturizers, cosmetics, shampoos, lip products, and oral vitamin supplements	Agents with oxybenzone, sulisobenzone, cinnamates, dibenzoylmethanes, and salicylates
Benzophenones Sulisobenzone, oxybenzone	All benzophenones	Sunscreens with PABA, padimate, cinnamate, salicylates, and dibenzoylmethanes
Cinnamates Cinoxate	All cinnamates in sunscreens, fragrances and flavoring agents, toothpastes and mouthwashes	Sunscreens with PABA, padimate, benzophenones, salicylates, and dibenzoylmethanes
Dibenzoylmethanes Butyl methoxydibenzoylmethane (avobenzone) 4-Isopropyl-dibenzoylmethane	Sunscreens containing any di-benzoylmethane	Sunscreens with PABA, padimate, benzophenones, salicylates, and cinnamate

reactions or chronic actinic dermatitis. The International Fragrance Association recommends that musk ambrette not be used in cosmetics and toiletries coming in contact with the skin. A concentration of 4% is recommended in other products.

6-METHYLCOUMARIN. A synthetic fragrance ingredient in cosmetics and in suntanning lotion in the 1980s, this agent was responsible for cases of PACD severe enough, in some instances, to require hospitalization. Identification of the photoallergen was made only when it was discovered that the agent becomes inactive as a photoallergen when applied to the skin. It is therefore recommended that the antigen be applied in duplicate 30 min prior to irradiation.

SANDALWOOD OIL. A rarely reported photoallergen.

Patients photoallergic or allergic to a fragrance product should be advised to use only fragrance-free cosmetics and personal care products.

Antibacterial Agents

Topical sulfonamides used to treat soldiers' wounds in World War II were responsible for the first major PACD epidemic. Among the most potent photosensitizers of the antimicrobial agents are tetrachlorosalicylanilide (TCSA) and tribromosalicylanilide (TBS). TCSA used in bar soaps was responsible for PACD in over 10,000 individuals in the 1960s. While use of TCSA and TBS in bar soaps and shampoos has been discontinued in the United States, these agents may be present in industrial cleaners in the United States and in products purchased abroad. Interestingly, persistent light reactors who were originally sensitized to these agents may still seek medical care.

TRICLOSAN. This antibacterial agent is contained in most deodorant and deodorant-type bar soaps in the United States. It is a rare photosensitizer.

DICHLOROPHENE. Widely used in the United States and Europe in shampoos, toothpastes, antiperspirants, and "athlete's foot" powder, this is a rare photosensitizer.

BITHIONOL. In the 1960s this chlorinated phenol was extensively used in soaps and shampoos in the United States and Japan. A potent photosensitizer, it is presently banned from United States-marketed products. However, it may still be used in veterinary medicine, in agriculture, and in industrial cleansers.

FENTICLOR. A phenolic antibacterial and antiseborrheic agent in hair-care products made in Canada, the United Kingdom, and the United States, this is a moderately potent photoallergen and may produce false-positive response in photopatch testing.

HEXACHLOROPHENE. Once a widely used ingredient in over-the-counter U.S. skin cleansers, pHisoHex is now used with much lower frequency following reports of neurotoxicity in the 1980s. It is a rarely reported photoallergen.

CHLORHEXIDINE. Chlorhexidine is a broad-spectrum antibacterial extensively used in the hospital setting as a surgical scrub and operative site cleanser, in gynecologic and urologic procedures, and in eyedrops and mouthwashes. In addition, it is a preservative in various topical medications and cosmetics.

Therapeutic Agents

Although many agents used in a medical setting induce photosensitivity when taken systemically, few cause PACD. The sulfanilamides have been previously mentioned; the other major group is the phenothiazines.

TABLE 8–4. Substitution Table for Fragrances, Antibacterials, and Therapeutic Agents

Allergen	Products to Avoid	Substitute
Fragrances Musk ambrette 6-Methyl-coumarin Sandalwood oil	All fragranced products including after-shave lotions and colognes	Use only fragrance-free cosmetics and personal care products. Household products and cosmetics used by close family members should be fragrance-free
Antibacterial agents Tribromosalicylanilide (TBS) Triclosan Dichlorophene Bithionol Fenticlor Hexachlorophene	Personal products-soaps, shampoos, deodorants Reactions may occur to other halogenated phenols used in foreign and domestically produced personal care products, detergents, and cleansers: hexachlorophene in pHisoHex, dibromosalicylanilide (DBS) in dibromsalan, multifungin (BCSA) in bromochlorosalicylanilide, trichlorocarbanilide (TCC) in trichlocarban, bithionol in thiobisdichlorophenol, fenticlor-thiobischlorophenol, buclosamide (Jadit), chloro-2-phenolphenol (Dowacide 32), tetrachlorosalicylanilide (TCSA), triclosan (Irgasan)	
Chlorhexidine	All chemically related chlorhexidines—chlorhexidine digluconate, chlorhexidine diacetate, chlorhexidine dihydrochloride.	
Therapeutic agents Sulfonylureas Chlorpromazine Promethazine	Avoid skin and systemic contact with these agents.	Wear gloves and other protective clothing if contact is unavoidable
Miscellaneous Thiourea	Avoid contact with photocopy paper and photographic developing. Reactions may occur to certain rubber products or adhesive agents.	Change to a nonthiourea-containing process

CHLORPROMAZINE HYDROCHLORIDE (THORAZINE). Chlorpromazine is a widely used tranquilizer, antiemetic, and sedative. Although a common systemic photosensitizer, chlorpromazine infrequently produces PACD and then usually in health care workers who experience skin contact when dispensing medication.

PROMETHAZINE (PHENERGAN). This agent is used as an antiemetic and antihistamine. The largest number of reports of photosensitization to it occurred when it was used as an antipruritic in promethazine cream in France in the 1950s. False-positive phototoxic responses are common with these agents.

Miscellaneous

THIOUREA (THIOCARBAMIDE). A component of photocopy paper and used in photography, thiourea induces PACD. Table 8-4 provides a list of products to be avoided and possible substitutes for patients with PACD to fragrances, various antibacterials, and therapeutic agents.

BIBLIOGRAPHY

Benezra C, Ducombs G, Sell Y, et al: *Plant Contact Dermatitis.* Toronto, Decker, 1985.

Cronin E: *Contact Dermatitis.* New York, Churchill Livingstone, 1980.

DeLeo VA, Harber LC: Contact photodermatitis, in Fisher AA (ed): *Contact Dermatitis,* 3d ed. Philadelphia, Lea & Febiger, 1986.

DeLeo VA, Suarez SM, Maso MJ: Photoallergic contact dermatitis: Results of photopatch testing in New York, 1985–1990. *Arch Dermatol* 128:1513–1518, 1992.

Droomgoole SH, Maiback HI: Contact sensitization and photocontact sensitization of sunscreening agents. *J Am Acad Dermatol* 22:1068–1078, 1990.

Emmett EA: Phototoxicity and photosensitivity reactions, in Adams RM (ed): *Occupational Skin Disease,* 2d ed. Philadelphia, Saunders, 1990, pp 184–194.

Faugi GJ, Storrs FT: Photosensitivity from men's cologne. *Arch Dermatol* 115:106, 1979.

Fisher AA: *Contact Dermatitis,* 3d ed. Philadelphia, Lea & Febiger, 1986.

Ham SK, Park YK, Im S, et al: Angelica-induced phytophotodermatitis. *Photoderm Photoimmunol Photomed* 8(2):84–85, 1991.

Ingber A: Primula photodermatitis in Israel. *Contact Dermatitis* 25:265–266, 1991.

International Fragrance Association: *Code of Practice,* October 1985.

Jackson RT, Nesbitt LT, DeLeo VA: 6-Methylcoumarin photocontact dermatitis. *J Am Acad Dermatol* 2:124–130, 1980.

Ljunggren B: Severe phototoxic burn following celery ingestion. *Arch Dermatol* 126:1334–1336, 1990.

Marks J, DeLeo VA: *Contact and Occupational Dermatology.* Chicago, Mosby Year Book, 1992.

Maso JM, Ruszkowski AM, Bauerle J, et al: Celery phytophotodermatitis in a chef. *Arch Dermatol* 127:912, 1991.

Menz MB, Sigfrid AM, Connolly SM: Photopatch testing: A six year experience. *J Am Acad Dermatol* 18:1047, 1988.

Nater JP, de Groot AC: *Unwanted Effects of Cosmetics and Drugs Used in Dermatology,* Amsterdam, Elsevier. 2d ed. 1985.

Schauder S: How to avoid phototoxic reactions in photopatch testing with chlorpromazine. *Photodermatology* 2:95–100, 1985.

Starke JC: Photoallergy to sandalwood oil. *Arch Dermatol* 96:62–63, 1967.

Thune P: Contact and photocontact allergy to sunscreens. *Photodermatology* 1:5–9, 1984.

Thune P, Jansen C, Wennersten G, et al: The Scandinavian multicenter photopatch study 1980–1985: Final report. *Photodermatology* 5:261–269, 1988.

Von der Leun TC, Dekreek EJ, Deensta-van Leeuwen M, et al: Photosensitivity owing to thiourea. *Arch Dermatol* 113:1611, 1977.

9

PHOTOPATCH TESTING

Deborah F. Mac Farlane
Vincent A. DeLeo

The photopatch test is a tool used to identify photoallergic contact dermatitis and is essentially patch testing with the addition of radiation to induce photoantigen formation. Topical application of the test substances is followed by irradiation, and thus photoxic/photoallergic reactions confined to the test area can be induced.[1]

LIGHT SOURCE REQUIREMENTS

The wavelength of light necessary to induce a reaction in sensitive subjects falls almost always within the UVA spectrum (320 to 400 nm). For photopatch testing, the ideal light source should produce UVA radiation in a continuous spectrum of sufficient irradiance and field size to allow radiation of 20 to 25 antigen sites with a dose of 5 to 10 J/cm^2 within a time interval of approximately 30 min. Such a source should possess both a filter to remove as much UVB radiation as possible and a photometer/radiometer to ensure proper dosimetry. The most readily available source to the dermatologist is the unit used for photochemotherapy (PUVA) (see Table 9-1).

Photopatch testing uses doses of radiation of 5 to 10 J/cm^2 of UVA.[2] In theory, the largest dose which does not alone induce erythema is most likely to yield production of the photoantigen and a positive test. In addition to photopatch testing, it is sometimes beneficial to determine the MED (minimal erythema dose) for patients undergoing photosensitivity evaluation. For a description of such testing, the reader is referred to DeLeo.[3]

PROCEDURE FOR PHOTOPATCH TESTING

The actual photopatch testing procedure varies between dermatologic centers both locally and internationally.[4] The photopatch testing format most widely used in the United States and described herein is that recommended by the North American Contact Dermatitis Group (NACDG) (see Table 9-2). Following this format, on day 1, two sets of photoantigens (see list in Table 9-3) in Finn chambers are applied, one set on either side of the upper back. Next, UVA at a dose which will be used for photopatch

TABLE 9–1. Light Sources for Photopatch Testing

UVA
Fluorescent black lights
Fluorescent PUVA lights
Mercury halide lamp with filter
Hot quartz lamp with filter [a]
Sunlight with filter

[a] Discontinuous spectrum; less desirable.

testing (5 to 10 J/cm^2) is delivered to an area of 1 cm^2 on one buttock. On day 2, the phototest site is assessed for erythema. Any erythema at the UVA site is considered abnormal, and the delivery of graded UVA doses (1 to 10 J/cm^2) is necessary for determination of the proper UVA photopatch dose.

If there is no erythema following UVA 5 to 10 J/cm^2, both antigen sets are removed and marked and all sites are assessed for contact allergy or irritancy. One antigen set (dark control) is covered with light-opaque material, such as gauze pads covered with aluminum foil or black felt, and the other set is exposed to UVA 5 to 10 J/cm^2. Following this, the irradiated site is also covered with light-opaque material. On day 4 and at one later time point up until a week after irradiation, the patient returns for a recommended two readings.

Alternatively, if 5 to 10 J/cm^2 of UVA produced erythema on day 2, a lower dose is necessary for photopatch testing. This dose is determined by reading the MED test on day 3 to graded UVA doses applied on day 2. A dose less than the MED should be used, but use of too low a dose may result in false-negative photopatch tests. A dose 1 J/m^2 less than the MED is recommended. With a lowered MED in the UVA range, patch irradiation will be on day 3; patches are in place for 48 rather than 24 h. There is no evidence that significant differences exist between these two different testing schedules.

The ability of one antigen, 6-methylcoumarin, to form a photoantigen rapidly disappears after its application to skin. It is therefore applied on the day of patch irradiation (usually day 2) in duplicate for a 30-min period prior to irradiation. Longer application times produce false-negative photopatch tests.[5]

Photopatch test reading is performed as for routine patch tests. The system used by the NACDG is outlined in Table 9-4. A positive response in the irradiated site and a

TABLE 9–2. Suggested Procedure for Photopatch Testing

Day 1	Apply UVA alone
	Apply two sets of antigens
Day 2	Read UVA dose site; if negative, proceed; if positive,
	determine MED in UVA range (see text)
Day 2 or 3	Remove antigen patches
	Irradiate one set of antigens
	Recover antigens
Day 4 or 5	Read patch and photopatch tests
	(48 h after patch irradiation)
Day 5 +	Second patch and photopatch reading

TABLE 9–3. Photopatch Test Antigens

1. Amyl dimethyl PABA	5% in pet or alcohol
2. Sulisobenzone (BZP-4)	10% in pet
3. Cinoxate	1% in pet
4. Thiourea (thiocarbamide)	0.1% in pet
5. Dichlorophen	1% in pet
6. Triclosan	2% in pet
7. Hexachlorophene	1% in pet
8. Chlorhexidine	0.5% H$_2$O
9. Sandalwood oil	As is
10. Chlorpromazine hydrochloride	0.1% in pet
11. Musk ambrette	1% in pet
12. Para-aminobenzoic acid	5% in pet or alcohol
13. Petrolatum control	
14. Tribromosalicylanilide	1% in pet
15. Octyl dimethyl PABA	5% in pet or alcohol
16. Oxybenzone (BZP-3)	3% in pet
17. Promethazine	1% in pet
18. Bithionol	1% in pet
19. Musk ambrette	1% in alcohol
20. Fenticlor	1% in pet
21. Butyl methoxydibenzoylmethane	5% in pet
22. 6-Methylcoumarin	1% alcohol[a]

[a] Apply 6-methylcoumarin 30 to 60 min before irradiation on the lit side and for regular time on the unlit side.

Abbreviations: pet = petrolatum.

negative response in the covered site is diagnostic of photoallergy. Equal positives in both irradiated and covered sites are diagnostic of contact allergy. With the North American system, the diagnosis of both allergy and photoallergy is made when both sites are positive but the irradiated is greater than the covered site. As in standard patch testing, false-positive and false-negative reactions can occur in photopatch testing. A common false-positive or photoirritant response is evoked by the phenothiazine agents chlorpromazine and promethazine. Some antigens produce an immediate photoirritant response which is not usually of clinical relevance and can be disregarded.

A list of conditions which can also result in further false-negatives and false-positives is provided in Table 9-5. In addition to the usual list of photoallergens, patients can be tested to their own products, such as sunscreens and fragrance-containing cosmetics. Industrial and personal care cleansers must be suitably diluted prior to such phototesting. Finally, it is suggested that patients about to undergo photopatch testing receive a patient information sheet explaining the procedure (see Table 9-6).

TABLE 9–4. Reading the Photopatch Test

Diagnosis	Reading	
	Irradiated Site	Nonirradiated Site
No sensitivity	−	−
Photocontact allergy	+	−
Contact allergy	+	+
Photocontact allergy and contact allergy	+ +	+

TABLE 9–5. Contraindications to Photopatch Testing

Do not perform photopatch testing when dermatitis is acute and/or severe. This can result in false-positive responses and can lead to a significant worsening of the patient's disease.

Do not photopatch test patients taking systemic steroids. To avoid false-negatives, it is preferable to test a patient after at least 1 week discontinuation of steroid therapy.

Do not test patients with sunburn. A recent sunburn to the back (1 to 2 weeks before testing) can also lead to false-negative results.

Do not test patients who give a history of an immediate urticarial type of disease without proper precaution. These patients could suffer a generalized urticarial response or even anaphylaxis with routine testing.

TABLE 9–6. Patient Information Sheet for Photopatch Testing

- Your doctor believes that your skin disease may be due to contact with chemicals in your environment followed by exposure to the sun. This is called photocontact dermatitis.
- The only way to obtain proof of photocontact dermatitis is by photopatch testing. This is different from scratch testing and does not identify food or inhalant allergies or allergies to oral medications.
- Chemicals will be taped to your back in small chambers. The skin will not be broken. The "patches" stay in place for 24 or 48 hours. They will be removed, irradiated and re-covered for another 48 hours. You cannot shower or do any form of work or exercise that will wet or loosen the patches.
- The coverings will be removed and a reading will be performed after 2 days. The patch sites will be marked with a felt pen and you will be asked to return for a final reading on another day. Between the two readings you can bathe, but you may not wash your back.
- You may develop itching under the patches. If it becomes very severe or if you develop pain, you should try to reach your physician. If he or she is unavailable, have someone carefully remove the painful patch. Try not to disturb the other patches.
- You may develop blisters at positive sites, and—very rarely—prolonged reactions or even scars may develop at these sites.
- You will be tested for your response to common chemicals. If you believe that your problem is aggravated by any agent or product, including medications, please bring it and its container with the ingredient list with you when you return for testing.
- You should not be tested if you are taking cortisone pills, have had a cortisone injection, are applying cortisone to your back, or have had sun on your back recently. Please tell your doctor if any of these have occurred or if you are pregnant. Please ask if you have any questions or call if you have any problems.
- Your tests may be completely negative. This probably means that an allergy is not the cause of your skin problem. As the test is not infallible, however, an allergy may be missed. Retesting may be indicated in the future.

REFERENCES

1. DeLeo VA: Workup of the photosensitive patient in DeLeo VA (ed): *Photosensitivity: Topics in Clinical Dermatology.* New York, Igaku-Shoin, 1992, pp 160–176.
2. DeLeo VA, Suarez S, Maso M: Photoallergic contact dermatitis: Results of photopatch testing in New York, 1985–1990. *Arch Dermatol* 128:1513–1518, 1992.
3. Marks J, DeLeo VA: *Contact and Occupational Dermatology.* Chicago, Mosby Year Book, 1992.
4. Menz MB, Sigfrid AM, Connolly SM: Photopatch testing: A six-year experience. *J Am Acad Dermatol* 18:1047, 1988.
5. Jackson RT, Nesbitt LT, DeLeo VA: 6-Methylcoumarin photocontact dermatitis. *J Am Acad Dermatol* 2:124–130, 1980.

II

STANDARD PATCH-TEST ANTIGENS

10

BENZOCAINE

Jere D. Guin

WHAT IS BENZOCAINE?

Benzocaine is a topical anesthetic agent for the skin and mucous membranes; it is found in both prescription and nonprescription medications. Products likely to contain benzocaine are those used to treat sunburn, poison ivy, itching rashes, and hemorrhoidal problems. It is commonly painted on by dentists just before a local anesthetic agent is injected. It is used on mucosal surfaces of the mouth, esophagus, pharynx, larynx, nasal cavity, and urethra for control of pain, the gag reflex, and so on.

About 1.8 to 2.0 percent of those patch tested for possible contact dermatitis react to benzocaine.[1] It is not a strong sensitizer in animal testing,[2] but it has been called a notorious allergen[3] in the United States, where it seems to be a more common sensitizer.[4,5] Perhaps the reason for this is its presence in over-the-counter products used to treat rashes such as the type of eczema that often appears over a swollen ankle.[6] Such use encourages the development of allergy to products containing benzocaine.

HOW IS CONTACT ALLERGY TO BENZOCAINE RECOGNIZED?

Contact dermatitis caused by benzocaine and many other topical medications can be suspected from the location, since it classically appears in and around the area where it is used and in a pattern seen with hand transfer.[6] When it has been applied to a rash, the eruption spreads around the lesions, which often become angrier and new areas may appear. This allergy can cause otitis externa, perianal eczema, vulvitis, and oral problems, among others. A classic presentation is a weeping, oozing dermatitis over a swollen ankle, perhaps with widespread patches of eczema.[7]

WILL ANY OTHER MEDICATIONS CAUSE A PROBLEM?

Persons allergic to one ester-type local anesthetic such as benzocaine may react to other related anesthetics as well, including butacaine, butamben, chloroprocaine, procaine, propoxycaine, or tetracaine. Patch testing for benzocaine is likely to uncover allergy

TABLE 10–1. Local Anesthetics with the PABA Structure That Benzocaine Allergic Persons Should Avoid

	Uses	Remarks
Topical Product		
Benzocaine (ethylaminobenzoate)	Topical skin, mucosal, genitourinary, proctologic	PABA ester, may cause rash in those allergic to hair dyes, PABA sunscreens, black rubber chemicals, etc.
Butacaine (Butyn)	Topical mucosal (denture pain)	PABA ester type
Butamben picrate (Butesin picrate)	Topical skin	PABA ester benzoate
Local (Injectable) Product		
Procaine (Novocain)	Skin, dental infiltration, local infiltration, peripheral nerve block, retrobulbar block	PABA ester, cross-reacts with group
Chloroprocaine (Nesacaine)	Caudal or lumbar epidural, dental infiltration, local infiltration, peripheral nerve block	PABA ester

Avoid in pregnancy |
| Tetracaine (Pontocaine) | Topical mucosal, eye, skin, transtracheal | PABA ester |
| Propoxycaine | Dental anesthesia | PABA ester; used in combination with procaine |

to this one class of anesthetic agent, but it may miss those with an unrelated chemical structure.[8,9] Therefore, one must learn which of these can and cannot be used safely, and patients should bring this information to the attention of prescribing physicians.

Several years back, benzocaine was found to be a contaminant in certain glyceryl para-aminobenzoic acid (PABA) sunscreens,[10] but this problem has largely been corrected. Such sunscreens tended to cause reactions in benzocaine-allergic persons, especially when the concentration was high.[11]

Another theoretical cross-reacting product is a pure food dye FD&C yellow #6, or sunset yellow. This azo dye has one component which is basically a sulfa and theoretically could cross-react with benzocaine, but there is no published proof that it does.

TABLE 10–2. Substitute Topical Anesthetics with Dissimilar Structure That Are Less Likely to Cross-React

Product	Uses	Remarks
Pramoxine HCl (Tronothane, Tronolane)	Topical use only—skin, anus, mucosa, larynx, trachea	Differs in structure from benzocaine
Dyclonine (Dyclone)	Topical, endoscopy episiotomy, dentistry. on mucous membranes (not in eyes); oral, bronchial, urologic, proctoscopic	Anesthetic 10–30 min after application for preinjection

Has been used as mouthwash |
| Dibucaine (Nupercainal) | Topical mucosal use | Long-acting amide with quinoline structure |

TABLE 10–3. Topical Agents with a Similar Structure (PABA and Benzoic Acid Derivatives) to Be Used with Caution

Product	Uses	Remarks
Benoxinate (Fluress)	Ophthalmic	Substituted PABA ester
Proparacaine (Alcaine, Ophthaine, Ophthetic, and others)	Ophthalmic	Said not to cross-react with procaine, but is m-amino benzoic acid
Cocaine	Topical to nasopharyngeal mucosa	Ester of benzoic acid (lacks amino group)

A rare problem with benzocaine is light sensitivity,[12–14] as a few sensitive persons break out only where the anesthetic is applied and exposed to the sun. To find such cases, one must expose the patch-test site to some form of light in order to produce a positive reaction, although sometimes a positive patch-test site may appear or become much worse following sun exposure.

WHAT KINDS OF PRODUCTS CONTAIN BENZOCAINE?

Benzocaine is commonly found in nonprescription medications used for poison ivy, hemorrhoids, itching rashes and burns, including sunburn.[15–17]

TABLE 10–4. Substitute Injectable Anesthetics for Benzocaine-Allergic Persons

Product	Uses	Remarks
Lidocaine (Xylocaine)	Caudal/epidural, subarachnoid, local infiltration, peripheral nerve block, retrobulbar block, transtracheal, sympathetic block	Amide-type anesthetic agent
Mepivacaine (Carbocaine)	Caudal/epidural, dental infiltration or nerve block, local infiltration, peripheral nerve block, transtracheal	Amide-type
Bupivacaine (Marcaine, Sensorcaine)	Caudal/epidural, subarachnoid, dental infiltration or nerve block, local infiltration, peripheral nerve block, retrobulbar block, sympathetic block, topical-respiratory mucous membranes.	Amide-type
Prilocaine (Citanest)	Dental infiltration or nerve block	Reportedly has not caused contact dermatitis Can cause urticaria and anaphylaxis May cause methemoglobinemia Amide-type
Etidocaine (Duranest)	Caudal/epidural	Amide-type

Benzocaine is a widely used topical anesthetic agent found in both prescription and nonprescription medications and even a few cosmetics. It is sometimes used by dentists and physicians especially on mucosal surfaces, as in the mouth, to prepare a site for an injection. The allergy is commonly seen as a flare and spread in a treated rash.

The data in this handout are provided for your information. However, it is impossible to guarantee safety, as it is impossible to predict perfectly whether or not someone will react to any medicine. However, knowing the probability of a reaction (based on the chemical structure of the medication) in advance should be helpful.

Perhaps the principal lesson to be learned is that persons allergic to this drug commonly break out to other "related" medications. These are similar in chemical structure, and the body's immune system can react to them just as it would to benzocaine. The skin lesions are likely to be weeping, oozing, itching, and crusting areas, although rarely sun allergy or hives may be seen.

One should check the labels of topical medications and even a few cosmetics for benzocaine, or ethyl-aminobenzoate, its chemical name.

POTENTIAL CROSS-REACTIONS MAY COME FROM sulfas, sulfones, thiazide-related diuretics, oral antidiabetes medicines, PABA sunscreens, and permanent (two-bottle) hair dyes.

LOCAL ANESTHETICS

CROSS-REACTING TOPICAL ANESTHETICS: Three topical anesthetics—benzocaine, butacaine (Butyn), and butesin picrate (Butamben)—are prone to cross react.

NONRELATED TOPICAL AGENTS: Pramoxine (Analpram, Fleetrelief, PrameGel, Pramosone, Prax, Procto Cream, Tronolane, Tronothane, Zone A) and dyclonine (Dyclone).

Dibucaine (Nupercainal) is said not to cross-react with benzocaine, but it may cross-react with other amide-type anesthetic agents.

OPHTHALMIC AGENTS: Benoxinate (Fluress) and tetracaine (Pontocaine, Cetylite) should be avoided.

Proparacaine (Alcaine, Ophthaine, AK-taine, I-paracaine, Kainair, Ophthetic, Spectrocaine) is said not to cross-react, but it has similar structural features, so patch testing before use is perhaps wise.

RELATED (CROSS-REACTING) INJECTABLES: For injection, procaine (Novocaine), chloro-procaine (Nesacaine), and tetracaine (Pontocaine) should not be used by benzocaine-sensitive persons.

UNRELATED INJECTABLES: Lidocaine (Xylocaine), mepivacaine (Carbocaine), bupivacaine (Marcaine, Sensorcaine), prilocaine (Citanest), and etidocaine (Duranest).

This information is provided to help persons with contact dermatitis in the understanding of their problem. The contents are subject to change as more information becomes available and are not intended as a substitute for medical treatment.

Local anesthetics are categorized by their allergic potential in Tables 10–1 to 10–4. Benzocaine can even be found in a few cosmetics, such as after-shave lotions. Benzocaine is also used in anesthetic eyedrops, in preparation for dental anesthesia, and to anesthetize the anogenital area.

Perhaps the most difficult problem for those allergic to benzocaine is the tendency to react to chemically related medicines including sulfa drugs, certain sulfa-related diuretic agents, sulfa-related hypoglycemics, procaine (Novocaine), chloroprocaine (Nesacaine), tetracaine (Pontocaine), procainamide (Pronestyl), paraaminosalicylic acid given as an antibiotic agent, sunscreens containing PABA, and permanent hair dyes (see "Benzocaine Reactors—Patient Handout").

WHAT SUBSTITUTES ARE AVAILABLE?

Persons allergic to ester-type agents (e.g., benzocaine) are likely to react to other ester-type anesthetic agents as well, including, for injectable use, tetracaine, procaine, chloroprocaine, tetracaine, and propoxycaine.[18] However they seem to tolerate the amide-type agents, e.g., lidocaine (Xylocaine), bupivacaine (Marcaine, Sensorcaine), Mepivacaine (Carbocaine), prilocaine (Citanest), dibucaine (Nupercaine), cinchocaine, and etidocaine (Duranest).[18] Rare cases of urticaria have been reported in response to some of these,[18] and while they can cross-react with each other, they usually do not cross-react with benzocaine. For topical use, pramocaine (Pramoxine or Tronothane), dyclonine, and dibucaine should not cross-react with benzocaine. A nonsulfa-related diuretic would be less likely to cross-react than thiazides, furosemide (Lasix), chlorthalidone (Hygroton), and metolazone (Zaroxolyn). Sunscreens which are PABA-free are usually labeled "PF," and they are widely available. Two-stage hair dyes usually contain a related chemical, but a number of other hair dyes may be tolerated. Patch testing over a 2- to 3-day period before using the dye on one's hair is recommended. Local anesthetic agents related to Xylocaine, Marcaine, Carbocaine, and other products of that group are usually tolerated without difficulty.

REFERENCES

1. Nethercott JR, Holness DL, Adams RM, et al: Patch testing with a routine screening tray in North America, 1985–9, No. 2. Gender and response. *Am J Contact Dermatitis* 2:130–134, 1991.
2. Maurer T, Thomann P, Weirich EG, Hess R: Predictive evaluation in animals of the contact allergenic potential of medically important substances: II. Comparison of different methods of cutaneous sensitization with "weak" allergens. *Contact Dermatitis* 5:1–10, 1979.
3. Fisher AA: *Contact Dermatitis,* 3d ed. Philadelphia, Lea & Febiger, 1986, p 220.
4. Fisher AA: Topical medicaments which are common sensitizers. *Ann Allerg* 49:97–100, 1982.
5. Durocher LP: Allergic reaction to topical drugs. *Can Med Assoc J* 118:162–164, 1978.
6. Fregert S: *Manual of Contact Dermatitis.* Copenhagen, Munksgaard, 1974.
7. Hogan DJ, Hill M, Lane PR: Results of routine patch testing of 542 patients in Saskatoon, Canada. *Contact Dermatitis* 19:120–124, 1988.
8. Beck MH, Holden A: Benzocaine—An unsatisfactory indicator of topical local anaesthetic sensitization for the UK. *Br J Dermatol* 118:91–94, 1988.
9. van Ketal WG, Bruynzeel DP: A forgotten topical anesthetic sensitizer: Butyl aminobenzoate. *Contact Dermatitis* 25:131–132, 1991.
10. Hjorth N, Wilkinson D, Magnusson B, et al: Glyceryl p-aminobenzoate patch testing benzocaine-sensitive subjects. *Contact Dermatitis* 4:46–48, 1978.

11. Fisher AA: The presence of benzocaine in sunscreens containing glyceryl PABA (Escalol 106). *Arch Dermatol* 113:1299–1300, 1977.

12. Kaidbey KH, Allen H: Photocontact allergy to benzocaine. *Arch Dermatol* 117:77–79, 1981.

13. Miyachi Y, Takigawa M: Mechanisms of contact photosensitivity in mice: III. Predictive testing. *Arch Dermatol* 119:736–739, 1983.

14. Fisher AA: *Contact Dermatitis,* 3d ed. Philadelphia, Lea & Febiger, 1986, p 859.

15. *Physicians' Desk Reference,* 46th ed. Montvale, NJ, Medical Economics Co, 1992.

16. *Physicians' Desk Reference for Nonprescription Drugs.* Montvale, NJ, Medical Economics Co, 1992.

17. Fisher AA: *Contact Dermatitis,* 3d ed. Philadelphia, Lea & Febiger, 1986, p 222.

18. *Drug Information for the Health Care Professional, USP DI.* U.S. Rockville, MD Pharmacopoeial Convention, Inc. 1992, pp 201–234.

11

2-MERCAPTOBENZOTHIAZOLE

Jere D. Guin

WHAT IS 2-MERCAPTOBENZOTHIAZOLE?

2-Mercaptobenzothiazole (MBT) is a chemical most often used in the rubber industry to help in the curing of rubber. Natural rubber comes from the rubber tree, *Hevea braziliensis,* largely in the form *cis*-1,4-polyisoprene, which must be cross-linked and polymerized to form usable rubber. The milky latex from the tree is gathered from incisions made into the bark of the tree and collected. Because this stimulates the tree, more sap is liberated as it is bled.[1,2] The unprocessed rubber may become solid, but it does not have the elastic or other necessary qualities to produce the forms we regard as typical or useful.[3] Therefore it must be treated, usually with certain chemicals, to give it the desired properties.[4] When the isoprene monomers are heated and treated chemically, they join into long-chain molecules or polymers. This can be accelerated and the rate of reaction controlled by chemical treatment, but the qualities of the end product depend upon many variables in this stage of manufacture.

Chemicals added are often listed in categories relating to their function, and MBT is considered an accelerator. It is also classed with chemicals known as benzothiazoles, which are similar in structure. There are so many rubber chemicals that four of the five rubber antigens in the standard tray are tested as mixes, which comprise three or four separate chemicals. However, MBT is the exception, as it was formerly in what is called the mercapto mix, but is now tested separately to allow use of a more optimal concentration. This is because irritancy is a problem when all of these (usually related) chemicals are used in optimum concentration. The remaining three structurally similar chemicals now make up the mercapto mix, but each is now used at 0.33% rather than at 0.25%, which was necessary for four antigens when MBT was included. This permits screening with a higher concentration of all four benzothiazole antigens. There is also a thiuram and a black rubber mix. The mixes are covered in other sections covering the standard patch-test antigens.

As a rubber accelerator, MBT gives fast, flat cures over a wide range of temperatures. It is used in the curing not only of natural rubber but of synthetic rubber as well. According to Adams,[2] styrene-butadiene rubber requires an even greater amount of MBT and other sulfur donors than natural rubber. Federal regulations allow the use of MBT in the manufacture of rubber utensils used for food preparation at a maximum concentration of 1.5 percent by weight of the rubber product.

2-Mercaptobenzothiazole is often used as a secondary accelerator (i.e., it is used with a primary accelerator such as a carbamate). Selection of rubber chemicals depends upon multiple factors, but thiazoles (MBT-related) account for over 90 percent of organic accelerators, activators, and vulcanizing agents.[4] About 6,531,000 lb of MBT were manufactured in the United States in 1984,[5] and this volume does not seem to be decreasing.[4] In addition, 198,414 lb were imported in 1981.[5]

The ultimate purpose of MBT as an accelerator is to cure the rubber, and its properties as an accelerator determine the physical properties of the end product. Selection of the specific chemical(s) is based on the particular industrial process and the end result desired. One cannot know whether a specific chemical is present in a rubber product without sophisticated laboratory methods, but some uses suggest a probable association. For example, foam rubber made from a combination of a carbamate accelerator and a (secondary) thiazole accelerator (e.g., MBT) is said to produce latex foam with a greater compression modulus and load-bearing capacity.[5] Therefore one might suspect shoe insoles as a source, and they usually are.

Is MBT a strong sensitizer? It certainly is a relatively potent sensitizer in guinea pigs,[6] and it is the cause of many cases of contact dermatitis to rubber. However, it causes far from all cases, and—despite the enormous amount used every year—it may not provide as good a patch-test screening antigen for rubber allergy as tetramethylthiuram disulfide.[6] In the United States, the prevalence in a population tested for contact dermatitis is about 2.1 percent,[7] which is lower than that found in previous years by the same group.[8,9] By age, positive responses are found in about 1.6 percent of persons under 40 and in 2.2 percent of those over 40 who were patch tested for investigation of a suspected contact dermatitis. The incidence is almost three times as great in occupational contact dermatitis,[10] and it is also high in some pediatric populations.[11]

The structure of MBT closely resembles that of many other rubber chemicals, and this allows significant cross sensitivity. The morpholinyl derivatives may be even more sensitizing, according to Wang and Suskind,[12] but MBT will probably pick up most of those sensitivities, as there is a prominent cross-reaction on challenge with MBT in animals allergic to morpholinylmercaptobenzothiazole (MMBT).

IS ALLERGY TO MBT CAUSED BY MBT OR A RELATED CHEMICAL?

This is not an easy question to answer. First, there is recent evidence that allergy felt to be caused by MBT might be caused by dibenzothiazyldisulfide (DBTD).[13] One group has even postulated that DBTD is the actual allergen in MBT-allergic persons, as MBT is converted to its dimer with heat and oxidation[13] and reduced back to MBT by glutathione.[14] Furthermore, there is cross-reactivity between members of the benzothiazole group, such as those in the mercapto mix. Foussereau et al.[15] found that N-cyclohexyl-2-benzothiazylsulfenamide, MMBT, and other substituted benzothiazoles cross-reacted with MBT. Wang and Suskind[12] ranked the order for sensitization for such agents as 4,4'-dithiodimorpholine (DTDM), MMBT, and then MBT. The reasons for differences have to do with absorption and affinity for protein, but one would expect such mixtures to produce as many or more reactions as did MBT from the data of Foussereau et al.[15] and from those of Wang and Suskind.[12] Allergy to mercapto mix has about the same incidence as MBT sensitivity,[7] but Mitchell's[16] data on mixes shows that of 171 persons allergic to either or both MBT and Mercapto mix, 48 reacted to MBT but failed to react to the mix, while only 14 responded to the mix and did not react to MBT.

RECOGNITION OF MBT SENSITIVITY

It is possible to suspect allergy to MBT in cases of insole dermatitis to shoes where the eczema is located on the plantar surface and typically spares protected areas such as the proximal toes and the longitudinal arch (Figs. 11-1 and 11-2). It may also involve other areas of the foot, of course, depending upon the construction and materials used. It may also be associated with a hand eczema in a glove distribution if rubber gloves have been worn. Rarely depigmentation has been reported.[17] Common sense will be one's most valuable ally in locating the cause, especially when there is a positive patch test. Eruptions from rubber products typically parallel the location of the contact, such as under a prosthesis, or the hands may break out where a rubber object has been handled even when rubber gloves have not been worn (Figs. 11-3 and 11-4). One may see an eruption from rubber bands or finger cots on the fingers, over the breast from a brassiere cup, or anywhere according to the source of contact. The severity varies enormously, probably due both to the level of sensitivity and the degree of exposure. Exposure to this chemical can occur from sources other than rubber, and the percentage of cases is higher among those seen for occupational contact dermatitis. A partial list of reported sources is included below.

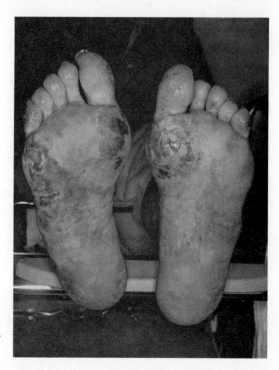

FIG. 11–1. Shoe dermatitis from MBT in athletic shoes.

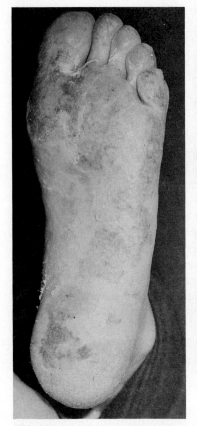

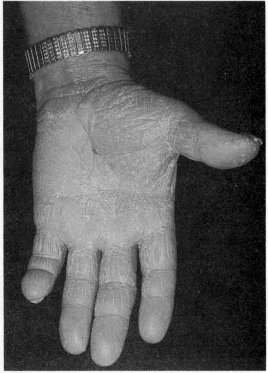

FIG. 11-3. Hand dermatitis in worker regularly holding a sponge rubber handle.

FIG. 11-2. Shoe dermatitis from MBT.

PATCH-TESTING CONSIDERATIONS

Patch testing is normally done with 2% MBT in petrolatum. That vehicle may not be ideal, as both MBT and DBTD in high-molecular-weight polyethylene glycol cause a more dramatic reaction in the same concentration in petrolatum.[13] The concentration used (in a different vehicle) for the True test has been adjusted so that result compares favorably with the 2% in petrolatum used as a control standard.[18] For this antigen, positive results are regularly confirmable with standard testing methods and on replicate testing.[18,19] As with any allergen, a positive test may be related to previous allergy or to the present problem; or it may be of unknown relevance. Whatever the reason, if the test is positive, the patient would do well to avoid contact with rubber which has not been proved to be of safe composition.

WHERE DOES ONE COME INTO CONTACT WITH 2-MERCAPTOBENZOTHIAZOLE?

The leading source is in shoes and boots, and especially the insole area[20] (Figs. 11-1 and 11-2), where 2-mercaptobenzothiazole is the most common allergen. This may be

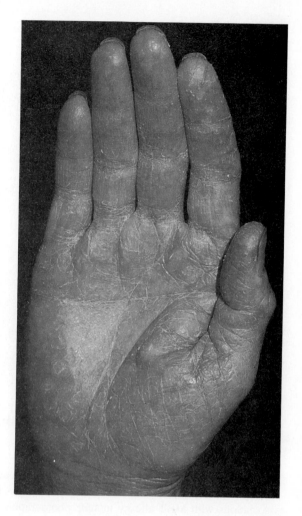

FIG. 11–4. Hand dermatitis in MBT-positive carpet maker. (See color Plate 2.)

in many kinds of shoes, even safety shoes,[21] but the leading source may be athletic shoes (Fig. 11-1). When the antigen was extracted and examined in one case, the actual sensitizer was found to be a dimer of MBT produced easily by heat and oxidation.[13] Some now claim that the latter chemical is the actual sensitizer, as MBT is easily oxidized to the dimer in the skin and reduced rapidly to MBT by glutathione.[14]

Many cases of exposure to MBT occur through contact with rubber products (Figs. 11-5 and 11-6), including brassiere cups,[22] rubber swim caps and face masks,[23] rubber bands (MBT weaker),[24] rubber banknote counters,[23] finger stalls,[23] Foley catheters,[25] medical prostheses,[26,27] elastic bandages,[28] rubber stoppers in medical syringes,[29] and baby bottle nipples.[30]

For a brief time, MBT was found in some spandex (polyurethane) elastomers,[31–33] but that has not been a problem for many years. Also, MBT has been found in nonrubber sources such as an anticorrosive agent,[34] in an antifreeze mixture,[15,23] and as a contaminant in digoxin injectable solution.[35] It occasionally causes allergy in condoms.[36,37]

In general, MBT can cause occupational contact dermatitis in many forms. For

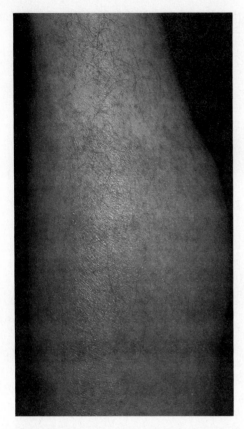

FIG. 11–5. Contact allergic reaction to rubber in socks in MBT-allergic individual.

example, it seems to be the most likely additive to cause reactions in "elastic threads" workers,[23] cement tube workers,[38] and those who use a Lycra conveyer belt.[39] Other associations with MBT allergy include photographic film,[40] veterinary medications,[41] a "releasing" fluid,[42] antifreeze, soluble oils, clothing, tools, cements and adhesives, cleansers, detergents, paints, black tires, fungicides, slimicides, greases, insecticides,[3,43] and even earrings.[44]

When a patient is allergic to one of the rubber accelerators, the physician must be suspicious of many items that are not listed. For example, an employee of a carpet manufacturer had problems with hand eczema (Fig. 11-4), which was located in areas where he used his hands with pressure, probably by gripping some item. His palms were so hyperkeratotic that he was considered by some very capable people to perhaps have psoriasis. Patch testing showed a reaction to MBT and an investigation of usage showed that carpet backing is commonly made of carboxylated styrene butadiene latex, which may well contain zinc salt of mercaptobenzothiazole.[45] Interestingly, MBT is also used as a secondary accelerator in EPDM (ethylene propylene) latex (as well as butyl rubber), which has an affinity for synthetic fibers used in the manufacture of hoses, tire cords, and conveyor belts. The limiting factor is lack of understanding of what is done in industry, and there are no good references to make it easier to develop such understanding.

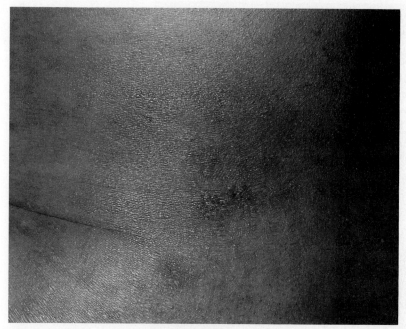

FIG. 11–6. Waistband dermatitis in MBT-allergic patient.

PREVENTION

Obviously the principal method of preventing eruptions from MBT is avoidance. This may involve staying away from rubber materials of unknown composition, which is difficult at best. Antigen substitution,[46] if contents can be discovered, often allows a sensitive person to maintain a normal lifestyle without jeopardizing safety.

The testing of rubber objects for MBT allergy is, for most patients, more convenient and much less expensive than the analytical methods necessary to determine the presence of MBT and related materials. The basic structure of these rubber chemicals is a thiazole structure, which is present on the benzothiazole group. Substitution within that group does not help as there is generous cross-reactivity.[15] The patch test to a piece of shoe or a square from a rubber glove will also tend to detect the presence of minor allergens that may not have been in the tray. In other words, the patch test often provides a better evaluation of safety than testing to standard rubber antigens, particularly in cases of shoe dermatitis.

Shoe dermatitis is covered in a separate chapter, but generally all leather shoes are tolerated provided that the patient is not allergic to other allergens such as chromates, which would probably be in the leather.

Another problem is allergy to socks and stockings, especially elastic stockings. Rietschel[47] found that MBT tends to contaminate socks that have been worn in shoes which have the chemical—and, worse yet, it does not wash out! This means that new socks and pantyhose must be substituted for those that have been contaminated. Since MBT may also be in the elastic threads of stockings, the safest substitute, at least on a temporary basis, is the type of athletic sock that is free of elastic. For those wearing

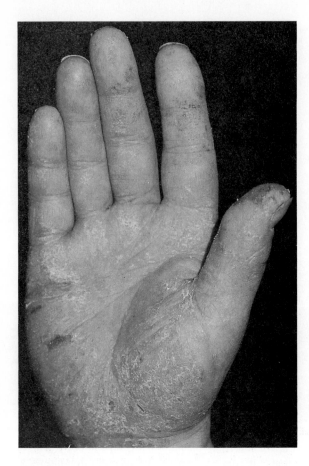

FIG. 11–7. Rubber dermatitis of the hands in MBT-sensitive person with shoe dermatitis. (See color Plate 3.)

support stockings, Jobst (1-800-221-7570) has surgical-weight elastic stockings that contain spandex, a polyurethane elastomer which (today at least) should be free of MBT.[48]

Allergy to rubber gloves (Fig. 11-7) is more often caused by sensitivity to thiurams rather than MBT, although one cannot assume that MBT is not present. There are two publications listing surgical and examination gloves and their chemical content. One should be warned, however, that substitution of an MBT-free rubber is not necessarily safe, as many persons allergic to one rubber chemical will also be allergic to others, some of which are not chemically related. To be safe, one must test to the product itself. If the test is negative, the product is much less likely to cause a problem. To test to gloves, we cut a small piece of the index fingertip of the glove and apply the palmar side of it to the skin of the upper arm. This is marked (with a fluorescent highlighter) and tacked into place with paper tape (Scanpor or Micropor). For some allergens, an elastic wrap is used, but this should be avoided in a rubber-sensitive patient. We have recently used petrolatum to cause deterioration of the rubber and the index fingertip because latex gloves are chemically treated there to improve traction.

Rubber-glove allergy is a problem especially for medical and dental workers. Often a "plastic" glove can be substituted. This often solves the immediate problem, but sometimes it does not. Patch testing is indicated to rule out sensitivity to the new glove before it is worn. Furthermore, testing to the routine screening series is indicated, as glove-allergic patients may be allergic to many other antigens as well. In the case of glove-allergic health care workers, additional allergy to glutaraldehyde is not infrequently a problem, although such patients are more likely to be allergic to thiuram than to MBT.[49]

REFERENCES

1. Rogers TH, Jr: Natural rubber, in Considine DM (ed): *Chemical and Process Technology Encyclopedia,* New York, McGraw Hill, 1974, p 298.
2. Adams RM: *Occupational Skin Disease.* New York, Grune & Stratton, 1983, pp 298–312.
3. Taylor JS: Rubber, in Fisher AA (ed): *Contact Dermatitis,* 3d ed. Philadelphia, Lea & Febiger, 1986, pp 603–643.
4. Greek BF: Rubber chemicals face more demanding market. *Chem Eng News,* April 17, 1989, pp 25–54.
5. Mausser RF: *The Vanderbilt Latex Handbook.* 3d ed. Norwalk, Conn, Vanderbilt, 1987.
6. Ziegler V, Suss E: The allergenic effect of rubber accelerators tetramethyl thiuram disulfide (TMTD) and mercaptobenzothiazole (MBT). *Allerg Immunol* 20–21:281–285, 1974–1975.
7. Nethercott JR, Holness DL, Adams RM, et al: Patch testing with a routine screening tray in North America, 1985–1989: I. Frequency of response. *Am J Contact Dermatitis* 2:122–129, 1991.
8. Rudner E, Clendenning WE, Epstein E, et al: Epidemiology of contact dermatitis in North America. *Contact Dermatitis* 6:309–315, 1980.
9. Storrs FJ, Rosenthal LE, Adams RM, et al: Results of patch tests in North America. *J Am Acad Dermatol* 20:1038–1044, 1989.
10. Nethercott JR, Holness DL, Adams RM, et al: Patch testing with a routine screening tray in North America 1987 through 1989: IV. Occupation and response. *Am J Contact Dermatitis* 2:247–254, 1991.
11. de la Cuadra Oyanguren J, Marquine Vila A, Martorell Aragones A, et al: Contact allergic dermatitis in childhood: 1972–1987. *Ann Espan Pediatr* 30:363–366, 1989.
12. Wang XS, Suskind RR: Comparative studies of the sensitization potential of morpholine, 2-mercaptobenzothiazole and 2 of their derivatives in guinea pigs. *Contact Dermatitis* 19:11–15, 1988.
13. Jung JH, McLaughlin JL, Stannard J, Guin JD: Isolation, via activity-directed fractionation, of mercaptobenzothiazole and dibenzothiazyl disulfide as 2 allergens responsible for tennis shoe dermatitis. *Contact Dermatitis* 19:254–259, 1988.
14. Hansson C, Agrup G: Stability of the mercaptobenzothiazole compounds. *Contact Dermatitis* 28:29–34, 1993.
15. Foussereau J, Menezes-Brandao F, Cavelier C, Herve-Bazin B: Allergy to MBT and its derivatives. *Contact Dermatitis* 9:514–516, 1983.
16. Mitchell JC: Patch testing with mixes: Note on mercaptobenzothiazole mix. *Contact Dermatitis* 7:98–104, 1981.
17. Achromatizing contact dermatitis caused by rubber sandals. *Med Cutan Ibero-latino-Americana* 15:1–7, 1987.
18. Wilkinson JD, Bruynzeel DP, Ducombs G, et al: European multicenter study of True Test panel 2. *Contact Dermatitis* 22:218–225, 1990.
19. Belsito DV, Storrs FJ, Taylor JS, et al: Reproducibility of patch tests: A United States multicenter study. *Am J Contact Dermatitis* 3:193–200, 1992.
20. Correia S, Brandao FM: Contact dermatitis of the feet. *Derm Beruf Umwelt* 34:102–106, 1986.
21. Foussereau J, Muslmani M, Cavelier C, Herve-Bazin B: Contact allergy to safety shoes. *Contact Dermatitis* 14:233–236, 1986.
22. Verbov J: Rubber in brassiere cups. *Contact Dermatitis Newsletter* 5:98, 1969.
23. Cronin E: *Contact Dermatitis.* Edinburgh, Churchill Livingstone, 1980, pp 714–770.
24. Kirton V, Williamson DS: Rubber band dermatitis in post office sorters. *Contact Dermatitis Newsletter* 11:257, 1972.

25. Petersen MC, Vine J, Ashley JJ, Nation RL: Leaching of 2-(2-hydroxyethyl-mercapto) benzothiazole into contents of disposable syringes. *J Pharm Sci* 70:1139–1143, 1981.

26. Correcher BL, Perez AG: Dermatitis from shoes and an amputation prosthesis due to mercaptobenzthiazole and paratertiary butyl formaldehyde resin. *Contact Dermatitis* 7:275, 1981.

27. Conde-Salazar L, Llinas Volpe MG, Guimaraens D, Romero L: Allergic contact dermatitis from a suction socket prosthesis. *Contact Dermatitis* 19:305–306, 1988.

28. Malten KE: Sensitizers in leg bandages. *Contact Dermatitis* 3:217–218, 1977.

29. Salmona G, Assaf A, Gayte-Sorbier A, Airaudo CB: Mass spectral identification of benzothiazol derivatives leached into injections by disposable syringes. *Biomed Mass Spectrom* 11:450–454, 1984.

30. Blosczyk G, Doemling HJ: HPLC determination of 2-mercaptobenzothiazole in rubber baby bottle nipples (abstract). *Lebensmittelchemie und gerichtliche Chemie* 36(3):90, 1982.

31. Joseph HL, Maibach HI: Contact dermatitis from spandex brassieres. *JAMA* 201:880–882, 1967.

32. Tannenbaum MH: Spandex dermatitis. *JAMA* 200:899, 1967.

33. Allenby CF, Crow KD, Kirton V, Munro-Ashman D: Contact dermatitis from Spandex yarn. *Br Med J* 1:624, 1966.

34. Fregert S, Skog E: Allergic contact dermatitis from mercaptobenzothiazol in cutting oil. *Acta Derm Venereol* 42:235–238, 1962.

35. Reepmeyer JC, Juhl YH: Contamination of injectable solutions with 2-mercaptobenzothiazole leeched from rubber closures. *J Pharm Sci* 72:1302–1305, 1983.

36. Wilson HTH: Rubber dermatitis: An investigation of 106 cases of contact dermatitis caused by rubber. *Br J Dermatol* 81:175–179, 1969.

37. Fisher AA: Condom dermatitis in either partner. *Cutis* 39:281–285, 1987.

38. Fregert S: "Cement dermatitis" caused by rubber packing. *Contact Dermatitis Newsletter* 6:123, 1969.

39. Fregert S: Dermatitis due to a conveyer belt of lycra: *Contact Dermatitis Newsletter* 12:325, 1972.

40. Rudzki E, Ostaszewski K, Grzya A, Kozlowska A: Sensitivity to some rubber additives. *Contact Dermatitis* 2:24–27, 1976.

41. Adams RM: Mercaptobenzothiazole in veterinary medications. *Contact Dermatitis Newsletter* 16:514, 1974.

42. Wilkinson SM, Cartwright PH, English JS: Allergic contact dermatitis from mercaptobenzothiazole in a releasing fluid. *Contact Dermatitis* 23:370, 1990.

43. Guin JD: The MBT controversy. *Am J Contact Dermatitis* 1:195–197, 1990.

44. Fowler JF, Adams RM: Earlobe contact allergy caused by rubber. *Am J Contact Dermatitis* 3:111, 1992.

45. Pole EG: Carboxylated styrene-butadiene latex, in Mausser RF (ed): *The Vanderbilt Latex Handbook,* 3d ed. Norwalk, Conn, Vanderbilt, 1987, pp 29–35.

46. Adams RM: Possible substitution for mercaptobenzothiazole in rubber. *Contact Dermatitis* 1:246, 1975.

47. Rietschel RL: Role of socks in shoe dermatitis. *Arch Dermatol* 120:398, 1984.

48. Fisher AA: Support hose for rubber-sensitive patients. *Am J Contact Dermatitis* 3:159, 1992.

49. Nethercott JR, Holness DL, Page E: Occupational contact dermatitis due to glutaraldehyde in health care workers. *Contact Dermatitis* 18:193–196, 1988.

12

COLOPHONY (ROSIN)

Jere D. Guin

WHAT IS COLOPHONY?

The patch test reagent called *colophony* is better known in the United States as *rosin*. It is the same rosin as that used by string musicians, who say "Rosin on your bow and here we go!" It is also the material used by baseball pitchers to improve their grip on the ball and by ballet dancers for added traction.[1]

Years ago certain pine wood materials were used principally for manufacture of turpentine, with rosin as a less valuable by-product, which was often discarded into rivers and streams.[2] Later, when it was found to be useful, reclamation efforts were begun, and many of these streams were dredged to recover the rosin. The name *colophony* comes from the ancient city of Colophon in Asia Minor, where rosin was manufactured.[2] In the United States, four species of pine are the dominant sources, loblolly pine, *Pinus taeda;* longleaf pine, *Pinus palustris;* shortleaf pine, *Pinus echinata;* and slash pine, *Pinus elliottii.*

IS ALL ROSIN THE SAME?

No, but if you are allergic to one type, you may break out to another as well. The composition of rosin varies with the species or variety of tree from which it comes, the method by which it is processed, and its handling and storage.[3] The main components are found in all rosins,[4] with abietic acid comprising some 25 to 50 percent. However, differences in composition cause differences in the allergic potential, and oxidation apparently increases the potential while hydrogenization reduces it.[5,6] Abietic acid is not a potent allergen until it oxidizes to form several sensitizers, including 15-hydroperoxyabietic acid.[2] Hydrogenation reduces the allergic potential of the product ostensibly by preventing formation of those allergens but also probably by producing stable products.

Rosin comes from three basic sources:

1. Gum rosin comes from the resinous tears obtained commercially by wounding and scarification of various species of *pine (Pinus)* and a few other members of the Pinaceae (family), but many other conifers may cause contact dermatitis in sensitive persons.[7] Today gum rosin comes mostly from China, Portugal, Honduras, Brazil,

and the former Soviet Union. However, the standard colophony patch-test antigen marketed by the American Academy of Dermatology in 1986 contained American rosin.[8] The patch test called colophony is usually 20% gum rosin in petrolatum (the generic name for Vaseline petroleum jelly). This test material will detect most but not all rosin reactions. It is a good screening test, however.

2. Wood rosin is manufactured from aged pine stumps, but production is decreasing. It has had considerably less press than the other two forms perhaps because we have run out of older pine-tree stumps. It is intermediate in cost between gum rosin and tall oil rosin.

3. Tall oil rosin gets its name from "tall," the Swedish word for pine. It is the least expensive of the three types because it is obtained from crude tall oil, a by-product of paper making. Crude tall oil comprises both resinous and fatty acids. The latter are separated, leaving the "tall oil bottom," with a high content of resinous acids. This can then be modified in various ways—i.e., with maleic anhydride—to make a product useful in paper sizing. The source is important, as the French tall oil rosin is more sensitizing than the Swedish product. The maleic acid derivative of Greek tall oil rosin is also potent.[9]

HOW COMMON IS THIS TYPE OF ALLERGY?

The incidence varies with the country studied as well as occupational and other factors. In Spain and Canada, it is low,[10,11] while in the United Kingdom it is 6 percent[12] and in China 7 percent.[13] Patient selection may influence the reported data, however. The same community in Germany reported an incidence of 2.8 and 11.9 percent in persons patch tested from two types of practice.[14] The incidence may be higher in those who carry HLAD-B27 histocompatibility antigen[15] and rosin is one of the allergens identified in pediatric patients.[16]

WHERE DOES ONE COME INTO CONTACT WITH ROSIN?

Some rosin exposure is occupational. In the electronics industry, rosin core solder can be a problem.[17] Other sources of work exposure includes varnishes, coolants,[18] and cutting oil[19]; ink, glues, and adhesives; dental cements and sealers[20]; and even the "rosin" musicians use on stringed instruments.[21,22] Rosin is also used as a tackifier or softener in synthetic rubber, including butyl, styrene-butadiene, and chloroprene latexes.[23,24] Occupations to suspect include electronics manufacture (solder), painting (paints and varnishes), forestry (plants), printing (inks and paper), and metalworking (cutting oils). However, the greatest opportunity for exposure may be in paper production.

Rosin can also be found in the home, in some forms of adhesive plasters[25] and tape,[26] paper products,[27] pine sawdust,[25] cosmetics[28] (mascara,[29] eyeshadow,[30] rouge,[31] lipstick,[32] dirt remover used in laundering,[33] clear soaps, and even chewing gum.[34]

Health professionals can develop allergy at work, and allergy can be iatrogenic in their patients. Medical exposure from surgical dressings is known, as well as from tape and surgical sutureless closures,[35] collodion,[36,37] a gel used to treat warts,[38,39] a leg bandage,[40] periodontal dressings,[41] and drug delivery systems.[42] Contact allergy has even been transferred to a bone marrow recipient.[43]

WHAT INFLUENCE DOES THE TEST MATERIAL HAVE?

Testing to the gum colophony, which is usually used, will miss some persons allergic to other materials in "rosin,"[11] but it is a good screening test. Testing with abietic acid alone is less effective,[2,44] but the oxidative derivatives are good, as 1% 15-HPA seems to substitute nicely, suggesting that it is the principal allergen in rosin.[45]

The concentration is important. Some claim a 60% concentration is ideal,[46] but most studies find that a concentration of 20% colophony in petrolatum will detect as many reactors as a 60% concentration[47,48] or even more.[49]

Some recommend the use of additional test materials including Venice turpentine[50] (from the European larch, related to our tamarack), tall oil rosin, and the neutral fraction. The nonacid component seems to be more important in gum rosin, where it is known to be a sensitizer, than in the tall oil rosin neutral fraction, where it is not.[51] Testing to the same rosins used on the job is another important way to detect minor antigens.[52]

In some industrial cases, testing to solder may be necessary, according to Liden, who used the flux 25 to 50% in alcohol and solder, as is.[53] *Some solder fluxes are caustic, so one should not test with acid core solder or non-rosin fluxes this way!*

WHAT IS THE CHEMISTRY INFLUENCING REACTIVITY?

At one time the allergen in rosin was identified as abietic acid, but "pure" abietic acid is not allergenic,[54] as hydrogenation reduces reactivity and oxidation increases it.[2,55] The point may be academic, however, as those oxidative products come from air exposure of resinous acids of the abietic acid series.[2] Hydroxylation and esterification also reduce the sensitizing potential of resin acids,[56] but they do not eliminate it.[57]

Rosin can be separated into components with an acid fraction and a neutral fraction,[51,58] as well as a residue cross-reacting with hydrogenated abietyl alcohol and containing mostly esters, which will detect allergy in some subjects negative with 20% colophony.[57] This residue can also cause contact dermatitis.[59] According to Karlberg et al.,[51] the allergenicity of hydrogenated abietyl alcohol apparently depends upon the unreacted component. The source of nonacid components is also important, as the "neutral fraction" of gum colophony is allergenic, while that component of tall oil colophony is less active.

HOW IS THE CLINICAL PICTURE RECOGNIZED?

Obviously someone with contact dermatitis after sawing pine wood or a Christmas tree would be suspect. Some cases are not so obvious. Rosin is associated with contact dermatitis in some cases of hand eczema,[60,61] perhaps at times from the newspaper.[62]

HANDOUT FOR PERSONS ALLERGIC TO ROSIN

WHAT IS ROSIN?

Colophony is the old-world name for rosin. It comes from the city of Colophon in Asia Minor, where rosin was produced in ancient times. It is a sticky, amber, resinous substance from pine and related conifers; the composition varies with the source. Persons allergic to one rosin chemical may not react to another.

WHERE IS ROSIN USED?

The tacky quality of rosin and its low price have made it a favorite ingredient of all sorts of varnishes, stains and coatings, sealers, putty and wood filler, dental cements, medications, paints, waxes and polishes, adhesive tape, cosmetics, (especially mascara, eye shadow, and lipstick), waterproofing and metal cutting fluids.

It is widely used in paper sizing, dental sealers, dressings and cements, adhesive tape, and medications, among other things. The solder used in electronics contains rosin as a flux. There are innumerable ways to use it to promote traction and decrease slippage.

WHAT DOES THE POSITIVE PATCH TEST MEAN?

A positive patch test to colophony demonstrates an allergy to rosin now or at some time in the past. It does not mean that it is or is not related to the present problem, but you should look for items that have had contact with the rash area and consider the possibility that one or more might contain rosin. Many persons who react to colophony have a history of allergy to Christmas trees, adhesive tape, eye makeup, or a variety of pine and other wood products.

HOW CAN REACTIONS BE PREVENTED?

Some things are high-risk exposures, e.g., a rosin bag, pine wood and products made from pine, as well as materials intended to promote tackiness and prevent slipping. Often, the ingredients of such material are not known. To see whether or not you are allergic to a specific product, it is sometimes possible to do a "usage" test, applying a nonirritating material twice daily for a week. The site of application should be one that absorbs well—e.g., the tender skin in front of the elbow, or perhaps a small spot on the neck (the site must not be broken out). If there is no reaction in a week, you may well be able to tolerate its use.

Tape or adhesive-plaster allergy requires the use of Micropore or Scanpor with sterile gauze rather than a commercial adhesive plaster. You can also do patch testing by applying several brands of tape to the back or (upper) arm for 2 days and then removing it. If there is no response, you may tolerate the tape.

Here are a few special considerations:

1. If you have both cosmetic and rosin allergy, consider especially mascara, lipstick, eye shadow, and rouge as sources.
2. If you have hand eczema, look for contact with spices (used in cooking), perfumes and flavors, and paper. Exposure may also be occupational, e.g., carpentry, where there is contact with pine boards or sawdust; electronics manufacture and repair where rosin-core solder is used; and paper manufacture, where rosin is both produced and used. Of course, the list is very long, so be on the alert.
3. Rashes suggesting sensitivity to light may require a patch test followed by light exposure. Light sensitivity, with a burning sensation, can cause a reaction immediately after exposure.
4. Facial rashes may mean either light sensitivity or exposure to rosin sprayed into the air.
5. Avoid contact with pine, juniper, tamarack, and other conifers until you can be tested. This can be done with sawdust, but let us help you. Don't try to do it yourself, as some sawdust is irritating.
6. Sometimes a positive patch-test reaction to rosin is a marker for allergy to perfumes, flavors, spices, and even plants—e.g., chrysanthemum. Be suspicious of things contacting the area where the rash has been located. Further testing may help to prove or disprove an association.
7. Last, the answer is avoidance, not treatment. While treatment will make the rash feel better, failure to remove the contact allergen from your environment will not only keep the rash active but could be followed by a *new* allergy to products applied to treat the rash.

Along with perfume mix, Peruvian balsam, and wood tars, rosin may be associated with allergy to spices used in cooking.[63] Of those who were positive to one of the four "indicator" antigens, 47 percent were allergic to one or more spices, chiefly nutmeg, paprika, and cloves.[62] Rosin is also an "indicator" or screening agent for fragrance reactions. As many as 60 percent of colophony-allergic patients react to one or more fragrance ingredients.[64]

For rosin, the area of contact will, of course, depend upon the source. For example, mascara causes eyelid dermatitis.[29] Rosin in occlusive dressings[65,66] and tape causes reactions where the tape is applied. Use of cosmetics other than those mentioned

TABLE 12–1. Products That May Contain Rosin

Adhesive and insulating tapes[2]	Musician's rosin[2,65]
Adhesives and glues[2,8]	Newspapers[66]
Antidust agents[24]	Ostomy devices[8,2]
Brown soaps[2]	Paints[8,2]
Caulking[24]	Paper and paperboard[2]
Chewing gum[2]	Paper sizing[24]
Cleansing agents[2]	Periodontal dressings
Coating of price labels[74]	Phenolic resin[24]
Core oils[24]	Pigments[24]
Corrosion inhibitors[8]	Plastics[8]
Cosmetics (eye shadow, makeup, mascara, depila-	Polishes[2,24]
tories)[2,8]	Pressure-sensitive tapes[24]
Cutting fluids[2]	Printing inks[2,8]
Dentistry products[2]	Rubber[24,66]
Detergents[24]	Sawdust[2]
Disinfectants[24]	Sealers and fillers[8]
Driers[24]	Shoes and clothing[8]
Emulsions[24]	Soaps[2,8,24]
Elastomers[24]	Solder,[8] soldering fluxes[2,24]
Esters and ester gums[24]	Solvents[8]
Floor-tile binders, wax[24]	Stains and varnishes[2,18]
Fungicides[24]	Substances promoting traction and preventing
Furniture polish, gloss oils[24]	slipping[65]
Greases[24]	Surface coatings[2]
Hot-melt adhesives and coatings[24]	Surfaces[8]
Insecticides[24]	Surgical dressings
Linoleum[24]	Tackifiers[2,24]
Lubricants[8]	Tapes[8]
Matches[8]	Waterproofing[8,24]
Medications (flexible collodion especially)[8]	Waxes and shoe polish[8,24]
Metal cleaners[24]	Wire drawing[24]

includes hair dressing or brilliantine and depilatories. For a very long list of other potential sources, see Table 12-1.

Airborne contact dermatitis of the face, neck, and forearms can occur from rosin core solder fumes. (All solder is not the same. Rosin core solder is used in the electronics industry, while a very different acid core solder is used in plumbing.)

Rosin has also been associated with a phototoxic reaction[67] and photosensitivity to lichens.[68,69] Contact urticaria has also been reported,[69] and rosin has antibacterial activity.[70]

WHAT IS THE BEST WAY TO PREVENT A REACTION?

Avoidance of colophony presents a number of problems, because the number of sources is large. Anything of pine origin is suspect. A long (but incomplete) list is given in Table 12-1 (see also the "Handout for Persons Allergic to Rosin", above).

SEVERAL CATEGORIES MAY REPRESENT AN UNSUSPECTED PROBLEM

1. Rosin is an "indicator" for allergy to fragrance materials, as positive patch test reactions to colophony (as well as fragrance mix, balsam of Peru, and wood tar) are associated with increased risk for allergy to essential oils.[63]

2. Colophony allergy may also be associated with sensitivity to spices used in cooking, especially in cases of hand eczema, cheilitis, gingivostomatitis (here also look for dental cements and sealers), and gastrointestinal and perianal problems.[62] Some recommend testing for spice sensitivity (e.g., nutmeg, paprika, mace, and cloves).

3. Paper products may aggravate some cases of hand eczema in persons allergic to rosin. Paper sizing material may also contain modified tall oil rosin, and some persons allergic to this are negative to the standard gum colophony used for testing.

4. Colophony responses are associated with an increased number of responses to plant materials including *Chrysanthemum*.[71]

5. Look for unusual sources of contact: colophony is used as a plasticizer in many synthetic products, and the incidence of allergy is higher in those allergic to phenol-formaldehyde plastics.[72]

6. Allergy can occur to conifers other than pine,[5,73] so it would seem wise to patch test colophony-sensitive patients before permitting them to handle those species.

7. Look for occupational exposure,[50] as to rosin-core solder (in the electronics field), wood, paints, varnishes, etc., in construction, and to rosin and paper sizing in paper making, to name a few.

8. In specific cases, avoiding environmental situations where airborne inhalation or contact can occur, and sun avoidance in cases of photoallergy and phototoxicity, are obvious.

REFERENCES

1. Aberer W: Allergy to colophony acquired backstage. *Contact Dermatitis* 16:34–36, 1987.
2. Karlberg AT: Contact allergy to colophony: Chemical identifications of allergens, sensitization experiments and clinical experiences. *Acta Derm Venereol Suppl* 139:1–43, 1988.
3. Karlberg AT, Boman A, Wahlberg JE: Allergenic potential of abietic acid, colophony and pine resin-HA: Clinical and experimental studies. *Contact Dermatitis* 6:481–487, 1980.
4. Zinkel D, Russell J (eds): *Naval Stores: Production, Chemistry, Utilization.* New York, Pulp Chemicals Association, 1989.
5. Karlberg AT, Boman A, Nilsson JL: Hydrogenation reduces the allergenicity of colophony (rosin). *Contact Dermatitis* 19:22–29, 1988.
6. Karlberg AT: Air oxidation increases the allergenic potential of tall oil rosin: Colophony contact allergens also identified in tall oil rosin. *Am J Contact Dermatitis* 2:43–49, 1991.
7. Dooms-Goossens A, Maertens M, van Lint L, et al: Colophony-induced sensitivity to Juniperus chinensis L. "Hetzii"? *Contact Dermatitis.* 10:185–187, 1984.
8. Fisher AA: *Contact Dermatitis,* 3d ed. Philadelphia, Lea & Febiger, 1986.
9. Hausen BM, Hessling C: Contact allergy due to colophony: VI. The sensitizing capacity of minor resin acids and 7 commercial modified-colophony products. *Contact Dermatitis* 23:90–95, 1990.
10. Hogan DJ, Hill M, Lane PR: Results of routine patch testing of 542 patients in Saskatoon, Canada. *Contact Dermatitis* 19:120–124, 1988.

11. Camarasa JM: First epidemiological study of contact dermatitis in Spain—1977: Spanish Contact Dermatitis Research Group. *Acta Derm Venereol Suppl* 59:33–37, 1979.

12. Shehade SA, Beck MH, Hillier VF: Epidemiological survey of standard series patch test results and observations on day 2 and day 4 readings. *Contact Dermatitis* 24:119–122, 1991.

13. Fan WX, Zhao B: Study on Chinese common allergens of contact dermatitis. *Derm Beruf Umwelt* 38:158–161, 1990.

14. Hausen BM, Mohnert J: Contact allergy due to colophony: V. Patch test results with different types of colophony and modified-colophony products. *Contact Dermatitis* 20:295–301, 1989.

15. Liden S, Beckman L, Cedergren B, et al: HLA antigens in allergic contact dermatitis. *Acta Derm Venereol Suppl* 58:53–56, 1978.

16. Kuiters GR, Smitt JH, Cohen EB, Bos JD: Allergic contact dermatitis in children and young adults. *Arch Dermatol* 125:1531–1533, 1989.

17. Widstrom L: Contact allergy to colophony in soldering flux. *Contact Dermatitis* 9:205–207, 1983.

18. Hendy MS, Beattie BE, Burge PS: Occupational asthma due to an emulsified oil mist. *Br J Indust Med* 42:51–54, 1985.

19. Fregert S: Colphony in cutting oil and in soap water used as cutting fluid. *Contact Dermatitis* 5:52, 1979.

20. Wennberg A, Orstavik D: Adhesion of root canal sealers to bovine dentine and gutta-percha. *Int Edodont J* 23:13–19, 1990.

21. Angelini G, Vena GA: Allergic contact dermatitis to colophony in a violoncellist. *Contact Dermatitis* 15:108, 1986.

22. Fisher AA: Allergic contact dermatitis in a violinist: The role of abietic acid—a sensitizer in rosin (colophony)—as the causative agent. *Cutis* 27:466, 468, 473, 1981.

23. *Vanderbilt Latex Handbook*. Norwalk, Conn, Vanderbilt, 1987.

24. *Rosins*. Arizona Chemical Company, 1968.

25. Burry JN: Contact dermatitis from radiata pine. *Contact Dermatitis* 2:262–263, 1976.

26. Schlewer G, Chabeau G, Reimeringer A, Foussereau J: Investigation of the allergens of colophony and its derivatives used in the manufacture of sticking plasters. *Derm Beruf Umwelt* 27:170–172, 1979.

27. Burry JN: Colophony, perfumes and paper handkerchiefs. *Contact Dermatitis* 15:304–305, 1986.

28. de Groot AC, Beverdam EG, Ayong CT, et al: The role of contact allergy in the spectrum of adverse effects caused by cosmetics and toiletries. *Contact Dermatitis* 19:195–201, 1988.

29. Karlberg AT, Liden C, Ehrin E: Colophony in mascara as a cause of eyelid dermatitis: Chemical analyses and patch testing. *Acta Derm Venereol* 71:445–447, 1991.

30. Fisher AA: Allergic contact dermatitis due to rosin (colophony) in eyeshadow and mascara. *Cutis* 42:507–508, 1988.

31. Foussereau J: A case of allergy to colophony in a facial cosmetic. *Contact Dermatitis* 1:259, 1975.

32. Rademaker M, Kirby JD, White IR: Contact cheilitis to shellac, Lanpol 5 and colophony. *Contact Dermatitis* 15:307–308, 1986.

33. Kirk J: Colophony collar dermatitis. *Contact Dermatitis* 2:294–295, 1976.

34. Satyawan I, Oranje AP, van Joost T: Perioral dermatitis in a child due to rosin in chewing gum. *Contact Dermatitis* 22:182–183, 1990.

35. Sjoborg S, Fregert S: Allergic contact dermatitis from a colophony derivative in a tape skin closure. *Contact Dermatitis* 10:114–115, 1984.

36. O'Brien TJ: Colophony in collodion [letter]. *Australasi J Dermatol* 27:142–143, 1986.

37. Barth JH: Colophony sensitivity—A regional variant. *Contact Dermatitis* 7:165–166, 1981.

38. Veraldi S, Schianchi-Veraldi R: Allergic contact dermatitis from colophony in a wart gel. *Contact Dermatitis* 22:184, 1990.

39. Monk B: Allergic contact dermatitis to colophony in a wart remover. *Contact Dermatitis* 17:242, 1987.

40. Dahlquist I: Contact allergy to colophony and formaldehyde from sand cores. *Contact Dermatitis* 7:167–168, 1981.

41. Lysell L: Contact allergy to rosin in a periodontal dressing: A case report. *J Oral Med* 31:24–25, 1976.

42. Sheorey DS, Dorle AK: Effect of solvents on the characteristics of rosin walled microcapsules prepared by a solvent evaporation technique. *J Microencapsulation* 8:71–78, 1991.

43. Olaguibel J, Almodovar A, Giner A, et al: Passive transfer of contact sensitivity to colophony as a complication of an allogenic bone-marrow transplant. *Contact Dermatitis* 20:182–184, 1989.

44. Wahlberg JE: Abietic acid and colophony. *Contact Dermatitis* 4:55, 1978.

45. Karlberg AT, Bohlinder K, Boman A, et al: Identification of 15-hydroperoxyabietic acid as a contact allergen in Portuguese colophony. *J Pharm Pharmacol* 40:42–47, 1988.

46. Bruze M, Dahlquist I, Fregert S: Patch testing with colophony at 60% concentration. *Contact Dermatitis* 15:193, 1986.

47. Karlberg AT, Liden C: Comparison of colophony patch test preparations. *Contact Dermatitis* 18:158–165, 1988.

48. Hausen BM, Jensen S, Mohnert J: Contact allergy to colophony: IV. The sensitizing potency of commercial products. An investigation of French and American modified colophony derivatives. *Contact Dermatitis* 20:133–143, 1989.

49. Nethercott JR, Holness DL, Adams RM, et al: Patch testing with a routine screening tray in North America 1985–1989. III. Age and response. *Am J Contact Dermatitis* 2:198–201, 1991.

50. Karlberg AT, Liden C: Clinical experience and patch testing using colophony (rosin) from different sources. *Br J Dermatol* 113:475–481, 1985.

51. Karlberg AT, Boman A, Holmbom B, Liden C: Contact allergy to acid and neutral fractions of rosins: Sensitization experiments in guinea pigs and patch testing in patients. *Derm Beruf Umwelt* 34:31–36, 1986.

52. Karlberg AT: Is unmodified gum rosin the best screening material for rosin allergy? *Am J Contact Dermatitis* 1:189–194, 1990.

53. Liden C: Patch testing with soldering fluxes. *Contact Dermatitis* 10:119–120, 1984.

54. Karlberg AT: Pure abietic acid is not allergenic (letter, comment). *Contact Dermatitis* 21:282–285, 1989.

55. Karlberg AT, Boman A, Hacksell U, et al: Contact allergy to dehydroabietic acid derivatives isolated from Portuguese colophony. *Contact Dermatitis* 19:166–174, 1988.

56. Hausen BM, Krohn K, Budianto E: Contact allergy due to colophony: VII. Sensitizing studies with oxidation products of abietic and related acids. *Contact Dermatitis* 23:352–358, 1990.

57. Foussereau J, Schlewer G, Chabeau G, Reimeringer A: Allergologic studies of intolerance to rosin. *Derm Beruf Umwelt* 28:14–15, 1980.

58. Fregert S, Gruvberger B: Patch testing with colophony. *Contact Dermatitis* 11:141–143, 1984.

59. Dooms-Goossens A, Degreef H, Luytens E: Dihydroabietyl alcohol (Abitol): A sensitizer in mascara. *Contact Dermatitis* 5:350–353, 1979.

60. Meding B, Swanbeck G: Occupational hand eczema in an industrial city. *Contact Dermatitis* 22:13–23, 1990.

61. Meding B. Epidemiology of hand eczema in an industrial city. *Acta Derm Venereol Suppl* 153:1–43, 1990.

62. Karlberg AT, Liden C: Colophony (rosin) in newspapers may contribute to hand eczema. *Br J Dermatol* 126:161–165, 1992.

63. van den Akker TW, Roesyanto-Mahadi ID, van Toorenenbergen AW, van Joost T: Contact allergy to spices. *Contact Dermatitis* 22:267–272, 1990.

64. Nater JP: Cosmetic allergy reactions to fragrance chemicals. *Br J Dermatol* 102:476–477, 1980.

65. Brandrup F, Menne T, Agren MS, et al: A randomized trial of two occlusive dressings in the treatment of leg ulcers. *Acta Derm Venereol* 70:231–235, 1990.

66. Jelen G, Schlewer G, Chabeau G, Foussereau J: Eczemas due to plant allergens in manufactured products. *Acta Derm Venereol Suppl* 59:91–94, 1979.

67. Krutmann J, Rzany B, Schopf E, Kapp A: Airborne contact dermatitis from colophony: Phototoxic reaction? *Contact Dermatitis* 21:275–276, 1989.

68. Thune PO, Solberg YJ: Photosensitivity and allergy to aromatic lichen acids, *Compositae* oleoresins and other plant substances. *Contact Dermatitis* 6:81–87, 1980.

69. Rivers JK, Rycroft RJ: Occupational allergic contact urticaria from colophony. *Contact Dermatitis* 17:181, 1987.

70. Soderberg TA, Gref R, Holm S, et al: Antibacterial activity of rosin and resin acids in vitro. *Scand J Plas Reconstr Surg Hand Surg* 24:199–205, 1990.

71. Bleumink E, Mitchell JC, Geismann TA, Towers GH: Contact hypersensitivity to sesquiterpene lactones in *Chyrsanthemum* dermatitis. *Contact Dermatitis* 2:81–88, 1976.

72. Bruze M: Simultaneous reactions to phenol-formaldehyde resins colophony/hydroabietyl alcohol and balsam of Peru/perfume mixture. *Contact Dermatitis* 14:119–120, 1986.

73. Lovell CR, Dannaker CJ, White IR: Dermatitis from X *Cupressocyparis leylandii* and concomitant sensitivity to colophony. *Contact Dermatitis* 13:344–345, 1985.

74. Hausen BM, Kuhlwein A, Schulz KH: Colophony allergy: A contribution to the origin, chemistry, and uses of colophony and modified colophony products, 1. *Derm Beruf Umwelt* 30:107–115, 1982.

13

PARAPHENYLENEDIAMINE

Jere D. Guin

WHAT DOES A POSITIVE PATCH TEST TO PARAPHENYLENEDIAMINE MEAN?

Positive patch tests to paraphenylenediamine (PPD) suggest an allergy to hair dyes or fur dyes, but chemicals with closely related structures may cause reactions in persons allergic to PPD, even though they have not been previously exposed. The sources for such reactions are too diverse to be named, but arranging many potential sources into categories should help. Such chemicals are said to include sulfas, sulfones, oral antidiabetes medications, *para*-aminobenzoic acid (PABA) sunscreens, some but not all "-caine" drugs (both topical and injectable), the antituberculosis drug para-aminosalicylic acid, non-PPD hair dyes, certain clothing dyes, black rubber products, and some inks. This is a long list, but it is still not complete, as there are numerous other agents with a chemical structure so close to PPD that they can cause the immune system to react in persons already allergic to PPD.

HAIR DYES

There are many kinds of hair dyes, not all of which contain the PPD group. PPD-type hair dyes come with two bottles to be mixed. Generally one bottle will contain PPD and additives (called *couplers*) in a soap or detergent solution. Into this an oxidizer is mixed, and the solution is then applied to the hair, where it remains for about 20 min before being rinsed out. The peroxide activates PPD, which binds to the couplers to produce the desired color.[1] Paraphenylenediamine dyes are stable products which collect in the outside layer of the hair, causing a permanent color change. They can also be used to dye the hair a lighter-than-natural color, because the peroxide component of the tint process also lightens the natural hair color. Hair dyes of the PPD type are popular because they produce long-lasting, more natural colors, and the percentage of allergic persons is not great. However, once people are allergic, they should either avoid hair dyes or substitute a product which is unrelated or perhaps not closely related and that produces a negative patch test. Hairdressers are often told in the labeled instructions to do a patch test before using the product. Such tests should be done as open patch tests to the mixture of the PPD-related materials and the oxidizer. This is read after 3 days or more to be safe, with a raised, itchy red rash being a positive test. Sometimes the test is read at the same sitting, but this will not pick up the allergic contact dermatitis, which does not appear immediately. Persons with a weakly reactive test to PPD, such as a 1 + reaction, will often tolerate dying of their hair with PPD-type dyes without a severe reaction.[2] There is sometimes a mild dermatitis on the forehead in a few, but it may not represent a severe problem. Furthermore, mild (1 +) reactors do not tend to become more allergic when their hair is dyed.[2]

Some hair dyes do not contain PPD, and in some countries government regulations forbid the use of PPD-related hair dyes.[3] There, the dyes used for permanent hair color have been changed chemically to try to get away from the allergy related to PPD-type dyes.[4] These substituted dyes are less natural and perhaps not any safer, according to some experimental work.[5] Semipermanent substitutes may or may not contain PPD-related chemicals, so it is important to read labels. Certainly anyone already allergic to PPD should be carefully and correctly patch tested to these "semipermanent" dyes before using them. Another low-risk way to tint hair is with a non-PPD hair coloring "mousse."[6]

Hairdressers allergic to PPD have a special problem because their livelihood depends upon being able to work where this chemical is used. Fortunately, handling dyed hair 24 h after it has been dyed should not cause a problem for a PPD-allergic hairdresser. There are a few isolated reports of reactions to dyed hair[7] on other persons[8,9] which have been attributed to incomplete curing,[10,11] but this seems to be rare. This has been blamed on incomplete oxidation, perhaps due to the inexpert methods used by the lay public with over-the-counter preparations. Vinyl gloves and a Danish product, 4-H gloves, seem to protect hairdressers from direct contact. Despite these precautions and sound instructions, some still have difficulty when continuing to work in that environment.[12] Hairdressers are at greater risk than their customers to become allergic to dyes and other salon chemicals.[13,14] They not infrequently become sensitive to dyes other than PPD as well as other hairdressing chemicals such as acid permanent waving solutions and the booster materials used to create platinum blonde shades.[13,14] Such allergies, which can occur with or without allergy to PPD, would, if present, contribute to the symptoms experienced at work as well as the complexity of avoiding exposure. It is impossible to sort out the allergies without careful, thorough patch testing to every allergen to which the patient has been exposed.

SULFA DRUGS

Some persons allergic to PPD will also react with certain sulfas. The incidence apparently is not high,[15] although one center found that 1 of 3 PPD-allergic persons who were tested reacted to one specific sulfa.[16] Because allergy to related medications is relatively specific,[16] it is best that patch tests be negative to the specific medication to be used. Some writers recommend that persons known to be PPD-allergic be wary of exposure to sulfas in general.[17]

SULFONES

Dapsone is the main sulfone used in the United States, perhaps mainly by dermatologists. While one might suspect a possible cross-reaction, it would not be a common one.[16] Because of the similarity in structure, caution is recommended.

ANTIDIABETES MEDICATIONS (SULFONYLUREAS)

Some of these products when given orally can cause reactions in PPD-allergic persons. Tolbutamide and carbutamide are more likely to cause problems than chlorpropamide, although that medication too can sometimes cause a reaction.[16]

"-CAINES"

Allergy to PPD and the topical anesthetic benzocaine is not uncommonly seen in the same person.[18] Benzocaine is found in a wide variety of both prescription and nonprescription topical products from troches to treatments for poison ivy. Avoidance of other chemically related -caines is also recommended. Fortunately, substitute products are available which do not tend to cross-react.

Procaine (Novocaine), chloroprocaine (Nesacaine), and tetracaine (Pontocaine) given by injection and benzocaine, butacaine (Butyn), and butamben picrate (Butesin) used topically are cross-reacting medications, while lidocaine (Xylocaine), bupivacaine (Marcaine, Sensorcaine), and mepivacaine (Carbocaine) used by injection and dibucaine (Nupercaine) used topically are not likely to cross-react. For persons who have problems with anesthetic agents, the handout on benzocaine may be of benefit.

COLOR FILM DEVELOPING

Persons working with color film developing (e.g., the Kodak E-6 Process) sometimes become allergic to PPD-related chemicals (CD-2, CD-3,[19] and CD-4[20]). Should this become a question, patch-test materials to look for such allergy are commercially available. The rash usually appears in exposed sites and resembles a skin disease called lichen planus both clinically and on biopsy, but patch testing usually shows a typical contact dermatitis.

EPOXY RESINS

Epoxy resins are used in adhesives, paints (especially waterproof paints), castings, insulation (especially on electrical transformers), protective coverings to prevent corrosion, aircraft and boat manufacture, and in many other ways. Usually the components include the resin or monomer, a hardener, and reactive diluents. While most allergy is to the resin, some persons are allergic to the hardener.[20,21] The finished resin is not usually a problem, but it can be if it is not completely cured. Cross-reactions to certain hardeners such as metaphenylenediamine or diaminodiphenylmethane will occur in 40 percent of PPD-allergic patients. The first is essentially the same chemical in a slightly different configuration, while the second contains common molecular structures. Some persons allergic to PPD will react to epoxy resins containing those hardeners. Contact allergy to hardeners is often not suspected, but when a dermatitis due to epoxy involves the face and especially the eyelids, one should suspect the hardener or active diluent.[22] Because epoxy chemicals readily penetrate rubber gloves,[23] protective gloves should be layered plastic (4-H)[15] if they must be thin or heavy-duty vinyl.[23]

PARAPHENYLENEDIAMINE (PPD)—
PATIENT HANDOUT

Because there is so much variation in the reaction patterns in the general population, there are no absolute rules, and there is no such thing as absolute safety. However, taken as a group, there is some reason to the patterns of allergy and the products tolerated. The information that follows below is provided to help you understand the meaning of a positive patch test to this chemical.

WHAT DOES A POSITIVE PATCH TEST TO PARAPHENYLENEDIAMINE (PPD) MEAN?

Most persons with prominent patch-test reactions to PPD are allergic to permanent hair dyes or the dyes in furs. Persons with mild (1 +) reactions often tolerate having their hair dyed without a severe reaction. A 2 + and 3 + patch-test response requires caution, as such persons are likely to break out to a wide variety of permanent hair dyes and other chemically related products.

Permanent hair dyes have a chemical structure similar to many medications and other products. Persons significantly allergic to PPD should be cautious about exposure to the following medications:

Sulfa drugs
Sulfonylurea (oral antidiabetes drugs)
Sulfones (used for skin disease, leprosy)
Para-aminosalicylic acid (for tuberculosis)
Benzocaine (topical anesthetic)
Procaine (injectable anesthetic)
PABA sunscreens

Nonmedications which may cross-react include the following:

Color film developer
Epoxy resin (hardener)
Stamp-pad ink
Black rubber products

ARE THERE SUBSTITUTE HAIR DYES FOR THE PPD-ALLERGIC?

Persons who break out to PPD hair dyes may or may not break out to the dyes in semipermanent hair dyes. They usually tolerate the temporary dyes, which are

This information is provided to help persons with contact dermatitis in the understanding of their problem. The contents are subject to change as more information becomes available and are not intended as a substitute for medical treatment.

pigments deposited on the hair. Metallic dyes such as Grecian formula should not cross-react, but they are less suitable for women who permanent wave their hair. Natural dyes, e.g., henna, do not cross-react, but they do not produce the more natural, desired colors either. There is also a non-PPD hair coloring "mousse," which can be used.

CAN YOU ESTABLISH THE SAFETY OF A DYE IN ADVANCE?

Persons who break out severely to PPD dyes should avoid the two-bottle permanent dyes. For the dyes such as semipermanent dyes, the best way to check for allergy is to do a patch test to the dye in advance. This is applied, as it will be put on the hair, to an area which absorbs well, e.g., a quarter-sized spot on the neck (behind the ear) or the tender skin in the bend of the arm. The test site is left open and should not be covered with a bandage. If the test is negative when it is read two to three days later, the risk of breaking out is much less, but one can never be certain. Tests that turn positive immediately are more likely to be caused by a (nonallergic) irritation.

IS PPD ALLERGY EVER OCCUPATIONAL?

Yes, positive patch tests to PPD are not uncommon in hairdressers, where such allergy is usually seen causing or aggravating hand eczema. Often plastic gloves help prevent contact.

ARE THERE SAFE SUNSCREENS?

Sunscreens labeled "P.F." should not contain PABA, the cross-reacting sunscreen.

ARE THERE SUBSTITUTE LOCAL ANESTHETICS?

Dyclonine, pramoxine, and dibucaine are topical anesthetics which should not cross-react. Injectable local anesthetics (such as used by a dentist)—lidocaine, mepivacaine, bupivacaine, and prilocaine—have a different (amide-type) structure, and normally they should not cross-react with benzocaine or PPD.

STAMP-PAD INK

An azo dye chemically related to PPD has been reported to cause a reaction; avoidance of the product solved the problem.[24]

BLACK RUBBER PRODUCTS

Rubber products tend to deteriorate in the atmosphere unless antioxidants are added in their manufacture, and the PPD derivatives (which account for the black color) are among the very best. This special quality has made black rubber products extremely common in our environment. Products such as eyelash curlers,[25] handlebar grips,[26] escalator railings,[27] watch straps,[28] the wishbone on a sailboat mainsail.[29] and the black rubber feet of staplers[30] are known to have caused contact dermatitis directly or by hand transfer. Although more than half of the persons allergic to PPD also break out to black rubber chemicals, they are usually unaware of their intolerance to black rubber.[31] The number of potential sources of exposure is legion, and the unsuspecting patient generally touches such objects with the hands. Oily materials cause degradation of rubber and perhaps aid in hand transfer of the allergy-causing rubber chemicals contained in black rubber products. Exposure can also occur in industry.[32]

OTHER DYES

Persons allergic to PPD may or may not react to clothing dyes. This has been reported[33] in stockings[34] and shoes.[35,36] Cross-reactions are especially likely with Disperse Orange Number 3, a lighter textile dye.

Azo dyes, used in foods, hair dyes, and other applications, sometimes cross-react with PPD, but the chance increases in the presence of oxidizing agents.[37]

SUNSCREENS CONTAINING *PARA*-AMINOBENZOIC ACID

Sunscreens containing PABA and related products may cause either an allergic contact dermatitis or a photocontact dermatitis.[38] The difference is that the latter occurs only after sun or light exposure. When one is allergic to PABA or related chemicals such as PPD, very good sunscreens labeled "PF" (for PABA-free) are available.

UNUSUAL REACTIONS OTHER THAN CONTACT DERMATITIS

Hives can be caused by allergy to PPD, sometimes with severe systemic symptoms.[39,40] This reaction comes on immediately, unlike the more common delayed reaction of contact dermatitis. While hives of this kind are rare, they can be serious. Should there be any question, therefore, testing should be done in a physicians office or in a hospital setting where proper equipment and specialty support are available.

Cataract formation has been reported in persons regularly exposed to PPD-containing hair dyes,[41] but, judging from the data available, this problem is probably not serious. Loss of skin pigmentation and bleeding into the skin (purpura) may be due to PPD-related rubber chemicals,[42] and photosensitivity (allergy to the chemical after sun exposure) can occur to this chemical or to PABA sunscreens.[43]

Related oral medications can sometimes cause a flare where contact dermatitis has occurred previously.[16] This is called *systemic contact dermatitis*. Drugs to suspect might include sulfas, sulfones, para-aminosalicylic acid, and perhaps even FD&C Yellow Dye Number 6, which contains a sulfanilamide component. Cross-reaction with benzocaine is known, and the risk seems to be greater for some oral antidiabetes medications than others. For example, about one-third of allergic persons given an oral antidiabetes medication reacted to carbutamide and tolbutamide, while only 1 or 2 of 20 reacted to chlorpropamide and none broke out when challenged with salicylazosulfapyridine (Azulfadine), a sulfa, or dapsone (a sulfone), saccharin, or the "pure food" dye FD&C Yellow Number 5 (tartrazine).[16]

PREVENTION

For those highly allergic to PPD, prevention of contact dermatitis to PPD requires that one either avoid hair dyes or use some other product that does not contain related dyes. This often necessitates the elimination of permanent dyes. Sometimes hair coloring is possible with semipermanent or temporary dyes, but patch testing to such products is necessary to determine safety before they are applied to the hair. Hairdressers should wear protective gloves such as 4-H or vinyl gloves,[15] but even then the prognosis is guarded.[12] Hairdressers should normally be able to handle hair dyed 24 h previously,[44] but there are exceptions. For the allergic client, semipermanent dyes sometimes can be used, but these products are less desirable. Before application of event his type of dye to the hair, patch testing should be done according to the manufacturer's instructions.

REFERENCES

1. Corbett JF: Changing the color of hair, in Frost P, Horwitz SN (eds): *Principles of Cosmetics for the Dermatologist*. St. Louis, Mosby, 1982, pp 160–163.
2. Fisher AA, Dorman RI: The clinical significance of weakly positive patch test reactions to certain antigens. *Cutis* 11:450–453, 1973.
3. Fisher AA: *Contact Dermatitis* 3d ed. Philadelphia, Lea & Febiger, 1986, pp 600–601.
4. Dooms-Goossens A: Reducing sensitizing potential by pharmaceutical and cosmetic design. *J Am Acad Dermatol* 10:547–553, 1984.
5. Magnusson B: The allergenicity of paraphenylene versus that of paratoluenediamine. *Contact Dermatitis Newsletter* 15:432, 1974.
6. Maibach HI: Paraphenylenediamine-free hair coloring "mousse." *Contact Dermatitis* 15:103, 1986.
7. Hindson C: O-nitro-paraphenylenediamine in hair dye—An unusual dental hazard. *Contact Dermatitis* 1:333, 1976.
8. Cronin E: Dermatitis from wife's dyed hair. *Contact Dermatitis Newsletter* 13:363, 1973.
9. Warin AP: Contact dermatitis to partner's dyed hair. *Clin Exp Dermatol* 1:283, 1976.
10. Foussereau J, Reuter G, Petitjean J: Is hair with PPD dyes allergenic? *Contact Dermatitis* 6:143, 1980.
11. Mitchell JC: Allergic contact dermatitis from paraphenylenediamine presenting as nummular eczema. *Contact Dermatitis Newsletter* 11:270, 1972.

12. Nethercott JR, MacPherson M, Choi BC, Nixon P: Contact dermatitis in hairdressers. *Contact Dermatitis* 14:73–79, 1986.
13. Guerra L, Tosti A, Bardazzi F, et al: Contact dermatitis in hairdressers: The Italian experience. *Contact Dermatitis* 26:101–107, 1992.
14. Guerra L, Bardazzi F, Tosti A: Contact dermatitis in hairdressers' clients. *Contact Dermatitis* 26:108–111, 1992.
15. Fisher AA: Management of hairdressers sensitized to hair dyes or permanent wave solutions. *Cutis* 43:316–318, 1989.
16. Angelini G, Meneghini CL: Oral tests to contact allergy to para-amino compounds. *Contact Dermatitis* 7:311–314, 1981.
17. Fisher AA: *Contact Dermatitis,* 3d ed. Philadelphia, Lea & Febiger, 1986, p 381.
18. Edman B: Computerized analysis of concomitant contact allergens. *Contact Dermatitis* 24:110–113, 1991.
19. Liden C, Brehmer-Andersson E: Occupational dermatoses from colour developing agents. *Acta Derm Venereol* 68:514–522, 1988.
20. Liden C, Bowman A: Contact allergy to colour developing agents in the guinea pig. *Contact Dermatitis* 19:290–295, 1988.
21. Rudzki E, Krajewska B, Grzywa Z: Sensitivity to meta-phenylenediamine. *Berufs-Dermatosen* 25:85–88, 1977.
22. Dahlquist I, Fregert S: Allergic contact dermatitis from volatile epoxy hardeners and reactive diluents. *Contact Dermatitis* 5:406–407, 1979.
23. Pegum JS: Penetration of protective gloves by epoxy resin. *Contact Dermatitis* 5:281–283, 1979.
24. Fowler JF: Occupational dermatitis from stamp pad ink. *Contact Dermatitis* 16:38, 1987.
25. Vestey JP, Buxton PK, Savin JA: Eyelash curler dermatitis. *Contact Dermatitis* 13:274–275, 1985.
26. Goh CL: Hand dermatitis from rubber motorcycle handle. *Contact Dermatitis* 16:40–41, 1987.
27. Dooms-Goossens A, Degreef H, de Veylder H, Maselis T: Unusual sensitization to black rubber. *Contact Dermatitis* 17:47–48, 1987.
28. Romaguera C, Aguirre A, Diaz Perez JL, Grimalt F: Watch strap dermatitis. *Contact Dermatitis* 14:260–261, 1986.
29. Tennstedt D, Lachapelle JM: Windsurfer dermatitis from black rubber components. *Contact Dermatitis* 7:160–161, 1981.
30. Guin JD: Delayed hypersensitivity. Rubber minisymposium, Sixteenth Hawaii Dermatology Seminar, Maui, Hawaii, February 18, 1992.
31. Rudzki E, Ostaszewski K, Grzywa Z, Kozlowska A: Sensitivity to some rubber additives. *Contact Dermatitis* 2:24–27, 1976.
32. Herve-Bazin B, Gradiski D, Duprat P, et al: Occupational eczema from N-isopropyl-N'-phenylparaphenylenediamine (IPPD) and N-dimethyl-1,3butyl-N'-phenylparaphenylenediamine (DMPPD) in tyres. *Contact Dermatitis* 3:1–15, 1977.
33. Massone L, Anonide A, Isola V, Borghi S: Two cases of multiple dye sensitization. *Contact Dermatitis* 24:60–62, 1991.
34. Kousa M, Soini M: Contact allergy to a stocking dye. *Contact Dermatitis* 6:472–476, 1980.
35. Romaguera C, Grimalt F, Vilaplana J: Shoe contact dermatitis. *Contact Dermatitis* 18:178, 1978.
36. Correia S, Brandao FM: Contact dermatitis of the feet. *Derm Beruf Umwelt.* 34:102–126, 1986.
37. Picardo M, Cannistraci C, Cristaudo A, et al: Study on cross-reactivity to the *para* group. *Dermatologica* 81:104–108, 1990.
38. Thune P: Contact and photocontact allergy to sunscreens. *Photo-Dermatology* 1:5–9, 1984.
39. Goldberg BJ, Herman FF, Hirata I: Systemic anaphylaxis due to an oxidation product of p-phenylene in a hair dye. *Ann Allerg* 58:205–208, 1987.
40. Temesvari E. Contact urticaria from paraphenylenediamine. *Contact Dermatitis* 12:21–23, 1984.
41. Jain IS, Jain GC, Kaul RL, Dhir SP: Cataractogenous effect of hair dyes: A clinical and experimental study. *Ann Ophthalmol* 11:1681–1686, 1979.
42. Zaitz ID, Proenca NG, Droste D, Grotti I: Achromatizing contact dermatitis caused by rubber sandals. *Med Cutan Iber Lat Am* 15:1–7, 1987.
43. LeVine MJ: Idiopathic photodermatitis with a positive paraphenylenediamine. *Arch Dermatol* 120:1488–1490, 1984.
44. Reiss F, Fisher AA: Is hair dyed with *para*-phenylenediamine allergenic? *Arch Dermatol* 109:221–222, 1974.

14

IMIDAZOLIDINYL UREA

Anthony F. Fransway

WHAT IS IMIDAZOLIDINYL UREA?

Imidazolidinyl urea is a preservative marketed under the trade name Germall 115 (Sutton Laboratories, Inc., Chatham, NJ) and a member of a family of biocides that notably includes diazolidinyl urea. Introduced in 1970, imidazolidinyl urea has become a preservative of choice for "hypoallergenic" cosmetic and pharmaceutical formulations. A stable, odorless, white powder with high water and low oil solubility, the vast majority of the microbicidal activity of imidazolidinyl urea is directed against bacterial contamination of the aqueous compartment of cosmetics; fungal inhibition is limited. The addition of paraben esters to the final formulation not only increases antibacterial activity but improves yeast and mold coverage as well.[1] The utility of imidazolidinyl urea as a biocide has been duly recognized by the industry, since it is rapidly becoming the second most frequently used class of preservative behind the paraben family.[2]

SOURCES OF EXPOSURE TO IMIDAZOLIDINYL UREA

OCCUPATIONAL

Unlike several other biocides capable of formaldehyde release, imidazolidinyl urea is generally not used in cutting oils. Occupational sensitization to imidazolidinyl urea has not been specifically reported, but it is anticipated that this agent, incorporated into lotions or soaps used in the workplace, could be a source of primary sensitization in individuals with disrupted barrier function.

COSMETIC AND THERAPEUTIC

The vast majority of specific reactions to imidazolidinyl urea relate to its use in topical cosmetic and pharmaceutical products. Cosmetics, moisturizing creams and lotions, body powders, sunless tanning creams and lotions, mascaras, eye shadows, cuticle removers, shampoos, sunscreens, burn remedies, and prescription and over-the-counter pharmaceutical products all may contain imidazolidinyl urea. Many of these products are marketed as "hypoallergenic," arguably appropriately so, as experience has revealed this biocide to be an infrequent sensitizer. Imidazolidinyl urea is rated a weak sensitizer by repeat open application testing,[3] although Andersen et al.[4] found it to be a strong sensitizer by guinea pig maximization testing.

Dooms-Goosens and colleagues[5] found only 8 patients sensitive to imidazolidinyl urea in 1175 tested using a cosmetic series, while other investigators have offered case reports.[6,7] The North American Contact Dermatitis Group determined preservatives to be causative of allergic reaction to cosmetics in 28 percent of patients tested, with 4 percent of these patients being sensitive to imidazolidinyl urea.[8]

CLINICAL PRESENTATIONS OF IMIDAZOLIDINYL UREA ALLERGY

The distribution of allergic contact dermatitis upon presentation is dependent upon the sensitizing cosmetic product utilized. Common presentations include malar distribution (from foundation), eyelid dermatitis (from mascara), patchy head and neck dermatitis (from cosmetics and moisturizers), and hand dermatitis (from moisturizers). Dermatitis may manifest as papular dermatitis or, less frequently, weeping or eczematous dermatitis. The picture of "violaceous dermal erythema," which may be seen with other formaldehyde-releasing biocides such as quaternium-15, may also occur in imidazolidinyl urea-sensitive patients.

A more common scenario is that of imidazolidinyl urea sensitivity with multiple allergies to this and other formaldehyde-releasing biocides, often in patients with widespread chronic dermatitis (Fig. 14-1). Imidazolidinyl urea is believed to be a weak

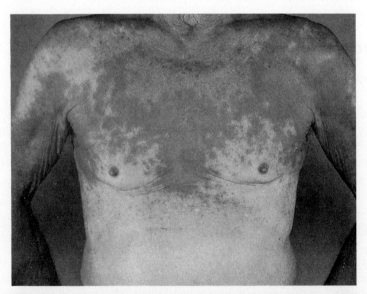

FIG. 14–1. Severe generalized dermatitis of over 10 years' duration in a patient with brisk patch-test responses to formaldehyde, quaternium-15, and imidazolidinyl urea. (See color Plate 4.)

formaldehyde donor, with roughly 90 parts per million formaldehyde released into a 2% aqueous imidazolidinyl urea solution[9]; quaternium-15 and bromonitropropane diol (two other formaldehyde donors) release 100 ppm formaldehyde at 0.1% concentration and 15 ppm at 0.02% concentration, respectively.[9,10] This would suggest that quaternium-15 is 20 times as potent a formaldehyde donor as imidazolidinyl urea. The probability of a positive patch test or clinical reaction to imidazolidinyl urea in formaldehyde-sensitive individuals is dependent upon the degree of sensitivity. Only one-third of Ford's 16 imidazolidinyl urea-sensitive patients were formaldehyde allergic with 5 of these also allergic to quaternium-15.[11] We have studied 87 individuals with imidazolidinyl urea sensitivity, with nearly half responding only to imidazolidinyl urea and over 40 percent responding to formaldehyde as well.[12]

FREQUENCY OF ALLERGIC REACTIONS IN SCREENING SERIES

Imidazolidinyl urea is not a frequent reactor in the standard series, ranging from 0.1 to 2.2 percent (mean, 1.3 percent) in seven major series (Table 14-1).[11,13–15] When positive, particularly with coexisting formaldehyde-releasing biocide sensitivity, the response is generally considered relevant. Indeed, imidazolidinyl urea may function as an anti-irritant in formulations with a concentration of 0.1 to 0.5%, and irritant patch-test responses to imidazolidinyl urea are rare. The difficulty arises when multiple formaldehyde-releasing biocides are positive, most frequently quaternium-15 and formaldehyde but also occasionally bromonitropropane diol, DMDM hydantoin, and diazolidinyl urea (10 percent of diazolidinyl urea patients being allergic to imidazolidinyl urea as well).[16] In this setting, with so many different preservatives in so many potential contactants, the relative contribution to existent dermatitis of each biocide may be difficult to ascertain, but it should be attempted. Many times the broad picture of allergy is, in essence, based upon and due to formaldehyde release from these preservatives and the presence of free formaldehyde in the cosmetic formulation. When such broad-spectrum allergy is present, ideally one should avoid the entire family of potential formaldehyde-releasing biocides, but it may not necessarily be essential (once again, depending on the degree of sensitivity exhibited by the patient).

TABLE 14–1. Imidazolidinyl Urea Sensitivity in Screening Series

Investigator	Country	Vehicle and Concentration[a]	Number Tested	Percent Positive
NACDG[13]	USA	2% aq.	7000–9000	0.9
NACDG[13]	USA	2% aq.	7001	1.7
NACDG[13]	USA	2% aq.	4193	1.9
NACDG[13]	USA	2% aq.	4663	2.1
Ford and Beck[11]	UK	2% pet.	2298	0.7
Broeckx et al.[14]	Belgium	NS	5202	0.1
Fransway[15]	USA	2% aq.	3415	2.2

[a]NS = Not specified by authors.

IMIDAZOLIDINYL UREA—PATIENT INSTRUCTIONAL MATERIAL

Imidazolidinyl urea is a preservative commonly found in a variety of cosmetics and pharmaceutical topical preparations. By law, all products made in the United States for topical use must have the ingredients listed on either the product package or the box that contains it. To determine whether you are exposed to this preservative to which you have been proven allergic, be sure to check the labeling of ingredients on the package.

Imidazolidinyl urea is frequently found in products that carry the "hypoallergenic" label. This is because this particular preservative is not a common cause of contact allergy when compared with a number of other preservatives that the manufacturer could have used. Obviously, for anyone allergic to this ingredient, these products are far from hypoallergenic. Now that you know you are allergic to this particular ingredient, you must avoid all products that contain it.

The following is a detailed but not all-inclusive list of products that may contain imidazolidinyl urea:

Cosmetics
Moisturizing creams and lotions
Powders used on face or body
Sunless tanning creams and lotions
Mascaras and eye shadows
Cuticle removers
Shampoos
Sunscreens
Burn remedies
Over-the-counter pharmaceuticals
Prescription topical medicaments

Discontinuation of use of these products should result in improvement and/or resolution of your dermatitis difficulty.

A number of products may also react because they are similar to imidazolidinyl urea or because such allergies often occur together. You should consult with your physician regarding which (if any) of these products need to be avoided as well. The following is again a detailed but not all-inclusive list of potential coreactive substances:

Diazolidinyl urea
Formaldehyde
Quaternium-15
DMDM hydantoin
Bromonitropropane diol

This information is provided to help persons with contact dermatitis in the understanding of their problem. The contents are subject to change as more information becomes available and are not intended as a substitute for medical treatment.

There are a number of preservatives that are also incorporated into cosmetic products that you may be safely exposed to (assuming you have not shown an allergic reaction to these on patch testing as well); one should substitute such cosmetic products for those containing problem ingredients. Acceptable preservatives include methylparaben, ethylparaben, propylparaben, butylparaben, methylchloroisothiazolinone/methylisothiazolinone, methyldibromoglutaronitrile/phenoxyethanol, sorbic acid, and propylene glycol.

If you are concerned whether a particular cosmetic product is safe to use on your skin, a use test is advised. You can do this yourself by applying a small amount of the cosmetic product (particularly moisturizers, lotions, and cosmetics) to an area opposite the elbow on the arm or over the upper arm twice a day for one week. If no redness or itching develops in the area, the same procedure is repeated over a small area in front of the ear on one of your cheeks. If still no response is noted, the product is probably safe for use, although you should continue to exercise caution regarding widespread use until you are certain it is well tolerated. *Note:* The use test is not acceptable for detergents, soaps, hair care products such as shampoos and conditioners, and mascaras or eyeliners. Again, consult your physician regarding which of these products, if any, would be safe for you to use.

Do imidazolidinyl urea–containing cosmetics need to be avoided in individuals who are patch-test negative to imidazolidinyl urea but positive to formaldehyde and other formaldehyde-releasing biocides? No double-blind studies have been performed in formaldehyde-sensitive patients to determine whether individuals who are not reactive to imidazolidinyl urea can use products containing this particular preservative. Several variables could influence the answer. It is the author's personal bias that such patients should exercise caution in using products containing any formaldehyde-donating preservative. The use test is extremely helpful in separating topical products which will and will not be tolerated.

CROSS-REACTING SUBSTANCES

As previously stated, imidazolidinyl urea may be an allergen reactive alone or in combination with other formaldehyde-releasing biocides (see "Imidazolidinyl Urea—Patient Instructional Material", above). Imidazolidinyl urea–sensitive patients may respond only to other members of the same family, such as diazolidinyl urea; in this setting, avoidance of this agent as well would be advised. If only imidazolidinyl urea is positive in the standard screening series but quaternium-15 and formaldehyde are negative, products containing quaternium-15 or other formaldehyde donors can probably be used safely. However, in patients who are allergic to both formaldehyde and imidazolidinyl urea, any of the formaldehyde donors may be a problem. These include quaternium-15, bromonitropropane diol, diazolidinyl urea, DMDM hydantoin, and other less frequently encountered biocides such as tris-nitro and bromonitrodioxane. Other less frequently encountered preservatives, such as polymethoxy bicyclic oxazolidine also may be, in certain circumstances, capable of formaldehyde release.[17] All of these antigens deserve scrutiny when a patient with imidazolidinyl urea sensitivity is being evaluated.

PATCH-TEST CONSIDERATIONS

The patch test concentration for imidazolidinyl urea in the standard series is 2% aqueous. Initially, 2% imidazolidinyl urea in petrolatum was used by several investigators reporting early cases of sensitivity,[5,14,18] while Foussereau and Carelier[19] reported two cases sensitive only to the aqueous formulation. As imidazolidinyl urea is more soluble in water than oil and as biocides incorporate into the aqueous compartment of cosmetics, the aqueous vehicle is the logical selection.

PREVENTION AND MANAGEMENT

Avoidance of imidazolidinyl urea in all cosmetic formulations is necessary for patients exhibiting sensitivity. With a low level of sensitivity, minor or minute degrees of reexposure may be well tolerated. Patients with positive responses to other formaldehyde-releasing biocides and formaldehyde generally must avoid this entire class of preservatives. Patients with coexistent sensitivity to diazolidinyl urea must avoid it as well. Cosmetic products containing paraben esters, methylchloroisothiazolinone/methylisothiazolinone, methyldibromoglutaronitrile/phenoxyethanol, propylene glycol, and sorbic acid may generally be substituted once dermatitis is controlled.

REFERENCES

1. Rosen WE, Berke PA: Germall 115: A safe and effective preservative, in Kabara JJ (ed): *Cosmetic and Drug Preservation: Principles and Practice.* New York, Dekker, 1984, pp 191–208.
2. Frequency of preservative use in corrective formulations as disclosed to FDA—1990. *Cosmet Toilet* 105:45, 1990.
3. Ziegler V, Ziegler B, Kipping D: Dose-response sensitization experiments with imidazolidinyl urea. *Contact Dermatitis* 19:236, 1988.
4. Andersen KE, Bowman A, Hamann K, et al: Guinea pig maximation tests for formaldehyde releasers: Results from two laboratories. *Contact Dermatitis* 10:257, 1984.
5. Dooms-Goosens A, Boulle K, Dooms M, et al: Imidazolidinyl urea dermatitis. *Contact Dermatitis* 14:322, 1986.
6. Fisher AA: Allergic contact dermatitis from Germall 115, a new cosmetic preservative. *Contact Dermatitis* 1:126, 1975.
7. DeGroot AL, Weyland JW: Hidden contact allergy to formaldehyde in imidazolidinyl urea. *Contact Dermatitis* 17:124, 1987.

8. Adams RM, Maibach HI, Clendenning WE, et al: A five-year study of cosmetic reactions. *J Am Acad Dermatol* 13:1062, 1985.

9. Jordan WP Jr, Sherman WT, King SE: Threshold responses in formaldehyde-sensitive subjects. *J Am Acad Dermatol* 1:44, 1979.

10. Storrs FJ, Bill DE: Allergic contact dermatitis to 2-bromo 2-nitropropane-1,3-diol in a hydrophilic ointment. *J Am Acad Dermatol* 8:157, 1983.

11. Ford GP, Beck MH: Reactions to quaternium-15, bronopol, and Germall 115 in a standard series. *Contact Dermatitis* 14:271, 1986.

12. Fransway AF, Schmitz NA: The problem of preservation in the 1990s: II. Formaldehyde and formaldehyde-releasing biocides: Incidences of cross-reactivity and the significance of the positive response to formaldehyde. *Am J Contact Dermatitis* 2:78, 1991.

13. Feinman SE: Frequency of allergic contact dermatitis from formaldehyde, in Feinman SE (ed): *Formaldehyde Sensitivity and Toxicity,* Boca Raton, FL, CRC Press, 1988, pp 73, 85.

14. Broeckx W, Blondeel A, Dooms-Goosens A, et al: Cosmetic intolerance. *Contact Dermatitis* 16:189, 1987.

15. Fransway AF: Isothiazolinine sensitivity. *Lancet* 1:910, 1989.

16. Hectorne K, Fransway AF: Diazolidinyl urea: incidence of sensitivity and significance. *Contact Dermatitis* 30:16, 1994.

17. Mansfield E, Thompson C: Personal communication.

18. Meynadier JM, Meynadier J, Colmas A, et al: Allergie aux conservateurs. *Ann Derm Vener* 109:1017, 1982.

19. Foussereau J, Carelier C: Water versus petrolatum for testing imidazolidinyl urea. *Contact Dermatitis* 21:54, 1989.

15

CINNAMIC ALDEHYDE

Jere D. Guin

WHAT IS CINNAMIC ALDEHYDE?

Cinnamic aldehyde is a flavoring and perfume chemical which gives the flavor to natural cinnamon. It is used both as a natural and a synthetic fragrance material. In its natural form, it can be obtained from any of several plants, but the commercial products are cinnamon from Sri Lanka (Ceylon), Madagascar, Japan, and China. The last is called *cassia*. It is an ingredient in several natural fragrance materials, including the biblical myrrh and the flower hyacinth.[1]

The synthetic form of cinnamic aldehyde, or cinnamaldehyde, is found in a wide range of scented and flavored products and is a common sensitizer. Some items normally not thought of as being cinnamon-flavored may well be so. A good example is toothpastes, especially those containing stannous fluoride; its metallic taste is difficult at best to cover. Perfumes which smell spicy often contain cinnamic aldehyde, and products from candy to dental floss are often flavored with cinnamic aldehyde along with other artificial flavors. Deodorants,[2] especially the spice-scented ones, may contain cinnamic aldehyde. Many perfumes used in consumer products contain it, along with numerous other fragrance synthetics, so it is something of a marker or indicator for at least one type of fragrance (flavor) allergy.

Persons who patch test positive to cinnamic aldehyde tend to have more responses to rosin and wood tars on patch testing; many fragrance mixes used in both the United States and Europe contain cinnamic aldehyde. Sensitivity to cinnamic aldehyde is also associated more specifically with allergy to ginger, benzoin, styrax, balsams of Peru and Tolu, hyacinth, Bulgarian rose, and patchouli, a perfume product.

Sources include perfumes and colognes, cinnamon used in cooking, bitters, soap, beverage flavoring, household deodorizers and other products, detergents and soaps, mouthwashes, candy, soft drinks, and chewing gum.[3-5]

Cinnamic aldehyde is an interesting chemical for many reasons. First, it is a well-known flavor and certain cinnamon-flavored dishes are favorites. Second, it is commonly used as a perfume ingredient both for personal use and in numerous items to add an esthetic odoriferous quality to one's impression of that item. Third, it is a common kitchen spice, occasionally associated with hand eczema. As such, it is tested *as is* without noticeable irritancy. The chemical itself in certain vehicles is irritant at a 2 percent concentration.[6] Fourth, it is the cause of a significant number of cases of contact dermatitis; as such, it causes cross-reactions with a wide range of other fragrance products. Opdyke[1] quotes Majeti and Suskind in unpublished reports to industry that a wide variety of alpha-alkyl cinnamic aldehydes (e.g., alpha-methyl cinnamic aldehyde) will cross-react with cinnamic aldehyde. Fifth, it causes contact urticaria. While a rare case of contact urticaria may be allergic, almost everyone will develop nonimmunologic contact urticaria from this in adequate concentration. Test materials for contact dermatitis are in petrolatum, but for contact urticaria alcohol is a much better vehicle. One can optimize that vehicle by using a solution of just enough alcohol in water to totally dissolve all of the cinnamic aldehyde.[7]

WHAT IS THE USUAL CLINICAL PICTURE?

The clinical picture depends upon the route and method of exposure. Following below are several definite patterns that have been described which should make one suspicious or at least wary.

1. Dermatitis where perfume or cologne is applied makes the diagnosis fairly obvious, and the patient usually immediately associates the rash with the cause. Reactions may occur on the neck and not the wrist, which can be confusing to the uninitiated, but the differences in absorption explain the difference. Perfume or cologne may contain cinnamic aldehyde either as a single chemical or as a component of a natural fragrance material.

2. Eczema where cosmetics are used is another typical pattern (Fig. 15-1). Fragrance reactions are the single most common cause of allergic reactions to cosmetics, so they are seen where cosmetics are used. Cosmetic dermatitis of the eyelids is not uncommon, but none of Nethercott's 79 patients with eyelid dermatitis were allergic to cinnamic aldehyde.[8] These allergic reactions should not be considered monolithic, as they are often associated with multiple allergies to perfume chemicals or other ingredients. However, cinnamic aldehyde is particularly problematic, causing more reactions than many other perfume components.

3. Cinnamic aldehyde can also cause a dermatitis where lotions are used (Fig. 15-1A), which can complicate stasis or hand eczema, and where treatment is given with a perfumed product. A corticosteroid-containing a fragrance has sensitized a number of patients, and essential oils used therapeutically can cause contact dermatitis. This is usually seen in and around the treatment site, sometimes with hand transfer to other sites (Fig. 15-1B). A rash developed where a wart was treated with cinnamon oil over the longitudinal arch of the plantar surface,[9] and the patient also broke out to cinnamon pastries and bitters in mixed drinks.

4. Reactions can also cause or aggravate hand eczema through exposure to fragrances in many products but especially in spices used in cooking (Fig. 15-2). Allergy to perfume mix, colophony, wood tars, and balsam of Peru in patients with hand eczema may indicate a problem with the handling of kitchen spices. Patch testing to these can be done with the spices as is, although garlic and onion must be diluted. Malten[10] described two bakers with hand eczema resembling dyshidrotic eczema of the fingers who had positive patch tests to cinnamon powder. Reactions in some areas of application, can be deceiving, as the sources may be unexpected, such as paper products[11,12] or toothpaste.

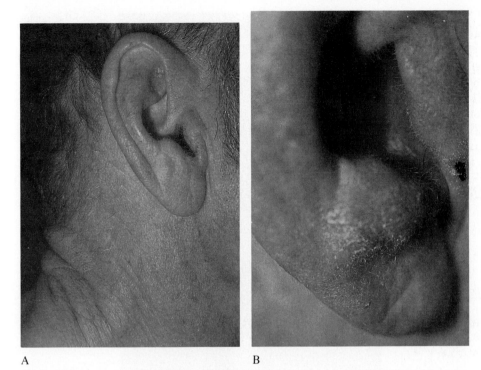

A   B

FIG. 15–1. *A.* Reaction to lotion applied to the face in a man sensitive to cinnamic aldehyde. *B.* Closeup of the ear of the same patient. This was probably caused by hand transfer.

5. Another characteristic pattern from this fragrance chemical is deodorant dermatitis which involves the peak of the axillae, usually without areas of sparing (Fig. 15-3). Spice scents are likely to be a cause in those allergic to cinnamic aldehyde.

6. Exposure in and around the mouth (Fig. 15-4) can produce any of several pictures, including contact stomatitis,[13] cheilitis, and burning mouth syndrome.[5,14] Some of such patients have problems in other areas as well. Perioral leukoderma has also been reported.[15] Another patient had purpura in addition to stomatitis.[16] Another had a recurrence after eating cinnamon.[17] Reactions to toothpaste containing cinnamic aldehyde are likely to show up as buccal ulcers, sore mouth, perioral dermatitis, or angular cheilitis.[18,19] Maibach[20] called lipstick cheilitis from cinnamic aldehyde an occult allergy because the patch test to the lipstick was negative, although it contained cinnamic aldehyde, and the patch test to cinnamic aldehyde was positive.[25] Some patients allergic to toothpaste may tolerate cinnamon in food, perhaps because the detergent in the dentifrice causes more irritation or absorption. Patch tests to the toothpaste may be negative, even though it contains cinnamic aldehyde and the patient is allergic to it.

7. Angular cheilitis is described especially from toothpaste, and it is much more common than recognized. Wilkinson[18] described several cases of toothpaste allergy from cinnamic aldehyde in 1975, but it seem still to go largely unrecognized. Notice the patient in Fig. 15-5 with allergy to cinnamic aldehyde and alcohol who reacted to perfumed paper products on the face but also had angular cheilitis.

8. Burning mouth syndrome can be caused by this chemical both as a local irritant,

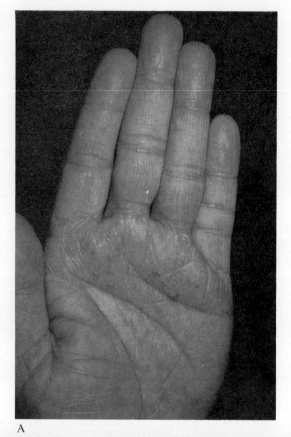

A

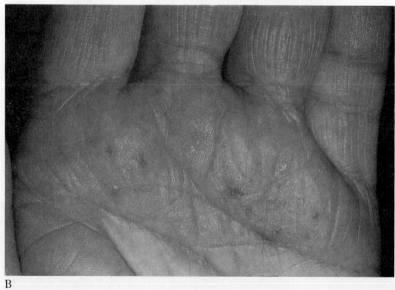

B

FIG. 15–2. *A*. Hand eczema in doughnut maker exposed to cinnamon. *B*. Closeup of the finger-web area. (See color Plate 5.)

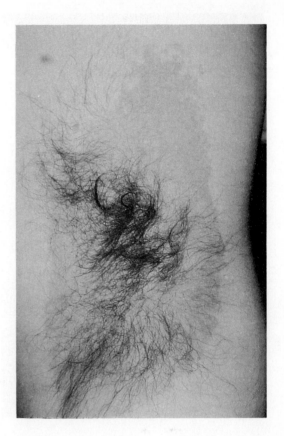

FIG. 15–3. Contact dermatitis to spice-scented deodorant in cinnamic aldehyde-allergic patient. (See color Plate 6.)

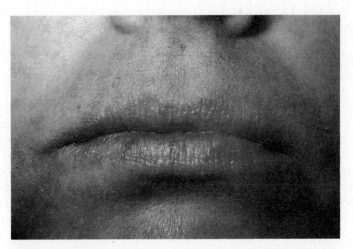

FIG. 15–4. Perioral eczema from oral exposure to cinnamic aldehyde in food and toothpaste.

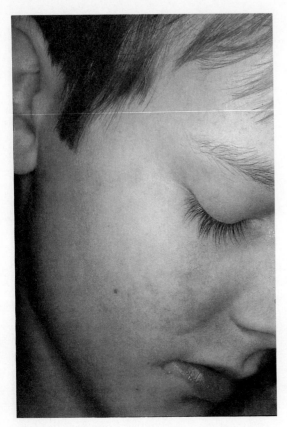

FIG. 15–5. Reaction to perfumed facial tissue and toothpaste in a 10-year-old boy allergic to both cinnamic aldehyde and cynnamic alcohol. The toothpaste contained cinnamic aldehyde. (See color Plate 7.)

from contact urticaria, and from allergic contact dermatitis. One should, in examining such patients, look for every possible cause as one almost always finds two or more known causes in such patients. Fragrance sensitivity is not uncommon, and patch testing to fragrances, colophony, wood tars, balsam of Peru, and—if positive—spices can be helpful.

9. Unusual presentations are always a problem with fragrance antigens. Goh and Ng[21] described a patient with an eruption so severe that the clinical presentation resembled bullous pemphigoid. Lichenoid oral lesions have also been reported.[22]

10. Contact urticaria can also occur, including swelling of the lips.[23] This is a form of irritation and may be regarded as such without anyone associating it with urticaria.

Unexpected sources of contact can also cause unusual pictures. Note, in Fig. 15-5, the reaction on the face to perfumed facial tissue. This appeared whenever the patient used such a tissue. Regular-size boxes of Kleenex should be safe, although the boutique boxes may be perfumed. Cinnamic aldehyde can actually cause an aggravation of rhinitis, as it can trigger mast cell release nonspecifically,[24] so avoidance is in order for a person with rhinitis. Perfumed hair spray has also caused aggravation of respiratory inflammation nonspecifically, while normals are not affected.[25] For a review of fragrance reactions, see Ref 26.

CINNAMIC ALDEHYDE—PATIENT HANDOUT

Cinnamic aldehyde is a commonly used flavoring and perfume chemical. It is the main flavoring agent in natural cinnamon, used as a kitchen spice. It is also found in many products which require a fairly strong flavor to cover an undesirable taste, such as the metallic flavor of the fluoride or stannous fluoride in toothpaste. It is also used as a scent in bathroom deodorants, in personal care products, and in foods.

Cinnamic aldehyde not only causes allergic reactions in certain people but cross-reacts with some other perfume chemicals, spices, and flavors. This is because the immune system does not distinguish this chemical from other allergy-causing substances with similar structures. Also, cinnamic aldehyde can be converted to related perfume chemicals in and on the skin, and vice versa. The implication is that a person who is highly allergic may not tolerate exposure to many scented and flavored items.

Spice-scented perfumes are especially a problem, and it may be worthwhile to test yourself by placing a small amount on a nickel- or quarter-sized area on your neck or the tender skin in the bend of your arm. If there is no reaction in 3 days, try doing it twice daily on the neck for a week. If there is no response, you may be able to tolerate normal usage. Remember, however, that this can change, as you may develop allergy to a related chemical more easily than someone who has not had a problem.

Another approach is to put the perfume or cologne on your clothing. Be sure that the quantity used is small, so that it does not soak through, as this can cause a reaction. Also use it on an area which does not show, as some perfumes (especially foreign ones) can stain clothing. Changing scents may also work, but you should do the usage test, as an allergic reaction may not show up immediately. Sometimes a person will break out on the neck and not on the wrist because the skin of the wrist does not absorb as well.

Persons with hand eczema may break out to perfumed lotions, household products with fragrance, and spices used in the kitchen. Soap with cinnamic aldehyde is usually colored, and the manufacturers of several soaps say that their products (Tone, Dial, Spirit, Mountain Fresh, and Pure & Natural), while scented, do not contain cinnamic aldehyde. The safest path is to use a fragrance-free product, as perfume allergy is often multiple. Basis soap is available fragrance-free, and there are a number of others. Many unscented products will be tolerated, as these contain only a masking fragrance, which is often not sensitizing. However, unscented products are not as reliable as the fragrance-free ones, so you must confirm your tolerance by a usage test.

Laundry products are no longer a problem, as quality fragrance-free products are available (e.g., Cheer Free and Tide without fragrance). (There is also a

---

This information is provided to help persons with contact dermatitis in the understanding of their problem. The contents are subject to change as more information becomes available and are not intended as a substitute for medical treatment.

perfumed form of Tide, which may be a problem.) Bounce makes an unscented fabric softener with masking fragrance but no cinnamic aldehyde. Paper products without perfume are freely available. Kleenex is not scented, and several brands of toilet tissue are not scented (e.g., Northern and Charmin Free). You should smell any new product as a routine to detect possible problem products, as it is easy to pick up two packages which superficially look alike until you use them and discover they are not.

Shampoos remain a problem for those who are perfume- and flavor-allergic. Sometimes a different scent is tolerated. Some herbal products will sometimes be tolerated by those allergic to cinnamates, although these contain sensitizers. You can use soft water with the fragrance-free soaps as a shampoo. Tincture of green soap has been used for hospitalized patients allergic to perfume, but fragrance-free Basis soap is much nicer. Ivory makes an unscented product, but it contains a masking fragrance.

Avoid artificial flavors in candy, mouthwashes, toothpastes, and even dental floss. You should also watch what is used at the dentist's office. He or she may have to call the manufacturer to find out what kind of flavoring agent is used in fluoride treatment.

Some persons allergic to cinnamic aldehyde are also allergic to rosin and balsam of Peru, but these are part of the standard patch-test series. If you do react to these, look at handouts for those as well.

Cinnamic aldehyde may be found in a wide range of scented and flavored products, including, among other things, cosmetics, perfumes, deodorizers, detergents, soaps, shampoos, candy, gum, toothpaste, mouthwash, baked goods, condiments, meats, and soft drinks. There may also be a problem with mixed drinks. Other plants, such as hyacinth and certain roses, may also cause a problem. Wart treatments and the tincture of benzoin used to make tape stick better can also cause reactions.

For those with problems of the mouth and lips, eating out should be deferred until the problem is controlled. Once dining out is restarted, it is vital to take the usual care and be alert to possible problem sources. Remember, it is important to *you,* but to most other people serving food and selling cosmetics, it may be more annoying than important. Don't let them dictate to you.

TOOTHPASTES CONTAINING CINNAMIC ALDEHYDE INCLUDE THE FOLLOWING:

Aim	Crest
Aqua-Fresh Tartar Control	Denquel
Close-up	Gleem

(Continued)

TOOTHPASTES FREE OF CINNAMIC ALDEHYDE INCLUDE THE FOLLOWING:

Aqua-Fresh Extra Fresh
Aqua-Fresh Triple Protection
Colgate (all flavors and tartar control)
Dent-A-Gard
MacLean's (mild mint and peppermint)
Mentadent (cool and fresh mint)
Pepsodent
Pique
Ultrabrite

WHAT IS THE SIGNIFICANCE OF A POSITIVE PATCH TEST?

Irritant responses can be seen from a concentration of 2% cinnamic aldehyde, and most now recommend a patch test concentration of 1% in petrolatum. Suboptimal concentrations may cause responses when combined in mixtures.[27] The details for such test materials still need work to understand what is happening. Perfume mix seems to work well even at 1% concentrations, although even when the mix is positive individual components may be negative on patch testing,[28] and vice versa,[29] perhaps because of the additive effect of multiple allergies in a test mixture[23] as well as the effect of a higher concentration. Patch-test positives are rare at 0.008% concentration.[30]

HOW CAN ONE AVOID CONTACT WITH THIS CHEMICAL?

Bakers and cooks are probably more at risk for exposure,[5,21] and the list of sources is large. Perfume, cosmetics,[21] household deodorizers (colored), detergents and soaps, mouthwashes, toothpastes, candy, gum,[3,4] ice cream, baked goods, condiments, meats,[31] and soft drinks.[21] It is contained in oil of hyacinth, myrrh, Bulgarian rose, and patchouli and is related to the contents of the balsam group (Peru, Tolu, Styrax). Cross- or concomitant reactions are seen with wood tar, eugenol, colophony, and ginger.[32] It is said to cross-react with cinnamic alcohol and balsam of Peru, although this is hardly automatic.[33]

WHAT IF THE PRODUCT IS NOT LABELED?

Fragrance ingredients were excluded from the law requiring labeling of cosmetics. A call to a responsible manufacturer helps, but there can be problems in proving presence or absence, especially in occult allergy. Where equipment is available a fluorometric method and high-pressure liquid chromatography (HPLC) can be used to confirm presence of cinnamic aldehyde in unknown sources.[34,35] Gas chromatography can be used for simpler mixtures.

THE QUENCHING PHENOMENON

When Opdyke was at the Research Institute for Fragrance Materials, he investigated an enigma in the industry: the tendency for cinnamic aldehyde to sensitize in some natural products but less so in others. It was found that either eugenol or limonene would reduce the tendency for cinnamic aldehyde to sensitize, and this was called "quenching."[36] Because of this, the use of the two components together was recommended. However, not all reactions are similarly controlled. The reactivity in contact urticaria is reduced with eugenol but not limonene.[37] However, the mechanisms are probably not the same and more recently the quenching effect has been questioned in sensitization and elicitation reactions.[38] It needs to be studied further in sensitization reactions.

REFERENCES

1. Opdyke D: Fragrance raw material monographs: Cinnamic aldehyde. *Foods Chem Toxicol* 17:253–258, 1979.
2. Nethercott JR, Pilger C, O'Blenis L, Roy A-M: Contact dermatitis due to cinnamic aldehyde induced in a deodorant manufacturing process. *Contact Dermatitis* 9:241–242, 1983.
3. Arctander S: *Perfume and Flavor Materials of Natural Origin.* Published by the author, Elizabeth, NJ, 1960.
4. Arctander S: *Perfume and Flavor Chemicals: Aroma Chemicals.* Published by the author, Montclair, NJ, 1969.
5. Collins FW, Mitchell JC: Aroma chemicals: Reference sources for perfume and flavour ingredients with special reference to cinnamic aldehyde. *Contact Dermatitis* 1:43–47, 1975.
6. Fergurson J, Sharma S: Cinnamic aldehyde test concentrations (letter). *Contact Dermatitis* 10:191–192, 1984.
7. Guin JD, Meyer BN, Drake RD, Haffley P: The effect of quenching agents on contact urticaria caused by cinnamic aldehyde. *J Am Acad Dermatol* 10:45–51, 1984.
8. Nethercott JR, Nield G, Holness DL: A review of 79 cases of eyelid dermatitis. *J Am Acad Dermatol* 21(2, part 1):223–230, 1989.
9. Schorr WF: Cinnamic aldehyde allergy. *Contact Dermatitis* 1:108–111, 1975.
10. Malten KE: Four bakers showing positive patch tests to a number of fragrance materials which can also be used as flavors. *Acta Derm Venereol* 59 (suppl 89): 117–121, 1979.
11. Guin JD: Sensitivity to perfumes in paper products: A case report in a 10-year-old-boy (correspondence). 4:733–734, 1981.
12. Larsen WG: Sanitary napkin dermatitis due to the perfume. *Arch Dermatol* 115:363, 1979.
13. Thyne G, Young DW, Ferguson MM: Contact stomatitis caused by toothpaste. *NZ Dent J* 85:124–126, 1989.
14. Drake TE, Maibach HI: Allergic contact dermatitis and stomatitis caused by a cinnamic aldehyde-flavored toothpaste. *Arch Dermatol* 112:202–203, 1976.
15. Mathias CG, Maibach HI, Conant MA: Perioral leukoderma simulating vitiligo from use of a toothpaste containing cinnamic aldehyde. *Arch Dermatol* 116:1172–1173, 1980.
16. Silvers SH: Stomatitis and dermatitis venenata with purpura resulting from oil of cloves and oil of cassia. *Dental Items of Interest* 61:649–651, 1939.

17. Leifer W: Contact dermatitis due to cinnamon: Recurrences of dermatitis following oral administration of cinnamon oil. *Arch Dermatol Syphilis* 64:52–55, 1951.
18. Magnusson B, Wilkinson DS: Cinnamic aldehyde in toothpaste: 1. Clinical aspects and patch tests. *Contact Dermatitis* 1:70–76, 1975.
19. Kirton V, Wilkinson DS: Sensitivity to cinnamic aldehyde in a toothpaste: 2. Further studies. *Contact Dermatitis* 1:77–80, 1975.
20. Maibach HI: Cheilitis: Occult allergy to cinnamic aldehyde. *Contact Dermatitis* 15:106–107, 1986.
21. Goh CL, Ng SK: Bullous contact allergy from cinnamon. *Derm Beruf Umwelt* 36:186–187, 1988.
22. Todd P, Garioch J, Lamey PJ, et al: Patch testing in lichenoid reactions in the mouth and oral lichen planus. *Contact Dermatitis* 23:300–301, 1990.
23. Mathias CG, Chappler RR, Maibach HI: Contact urticaria from cinnamic aldehyde. *Arch Dermatol* 116:74–76, 1980.
24. Nater JP, de Jong MCJM, Baar AJM, Bleumink F: Contact urticarial skin responses to cinnamaldehyde. *Contact Dermatitis* 3:151–154, 1977.
25. Schleuter DP, et al: Airway response to hairspray in normal subjects and subjects with hyperreactive airways. *Chest* 75:544, 1978.
26. Guin JD: History, manufacture, and cutaneous reactions to perfumes, in Frost P, Horwitz SN (eds): *Principles of Cosmetics for the Dermatologist.* St Louis, Mosby, 1982.
27. McLelland J, Shuster S: Contact dermatitis with negative patch tests: The additive effect of allergens in combination. *Br J Dermatol* 122:623–630, 1990.
28. Enders F, Przybilla B, Ring J: Patch testing with fragrance mix at 16% and 8% and its individual constituents. *Contact Dermatitis* 20:237–238, 1989.
29. Melanin G, Ohela K: Allergic reactions to fragrance mix and its components. *Contact Dermatitis* 21:62–63, 1989.
30. Danneman PJ, Booman KA, Dorsky J, et al: Cinnamic aldehyde: A survey of consumer patch-test sensitization. *Food Chem Toxicol* 21:721–725, 1983.
31. Fenaroli G: *Fenaroli's Handbook of Flavor Ingredients.* Cleveland, Ohio, Chemical Rubber Company, 1971.
32. Calnan CD: Oil of cinnamon. *Contact Dermatitis Newsletter* 8:181, 1971.
33. Calnan CD: Cinnamon dermatitis from an ointment. *Contact Dermatitis* 2:167–170, 1976.
34. Wisneski HH, Yates RL, Davis HM: High-performance liquid chromatographic-fluorometric determination of cinnamaldehyde in perfume, cologne and toilet water. *J Chromatog* 317:421–426, 1984.
35. Tsai SY, Chen SC: A fluorometric assay of trans-cinnamaldehyde in cinnamon. *J Natural Products* 47:536–538, 1984.
36. Opdyke D: Inhibition of sensitization reactions induced by certain aldehydes. *Food Cosmetics Toxicol* 14:197–198, 1976.
37. Guin JD, Meyer BN, Drake RD, Haffley P: The effect of quenching agents on contact urticaria by cinnamic aldehyde. *J Am Acad Dermatol* 10:45–51, 1984.
38. Basketter DA, Allenby CF: Studies of the quenching phenomenon in delayed contact hypersensitivity reactions. *Contact Dermatitis* 25:160–171, 1991.

16

LANOLIN (WOOL) ALCOHOLS

Jere D. Guin

Simply speaking, sensitivity to wool alcohols means an allergy to "lanolin" products. Obviously, persons allergic to lanolin need to know where one finds it and under what names, but that can be difficult to answer. However, the problem is perhaps not as severe as some in contact dermatitis, because many persons—if not most—lose their allergy within 3 to 4 years, and for some unknown reason some, despite positive patch tests, can apply lanolin to their skin without any hint of itching or a rash. While this is definitely not recommended, there are possibly some products which would be tolerated if one were willing to do a usage test, repeatedly applying the product to the skin of an area which absorbs well, over a period of several days.

WHAT IS LANOLIN?

Lanolin is a sticky substance which comes from sheep hair when sheep are sheared. This ingredient produced from the skin and oil glands of the sheep protects the wool from the sun, wind, and rain; it may represent as much as 5 to 25 percent of the weight of the unprocessed wool.[1] It differs in composition from one source to another, but it is made up mostly of esters of wool alcohols and fatty acids, some free alcohol, and small components of free acids and other hydrocarbons.[1] The sterol content, mostly cholesterol and lanosterol, is also high.[2] Lanolin is a good emulsifier and it binds water well, making it valuable in cosmetic formulations. It also blends well with skin and hair. Since it is not uniform in composition, both liquid and solid fractions can be derived by fractional distillation, with different applications. Hydrogenation produces the high percentage of free alcohols[1,3] and as a result a more allergenic product.[3] The hydrogenated form has a less sticky feel, less color and odor, and few if any esters, but it retains its affinity for water and its emollient properties. The hydrogenation is said to increase allergenicity, but following "purification," a process combining distillation and solvent extraction, the allergic potential is reduced.[3]

LANOLIN ALLERGY

Lanolin allergy is extremely complex. Much of the lanolin used in the cosmetics industry is made from hydrogenated lanolin, which is an altered product, probably with additional (new) allergens. Attempts to identify "the" allergen in lanolin[3] have been futile, perhaps because there is no single agent. In 1953 it was reported that the alcohol fraction was mainly responsible for sensitivity,[4] and this is felt to be due to the alkali-derived free aliphatic alcohols.[5-7] The reason "wool alcohols" are used for patch testing is that this fraction produces more positive reactions than whole lanolin.[8] Clark et al.[9] found 71 percent of their lanolin-allergic population to be sensitive to the free alcohol fraction; but after removal of the free fatty alcohols and detergent, the incidence of patch test reactivity was only 1 percent of the previous level.[9] Using the patient's product, if available, would be a useful addition to testing with the wool alcohols standard.[9] Sometimes more than one fraction causes a reaction in the same subject, proving the nonuniformity.[10]

Testing to one product may not be adequate to detect all "lanolin" allergic persons; some investigators recommend two or even three test materials to screen for allergy to lanolin. An emulsifier, Amerchol 101, has been recommended as an additional antigen for testing, with differing results. Edman and Moller[11] found that three reagents were necessary to confirm all of their known lanolin-allergic patients. Only 75 percent reacted to either wool alcohols alone or Amerchol 101, but by testing to both, 90 percent would have been found.[11] With those two materials plus the alcohol soluble fraction of Amerchol, "Ameralc," they found positive tests in all of their known lanolin-allergic population. However, in a study of emulsifiers done elsewhere, every subject allergic to Amerchol 101 was also picked up with the screening test with wool alcohols.[12]

THE CLINICAL PICTURE

Most patients are older women with eczema, especially leg eczema, and ulcers of various types.[3,8,13,14] Of 81 patients with venous leg ulcers, two-thirds had positive patch tests; lanolin and topical antibiotics were high on the list of offenders.[14]

Medication allergy is another leading cause,[15] as lanolin is used in the vehicle of applied lotions and medicaments. Such allergy is very common in patients with stasis eczema.[16] In a large U.S. series of medication-induced allergy, testing with whole lanolin also showed about a 6 percent reactivity in this very special population.[17]

The incidence of reactors to cosmetics is more controversial as the incidence in the healthy population is probably very low.[2] However, of 487 cases of suspected "cosmetic" allergy, 11 cases attributed to lanolin were found. These patients were different from the European (medication-induced) group, where many had dermatitis of the lower extremities, while less than 1 percent of the American cosmetic series had eczema of the feet or legs. Rather, most lesions were located on the face.[18]

Many of those reacting to emulsifiers have multiple sensitivities[19]; some of this may be a concomitant allergy caused by broadening of the allergic base. Finding the sources by reading the label is not easy either. Even cetyl and stearyl alcohols, which are in the alcohol fraction, may occasionally be a cause of allergy.[20] The total number of potential sources is legion. Lanolin can even be found in chewing gum![21]

LANOLIN—PATIENT HANDOUT

WHAT EXACTLY IS LANOLIN?

Lanolin is a sticky substance which comes from wool when sheep are sheared. This ingredient, produced from the skin and oil glands of the sheep, protects the wool from sun, wind, and rain; it may represent as much as 5 to 25 percent of the weight of unprocessed wool. It differs in composition from one source to another, but it is made up mostly of esters of wool alcohols and fatty acids and some free alcohol with small components of free acids and other hydrocarbons. The sterol content, mostly cholesterol and lanosterol, is also high. Lanolin is a good emulsifier, and it binds water well, making it valuable in cosmetic formulations. It also blends well with skin and hair. Since it is not uniform in composition, one can get both liquid and solid fractions by a process called fractional distillation, and these have different applications. In short, lanolin can be treated to produce a wide variety of cosmetic ingredients used in many cosmetics, creams, lotions, and other products.

ARE ALL LANOLIN PRODUCTS A PROBLEM FOR SOMEONE ALLERGIC TO LANOLIN?

Lanolin varies somewhat with the source, but it can be very different after undergoing industrial treatment. Specific derivatives are made to produce a product with the specific qualities needed for an intended use. Some of these are less likely to sensitize, while others are much more likely to be a problem. For example, hydrogenation (which has been used to convert cooking oil into the solid forms of shortening) produces a high percentage of free alcohols, which are more likely to cause allergy. The hydrogenated form has a number of cosmetically desirable qualities. It has a less sticky feel, less color and odor, and few if any esters, but it retains its affinity for water and its emollient properties. Unlike hydrogenation, "purification," a process combining distillation and solvent extraction, is said to reduce the allergic potential.

Products containing whole lanolin will probably have it on the label. However, there are many derivatives which may not be so easily identified.

HOW DOES ONE BECOME ALLERGIC TO LANOLIN?

No one can be sure how someone becomes allergic to a substance, but much lanolin allergy is associated with use of lanolin-containing products on chronic eczemas. Perhaps the archetypal patient is a mature woman with hand eczema or perhaps with an eczema around a leg ulcer. Lanolin allergy should be considered when there is a rash were cosmetics, lotions, or medication have been applied.

This information is provided to help persons with contact dermatitis in the understanding of their problem. The contents are subject to change as more information becomes available and are not intended as a substitute for medical treatment.

One unsuspected source is lanolin derivatives contained in *some* cortisone salves being used to treat the eczema.

Uncommon sources include furniture and shoe polishes, corrosion inhibitors, or, in the case of sheep farmers, exposure to the animals themselves. In a few patients, even Aquaphor, which contains lanolin-derived emulsifiers, can be a problem.

WHAT IS THE PROGNOSIS IN LANOLIN-ALLERGIC PEOPLE?

This is a bit of good news, as many no longer have the allergy after a few years. One-third lose the allergy in less than a year, and only 41 percent are still allergic after a year.

HOW CAN EXPOSURE BE AVOIDED?

Avoidance is perhaps not as simple as it might be were the antigen in one form and clearly labeled. Labeling is not available in some countries, but avoidance is perhaps best achieved by staying away from all products not known to be free of lanolin-related ingredients until usage tests can be done. In a usage test, you apply the product daily for 5 to 7 days to a specific area of the neck, upper arm, or bend of the arm. Do not do this with soaps, shampoos, solvents, cleansers, or other irritating substances. If a reaction occurs, one must do this in volunteers to be sure it is not an irritation.

Some seemingly unrelated products, such as cetyl or stearyl alcohols, Eucerin, and Aquaphor, may cause a reaction. Persons allergic to one product may tolerate another. In fact, some who react on patch testing will tolerate direct application of lanolin, so usage tests or repeat open application tests are in order.

IS THERE A LISTING OF LANOLIN-CONTAINING PRODUCTS?

Such a list would, if available be impossibly long. At least some brands of the following things are known to contain lanolin:

Baby oil
Bath oil
Blush
Diaper lotion
Eyeliner

(*Continued*)

Face creams
Fluorescent dyes
Furniture polish
Hair dressing
Hair spray
Hemorrhoidal suppositories and ointments
Home permanents
Liniment
Lipstick
Lubricating cream
Makeup
Medications
Ointments
Shampoo
Shaving cream
Shoe polish
Soap
Sunscreen
Tanning lotions
Topical corticosteroids
Veterinary products
Waterless hand cleanser

WHAT CAN ONE SAFELY USE IF ONE IS LANOLIN-ALLERGIC?

Theraplex makes three lotions which contain no lanolin or lanolin derivatives: Theraplex ClearLotion, Theraplex HydroLotion, and Theraplex Emollient.

Moisturel cream and lotion, Neutrogena Norwegian formula emulsion and Hand Cream, and Nutraderm cream and lotion have no lanolin, but they contain cetyl alcohol, to which some lanolin-allergic persons react. The term *cetearyl alcohol* used in some products is a mixture which contains, among other things, cetyl alcohol. Lanolin-allergic individuals should rule out the presence of lanolin and its derivatives as best they can and then use what seems to be a safe product in a limited area for a week or so to be sure they are not allergic to it. The application site should be one which absorbs well, such as the neck.

TABLE 16–1. Lanolin Cosmetics Ingredients

Lanolin	Refined wool fat (wax) which has been purified, alkali-treated, bleached, and deodorized to meet (or exceed) USP specifications. It is an amber-yellow, tenacious, unctuous mass with a mild, distinct odor and emollient qualities.
Lanolin acid	Organic acids from hydrolysis of lanolin. About half are normal and iso acids and half are hydroxy acids.
Lanolin alcohol	Mixture of organic alcohols from hydrolysis of lanolin. Lanolin alcohols are 90 percent monohydric and 10 percent dihydric. Lanolin alcohols are a mixture of about 31 percent sterols (mostly cholesterol), 15 percent triterpene alcohols (mostly lanosterol), 23 percent long-chain aliphatic alcohols (normal, branched, and dihydroxy), 1 percent hydrocarbons, and 20 percent unclassified.
Lanolinamide	Ethanolamide of lanolin acid.
Acetylated lanolin	Acetyl ester of lanolin from hydroxy acid and alcohols in esters.
Acetylated lanolin alcohol	Acetyl ester of lanolin alcohols.
Acetylated lanolin ricinoleate	Acetyl of ricinoleate.
Lanolin linoleate	Ester of lanolin alcohol and oleic acid.
Lanolin oil	Liquid fraction on separation by physical means, e.g., vacuum distillation and solvent crystallization. Product is less sticky but retains emollient quality and substitutes for whole lanolin. Improved drug release. It is odorless, tasteless, and has low irritancy.[1]
Lanolin wax	Semisolid fraction of lanolin obtained by physical means. Water in oil emulsifier with waxlike qualities. Also odorless and tasteless. Useful in lipstick, lip gloss, etc.
Lanosterol	Triterpene alcohol obtained from lanolin with sterol structure.
Laneth-(n)	Polyethylene glycol ether of lanolin alcohol with ethoxylation value of n. Ethoxylation gives high hydroalcoholic solubility.
Laneth-(n) acetate	Acetate ester of polyethylene glycol ether of lanolin alcohol with ethoxylation value of n.
Lanolinamide	Ethanolamide of lanolin acid.
PEG (n) Lanolinamide	Polyethylene glycol amide of lanolin acid from ethylene oxide treatment (ethoxylation) with n average moles of ethylene (oxide) added.
PEG (n) lanolin oil	Ethylene oxide derivative of lanolin oil from ethylene oxide treatment with n average moles of ethylene oxide added.
PEG (n) lanolin wax	Ethylene oxide derivative of lanolin wax from ethylene oxide treatment with n average moles of ethylene oxide added.
(Alcohol) lanolate	Ester from (alcohol) transesterification to produce lanolin acid ester of alcohol used, e.g. isopropyl lanolate.
Hydrogenated lanolin	Reduced lanolin with saturated bonding and few esters but abundant free alcohols and acids and increased potential for sensitization.

Sources: Adapted from Refs. 1 and 3; also Nikitakis JM, McEwen GN, Wenninger JA: *CTFA International Cosmetic Ingredient Dictionary,* 4th ed. Washington, DC, Cosmetic, Toiletry, and Fragrance Association, 1991.

Occupational exposure to sheep is reported[22] but must be rare. Metal workers exposed to coolant may also become allergic,[23] but treatment of eczemas and ulcers, and especially stasis eczema, is the leading cause worldwide.

HOW BIG IS THE PROBLEM?

Kligman[2] feels that it is blown out of proportion, as very few of the normal population are allergic and it is difficult to sensitize anyone to the antigen. Another bit of good news is that the allergy tends to disappear spontaneously in 3 or 4 years, at least in many persons. One-third seem to lose their reactivity in less than a year, and only 41 percent are positive after a year.[24]

HOW CAN EXPOSURE BE AVOIDED?

Avoidance is perhaps not as easy as it might be were the antigen in one form and clearly labeled. Table 16-1 lists a number but not all of cosmetic ingredients derived from lanolin. Labeling is not available in some countries, but avoidance is perhaps best achieved by staying away from all products not known to be free of lanolin-related ingredients until usage tests can be done. Some seemingly unrelated products such as cetyl or stearyl alcohols,[20] Eucerin, and Aquaphor may cause a reaction.[25]

Persons allergic to one product may tolerate another.[3] In fact, some who react on patch testing will tolerate direct application of lanolin,[2] so usage tests or repeat open application tests are in order. It is also possible for industry to produce products that are unlikely to cause a reaction, even in sensitive persons. Hydroxylation reduces and acetylation eliminates the allergy. Acetic anhydride can be used to esterify (bind acetate to) hydroxyl groups. Transesterification also eliminates reactivity.[26] Perhaps a relatively harmless form is possible.[111] Just removal of the alcohol fraction and detergents will eliminate 99 percent of the reactors,[9] and many products of distillation and extraction are not highly allergenic.[3] Lanolin represents an ideal model to provide product safety from using the information available in product design.[28] Contact urticaria can also be produced by lanolin,[30] which is not unsuspected, as many animal products are known to do this.

An extensive list of lanolin products and their categorization, chemistry, and manufacture can be found in a review by Barnett.[30]

REFERENCES

1. Schlossman ML, McCarthy JP: Lanolin and derivatives chemistry: Relationship to allergic contact dermatitis. *Contact Dermatitis* 5:65–72, 1979.
2. Kligman AM: Lanolin allergy: Crisis or comedy. *Contact Dermatitis* 9:99–107, 1983.
3. Sugai T, Higashi J: Hypersensitivity to hydrogenated lanolin. *Contact Dermatitis* 1:146–57, 1975.
4. Sulzberger MB, Lazar MP: A study of the allergenic constituents of lanolin (wool fat). *J Invest Dermatol* 15:453–458, 1950.
5. Sulzberger MB, Warshaw T, Herrmann F: Studies of skin hypersensitivities to lanolin. *J Invest Dermatol* 20:33–43, 1953.
6. Cronin E: Lanolin dermatitis. *Br J Dermatol* 78:167–171, 1966.
7. Peter G, Schropl F, Franzwa F: Experimentelle Untersuchungen uber die allergene Wirkung von Wollwachsalkoholen. *Hautarzt* 20:450, 1969.
8. Hjorth N, Trolle-Lassen C: Skin reactions to ointment bases. *Trans St Johns Dermatol Soc* 49:127–139, 1963.
9. Clark EW, Cronin E, Wilkinson DS: Lanolin with reduced sensitizing potential: A preliminary note. *Contact Dermatitis* 3:69–74, 1977.
10. Fregert S, Dahlquist I, Trulsson L: An attempt to isolate and identify allergens in lanolin. *Contact Dermatitis* 10:16–19, 1984.
11. Edman B, Moller H: Testing a purified lanolin preparation by a randomized procedure. *Contact Dermatitis* 20:287–290, 1989.

12. Tosti A, Guerra L, Morelli R, Bardazzi F: Prevalence and sources of sensitization to emulsifiers: A clinical study. *Contact Dermatitis* 23:68–72, 1990.

13. Blondeel A, Oleffe J, Achten G: Contact allergy in 330 dermatological patients. *Contact Dermatitis* 4:270–276, 1978.

14. Wilson CL, Cameron J, Powell SM, et al: High incidence of contact dermatitis in leg-ulcer patients— Implications for management. *Clin Exp Dermatol* 16:250–253, 1991.

15. Oleffe JA, Blondeel A, Boschmans S: Patch testing with lanolin. *Contact Dermatitis* 4:233–247, 1978.

16. Wilkinson JD, Hambly EM, Wilkinson DS: Comparison of patch test results in two adjacent areas of England: II. Medicaments. *Acta Derm Venereol* 60:245–249, 1980.

17. Fisher AA, Pascher F, Kanof NB: Allergic contact dermatitis due to ingredients of vehicles: A "vehicle tray" for patch testing. *Arch Dermatol* 104:286–290, 1971.

18. Eiermann HJ, Larsen W, Maibach HI, Taylor JS: Prospective study of cosmetic reactions: 1977–1980. North American Contact Dermatitis Group. *J Am Acad Dermatol* 6:909–917, 1982.

19. Hannuksela M, Kousa M, Pirila V: Contact sensitivity to emulsifiers. *Contact Dermatitis* 2:105–110, 1976.

20. Marston S: Contact dermatitis from cetostearyl alcohol in hydrocortisone butyrate lipocream, and from lanolin. *Contact Dermatitis* 24:372, 1991.

21. Mitchell JC: The skin and chemical additives to foods. *Arch Dermatol* 104:329–330, 1971.

22. Sirieix-Sorhouet M, Sirieix P, Ducombs G: Ewe milkers and hand eczema. *Contact Dermatitis* 25:135–136, 1991.

23. Van Hecke E: Contact allergy in metal workers. *Contact Dermatitis* 23:241–242, 1990.

24. Carmichael AJ, Foulds IS, Bransbury DS: Loss of lanolin patch-test positivity. *Br J Dermatol* 125:573–576, 1991.

25. Epstein E: The detection of lanolin allergy. *Arch Dermatol* 106:678–681, 1972.

26. Giorgini S, Melli MC, Sertoli A: Comments on the allergenic activity of lanolin. *Contact Dermatitis* 9:425–426, 1983.

27. Clark EW, Blondeel A, Cronin E, et al: Lanolin of reduced sensitizing potential. *Contact Dermatitis* 7:80–83, 1981.

28. Blondeel A: Allergy in cosmetology. *Ann Dermatol Venereol* 110:513–522, 1983.

29. Foussereau J: Allergy to turpentine, lanolin and nickel in Strasbourg. *Contact Dermatitis* 4:300, 1978.

30. Barnett G: Lanolin and derivatives. *Cosmetics and Toiletries* 101:21–44, 1986.

17

CARBA MIX (RUBBER)

Jere D. Guin

WHAT IS CARBA MIX?

Carba mix is a mixture of three rubber chemicals. Two are "carbamates," which are activators and/or accelerators (i.e., they are used in curing both natural and many types of synthetic rubber). The third chemical is diphenylguanidine, a "medium" accelerator. It is often used as an activator with benzothiazole or sulfenamide accelerators in curing rubber, especially the heavier, industrial types. It can also be used as a primary accelerator with natural rubber but is a bit slow for the synthetic rubbers. This chemical is also found to be the cause of some cases of shoe dermatitis,[1,2] and it is used as a laboratory reagent.

The term *mix* is used when more than one chemical is included in a patch-test antigen or material. In this case the three chemicals are zinc diethyldithiocarbamate, zinc dibutyldithiocarbamate, and diphenylguanidine, each in a 1% concentration in petrolatum.

HOW COMMON IS THIS TYPE OF ALLERGY?

The percentage varies with the person or group doing the testing, but carba mix is one of the allergens likely to be have a greater than 1 percent prevalence in persons being patch tested, and it is the second most commonly positive rubber allergen (after thiuram mix). When tests positive on either the first or second reading are included, the prevalence reaches the 4 percent level, and the accepted prevalence for the United States is probably at the 3 percent level.[3,4] Allergy to carba mix is more common in persons with stasis eczema, more likely to be positive with increasing age,[5] more common in men,[6] and more likely to be occupationally induced.[7]

This is also one of the standard allergens commonly positive in a pediatric population.[8] Carbamates are structurally related to the thiurams, and there is a significant association of the two standard text mixes.[9] In fact, most of the reactors to carba mix who do not react to thiuram mix as well, are allergic to diphenylguanidine.

The overlap in one series was so great that the authors considered carba mix to be a superfluous test where thiuram mix was being used.[10] This may be related to the location of that study. Cronin[11] found that most of those allergic only to carba mix

161

were sensitive to the diphenylguanidine component. This is a less common sensitizer in the United Kingdom, which would influence the need for carba mix as a separate test in that country. The mercapto mix is not chemically related, but reactions to it are also linked to carba mix.[9] Because carbamates are commonly used with other accelerators, some of these are perhaps concomitant sensitivities. However, there are documented cases where strong reactions to thiuram mix can be found in persons reacting to carbamates and many associate this with cross-reactivity.

WHY IS A MIXTURE USED?

Mixtures introduce a number of variables in testing, but overall they have proved to be a convenient way to test to multiple chemicals as a screening procedure. This was discussed by Mitchell,[12] and it is discussed in Chap. 25, on the mercapto mix.

Briefly, a mixture is a practical way to save time and money when screening multiple chemicals for allergy. In some cases mild allergic reactions to more than one may have an additive effect, allowing us to find what would otherwise be subclinical allergy to one. The disadvantage is that the concentration of each antigen is reduced, and the possibility of both a false-negative response and an irritant effect is increased.

Manufacturing methods vary, and so many rubber chemicals are available that the chemical contents of a specific finished product may not be known even to the manufacturer. Commercial-grade chemicals are seldom pure when added, and they are subject to change during the manufacturing process. Also, many products such as shoes are assembled from components, and the methodology and composition may not be under the supervision of the final manufacturer.

Rubber chemicals are routinely added to the latex gathered from the tree, which would not be known unless an analysis were made of each lot of the raw material. Therefore, it is often less important to know what specific chemical caused the allergy and where it is likely to be found. In such an environment use of mixtures provides the physician with more individual chemicals in the test series than would be available if individual reagents were used.

WHAT ARE THE SOURCES OF EXPOSURE FOR THE CHEMICALS IN CARBA MIX?

Many types of rubber, both natural and synthetic, are likely to contain carbamates. The list is very long, and anyone allergic to carbamates should be wary of rubber in general and limit exposure to those objects and materials which do not elicit a positive patch or usage test. Diphenylguanidine is more likely to be used in heavier industrial rubber products than in consumer products.[11,13] This rubber chemical can be used in a wide variety of both natural and synthetic rubbers, and many of the latter are used industrially. Cronin[14] listed mats, face masks, and rubberized hose pipes as possible sources.

Wilson[15] found that boots (shoes), underclothing, and condoms may contain carbamates. Carbamates are also commonly found in latex gloves,[16–18] which can, in the presence of sweat, release as much antigen as patch testing materials.[19] Rubber in a prosthesis caused allergic contact dermatitis on an amputation stump.[20] At one time, carbamates were found in some adhesive tapes.[21] Occupational exposure can occur in the rubber[22] and chemical industries. Hyperpigmentation has been associated with carbamates, but the reason for this is unclear.[23]

Prevention of reactions usually means avoiding rubber products. While one can find carbamates by a qualitative chemical analysis, the potential list of sources makes this impractical for everyday exposure. For some sources (e.g., latex gloves), there are published reports of chemical content. However, one would be well advised to test to the object itself, as minor antigens not in the standard series can be a problem, and some lists contain inaccurate information.

Elastyren gloves, a hypoallergenic product often recommended for persons who are sensitive to thiurams and cannot wear latex gloves, contain small amounts of carbamates,[24] so these are probably not an option for those who are also carbamate-allergic. Vinyl gloves can often be substituted if the patient is not allergic to vinyl, and Tactylon gloves seldom cause a reaction in anyone not allergic to glove powder.

Another reaction to carbamates in clothing is usually not accompanied by a reaction to rubber chemicals in the standard tray. Jordan and Bourlas[25] reported six persons who were found to be allergic to underwear which had been bleached, but not to new underwear. The cause was a new chemical produced when the elastic in underwear was bleached, converting the rubber chemical present, zinc dibenzyldithiocarbamate, to N,N'-dibenzylcarbamyl chloride. One can produce patch-test material for this by repeatedly pouring a chlorine laundry bleach over zinc dibenzyldithiocarbamate held in filter paper in a funnel and placed in an empty container such as a beaker. By using two beakers, the same bleach can be used repeatedly. The treated chemical is dried, weighed, and mixed with petrolatum in a 2% concentration. Patch testing to this chemical should be routine in persons with waistband dermatitis. Unfortunately, I am not aware of its being commercially available. However, commercial-grade zinc dibenzyldithiocarbamate is available and can easily be treated to make the antigen.

Agricultural chemicals are another source of exposure to carbamates. According to Cronin,[26] the methyl carbamates are weak choline esterase inhibitors and are more toxic than the phenyl carbamates which are used as herbicides. The best-known of the former group are perhaps the fungicides Maneb[27–29] and Zineb. These chemicals are used on seeds and bulbs and may also be applied to plants. Zineb and Mancozeb are similarly used to protect against perenosporosis on vines, phytophtoriosis in potatoes, cladiosporosis in tomatoes, and fusariosis in tulips.[30] The allergic contact reactions are well known. Sharma and Kaur[31] found that of 30 farmers with contact dermatitis, 7 were allergic to carbamate pesticides. These chemicals are also common sensitizers among Spanish agricultural workers.[32] Benomyl, a commonly used garden chemical of this class, can also cause contact dermatitis.[33,34] There is also a report of allergy to a thiocarbamic acid derivative used as a fungicide.[35] Sometimes sensitivity is found to multiple agents of the same class,[36] although this is not what most reports show. One report suggested that a chemical derivative in some cases might be the allergen.[37]

Slimicides may also be related to the dithiocarbamates. Fregert[38] listed potassium-hydroxymethyl-N-methyl-dithiocarbamate, sodium dimethyl-dithiocarbamate, and di-sodium-methylene-bis-dithiocarbamate among the slimicides used in the inhibition of bacteria, mildew fungus, yeast fungus, protozoa, and algae.

The morphology of the reactions to agricultural chemicals varies, but several patterns are reported. A hand eczema resembling dyshidrotic eczema was found in a retail florist,[39] and the presenting rash in agricultural workers can be an eczema of the hands,

CARBA MIX—PATIENT HANDOUT

WHAT IS "CARBA MIX"?

Carba mix is a mixture of three chemicals used in curing rubber, both natural and synthetic, and a positive patch test to carba mix can be caused by any one or more of the three chemicals. In the United States, about 3 percent of persons tested for suspected contact allergy are positive to carba mix, and such allergy also occurs frequently in children. Often chemicals in this group are used with other rubber chemicals, and when one is allergic to carbamates one may well be allergic to other rubber chemicals.

WHO IS LIKELY TO BE ALLERGIC TO CHEMICALS IN CARBA MIX?

Anyone suspected of being allergic to rubber should be suspected of possibly being allergic to carbamates of carba mix. Allergy to this group of rubber chemicals occurs in children, but prevalence increases with age. This allergy not infrequently is associated with eczema over a swollen ankle. Carbamates are similar in chemical structure to the chemical used to make latex gloves, and persons allergic to rubber gloves often react to carba mix.

HOW DOES ONE AVOID CONTACT WITH THE CHEMICALS IN CARBA MIX?

This may not be easy, as carbamates are widely used, and success may even require avoiding rubber products in general. If you are also allergic to thiuram mix, then following directions for avoiding that group is important (there is a handout for that mix as well). In any event, one should probably be tested to any rubber object with which contact is likely, as there are many rubber chemicals to which you were not tested, and this is the best way to find such allergy. Occupational exposure can also occur, especially in the rubber and chemical industries.

Published sources of rubber products known at one time to contain carbamates include face masks, rubberized hose, pipes, boots (shoes), underclothing, condoms, latex gloves, rubber in a prosthesis for an amputation stump, tapes, and certain agricultural or garden chemicals including carbamate fungicides, herbicides, and pesticides. Look on the label and avoid any containing the words "carbamate," "carbanilate," or "thiuram."

For those allergic to latex gloves, vinyl or Tactylon can be substituted provided patch testing to these is negative. Elastyren gloves, often recommended for persons sensitive to latex gloves, contain small amounts of carbamates and probably not an option for carbamate-allergic persons. Agricultural chemicals, e.g., pesticides, herbicides and all the fungicides, benomyl, maneb, and zineb as well as carbamates used on seeds and bulbs can cause allergy. Another potential source is slimicides, used in the inhibition of bacteria, mildew fungus, yeast fungus, protozoa, and algae.

trunk, or face and upper arms.[40,41] Widespread eczema may also occur.[30] A pellagra-like rash was caused by sensitivity to Mancozeb.[42] Carbamates may also cause contact urticaria.[41,43]

Recently a large number of cases of allergic contact dermatitis followed what was probably a high level of exposure. In 1991, a train tanker car derailed in California, causing a chemical spill of the soil fumigant sodium methyldithiocarbamate into the Sacramento River nearby. There was an outbreak of dermatitis in the jail inmates and crew leaders who helped in removing dead fish. Concentration of the chemical in the river water was measured at 20 to 40 ppb.[44]

There is also the potential for toxicity from cutaneous absorption, and this is greater from "dermal" exposure than from inhalation.[45] One can also absorb these products from clothing, especially where sebum contaminates clothing.[46] Another activity is the tendency to augment certain phototoxic reactions, at least in laboratory animals.[47]

Fisher[48] lists the following as carbamate (and chemically related thiuram) fungicides: 4-chloro-2-butynyl m-chlorocarbanilate (barban); cuprous dimethyldithiocarbamate, cuprous chloride complex (cuprobam); ferric dimethyldithiocarbamate (ferbam); manganous and zinc ethylenebis (dithiocarbamate) (mancozeb); manganous ethylenebis (dithiocarbamate) (maneb); methyl-butylcarbamoyl-benzimidazole-carbamate (benomyl); mixture of polyethylenebis (thiuram sulfides) (Carbatene); sodium methyldithiocarbamate (sodium metham); tetramethylthiuram disulfide (thiram); tetraethylthiuram monosulfide (Tetmosol); zinc dimethyldithiocarbamate (ziram); zinc ethylenebis (dithiocarbamate) (zineb); and zinc propylenebis-(dithiocarbamate) (antracol).

REFERENCES

1. Bajaj AK, Gupta SC, Chatterjee AK, Singh KG: Shoe dermatitis in India. *Contact Dermatitis* 19:372, 1988.
2. Saha M, Srinivas CR, Shenoy SD, et al: Footwear dermatitis. *Contact Dermatitis* 28:260, 1993.
3. Nethercott JR, Holness DL, Adams RM, et al: Results of first and second readings with standard screening tray in North America. *Am J Contact Dermatitis* 2:255, 1991.
4. Nethercott JR, Holness DL, Adams RM, et al: Patch testing with a routine screening tray in North America, 1985 through 1989: I. Frequency and response. *Am J Contact Dermatitis* 2:122, 1991.
5. Christophersen J, Menne T, Tanghoj P, et al: Clinical patch test data evaluated by multivariate analysis. Danish Contact Dermatitis Group. *Contact Dermatitis* 21:291, 1989.
6. Nethercott JR, Holness DL, Adams RM, et al. Patch testing with a routine screening tray in North America, 1985 through 1989: I. Gender and response. *Am J Contact Dermatitis* 2:130, 1991.
7. Nethercott JR, Holness DL, Adams RM, et al: Patch testing with a routine screening tray in North America, 1987 through 1989: Occupation and response. *Am J Contact Dermatitis* 2:247, 1991.
8. Kuiters GR, Smitt JH, Cohen EB, Bos JD: Allergic contact dermatitis in children and young adults. *Arch Dermatol* 125:1531, 1989.
9. Edman B: Computerized analysis of concomitant contact allergens. *Contact Dermatitis* 24:110, 1991.
10. Logan RA, White IR: Carbamix is redundant in the patch test series. *Contact Dermatitis* 18:303, 1988.
11. Cronin E: *Contact Dermatitis.* Edinburgh, Churchill Livingstone, 1980, pp 731–732.
12. Mitchell JC: Patch testing with mixes. *Contact Dermatitis* 7:98, 1981.
13. Taylor JS: in Fisher AA (ed): *Contact Dermatitis.* Philadelphia, Lea & Febiger, 1986, p 622.
14. Cronin E: *Contact Dermatitis.* Edinburgh, Churchill Livingstone, 1980, p 740.
15. Wilson HT: Rubber dermatitis: An investigation of 106 cases of contact dermatitis caused by rubber. *Br J Dermatol* 81:175, 1969.
16. Rich P, Belozer ML, Norris P, Storrs FJ: Allergic contact dermatitis to two antioxidants in latex gloves: 4,4'-thiobis(6-*tert*-butyl-*meta*-cresol) (Lowinox 44S36) and butylhydroxyanisole: Allergen alternatives for glove-allergic patients. *J Am Acad Dermatol* 24:37, 1991.

17. Hesse A, v Hinzenstern J, Peters KP, et al: Allergic and irritant reactions to rubber gloves in medical health services. *J Am Acad Dermatol* 25:831, 1991.

18. Frosch PJ, Born CM, Schutz R: Contact allergy to rubber, surgical and vinyl gloves. *Hautarzt* 38:210, 1987.

19. Knudsen BB, Larsen E, Egsgaard H, Menne T: Release of thiurams and carbamates from rubber gloves. *Contact Dermatitis* 28:63, 1993.

20. Baptista A, Barros MA, Azenha A: Allergic contact dermatitis on an amputation stump. *Contact Dermatitis* 26:140, 1992.

21. Calnan CD: Diethyldithiocarbamate in adhesive tape. *Contact Dermatitis* 4:61, 1978.

22. Rudzki E, Napiorkowska T: Sensitivity to carbamate accelerators in rubber processing. *Przeglad Dermatologiczny* 71:121, 1984.

23. Binder R: Letter: Hyperpigmentation caused by a fungicide. *Arch Dermatol* 112:880, 1976.

24. Guin JD: The doctor's surgical/examination gloves—Problems with and without them. *Int J Dermatol* 31:853, 1992.

25. Jordan WP Jr, Bourlas MC: Allergic contact dermatitis to underwear elastic: Chemically transformed by laundry bleach. *Arch Dermatol* 111:593, 1975.

26. Cronin E: *Contact Dermatitis*. Edinburgh, Churchill Livingstone, 1980, 410.

27. Piraccini BM, Cameli N, Peluso AM, Tardio M: A case of allergic contact dermatitis due to the pesticide maneb. *Contact Dermatitis* 24:381, 1991.

28. Nater JP, Terpstra H, Bleumink E: Allergic contact sensitization to the fungicide Maneb. *Contact Dermatitis* 5:24, 1979.

29. Adams RM, Manchester RD: Allergic contact dermatitis to Maneb in a housewife. *Contact Dermatitis* 8:271, 1982.

30. Kleibl K, Rackova M: Cutaneous allergic reactions to dithiocarbamates. *Contact Dermatitis* 6:348, 1980.

31. Sharma VK, Kaur S: Contact sensitization by pesticides in farmers. *Contact Dermatitis* 23:77, 1990.

32. Garcia-Perez A, Garcia-Bravo B, Beneit JV: Standard patch tests in agricultural workers. *Contact Dermatitis* 10:151, 1984.

33. Larsen AI, Larsen A, Jepsen JR, Jorgensen R: Contact allergy to the fungicide benomyl? *Contact Dermatitis* 22:278, 1990.

34. van Ketel WG: Sensitivity to the pesticide benomyl. *Contact Dermatitis* 2:290, 1976.

35. Veraldi S, Schianchi-Veraldi R: Allergic contact dermatitis from tolciclate. *Contact Dermatitis* 24:315, 1991.

36. Peluso AM, Tardio M, Adamo F, Venturo N: Multiple sensitization due to bis-dithiocarbamate and thiophthalimide pesticides. *Contact Dermatitis* 25:327, 1991.

37. Schubert H: Contact dermatitis to sodium *N*-methyldithiocarbamate. *Contact Dermatitis* 4:370, 1978.

38. Fregert S: Registration of chemicals in industries. Slimicides in the paper pulp industry. *Contact Dermatitis* 2:358, 1976.

39. Crippa M, Misquith L, Lonati A, Pasolini G: Dyshidrotic eczema and sensitization to dithiocarbamates in a florist. *Contact Dermatitis* 23:203, 1990.

40. Manuzzi P, Borrello P, Misciali C, Guerra L: Contact dermatitis due to Ziram and Maneb. *Contact Dermatitis* 19:148, 1988.

41. van Joost T, Naafs B, van Ketel WG: Sensitization to benomyl and related pesticides. *Contact Dermatitis* 9:153, 1983.

42. Lisi P, Caraffini S: Pellagroid dermatitis from mancozeb with vitiligo. *Contact Dermatitis* 13:124, 1985.

43. Helander I, Makela A: Contact urticaria to zinc diethyldithiocarbamate (ZDC). *Contact Dermatitis* 9:327, 1983.

44. Anonymous: Dermatitis among workers cleaning the Sacramento River after a chemical spill—California, 1991. [Published erratum appears in *MMWR* 40:862, 1991.] *MMWR* 40:825, 833, 1991.

45. Brouwer DH, Brouwer EJ, van Hemmen JJ: Assessment of dermal and inhalation exposure to zineb/maneb in the cultivation of flower bulbs. *Ann Occup Hyg* 36:373, 1992.

46. Nelson C, Braaten A, Fleeker J: The effect of synthetic dermal secretion on transfer and dissipation of the insecticide aldicarb from granular formulation to fabric. *Arch Environ Contam Toxicol* 24:513, 1993.

47. Wagai N, Tawara K: Important role of oxygen metabolites in quinolone antibacterial agent-induced cutaneous phototoxicity in mice. *Arch Toxicol* 65:495, 1991.

48. Fisher AA: Occupational dermatitis from pesticides: Patch testing procedures. *Cutis* 31:483, 492, 508, 1983.

18

NEOMYCIN SULFATE

Deborah K. Phillips

WHAT IS NEOMYCIN?

Neomycin sulfate is one of the most widely used topical antibiotics, well known for its sensitizing properties. It is available in various preparations for topical cutaneous, otic, and ophthalmologic use in both prescription and nonprescription forms (Table 18-1). Products containing neomycin are often used for postoperative wound care, minor cuts, burns, open sores, conjunctivitis, and secondarily infected skin conditions such as impetiginized dermatitis or insect bites.

Contact dermatitis to neomycin will typically present as an inflamed, weepy dermatitis in an area of prolonged or repeated use. Those affected will often note expansion of the original eruption or worsening of the underlying condition in association with their use of topical neomycin (Figs. 18-1 and 18-2). The involved skin may show eczematous changes such as increasing erythema, clusters of pinpoint blisters (Fig. 18-3), breakdown of the superficial skin, and even oozing of fluid with eventual crusting. This allergy may also involve the mucous membranes, including the conjunctiva, vaginal mucosa, or other moist surfaces. Less commonly, the reaction to neomycin may be noneczematous, in which case the skin changes are limited to the dermis and referred to as "dermal contact dermatitis."[1]

Patch-test sensitivity to neomycin in the general population is only about 1 percent,[2] whereas estimates for dermatologic clinic populations range from 3 to 7 percent.[3,4] These figures generally reflect testing to 20% neomycin applied to the back in the standard fashion. "Use" tests, on the other hand, utilize commercially available products with much lower concentrations of neomycin without occlusion. These tests are often used to look for allergy to whole products, but they can also be used to determine the clinical relevance of positive patch tests. They involve the application of commercially available products to an area of the skin such as the neck two to three times a day for about a week.[5] One study examining the relationship between patch-test reactions and clinical "use" testing noted that, although patch testing may be slightly more sensitive in detecting contact allergy to neomycin, use-test reactions were usually mild and remained localized.[5] Their findings suggest that use testing may be a helpful adjunct in evaluating the relevance of positive patch reactions, and that those individuals with positive patch tests and negative use tests are probably at a low risk for developing significant problems from the use of neomycin on a limited basis for minor skin lesions. Besides false-positive reactions that may be related to irritant effects, false-negative

TABLE 18–1. Products Containing Neomycin to Be Avoided by Neomycin-Allergic Persons

Cutaneous preparations
  Bactine First Aid Antibiotic ointment
  Campho-Phenique Triple Antibiotic ointment
  Cortisporin Cream or Ointment
  Myciguent Ointment
  Mycitracin Ointment
  NeoDecadron Topical Cream
  Neosporin Cream or Ointment
  Neosporin GU Irrigant, Sterile
  Neo-Synalar Cream
Ophthalmic preparations
  Cortisporin Ophthalmic Ointment or Suspension, Sterile
  NeoDecadron Sterile Ophthalmic Ointment or Solution
  Neosporin Ophthalmic Ointment or Solution Sterile
Otic preparations
  Coly-Mycin S Otic
  Cortisporin Otic Solution or Suspension, Sterile
  LazerSporin-C Solution
  PediOtic Suspension, Sterile

Source: From Refs. 43–46.

patch test results may also occur; these can be uncovered in some cases by the use of intradermal testing.[6]

HOW DOES ONE ACQUIRE SENSITIVITY?

Individuals at greatest risk for neomycin sensitivity appear to be those with atopic dermatitis or other chronic eczematous conditions.[7-10] Perhaps the most common skin condition associated with contact allergy results from the treatment of stasis dermatitis or stasis ulcers of the lower extremities with a topical neomycin-containing product. Up to 34 percent of individuals suffering from stasis dermatitis and leg ulcers will demonstrate sensitivity to neomycin, and of all the potential sensitizers used in the treatment of stasis dermatitis, neomycin appears to be the most common sensitizing agent.[9] Chronic otitis externa, an eczematous condition involving the external ear, is another potentially predisposing condition. The patient in Fig. 18-4, who had neomycin applied to treat external otitis, developed temporary depigmentation from the resulting contact dermatitis. The first report of neomycin sensitivity was actually that of a patient with otitis externa treated with neomycin in 1952,[11] and many such cases have appeared in the literature since that time.[12] Neomycin used for external otitis may even contribute to hearing loss.[13] Estimates of neomycin sensitivity in this disorder vary from 8 to 32 percent, and neomycin does appear to be the most common sensitizer.[10,14] Neomycin also causes prolonged or chronic conjunctivitis, blepharoconjunctivitis, and keratoconjunctivitis.[15] It may likewise play a role in persistent eyelid dermatitis.[16] Therefore, patch testing to identify relevant sensitizers should be considered in patients for whom standard therapy with topical ophthalmic preparations fails. Thus, sensitization appears

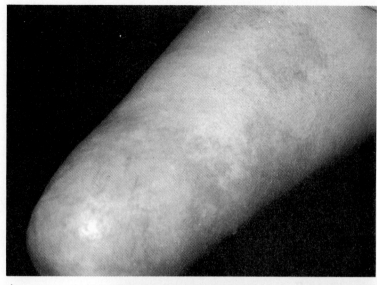

A

FIG. 18–1. *A.* Typical medication pattern of an eczema spreading around a treated lesion, in this case another eczema.   *B.* Closeup of *A.*

B

FIG. 18–2. Acute neomycin contact dermatitis of the chest.

to be enhanced by extended use for marked inflammatory conditions. Infrequent use for minor wounds, on the other hand, is not thought to pose a problem for most people.[17]

Allergic contact dermatitis to neomycin in postoperative wound care has been estimated to occur in 5.3 percent of cases.[18] Although this figure is low compared with the more eczematous skin conditions, neomycin-containing products should probably not be used on postsurgical wounds.

Medical, dental, and veterinary personnel may be at special risk for neomycin sensitivity because of their increased contact with neomycin-containing medications or with products that may cross-react with neomycin. This has been well documented

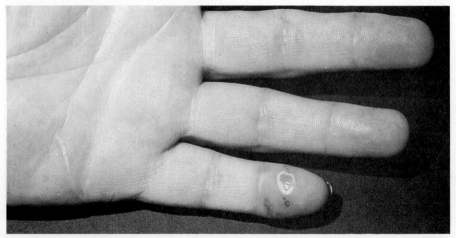

FIG. 18–3. Contact to an antibiotic ointment applied under an adhesive plaster. This sensitivity is deceiving in its appearance as it has the pattern of the agent used for occlusion.

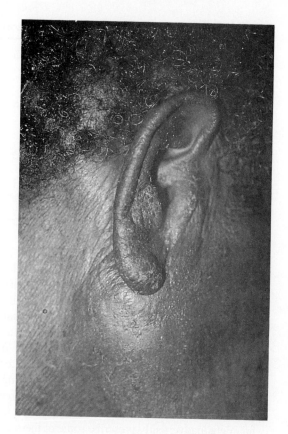

FIG. 18–4. Loss of pigment following a reaction to a neomycin topical applied to the ear canal.

in nurses, pharmacists, dentists, veterinarians, oculists, and other physicians who handle these medications.[19–23]

Additionally, neomycin is one of the allergens seen in the pediatric populations.[24] Severe allergic keratoconjunctivitis and erythema multiforme following eye instillation in a sensitive person has also been reported.[25] Sensitization appears to be increased in patients with Hailey-Hailey disease as well,[26] perhaps due to the chronic inflammatory nature of this disease and the common need for repeated topical antibiotic therapy.

A popular antibiotic preparation called Mycolog cream formerly contained both neomycin and ethylenediamine, two known sensitizers.[27] Many individuals may have acquired their sensitivity to neomycin through the use of this product, which has since been reformulated without either neomycin or ethylenediamine. However, as of August 1994, at least one generic product still contained ethylenediamine.

CAN OTHER MEDICATIONS CAUSE PROBLEMS?

Neomycin belongs to a family of antibiotics with similar structural features known as aminoglycosides. Other members of this group of antibiotics may cross-react with neomycin. For those who are sensitized to neomycin, this means that medications containing gentamicin, tobramycin, kanamycin, butirosin, amikacin, paromomycin,

TABLE 18–2. Products to Be Used with Caution in Neomycin-Allergic Persons

Cutaneous preparations
  Potential cross-reacting medications
    Garamycin Cream or Ointment
    G-myticin Creme or Ointment
  Bacitracin-containing products with the potential for concomitant allergic reactions
    Aquaphor Antibiotic Formula
    Polysporin Ointment or Powder
Ophthalmic preparations
  Potential cross-reacting medications
    Garamycin Ophthalmic Ointment or Solution, Sterile
    Tobrex Ophthalmic Ointment or Solution
  Bacitracin-containing products with the potential for concomitant allergic reactions
    Polysporin Ophthalmic Ointment, Sterile

Source: From Refs. 43–46.

spectinomyin, or streptomycin may likewise elicit contact reactions and should be avoided.[28–31] Of this group, streptomycin is the least likely to cross-react with neomycin, presumably because of the structural dissimilarities between these two aminoglycoside antibiotics.[32] Gentamicin and tobramycin ophthalmic preparations are therefore not ideal alternatives for neomycin-sensitive individuals.[31]

Neomycin-sensitive health care professionals may be repeatedly exposed to such cross-reacting antibiotics and require special precautions such as gloves as well as careful handling of the medications.[21] Patch testing can be a helpful tool in identifying related sensitizers.[31] Once these potential sensitizers are known to an individual, these products can be avoided (Table 18-2). The patient is then in a position to alert physicians who might inadvertently prescribe some of these cross-reacting antibiotics for other infections.

CONCOMITANT ALLERGIES

Many of the available topical antibiotics contain two or more unrelated antibiotics in combination. One of the more common combination preparations, Neosporin, contains neomycin, polymyxin, and bacitracin. Although neomycin and bacitracin are structurally distinct, the use of these products simultaneously may elicit a concomitant allergy.[33] This phenomenon is thought to represent independent yet simultaneous sensitization rather than actual cross-reactivity and is believed to occur when certain individuals are exposed to these popular combination antibiotic preparations.[34] Animal studies have supported this lack of true cross-sensitization.[35] Additional reports suggest that almost all of those who test positive for bacitracin sensitivity are reactive to neomycin[33,36,37]; however, a more recent report asserts that bacitracin sensitivity may occur more frequently without concomitant allergy to neomycin.[34] In any case, preparations such as Polysporin, which lack neomycin but contain bacitracin, may not be suitable alternatives for those sensitized to neomycin.[21]

Simultaneous contact allergies to all three of the antibiotics in Neosporin has also been reported.[38] The relationship between bacitracin and neomycin sensitization is thought to be concomitant, as they are often used together. However, there may be some degree of cross-sensitization between bacitracin and polymyxin, because they are produced from similar strains of bacteria.[39]

One additional feature of bacitracin sensitivity is that reactions are often delayed. Routine patch-test determinations are made at 48 and 72 h, but reactions to bacitracin may not be evident for at least 96 h. Bacitracin hypersensitivity may have been missed in some individuals because of this delayed reactivity, and the actual incidence of sensitivity may be much higher than previously estimated.[34] This problem of delayed sensitivity has also been described with neomycin.[3]

SYSTEMIC CONTACT DERMATITIS

Although the site of exposure in contact dermatitis is usually cutaneous, systemic exposure to neomycin may evoke a cutaneous reaction in sensitive persons. Such reactions to oral, intravenous, or intramuscularly administered medications manifest in a variety of ways, including a flare at the site of the original eruption[40] or a reaction at prior patch-test sites. A more diffuse eruption known as exfoliative erythroderma has also been described in a neomycin-sensitive individual who was given a cross-reactive antibiotic intravenously.[41] The cross-reacting aminoglycosides are used systemically for a wide array of infections and should be used with caution in neomycin-

---

TABLE 18–3. Antibiotic Substitutes for Neomycin-Allergic Persons

Cutaneous preparations
  Achromycin Ointment
  Akne-Mycin Ointment
  Aureomycin Ointment
  Bactroban Ointment
  Betadine Ointment
  Chloromycetin Cream
  Furacin Topical Cream
  Silvadene Cream
  Silver sulfadiazine cream
Ophthalmic preparations (suitable for both ocular and cutaneous use)
  Achromycin Ophthalmic Ointment or Suspension
  Chibroxin Sterile Ophthalmic Solution
  Chloromycetin Ophthalmic Ointment or Solution
  Gantrisin Ophthalmic Ointment
  Ilotycin Ophthalmic Ointment
  Polytrim Ophthalmic Solution, Sterile
  Sodium Sulamyd Ophthalmic Ointment or Solution
  Terra-Cortril Ophthalmic Suspension
  Terramycin Ophthalmic Ointment, Sterile
Otic preparations
  Castellani paint
  Chloromycetin Otic
  Otic Domeboro Solution
  VoSol Otic Solution
  VoSol HC Otic Solution

Source: From Refs. 43–46.

NEOMYCIN—PATIENT HANDOUT

Neomycin is one of the most widely used topical antibiotics, well known for its sensitizing (allergic) properties. Both prescription and nonprescription preparations are available for treating a variety of skin disorders as well as inflammatory or infectious processes involving the eyes or external ears. An allergic reaction to neomycin commonly presents as an inflamed, weepy rash in an area of prolonged or repeated use. Patients often note expansion of the original eruption or worsening of the underlying condition.

The information in this handout is provided to help you understand the meaning of a positive patch test and to offer suggestions for suitable alternative products. While patch tests for contact sensitivity are not perfect predictors of allergic reactions and negative reactions do not guarantee absolute safety, they do provide individuals with valuable information for avoiding potential allergens.

WHAT DOES A POSITIVE PATCH TEST MEAN TO YOU?

In general, a positive patch test means that neomycin-containing products or those with a comparable chemical structure should be avoided. These include the following:

A. Antibiotics containing *neomycin*
1. *Topical* (skin): Bactine, Campho-Phenique, Cortisporin, Myciguent, Mycitracin, NeoDecadron, Neosporin, Neo-Synalar
2. *Ophthalmic* (eyes): Cortisporin, NeoDecadron, Neosporin
3. *Otic* (ears): Coly-Mycin S, Cortisporin, LazerSporin-C, PediOtic
4. *Misc:* Neomycin Sulfate tablets (for oral intake) or Neosporin GU irrigant

B. Antibiotics with *similar chemical structures*
1. *Topical* (skin): Garamycin, G-myticin
2. *Ophthalmic* (eyes): Garamycin, Tobrex
3. *Systemic* (inside the body): Aminoglycoside antibiotics such as gentamicin, tobramycin, or amikacin

C. Bacitracin-containing products with *potential* for accompanying allergic reactions
1. *Topical* (skin): Aquaphor Antibiotic Formula, Polysporin
2. *Ophthalmic* (eyes): Polysporin

This information is provided to help persons with contact dermatitis in the understanding of their problem. The contents are subject to change as more information becomes available and are not intended as a substitute for medical treatment.

WHAT SUBSTITUTES ARE AVAILABLE?

A. *Topical* (skin) antibiotics: Achromycin, Akne-Mycin, Aureomycin, Bactroban, Betadine, Chloromycetin, Furacin, Silvadene, and Silver Sulfadiazine
B. *Ophthalmic* (eyes) antibiotics: Achromycin, Chibroxin, Chloromycetin, Gantrisin, Ilotycin, Polytrim, Sodium Sulamyd, Terra-Cortril, and Terramycin
C. *Otic* (ears) antibiotics: Castellani's paint, Chloromycetin, Otic Domeboro, and VoSol

OTHER PRECAUTIONS

Individuals with atopic dermatitis or other chronic eczematous conditions such as stasis dermatitis or otitis externa are at greatest risk for developing neomycin sensitivity. These individuals should carefully read the labels of all "over-the-counter" products for possible sensitizers and alert their physicians to potential problems with any prescription medications containing neomycin or related products, as listed above.

Medical, dental, and veterinary personnel are also at special risk for neomycin reactions if their work requires contact with neomycin or related antibiotics. These individuals should take precautions, such as using gloves, masks, protective eyewear, and gowns as needed, to prevent contact with the skin or mucous membranes.

sensitive individuals. Oral neomycin is occasionally used preoperatively for bowel surgery and hepatic cirrhosis,[38] and although oral absorption is poor, systemic contact dermatitis can be precipitated by oral neomycin.[42] Systemic administration should be avoided in those with known cutaneous sensitization. The exact mechanism for this phenomenon is unknown.

ARE SAFE ALTERNATIVES AVAILABLE?

Neomycin-sensitive individuals should avoid the many neomycin-based topical preparations available. In general, safe alternatives are erythromycin, mupirocin, tetracycline, or iodine-based products such as Betadine (Table 18-3). Cross-reacting antibiotics in the aminoglycoside family, as well as potential concomitant allergens, should also be avoided in these individuals.

Many preparations for the treatment of infections involving the external ear also contain neomycin. Alternatives include Castellani paint, an antifungal agent with drying properties, acetic acid preparations, and chloramphenicol-based medications.

Likewise, several antibiotics used for treating ophthalmic infections contain neomycin. Erythromycin, sulfa, chloramphenicol, tetracycline, or norfloxacin-based products are considered safe alternatives.

REFERENCES

1. Shouji A: Dermal contact dermatitis induced by neomycin. *Nippon Rinsho* 35:210–212, 1977.
2. Prystowsky SD, Allen AM, Smith RW, et al: Allergic contact hypersensitivity to nickel, neomycin, ethylenediamine, and benzocaine. *Arch Dermatol* 115:959–962, 1979.
3. Patrick J, Panzer JD: Neomycin sensitivity in the normal (nonatopic) individual. *Arch Dermatol* 102:532–535, 1970.
4. Rudner EJ, Clendenning WE, Epstein E, et al: Epidemiology of contact dermatitis in North America. *Arch Dermatol* 108:537–540, 1973.
5. Prystowsky SD, Nonomura JH, Smith RW, Allen AM: Allergic hypersensitivity to neomycin. *Arch Dermatol* 115:713–715, 1979.
6. Epstein E: Contact dermatitis to neomycin with false negative patch tests: Allergy established by intradermal and usage tests. *Contact Dermatitis* 6:219–220, 1980.
7. Epstein S: Neomycin sensitivity and atopy. *Dermatologica* 130:280–286, 1965.
8. Wereide K: Neomycin sensitivity in atopic dermatitis and other eczematous conditions. *Acta Derm Venereol* 50:114–116, 1970.
9. Fraki JE, Peltonen L, Hopsu-Havu VK: Allergy to various components of topical preparations in stasis dermatitis and leg ulcer. *Contact Dermatitis* 5:97–100, 1979.
10. Smith IM, Keay DG, Buxton PK: Contact hypersensitivity in patients with chronic otitis externa. *Clin Otolaryngol* 15:155–158, 1990.
11. Baer RL, Ludwig JS: Allergic eczematous sensitization to neomycin. *Ann Allerg* 10:136–137, 1952.
12. Jensen OC, Mordecai LR: Neomycin contact dermatitis superimposed on otitis externa. *JAMA* 195:175–177, 1966.
13. Podoshin L, Fradis M, Ben David J: Ototoxicity of ear drops in patients suffering from chronic otitis media. *J Laryngol Otolaryngol* 103:46–50, 1989.
14. Rasmussen PA: Otitis externa and allergic contact dermatitis. *Acta Otolaryngol* 77:344–347, 1974.
15. Hatinen A, Terasvirta M, Fraki JE: Contact allergy to components in topical ophthalmologic preparations. *Acta Ophthalmol* 63:424–426, 1985.
16. Nethercott JR, Nield G, Holness DL: A review of 79 cases of eyelid dermatitis. *J Am Acad Dermatol* 21:223–230, 1989.
17. Leyden JJ, Kligman AM: Contact dermatitis to neomycin sulfate. *JAMA* 242:1276–1278, 1979.
18. Gette MT, Marks JG, Maloney ME: Frequency of postoperative allergic contact dermatitis to topical antibiotics. *Arch Dermatol* 128:365–367, 1992.
19. Strauss MJ, Warring FC: Contact dermatitis from streptomycin. *J Invest Dermatol* 9:3, 1947.
20. Wilson HT: Streptomycin dermatitis in nurses. *Br Med J* 1:1378, 1958.
21. Fisher AA: *Contact Dermatitis,* 3d ed. Philadelphia, Lea & Febiger, 1986, pp 199–200.
22. Falk ES, Hektoen H, Thune PO: Skin and respiratory tract symptoms in veterinary surgeons. *Contact Dermatitis* 12:274–278, 1985.
23. Rebandel P, Rudzki E: Occupational contact sensitivity in oculists. *Contact Dermatitis* 15:92, 1986.
24. Barros MA, Baptista A, Correia TM, Azevedo F: Patch testing in children: A study of 562 school children. *Contact Dermatitis* 25:156–159, 1991.
25. Sherertz EF, Reed JW, Zanolli MD, Goldsmith SM: Severe allergic keratoconjunctivitis and erythema multiforme after a routine eye examination: Discerning the cause. *Ann Ophthalmol* 23:173–176, 1991.
26. Reitama S, Remitz A, Lauerma AI, Forstrom L: Contact allergies in patients with familial benign chronic pemphigus. *J Am Acad Dermatol* 21:506–510, 1989.
27. Hogan DJ, Hill M, Lane PR: Results of routine patch testing of 542 patients in Saskatoon, Canada. *Contact Dermatitis* 19:120–124, 1988.
28. Pirila V, Pirila L: Sensitization to the neomycin group of antibiotics. *Acta Derm Venereol* 46:489–496, 1966.
29. Forstrom L, Pirila V: Cross-sensitivity within the neomycin group of antibiotics. *Contact Dermatitis* 4:312, 1978.

30. Chung CW, Carson TR: Sensitization potentials and immunologic specificities of neomycin. *J Invest Dermatol* 64:158, 1975.
31. Schorr WF, Ridgway HB: Tobramycin-neomycin cross sensitivity. *Contact Dermatitis* 3:133–137, 1977.
32. Samsoen M, Metz R, Melchior E, Foussereau J: Cross-sensitivity between aminoglycoside antibiotics. *Contact Dermatitis* 6:141, 1980.
33. Bjorkner B, Moller H: Bacitracin: A cutaneous allergen and histamine liberator. *Acta Derm Venereol* 53:487–492, 1973.
34. Katz BE, Fisher AA: Bacitracin: A unique topical antibiotic sensitizer. *J Am Acad Dermatol* 17:1016–1024, 1987.
35. Epstein S, Wenzel F: Cross-sensitivity to various "mycins." *Arch Dermatol* 86:183–185, 1962.
36. Pirila V, Rouhunkosky S: On sensitivity to neomycin and bacitracin. *Acta Derm Venereol* 39:470–473, 1959.
37. Binnick AN, Clendenning WE: Bacitracin contact dermatitis. *Contact Dermatitis* 4:180–181, 1978.
38. Grandinetti PJ, Fowler JF: Simultaneous contact allergy to neomycin, bacitracin, and polymyxin. *J Am Acad Dermatol* 23:646–647, 1990.
39. Van Ketel WG: Polymyxin B sulfate. *Contact Dermatitis Newsletter* 15:445, 1974.
40. Elelund AF, Moller H: Oral provocation in eczematous contact allergy to neomycin and hydroxyquinolines. *Acta Derm Venereol* 49:422, 1969.
41. Guin JD, Phillips D: Erythroderma from systemic contact dermatitis: A complication of systemic gentamicin in a patient with contact allergy to neomycin. *Cutis* 43:564–567, 1989.
42. Menne T, Weismann K: Hematogenous contact eczema following oral administration of neomycin. *Hautarzt* 35:319–320, 1984.
43. *Physicians' Desk Reference,* 46th ed. Montvale NJ, Medical Economics Data, 1992.
44. *Physicians' Desk Reference for Nonprescription Drugs.* Montvale NJ, Medical Economics Data, 1992.
45. Scheman AJ: *Pocket Guide to Medications Used in Dermatology,* 3d ed. Baltimore, Williams & Wilkins, 1992, pp 32–33, 108–110.
46. Fisher AA: *Contact Dermatitis,* 3d ed. Philadelphia, Lea & Febiger, 1986, p 197.

19

THIURAM MIX

Jere D. Guin

WHAT ARE THIURAMS AND WHY ARE THEY IMPORTANT?

Thiurams are chemicals which contain a basic urea structure except that a sulfur is substituted for oxygen, making the basic structure similar to a thiourea. These chemicals are mostly used in the rubber industry as accelerators, but they also have a range of activities based on germ killing. Thiuram chemicals are important because they are the most common cause of allergy to rubber. This has become a major problem in health care because it alters the methodology for protective measures for both health care workers and their patients.[1] Perhaps of greatest importance is their tendency to cause contact dermatitis to latex gloves. The thiuram mix is a mixture of four rubber chemicals with a similar structure.

The mixture of thiurams comprises tetramethylthiuram disulfide (TMTD), tetraethyl-thiuram disulfide (TETD), dipentamethylenethiuram disulfide (PTD), and tetramethyl-thiuram monosulfide (TMTM) (Fig. 19-1). By far the most important in the group is TMTD. The components are usually equal in proportion, so that a 0.25% concentration of each agent is contained within the mix, to make a total of 1% thiuram chemical in petrolatum. The rank order of importance in this mixture is TMTD>TMTM>TETD> PTD based on the number of isolated reactions or TMTM>TMTD>TETD>PTD based on the number of positive reactions.[2]

HOW COMMON IS THE PROBLEM?

Approximately 5 percent of persons who are patch tested routinely in the United States are allergic to thiuram, according to Nethercott et al.,[3] and this has changed little since 1974.[4] Approximately 5 percent of individuals tested are allergic to thiuram at the first reading and 5.4 percent at the second reading, for a total of 5.5 percent with relevant reactions.[3] This is quite high, and the percentage seems to be increasing, perhaps because of the widespread use of latex gloves in health-related professions. Two studies in Europe in 1984–1987 and in 1989 showed response rates of 3.2 percent.[5] The rate was 3 percent[6] in a study done in 1989 in Belgium. About 4.5 percent of the individuals tested positive in a test to the thiuram mix in a similar 10-year study.[7] This test is more commonly positive than the other rubber mixes or mercaptobenzothiazole (MBT).[8]

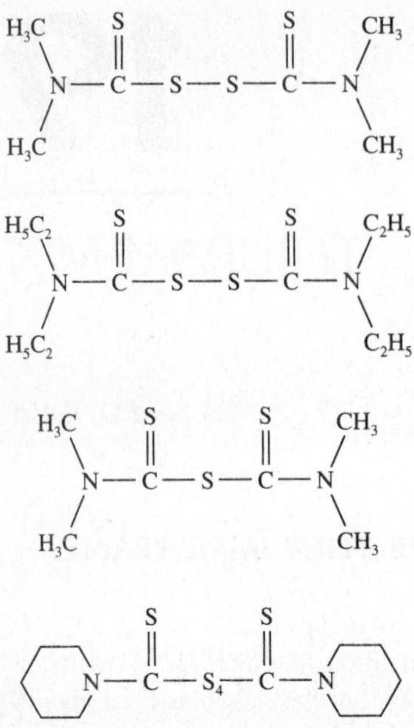

FIG. 19-1. Structure of the ingredients of thiuram mix. *From top to bottom:* tetramethylthiuram disulfide (TMTD), tetraethylthiuram disulfide (TETD), tetramethylthiuram monosulfide (TMTM), and dipentamethylenethiuram disulfide (PTD).

More than half of all rubber-sensitive persons are reactive to thiuram mix, which is somewhat higher than the next most frequent screening antigen,[9] and thiuram mix is a much better screening antigen for rubber sensitivity than either MBT[10] or carba mix, which may not be as regularly positive.[11,12]

HOW DOES ONE RECOGNIZE THIURAM CONTACT DERMATITIS?

THE GLOVE PATTERN

By far the most common area of contact dermatitis in individuals sensitive to thiuram is on the hands, because of the incidence of rubber glove dermatitis. The pattern in surgeons and surgical nurses varies, but one frequently sees a diffuse eruption of the palms and dorsa of the hands (Fig. 19-2) with a sharp cutoff at the wrists (Fig. 19-3). It may or may not be uniform and it may mimic pompholyx.[13] Not infrequently, contact dermatitis is superimposed upon another eczema, especially contact dermatitis as the patient tries to protect himself or herself from what is perceived to be a problem.[9,13] For example, hairdressers not infrequently become allergic to both glyceryl monothioglycolate and rubber gloves, as latex gloves are not adequate protection. One frequently sees allergy to glutaraldehyde[14,15] as well as to latex gloves in medical and dental personnel, as that allergen also penetrates what is thought to be a protective barrier. Therefore, in health care workers considered to have possible glove allergy, it is often rewarding to test to glutaraldehyde as well as rubber antigens.

Glove dermatitis[16,17] is not limited to surgeons, surgical scrub nurses,[18] and dentists,[19]

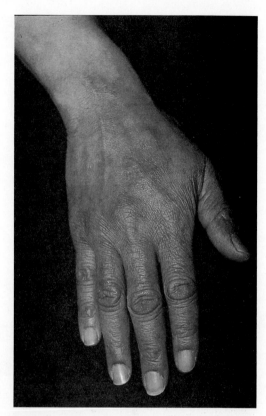

FIG. 19–2. Glove dermatitis in a dentist. Patch tests were positive to the glove and strongly reactive to thiuram mix.

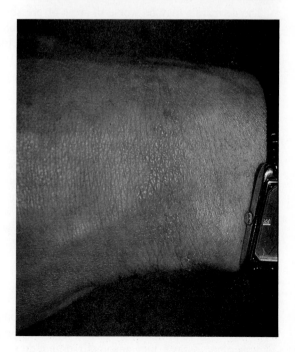

FIG. 19–3. Closeup of Fig. 19–2, demonstrating the sharp cutoff at the wrist.

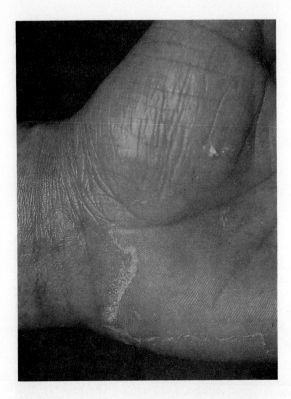

FIG. 19–4. Closeup of the palmar side of the lesion in Fig. 19–2. It is advisable to examine the feet in such patients, as they not infrequently also react to athletic shoes.

however, as one may also see it in housekeeping employees[20] and others, from hairdressers to housewives.

The dermatitis may be worse in areas of pressure or may have a typical glovelike distribution (Figs. 19-2, 19-3, and 19-4). While thiuram is not present in all latex, it is certainly the leading cause of sensitivity to latex gloves. Not infrequently, sensitivity is seen also on the plantar surface of the foot (Fig. 19-5), and sensitivity to other rubber chemicals may accompany thiuram sensitivity.

AIRBORNE PATTERN

The eruption from this is not limited to the hands, because many different rubber objects may contain thiurams and it may be sprayed on grass or other plants as a fungicide.[21] Thus an airborne contact dermatitis can occur from agricultural chemicals that are sprayed.[22] A fruit grower seen by Dooms-Goossens[23] broke out in exposed sites after walking near an area where fruit trees were being sprayed. Thiurams may also cause airborne contact in health care workers who apply spray dressings to surgical wounds.[24]

PHOTODERMATITIS

Thiuram sensitivity may be associated with photodermatitis,[25] perhaps as part of the extended antigen syndrome. While thiurams may produce a positive *Candida albicans* phototoxicity assay,[26] they apparently do not do so clinically, even in animal studies.

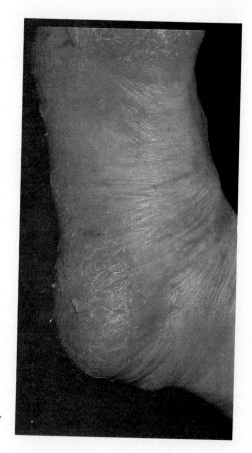

FIG. 19–5. Insole dermatitis to shoes caused by
thiuram sensitivity.

SYSTEMIC CONTACT DERMATITIS

Systemic contact dermatitis may be initiated in several ways, including the administration of disulfiram (Antabuse). Webb et al.[27] described a bartender who took disulfiram and, 5 h after the first dose, awoke with diffuse itching, swelling of the feet, and a vesicular eruption of the face, arms, and feet. He also had had a history of waistband dermatitis.

Disulfiram is tetraethylthiuramdisulfide. The systemic administration of this for prophylaxis of alcoholism and for the treatment of nickel dermatitis may, in sensitive individuals, cause a systemic reaction. Van Hecke's patient had pompholyx, acute nummular dermatitis of the extremities, and an old scar site.[28] This chemical can also be ingested as a preservative in jams and jellies, causing recrudescence of previous dermatitis of the hands and feet.[29]

Can "systemic" contact dermatitis be "local"? The same drug can be administered in pellet form as a skin implant; this is sometimes followed by an eczematous dermatitis in the area. When the disulfiram pellets are buried deeply, the drug does not tend to cause difficulty. However, it will produce a local dermatitis or a systemic dermatitis when implanted closer to the surface.[30]

PSEUDOSYSTEMIC CONTACT DERMATITIS

Another unusual form of systemic dermatitis has been attributed to rubber parts in hemodialysis equipment,[31,32] but a better explanation may be the rubber gloves of the personnel who administer the treatment[33] rather than the equipment used.

CONDOMS

Dermatitis from condoms[34] like that from latex gloves, is also most commonly due to thiuramic accelerators,[34] but it does not seem to be as serious a problem as that with rubber gloves.[1] The reason for this is not known, but the fact that condoms are coagulant-dipped and gloves are straight-dipped is often given as an explanation. Another reason may have to do with the fact that the type of lubricant used for condoms should be nonlipid, as lipid materials tend to degrade rubber.[35]

MEDICAL AND DENTAL RUBBER REACTIONS

Glove dermatitis may occur elsewhere than on the hand, not only on people who wear gloves but also in rubber-sensitive patients when exposed to the gloves of health care workers.[36] This may be in the form of either dermatitis or urticaria. Frequently lesions in and around the mouth are seen in the patients of dentists who employ rubber gloves or use rubber dams. Disulfiram may cause an alcohol flush when the patient is exposed to alcohol, a dyshidrotic and nummular eczema, and other forms of systemic contact dermatitis.[37-40] It may also cause contact dermatitis from implantation[30] and exposure during manufacture.[41]

Other medical causes include prostheses for amputees (Fig. 19-6),[42] surgical tape,[43] and dressing.[44]

OTHER SOURCES OF CONTACT

Sensitivity to thiuram may occur in a wide range of uses including balloons, clothing, protective aprons, pillows, sponges, applicators, pesticides, putty, tires, rubber bands, adhesives, plastic-treated seeds, fungicides, neoprene (chloroprene), germicides, insecticides, soluble oils, paints, animal repellants, soaps, shampoos, finger cots, gaskets, and many other applications.

HOW DO PATIENTS BECOME ALLERGIC TO THIURAM?

This is not easily answered. Not infrequently, health care workers who regularly wear rubber gloves are exposed to the chemical in quantity. Persons with hand dermatitis due to another cause commonly attempt to protect the sensitive area by wearing rubber gloves, only to find themselves suddenly allergic to rubber gloves. By far the most common sensitizer in rubber gloves is one of the thiurams. When Knudsen et al.[45]

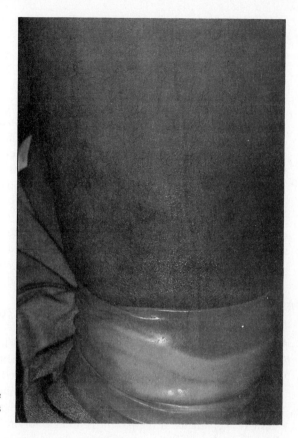

FIG. 19–6. Contact dermatitis to the rubber sleeve on a prosthesis. This was caused by thiuram allergy.

investigated the levels of thiuram and carbamates released from latex gloves exposed to "synthetic sweat," they were similar to those released by the patch-testing reagent, and the severity of patch tests to the gloves paralleled the amount of thiuram or carbamate released. Knudsen et al. also found that surgical gloves caused more problems with patch-test reactions than household gloves, even though both were made of natural rubber. Estlander et al.[46] reported 108 cases of rubber dermatitis; 68 of these were caused by gloves. Of these, 38 reacted to both the patch-test reagent and the glove, 11 only to the patch-test reagent, and 14 only to the gloves. There were 5 cases of sensitivity to polyvinylchloride in this group.

CONTACT URTICARIA

Contact urticaria to rubber gloves can be a severe problem. While this was reported in a few cases to be due to rubber chemicals, none of these chemicals were thiurams.[47] Contact urticaria from rubber is more often caused by a "protein" with molecular mass of 2000 to 30,000 daltons[48,49] or more. Interestingly, not all rubber condoms are equally allergenic, so it may be possible to reduce risk when we know how to manufacture rubber products without the presence of the allergen. Investigation requires testing for immediate hypersensitivity rather than patch testing. Methodology for this, including modified prick testing (with reduced antigen levels), is given in Table 19-1.

SOURCES OF THIURAM EXPOSURE

Tetramethylthiuramdisulfide may be present as a fungicide or an animal repellant. In neoprene adhesives—as in antioxidants and polyolefin plastics; the crepe soles of shoes; lubricating oils; putty; rubber accelerators; repellants for rabbits, rats, deer, and meadow mice; soaps and shoes[50]; rubber bands[51]; and rubber banknote counters.[52] Everyday exposure may occur from such innocuous items as shoes and boots,[34,53] elasticized underclothing,[34] tires,[54] eyelash curlers,[55] or even soap.[56] Unsuspected contacts may involve the use of these chemicals as pesticides[57] or fungicides[58] or in unsuspected areas of exposure, as in baking or cooking.[59]

Polychloroprene synthetic rubber, which often goes under the name of neoprene, may contain tetramethylthiuramdisulfide, which is added to control the level of polymerization. This type rubber is often used in oils, solvents, heat- and weather-resistant rubber products, gaskets, seals, water-protective coatings, putty, paint, and so on.[60]

MANAGEMENT OF THIURAM SENSITIVITY

Patients who are allergic to thiuram should be aware of their sensitivity to rubber gloves. They should inform a dentist or a doctor when they make an appointment that they are sensitive to rubber gloves, and this should be restated prior to any examination or operative procedure. It is also wise to know whether or not one is allergic to vinyl as well as rubber, because most physicians and dentists will use vinyl gloves in rubber-sensitive individuals. If the patient is allergic to vinyl, this could also be a problem. Some have advocated the use of rubber gloves free of the chemicals to which patients are sensitive on patch testing, and lists of the contents are given by manufacturers.[17,61] However, some products may contain rubber chemicals which are unknown to the manufacturer, as they may have been added prior to the time the glove manufacturer works with the product.[45] Therefore the safest pathway is to use a "safe" product but also to patch test to a finger of the glove prior to wearing it.

TABLE 19-1. Testing for Contact Urticaria to Rubber

1. Use the finger of a glove on a patient's wet finger as a first test and only do the prick test if the glove test is negative. Preparations to manage a potential anaphylactic reaction should be at hand.

2. Glove material (1 cm square or so), sterile glove material, and sterile saline (about 5 mL) are agitated from 1/2 h or less to a day or more and a drop of the solution is put on the skin (usually the forearm).

3. Through this, the epidermis is pricked with the bevel of a sterile 30-gauge needle angled so as not to cause bleeding. Both negative and positive controls are used.

4. Histamine to stimulate gastric acid secretion (about 2.75 mg/mL) is used as a positive control and sterile saline as a negative control. A drop of each is placed on an area clearly separate from but in plain view of the test site, and the skin is pricked similarly with a sterile needle.

5. Patch-test materials for the rubber chemicals in the standard tray are applied for 5 to 10 min, removed, and read after a few minutes. The area selected is one where contact urticaria has occurred previously.

6. Epinephrine, trained medical personnel, and rubber-free resuscitation equipment should be on hand, to be used in the event of systemic symptomatology.

For individuals who have contact urticaria, everyone familiar with the case should know about rubber during any hospitalization, laboratory procedure, or office examination. Untoward reactions to rubber products can occur from seemingly harmless exposures, as with an enema tube, a rubber mask, or elasticized bandages. In individuals who have urticarial and indeed anaphylactic reactions to rubber, prophylactic medication should be considered if there is any chance that they will be exposed to a rubber product inadvertently.

For those who have contact dermatitis to rubber gloves, patch testing should be done to any substitute glove before it is used. Vinyl gloves will be an effective substitute in many people. Sometimes, for nonsterile applications, polyethylene can be used. The 4-H glove, a layered glove with polyethylene surfaces, can be used by individuals who must protect their hands from external exposure to chemicals such as glutaraldehyde or formaldehyde. This is a valid consideration in health care workers who must work around Cidex, which contains glutaraldehyde. Glutaraldehyde will penetrate rubber and to a lesser degree vinyl, so protective gloves are in order, and 4-H gloves are available as sterile gloves.

Another possible type of sterile glove is the Elastyren glove, which contains a very low level of carbamates but no thiurams. These gloves are satisfactory substitutes unless one is extremely sensitive to carbamates. A relatively safe glove overall is the Tactylon glove (Smart Practice, Phoenix, AZ). From the data available, this product would probably be a problem only for individuals who are sensitive to glove powder. There are lists available, in two publications, of rubber gloves that do not contain thiuram.[17,61] Unfortunately, many individuals who are allergic to rubber will break out to latex materials even though these materials ostensibly do not contain the allergens to which the individual tests positive. There are many reasons for this. First of all, many rubber products are contaminated by rubber chemicals without the manufacturer's knowledge, but they can be found by qualitative analytical techniques. In addition, there may be antigens present in rubber to which an individual is allergic and which are not in the test tray. Furthermore, the fingertips of rubber gloves are often treated chemically in order to give traction to the areas where gripping is important, so as to make these gloves more functional during surgical procedures. Therefore, patch testing should be done with the tip of the index finger or thumb from a surgical glove. These are usually tested in the form of a 1-cm or smaller square which is held in place for a period of 48 h provided that there is no urticarial component. It is then marked carefully and removed. This is read twice, either at 48 or 72 h and once again later. Most individuals who are negative on testing can safely wear this rubber product. But false-negative tests do occasionally occur. In addition, testing to gloves which would be worn as an alternative would be a good idea, because it reduces the testing procedures to one test and two readings rather than a different test with each finding. In other words, one should test to the fingertip of a "safe" latex glove which one plans to wear as a substitute, to a vinyl which will be worn in the event the latex glove causes a positive reaction, and perhaps to Tactylon as well, so that there is always something available. All these are available both as sterile and nonsterile gloves. If there is a problem with gripping, it is sometimes possible to use a latex glove over a safe glove, but accidents do happen.

Shoes that contain sponge rubber insoles may also be a problem. Not infrequently, glove-sensitive professionals will, when their shoes and socks are removed, have a

(Text continues on p. 191)

THIURAM MIX—PATIENT HANDOUT

WHAT IS THIURAM MIX?

Thiurams are chemicals used in the rubber industry to help cure rubber. The quality of rubber depends on how it is processed. When Columbus came to America, he found Native Americans who played with rubber balls and who protected their clothing with a rubber-coated material. The discovery was largely a curiosity until Charles Goodyear, in the nineteenth century, learned how to "vulcanize" rubber so that the properties were more usable. At first, sulfur and heat were used, but later sulfur-containing chemicals were found to cross-link the chains of "rubber" molecules to produce the properties we now recognize as typical of rubber. The type of product largely determines which chemicals are used, but thiurams are commonly found, especially in latex gloves. Thiurams also have a germ-killing quality and they are used as fungicides and pesticides. Formerly a thiuram was added to Lifebuoy soap to impart a germ-killing quality.

The test material to which you reacted is a mixture of four different but similar chemicals commonly used to cure rubber. A mixture is employed as a practical matter, as this allows testing to four such chemicals with one test. One of these four will detect about 9 out of 10 persons allergic to thiuram mix, so testing with only one of these chemicals would miss some.

WHAT DOES A POSITIVE TEST MEAN?

Positive tests suggest that you are allergic to certain forms of rubber. Whether or not the current skin problem is due to your allergy to thiurams will depend upon the evidence. It may be related to your present problem, but since allergy tends to stay for a long time, it could be just an older allergy from a previous exposure.

HOW COMMON IS ALLERGY TO THIURAM MIX?

In the United States, about 5 percent of the population tested for contact allergy is allergic to this chemical, and this percentage seems to have been relatively stable since 1972–1974. In the United States, thiuram is the most commonly positive of the rubber chemicals. It may be a bit less common in Europe, but more than half of rubber-sensitive persons are reactive to this test alone.

WHAT DOES A THIURAM RASH LOOK LIKE?

Thiurams can cause rashes (eczemas) in many areas and in any of several patterns. By far the most common location is on the hands, where rubber gloves are worn.

This is often in a glovelike pattern, with a sharp cutoff at the wrist. It may also be worse in pressure areas, either due to rubber allergy or sometimes contact with a second material to which you are allergic. This would be especially true in orthopedic surgeons, who become allergic to a plastic material used in the operating room, and in hairdressers, who become allergic to acid perms. This type of allergy is seen not just in doctors, dentists and nurses, either, as many persons with hand eczema become allergic to rubber in trying to protect their hands from other allergens. Sometimes there is an eczema on the bottoms of the feet as well, as many shoes contain rubber.

Allergic persons working in agricultural environments where thiurams are sprayed to kill fungi can break out diffusely wherever they are exposed. Nurses have reacted similarly to a "spray-on" surgical dressing. This normally involves the face, neck, hands, and arms in what is called an airborne pattern. The rash can also come from the hands, when this chemical is inadvertently handled and transferred to other areas with the hands.

A medication taken to prevent alcoholism and to prevent nickel allergy is called Antabuse. This is a thiuram which may cause a drug rash in allergic persons. Such cases may show swelling of the hands and feet and water blisters on the hands and fingers. Antabuse may cause a local reaction when it is "implanted" in the skin. It may also be used as a preservative in jams and jellies; on ingestion, such foods can cause a flare of the allergy.

WHAT ARE SOME SOURCES?

There are many rubber objects which *may* contain thiurams, but rubber gloves are the chief source of exposure. Condoms are occasionally a problem, and almost any rubber object is suspect. Articles of clothing such as shoes, elastic in underwear, and protective aprons would be typical examples. Other items found around the house might include balloons, pillows, sponges, applicators, putty, rubber bands, soap (in some countries), and almost any rubber object.

Other sources include farm and garden exposure to pesticides (insecticides), fungicides, plastic-treated seed, animal repellants, and agricultural products. Exposures in health workers include finger cots, surgical spray-on dressings, rubber dams used by dentists, dialysis equipment, and, of course, gloves. Industrial exposure may occur from chemical or rubber manufacture, soluble oils, paints, banknote counters, neoprene rubber, tires, and, of course, rubber gloves. Occupational exposure may even be seen in bakers.

CAN PATIENTS BREAK OUT TO GLOVES USED BY PHYSICIANS AND DENTISTS?

Yes, they may. Dental patients typically break out around the mouth and surgery patients may break out in the area of the operation. This is a special problem for those with hives from rubber, but that problem seldom stems from thiurams. The amount of the chemical which comes out of the rubber gloves from exposure to sweat is as much as from the test done for allergy, so it can be a significant source of exposure.

HOW COULD I HAVE BECOME ALLERGIC TO THIURAM?

This is often impossible to know, but chronic exposure is a problem, especially when rubber gloves are used to protect another contact dermatitis. Sensitivity in nurses, physicians, and dental assistants not infrequently is accompanied by allergy to glutaraldehyde, a germ killer used to sterilize instruments, and hairdressers allergic to gloves may also be allergic to acid perms.

WHAT CAN BE DONE TO PREVENT EXPOSURE?

Rubber gloves free of thiurams are available, but often persons allergic to thiurams are also allergic to other rubber chemicals. Therefore you should be patch tested to any rubber object you intend to wear. Sometimes vinyl gloves are a suitable substitute, but some persons are allergic to both rubber and vinyl. If this is the case, Tactylon gloves are a good substitute for almost everyone. Elastyren gloves are acceptable if patch tests are negative. This product is not made of natural rubber, but it contains low levels of carbamates, a related group of rubber chemicals, which cause a problem in some persons who are allergic to thiurams. Patch tests to gloves should probably be done with the (index) fingertip area of the glove, and tests are read twice at two to three days and once again later.

You should inform any physician, dentist, or other health worker of your allergy far enough in advance to test you to the gloves they plan to use. Even examination gloves can be a problem, so warn physicians and dentists about this at any regular visit. Rubber oxygen and anesthesia masks, catheters, enema tubes, and other components of equipment can be a problem, especially with chronic use. Oral Antabuse should be avoided.

Shoes free of sponge-rubber insoles are recommended, but if there is already involvement of the soles of the feet, patch tests to any pair of shoes should be done to the part of the shoe which touches the worst area of the rash. You should not wear a pair causing a positive test. Persons allergic to condoms can purchase non-rubber condoms which are usually satisfactory for birth control, but these may not protect as well against AIDS. The contents are not standard, so patch testing is indicated if there is a question.

dermatitis on the plantar surface of the foot along with the glove dermatitis. Sometimes this problem is clinically significant and sometimes it is not.

Condom dermatitis has been reported to be due to thiurams in some cases. Why the incidence of dermatitis due to condoms does not seem to match that of rubber gloves is a question, but it is probably explained by the methods of dipping used in producing the glove or condom. Condoms are coagulant-dipped, whereas gloves are straight-dipped. Gloves are also used with oily materials which tend to degrade rubber. Oily lubricants are contraindicated with condoms because of the degradation and breakdown of rubber in the presence of any oily material such as mineral oil, petrolatum, or vegetable oil.[35] Of 9 individuals who were condom-sensitive in a series reported by Wilson,[34] all reacted to dipentomethylenethiuram disulfide, four were allergic to tetramethylthiuramdisulfide, one to mercaptobenzothiazole, and one to zinc diethyldithiocarbamate. An attempt has been made to produce hypoallergenic condoms, but this was not successful, in at least one trial.[62]

REFERENCES

1. Guin JD: The doctor's surgical/examination gloves—Problems with and without them. *Int J Dermatol* 31:853–855, 1992.
2. Themido R, Brandae FM: Contact allergy to thiurams. *Contact Dermatitis* 10:251, 1984.
3. Nethercott JR, Holness DM, Adams RM, et al: Patch testing with a routine screening tray in North America 1985–1989: I. Frequency of response. *Am J Contact Dermatitis* 2:122–129, 1991.
4. Anonymous: The frequency of contact sensitivity in North America, 1972–74. *Contact Dermatitis* 1:277–280, 1975.
5. Sertoli A, Gola M, Martinelli M, et al: Epidemiology of contact dermatitis. *Semin Dermatol* 8:120–126, 1989.
6. Dooms-Goossens A: Cited by Sober AJ, Fitzpatrick TB, in Statistics of interest to the dermatologist, *Year Book of Dermatology*. St Louis, Mosby Year Book, 1990, p xxx.
7. Dooms-Goossens A: Cited by Sober AJ, Fitzpatrick TB, in Statistics of interest to the dermatologist, *Year Book of Dermatology*. St Louis, Mosby Year Book, 1989, p 11.
8. Lammintausta K, Kalimo K: Sensitivity to rubber: Study with rubber mixes and individual rubber chemicals. *Derm Beruf Umwelt* 33:204–208, 1985.
9. Song M, Degreef H, De Maubeuge J, et al: Contact sensitivity to rubber additives in Belgium. *Dermatologica* 158:163–167, 1979.
10. Ziegler V, Suss E: The allergenic effect of rubber accelerators tetramethyl thiuram disulfide (TMTD) and mercaptobenzothiazole (MBT). *Allerg Immunol* 20-21:281–285, 1974–1975.
11. van Ketal WG, van den Berg WH: The problem of the sensitization to dithiocarbamates in thiuram-allergic patients. *Dermatologica* 169:70–75, 1984.
12. Logan RA, White IR: Carbamix is redundant in the patch test series. *Contact Dermatitis* 18:303–304, 1988.
13. Fisher AA: Management of dermatitis due to surgical gloves. *J Dermatol Surg Oncol* 11:628–631, 1985.
14. Hansen KS: Glutaraldehyde occupational dermatitis. *Contact Dermatitis* 9:81–82, 1983.
15. Nethercott JR, Holness DL, Page E: Occupational contact dermatitis due to glutaraldehyde in health care workers. *Contact Dermatitis* 18:193–196, 1988.
16. Frosch PJ, Born CM, Schutz R: Contact allergy to rubber, surgical and vinyl gloves. *Hautarzt* 38:210–217, 1987.
17. Heese A, van Hintzenstern J, Peters KP, et al: Allergic and irritant reactions to rubber gloves in medical health services: Spectrum, diagnostic approach, and therapy [published erratum appears in *J Am Acad Dermatol* 26(3 pt 2):403, 1992]. *J Am Acad Dermatol* 25(5 pt 1):831–839, 1991.
18. Agathos M, Bernecker HA: Hand dermatitis in medical personnel. *Derm Beruf Umwelt* 30:43–47, 1982.
19. Jokstad A: Contact dermatitis due to professional activity among dental health care personnel. *Norske Tannlaegeforenings Tidende* 99:48–57, 1989.
20. Hansen KS: Occupational dermatoses in hospital cleaning women. *Contact Dermatitis* 9:343–351, 1983.

21. Shelley WB: Golf course dermatitis due to thiuram fungicide. *JAMA* 188:415, 1964.

22. Cronin E: Pesticides, in *Contact Dermatitis*. Edinburgh, Churchill Livingstone, 1980, p 398.

23. Dooms-Goossens AE, Debusschere KM, Gevers DM, et al: Contact dermatitis caused by airborne agents: A review and case reports. *J Am Acad Dermatol* 15:1–10, 1986.

24. Pock-Steen B: Contact allergy to Nobecutan. *Contact Dermatitis* 18:52–53, 1988.

25. Hannuksela M, Suhonen R, Forstrom L: Delayed contact allergies in patients with photosensitivity dermatitis. *Acta Derm Venereol* 61:303–306, 1981.

26. Muller R, Mitchell JC: Psoralen-type phototoxicity of tetramethylthiuram-monosulphide for *Candida albicans,* not for mouse or man. *J Invest Dermatol* 56:340, 1971.

27. Webb PK, Gibbs SC, Mathias CT, et al: Disulfiram hypersensitivity and rubber contact dermatitis. *JAMA* 241:2061, 1979.

28. van Hecke E, Vermander F: Allergic contact dermatitis by oral disulfiram. *Contact Dermatitis* 10:254, 1984.

29. Goitre M, Bedello PG, Cane D: Allergic dermatitis and oral challenge to tetramethylthiuram disulphide. *Contact Dermatitis* 7:272–273, 1981.

30. Lachappelle JM: Allergic contact dermatitis from disulfiram implants. *Contact Dermatitis* 1:218–220, 1975.

31. Penneys NS, Edwards LS, Katsikas JL: Allergic contact sensitivity to thiuram compounds in a hemodialysis unit. *Arch Dermatol* 112:811–813, 1976.

32. Buxton PK, Going SM, Hunter JA, Winney RJ: Allergic reaction to rubber chemicals in haemodialysis equipment. *Br Med J Clin Res* 287:1513–1514, 1983.

33. Kruis-de Vries MH, Coenraads PJ, Nater JP: Allergic contact dermatitis due to rubber chemicals in haemodialysis equipment. *Contact Dermatitis* 17:303–305, 1987.

34. Wilson HT: Rubber dermatitis: An investigation of 106 cases of contact dermatitis caused by rubber. *Br J Dermatol* 81:175–179, 1969.

35. Can you rely on condoms? *Consumer Reports.* March 1989, pp 135–141.

36. Goh CL: Contact allergy to surgeons' gloves in their patients. *Contact Dermatitis* 20:223, 1989.

37. van Hecke E, Vermander F: Allergic contact dermatitis by oral disulfiram. *Contact Dermatitis* 10:254, 1984.

38. Fisher AA: Dermatologic aspects of disulfiram (Antabuse) use. *Cutis* 30:461–524 passim, 1982.

39. Webb PK, Gibbs SC, Mathias CT, et al: Disulfiram hypersensitivity and rubber contact dermatitis. *JAMA* 241:2061, 1979.

40. Larbre B, Larbre JP, Nicolas JF, et al: Bullous toxic dermatitis due to disulfiram: Apropos of a case. *Ann Dermatol Venereol* 117:721–722, 1990.

41. Rembadel P, Rudzki E: Occupational allergy in the production of drugs. *Polski Tygodnik Lekarski* 45:82–84, 1990.

42. Baptista A, Barros MA, Azenha A: Allergic contact dermatitis on an amputation stump. *Contact Dermatitis* 26:140–141, 1992.

43. Marks JG Jr, Rainey MA: Cutaneous reactions to surgical preparations and dressings. *Contact Dermatitis* 10:1–5, 1984.

44. Pock-Steen B: Contact allergy to Nobecutan. *Contact Dermatitis* 18:52–53, 1988.

45. Knudsen BB, Larsen E, Egsgaard H, Menne T: Release of thiurams and carbamates from rubber gloves. *Contact Dermatitis* 28:63–69, 1993.

46. Estlander T, Jolanki R, Kanerva L: Dermatitis and urticaria from rubber and plastic gloves. *Contact Dermatitis* 14:20–25, 1986.

47. Belseto BV: Contact urticaria caused by rubber. *Dermatol Clin* 8(1):61–66, 1990.

48. Turjanmaa K, Laurilak MA, Kinen-Kiljunen S, Reunala T: Rubber contact urticaria allergenic properties of 19 brands of latex gloves. *Contact Dermatitis* 19:362–367, 1988.

49. Turjanmaa K, Reunala T: Condoms as a source of latex allergen and cause of contact urticaria. *Contact Dermatitis* 20:360–364, 1989.

50. Fineman S: Sensitivity to rubber chemicals. *J Toxicol: Cutan Ocular Toxicol* 6:117–153, 1987.

51. Weinstein LH, Fellner MJ: Rubber band dermatitis. *Int J Dermatol* 18:558, 1979.

52. Eriksson G, Ostlund E: Rubber band note counters as a cause of eczema among employees at the Swedish post office. *Acta Derma Venereol* 48:212–214, 1968.

53. Lynde CW, Warshawski L, Mitchell JC: Patch test results with a shoewear screening tray in 119 patients, 1977–80. *Contact Dermatitis* 8:423, 425, 1982.

54. Varigos GA, Dunt DR: Occupational dermatitis: An epidemiological study in the rubber and cement industries. *Contact Dermatitis* 7:105–110, 1981.
55. Cabrita JC, Goncalo M, Azenha A, Goncalo S: Allergic contact dermatitis of the eyelids from rubber chemicals. *Contact Dermatitis* 24:145–146, 1991.
56. Dick DC, Adams RH: Allergic contact dermatitis from monosulfiram (Tetmosol) soap. *Contact Dermatitis* 5:199, 1979.
57. Jung HD, Honemann W, Kloth C, et al: Contact eczema caused by pesticides in East Germany. *Dermatol Monatsschr* 175:203–214, 1989.
58. Rudzki E, Napiorkowska T: Dermatitis caused by the Polish fungicide Sadoplon 75. *Contact Dermatitis* 6:300–301, 1980.
59. Nethercott JR, Holness DL: Occupational dermatitis in food handlers and bakers. *J Am Acad Dermatol* 21:485–490, 1989.
60. Adams RM: *Occupational Skin Disease.* New York, Grune & Stratton, 1983.
61. Rich P, Belozer ML, Norris P, Storrs FJ: Allergic contact dermatitis to two antioxidants in latex gloves: 4,4'-thiobis(6-tert-butyl-meta-cresol) (Lowinox 44S36) and butylhydroxyanisol—Allergen alternatives for glove-allergic patients [Erratum in *J Am Acad Dermatol* 26:144, 1992]. *J Am Acad Dermatol* 24:37–43, 1991.
62. Rademaker M, Forsyth A: Allergic reactions to rubber condoms, from the Contact Dermatitis Investigation Unit, Belvidere Hospital, Glasgow, Scotland. *GU Med* 65:194–195, 1989.

20

FORMALDEHYDE

Susan E. Feinman

WHAT IS FORMALDEHYDE, AND WHERE DOES ONE CONTACT IT?

Formaldehyde is a ubiquitous chemical which comes in various forms and causes a wide assortment of health effects. Formaldehyde itself is a colorless and highly soluble gas with a characteristic, unpleasantly pungent odor. It is present in air, water, gasoline emissions, and wood or cigarette smoke from incomplete combustion.

EXPOSURE

Formaldehyde exposure occurs through both consumer and occupational use. Consumers are commonly exposed through contact with products such as cosmetics or medicated creams which contain formaldehyde or formaldehyde releasers as a preservative and with resin-treated "drip dry" or "permanent press" clothing. Some other uses are shown in Table 20-1. Workers are exposed through the manufacture of textiles, formaldehyde resins, embalming fluid, microbiocidal solutions, deodorants, cooling solutions and cutting oils, and other products (see Table 20-2). Generally, formaldehyde is sold commercially as the liquid formalin (at least 37% aqueous formaldehyde by weight in the United States) with 10% to 15% methanol added to prevent polymerization.[1]

SOURCES OF FORMALDEHYDE

Formaldehyde is present in forms other than formaldehyde and formalin and is derived from other compounds. The solid *para*-formaldehyde, available in powder or flakes, slowly hydrolyzes to formaldehyde at pH 3 to 5.[2] The United States produced about 5.5 billion pounds of formaldehyde in 1983,[3] about 90 percent going through further processing and becoming such products as urea and phenol formaldehydes and hexamethylene tetramine. Various manufactured liquid compounds and resins act as formaldehyde releasers; in products such as textiles and cosmetics, these are especially important causes of contact dermatitis. In 1987, more than two million American workers were engaged in manufacturing formaldehyde or its by-products.[4]

TABLE 20-1. Products Containing Formaldehyde

Textiles and clothing
  Miracle fabrics (permanent press, drip-dry, no-iron, nonwrinkle), tanned leather, and furs

Cosmetics
  Baby shampoo, lotion, powder, cream, and oil
  Bath soaps and detergents
  Blusher or rouge
  Bubble and milk baths, bath oils, tablets, other bath preparations
  Deodorants (underarm)
  Dry-skin treatment lotion
  Facial masks
  Feminine hygiene deodorants and personal cleanliness products
  Hair tonic and hair grooming aids, setting lotion, hair thickener
  Hair dye and skin dye cleanser
  Makeup foundation and base
  Mascara, eyebrow pencil, makeup remover, other eye makeup
  Mouthwashes and breath fresheners (spray or liquid)
  Nail creams, lotions, cuticle softener
  Nail hardeners
  Permanent-wave lotion
  Sachets, powders, talcs, and perfumes
  Shampoo and hair rinses
  Skin cleanser (cold cream, eye and hand cream, lotion, liquid, pads)
  Tanning cream, after-tanning lotion
  Theatrical makeup and adhesives
  Waterless hand cleaner

Other products
  Adhesives (glues, pastes, cements)
  Agricultural chemicals (seed disinfectants)
  Antifreeze, anticorrosive agents
  Biocides and disinfectants
  Cleaners (rug, carpet, tire, toilet, window, brush)
  Corrosion inhibitors, cutting fluids
  Dishwasher detergents
  Disinfectants (beauty and barber shop, medical equipment, household sprays)
  Dental preparations and dentifrices
  Dry cleaning and spotting fluids
  Dyes and inks
  Embalming fluid and tissue fixatives
  Fumigants
  Hydrocarbons (e.g., oil)
  Latex rubber
  Medicine (hexamethylene diamine for urinary tract infections, drug preservative)
  Metal and tire cleaners
  Paper
  Paints, lacquers, varnishes, and paint removers
  Photographic chemicals (developers, stabilizers, hardeners)
  Polishes and finishes (automobile, windshield, floor, shoe, furniture, suede)
  Renal dialysis rinse in reused dialysers
  Room deodorizers/mildew preventives
  Silk screen preservatives
  Starch (spray and powdered)

(Continued)

TABLE 20–1 (*Continued*). Products Containing Formaldehyde

Formaldehyde releasers
  para-formaldehyde
  Hexamethylene tetramine
  DMDM hydantoin
  Polynoxyline
  Dimethylolurea
  Preventol D1
  Preventol D2
  Preventol D3
  Quarternium-15
  Bakzid
  Bakzid P
  Parmetol K50
  Grotan BK
  Imidazolidinyl urea
  Diazolidinyl urea
  2-Bromo-2-nitropropane-1,3-diol
  KM 103
  Biocide DS 5249 (Proxel T)

DETECTION

Exposure to formaldehyde may occur through its presence in the air, in liquids, or in fabrics; the level of exposure may be determined analytically. Formaldehyde in the air is measured by various tests after gas is trapped with a sampling device. These devices may measure area or personal exposure.[5–8] Formaldehyde can be detected in clothing or paper by a simple qualitative color test based on chromotropic acid.[9] Among the many quantitative procedures is a vapor extraction procedure standardized by the American Association of Textile Chemists and Colorists.[10,11] Many qualitative and quantitative tests are used for formaldehyde in liquids such as kidney dialysates or cosmetics, depending on the reliability and practicality of the application.[12]

WHAT TYPES OF REACTION OCCUR?

Formaldehyde reactions include irritant contact dermatitis, allergic contact dermatitis, contact urticaria, reactions in the mouth and respiratory system, and unusual reactions. These may be immunologically mediated, caused by irritation, or induced by unknown means.

IRRITANT CONTACT DERMATITIS

Irritant contact dermatitis is far more common than allergic contact dermatitis. About 75 percent of workers with occupational dermatitis develop irritant rather than allergic dermatitis. Irritant reactions do not usually occur with the low concentration of formaldehyde used for patch testing (e.g., 1%). Irritant dermatitis does not involve sensitization, so it can occur upon first exposure, often within a few minutes. It may also occur upon

TABLE 20–2. Some Occupations with Exposure to Formaldehyde

Agricultural workers
Anatomists
Attendants and taxidermists
Artists and silk screeners
Athletes, spa and health club attendants
Auto mechanics and body workers
Bakers and butchers
Barbers and beauticians
Bartenders
Biologists
Biology teachers and students
Botanists
Cabinet workers, caulkers, and carpenters
Cashiers
Cleaning personnel (domestic, hospital, industrial)
Dental, medical, surgical, and veterinary personnel
Dry cleaners
Electricians, electronics workers, workers in electrical insulation
Electron microscopists
Embalmers
Fertilizer makers
Fireproofers
Formaldehyde, formaldehyde resin, hexamethylene triamine, pentaerythritol producers
Foundry workers
Furniture dippers and sprayers
Glass etchers
Glue and adhesive makers
Greenhouse workers
Hide preservers and leather makers
Histologists
Lacquer workers
Medical students
Mirror workers
Morticians
Oil well workers
Machinists
Painters and paperhangers
Paper makers
Pathologists
Pest control workers
Photographers
Plumbers
Printers and lithographers
Rubber workers
Soil sterilizers
Solderers and welders
Stonemasons
Tattoo artists
Textile workers
Theatrical artists
Varnish and wood preservative workers

repeated exposure to the same site (cumulative irritation), but, conversely, the irritant response may be eliminated by a form of increased tolerance called "skin hardening." Allergic contact dermatitis may be difficult or impossible to distinguish from irritant dermatitis on the basis of clinical or morphological observations, especially in mild cases. Irritant reactions are often seen the first day of exposure instead of appearing after a period of delay. They are self-contained and may improve before the final patch-test reading. They have been described as burning rather than itching. The physician must take the time to evaluate the eruption, the history, and other patch-test data to determine relevance.[13]

IMMUNE REACTIONS

Formaldehyde sensitization can occur by both immediate and delayed immune mechanisms. Allergic contact dermatitis, contact urticaria, and respiratory reactions may all be immunologically mediated, primarily by two different mechanisms: antibody-mediated (immediate-type hypersensitivity) and cell-mediated (delayed-type hypersensitivity). Immunologically based formaldehyde contact urticaria (and asthma) occur through an antibody-mediated mechanism. In contrast, allergic contact dermatitis from formaldehyde occurs through a cell-mediated (delayed hypersensitivity) mechanism.[14,15]

Allergic contact dermatitis to formaldehyde can be induced in humans or animals by any of several published methods, and the concentration may influence the level of sensitivity.[13,16–18] In published studies using predictive methods, quantitative induction of formaldehyde sensitivity in guinea pigs could be produced by levels of formalin as low as 0.1%; in humans, sensitization could be induced at 1% formalin (0.37% formaldehyde). In a quantitative repeated use test, reactions to formaldehyde could be elicited at the lowest level tested, 30 ppm formaldehyde, in four highly sensitive human subjects from nine individuals tested. Six of the nine subjects gave positive reactions to 100 ppm formaldehyde.[19]

CROSS-REACTIONS

Formaldehyde probably does not cross-react with other aldehydes such as glutaraldehyde or cinnamic aldehyde. It does, however, produce concurrent reactions.[20–22] Individuals exposed to formaldehyde-releasing preservatives, such as quaternium-15[19,20,21], 2-bromo-2-nitropropane-1,3-diol,[22–24] imidazolinyl urea,[22,25,26] or diazolidinyl urea,[27,28] may be sensitive to formaldehyde alone, to the preservative alone, or to both.

HOW DOES ONE RECOGNIZE ALLERGIC CONTACT DERMATITIS FROM FORMALDEHYDE?

CLOTHING DISTRIBUTION

Allergic contact dermatitis reactions from formaldehyde often have a characteristic pattern; they may, for example, occur where clothing contacts the body (Fig. 20-1) or

FIG. 20-1. Clothing dermatitis in a formaldehyde-sensitive patient.

where liquids containing formaldehyde contact the hand (Fig. 20-2). Clothing dermatitis from upper-body garments may be distributed on the trunk at the back of the neck, chest, and elbows. Trousers may contact the inner thighs, gluteal folds, and the areas above or behind the knees.[29] Clothing dermatitis is especially predominant where skin is damp, as at the axillae, although it tends to spare the axillary apex, where direct contact is absent.[30]

OTHER PATTERNS OF ALLERGIC CONTACT DERMATITIS

The cause of allergic contact dermatitis from sources other than clothing is also suggested by the location and pattern of the eruption, as this reflects the area contacted. Allergic contact dermatitis, onycholysis, subungual keratosis, or hemorrhage may occur at the nail from nail hardeners used improperly at 5% or more.[31] Allergic contact dermatitis, facial swelling, urticaria, and cheilitis at the lips may occur from exposure to endodontal preparations.[32] Soap or cosmetics may cause facial reactions.[33] Shampoo rarely causes reactions, as it is quickly diluted and rinsed away.[34] It may occasionally affect the hands of apprentice hairdressers or the ears of clients.

Formaldehyde can be a primary cause of hand dermatitis.[35] The hands may be exposed domestically from cleaning supplies[36] or cosmetics; they may be exposed occupationally from hospital cleaning materials and biocides,[36] hairdressing preparations,[37] histology fluids,[38] coolants,[39] or metalworking fluid/cutting oil.[40] In a recent study of 117 patients with hand dermatitis, 88 percent had domestic exposure and only

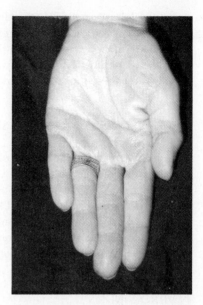

FIG. 20–2. Recalcitrant hand eczema in a patient allergic to formaldehyde. This improved with removal from each source but did not clear until the patient avoided shampoo containing formaldehyde and formaldehyde-releasing preservatives.

12 percent occupational exposure.[35] The use of medicated creams or lotions containing formaldehyde releasers may aggravate hand dermatitis.

Occupational exposure to fumes or emissions may occasionally cause eczema. Very sensitive individuals have been affected by emissions from paper,[41] textiles,[42] kidney dialyzers,[43] and glue.[44]

URTICARIA

Contact urticaria from formaldehyde may be immunologically or nonimmunologically mediated; urticaria also may result from topical or systemic exposure.[45] Prick tests with aqueous formaldehyde have been used occasionally in Europe to demonstrate urticaria.[46–48] They require careful controls and interpretation and must be used with caution to avoid possible anaphylactoid reactions. Examples of topical exposures reported as causing contact urticaria include formalin used occupationally,[49] vapor,[50,51] leather clothing,[52] and starch[53]; examples of systemic exposure include urticaria from hemodialysis,[47] ingestion,[6] or dental exposure.[54–57]

PATCH TESTING

Formaldehyde patch testing is usually performed as part of a standard screening series[58]; the methodology is described by Bruze in Chap. 5. Special considerations include the fact that reactions are often delayed and readings can be missed if not performed at 48 and 72 h and again after an additional 2 or 3 days.[59] The best vehicle is water and the concentration of 1% aqueous formaldehyde has evolved for the Finn chamber test, although the A1-test uses 2% formaldehyde. The concentration of 1% formaldehyde is slightly higher than the 2% formalin concentration (0.74% formaldehyde) once used. Dilutions have been used to determine level of sensitivity and to prove allergy as opposed to irritation. Weak concentrations should be fresh, since the potency of these formaldehyde solutions diminishes with time.[60] In a rare and unusual case, photoactivation[61] was required to elicit a positive test for formaldehyde.

PATCH-TEST RESULTS IN LARGE SURVEYS

Formaldehyde is about the fifth most common sensitizer in North America according to tests by a geographically diverse group of dermatologists.[62] Patch-test surveys in Britain, Europe, Canada, and the United States demonstrate that 1.0 to 9.0 percent of consecutive dermatitis patients react to formaldehyde.[21,63–66] Similar rates occur in Asia, Africa, and South America.[63,67] From 10 to 50 percent of formaldehyde reactions may be due to clothing dermatitis.[68] In one study, 4 percent of 84 funeral service workers were patch-test positive to formaldehyde.[38]

IN VITRO STUDIES

In vitro techniques are sometimes used to show delayed-type hypersensitivity. These tests have not yet demonstrated formaldehyde sensitivity despite their use in tuberculosis and tissue transplantation and their value in distinguishing immunologically mediated reaction from those of the irritant type.

OTHER HEALTH EFFECTS

Formaldehyde can cause health effects other than contact dermatitis and urticaria. Most of formaldehyde's respiratory effects are thought to be due to irritation rather than allergy. These effects include tearing, asthma-like bronchial disease, runny nose, coughing, and headache. Irritation from formaldehyde in air begins at levels as low as 0.1 ppm in air for some individuals; but the threshold of irritation for most persons lies at 0.8 ppm.[69]

There is little evidence to indicate that "formaldehyde asthma" is a true allergy. Allergy is demonstrated by the presence of immunoglobulin E, affirmative prick tests, and positive bronchial provocation tests. Only in a small number of cases with very high exposure levels, however, have IgE or positive bronchial provocation tests been demonstrated.[70–72] Other immune effects—including antigen-antibody reactions that change blood type and anaphylaxis—may also occur from the use of renal dialyzers and from dental procedures.[47,73–75]

PROTECTIVE MEASURES

REGULATION OF FORMALDEHYDE

The industrial air level of formaldehyde is carefully regulated. The OSHA 8-h time-weighted average for formaldehyde exposure is currently set at 1 ppm, with a 15-

min short-term limit of 2 ppm.[76] The American Council of Governmental Industrial Hygienists recommends a similar maximum level for worker exposure.[77]

Despite recommendations, formaldehyde is subject to only minimal regulations. The cosmetic ingredient review expert panel of the Cosmetic, Toiletry and Fragrance Association has recommended that cosmetics not exceed the level of 0.2% free formaldehyde and that no level be considered safe in aerosols.[78] Similarly, the European Economic Council has recommended labeling as a sensitizer for cosmetics at concentrations greater than 0.05%, with a maximum concentration of 0.2% free formaldehyde.[79] The U.S. Consumer Products Safety Commission, however, requires labeling of formaldehyde as a strong sensitizer only for products containing 1% or more.[80] The U.S. Food and Drug Administration (FDA) requires sensitizer labeling for nail hardeners up to 5% and provides that nail shields must be used to restrict use to the nail tip and that directions must be provided for safe use. The FDA requests voluntary registration of cosmetics. In 1981, only two products, a hair tonic and a wave set, contained more than 1% formaldehyde; these were intended for dilution before use. Seven products contained 1% to 5% formaldehyde, however. The majority of other cosmetics reported less than 1% formaldehyde present.[81] Cosmetics have ingredients listed in descending order of concentration on their labels.

The FDA and Environmental Protection Agency (EPA) have miscellaneous regulations ranging from use in tapping maple syrup to use in ruminant animal feed. Most are based on the concentration in a final product being no more than 1%. These regulations involve use of formaldehyde/para-formaldehyde in applications such as grain, seed, bulbs, aquaculture, fumigation, food packaging, food additives, and drug preservation.

AVOIDANCE

Formaldehyde exposure may be minimized by sensitive consumers through reading labels of cosmetics, washing new "drip dry" or "permanent press" clothing and sheets several times before use, and avoiding potential problems that may occur from items and occupations listed in Tables 20-1 and 20-2. Other products to be avoided include cigarettes, room deodorants, kitty litter, woodstoves, and any items with the characteristic formaldehyde odor.[82] Recently remedial measures (such as use of formaldehyde scavengers) have decreased annoyance from exposure to off-gassing from formaldehyde resins in urea formaldehyde foam insulation, clothing, and some plastic furniture.[83] Occupationally, engineering controls, periodic health screening, protective clothing, and barrier creams may be used[84]; in some cases of occupational exposure, however, as with hairdresser apprentices, dialysis nurses, or pathologists, a change of profession is necessitated.

A recent Danish study demonstrates that avoidance of exposure to formaldehyde may be difficult. Out of 285 cosmetic products, 85 (29.5 percent) contained more than 0.001% formaldehyde (10 ppm),[85] the detection level of the method used. Many of these products were made in the United States. In 27 (9.5 percent) of the products, the formaldehyde content was greater than 30 ppm, the human threshold level for formaldehyde sensitization found in Jordan's study.[19] In ten (3.5 percent) of the products examined, the total formaldehyde content was greater than the EEC limit of 0.05%, although they were not labeled "contains formaldehyde."[85] This study illustrates the difficulty of identifying the source of formaldehyde based on labeling.

FORMALDEHYDE—PATIENT HANDOUT

WHAT IS FORMALDEHYDE?

Formaldehyde is a chemical which is widely used as a germ killer, as a preservative (as for embalming), in the making of clothing, plastics, paper, fiberboard, and plywood, and in many, many other uses. In fact, formaldehyde is extremely widespread in our environment. Not only is the chemical itself added to manufactured materials, but it can also be formed by the breakdown of many products. Sometimes this is deliberate and sometimes it is unintended. For example, chemicals called preservatives are frequently added to a cosmetic to preserve the original form of the product, such as a makeup or a hand lotion. Some of these are added to kill germs and mildew and to keep the product from becoming rancid. Many of these preservatives release formaldehyde very slowly, so that there is a germ-killing level of the chemical at all times. Persons who are allergic to formaldehyde therefore would tend to break out to the formaldehyde which is formed by the breakdown of the preservative.

WHERE AM I MOST LIKELY TO BE EXPOSED TO FORMALDEHYDE?

The list of possibilities is very long, but permanent-press clothing, cosmetic items, and occupational exposure are all important.

HOW DO I KNOW WHETHER OR NOT A RASH I GET IS CAUSED BY MY FORMALDEHYDE ALLERGY?

Unfortunately, this is a very real problem, because one does not always know. Sometimes you can tell from the pattern. People who are exposed at work will break out in exposed areas. Those who break out to clothing will have a clothing distribution, sparing the armpits and breaking out where there is pressure, as over the rib cage, in front of and behind the armpits, and sometimes above the knees and other areas where clothing tends to produce pressure. When one breaks out to a cosmetic containing formaldehyde, the rash will usually be where the cosmetic is applied, but sometimes the fingers and finger webs will break out where you handle it to apply it. An unusual form of formaldehyde sensitivity is to shampoos, in which case the ears are sometimes involved as well as the fingers. One may also occasionally break out to plastic materials and leather containing formaldehyde where these touch the skin.

Not every rash you get will be caused by formaldehyde allergy. However, for those people who are prominently allergic to formaldehyde, it is very likely that any exposure will cause a problem, so they are well-advised to avoid it.

This information is provided to help persons with contact dermatitis in the understanding of their problem. The contents are subject to change as more information becomes available and are not intended as a substitute for medical treatment.

HOW CAN I AVOID FORMALDEHYDE?

There are a number of sources of exposure. People who work in industry—such as the paper industry, embalmers, morticians, and medical students who handle material preserved in formaldehyde—are obviously going to be exposed where they touch materials contaminated with it. When occupational exposure occurs, it may be possible to find the sources of formaldehyde by looking on material safety data sheets, which are kept in the work place. Also a job description in one of the books on occupational skin disease will sometimes give you a clue as to how you might be exposed.

A prominent source of formaldehyde exposure is in permanent-(durable-) press clothing. Many of the textile fabrics are treated with a finish to help maintain their shape, and these finishes frequently contain formaldehyde and release it. Another source is paper products. Makeup and many other cosmetic products may contain formaldehyde if a formaldehyde-releasing preservative is included in the formulation.

Individuals who work with metals, as with a grinder or a lathe, or who use coolants will probably be exposed to formaldehyde in their work. Formaldehyde is by far the most common allergen in coolant solutions. For persons working in coolants, it can be very difficult to avoid.

HOW CAN I KNOW WHICH PRODUCTS CONTAIN FORMALDEHYDE?

Clothing is probably a principal source, as many of the permanent-press textile materials contain fabric finishes that can release formaldehyde. To be absolutely certain, one can run a test for formaldehyde on a sample taken from the garment, but this usually has to be done in a laboratory where strong acids can be handled safely. Generally, polyester, nylon, and acrylates, which are not mixed with other textile fibers, do not contain such fabric finishes. According to one author, 100 percent cotton items may also be safe. Check the label for the words *permanent press* or *durable press* and for warnings against washing with a chlorine bleach, as such products usually contain finishes which can release formaldehyde. Products which are labeled not more than 4 to 5 percent shrinkage are also likely to contain a fabric finish which releases formaldehyde.

In questionable cases, testing the items first is safer. A laboratory test can be done from a small swatch from the lining of a garment to see whether or not there is free formaldehyde in it. One can also start with relatively safe materials and add one new garment a week, wearing it two or three times during the week to see whether or not a flare occurs (provided that the skin is clear at the time one starts). This type of test is called a usage test.

All polyester fabrics are generally safe, but those made from mixtures of fibers, such as polyester and cotton (Dacron and cotton) and the like are not. Certain

(*Continued*)

100 percent cotton knits may contain finishes with low levels of formaldehyde. Washing a new garment in hot, soapy water several times before wearing it tends to reduce the formaldehyde content, but it does not totally eliminate it.

To avoid exposure to formaldehyde in cosmetics, read the labels before purchasing a cosmetic and avoid anything containing any of the formaldehyde-releasing preservative such as quaternium-15, 2-bromo-2-nitropropane-1,3-diol, DMDM hydantoin, imidazolidinyl urea, diazolidinyl urea, tris-(hydroxymethyl)-nitromethane, and 5-bromo-5-nitro 1,3-dioxane. Of course, if formaldehyde is included in the list of ingredients, that product also should not be used.

Shampoos are another problem. Generally speaking, the same formaldehyde-releasing preservatives will be included in the ingredient list on the label. The products that contain methyl isothiazoline and chloromethyl isothiazoline and do not contain one of the formaldehyde-releasing preservatives may be acceptable provided you are not allergic to that chemical. Some of the shampoos which do not contain formaldehyde include Prell, Neutrogena, Polytar, Ionil, Silkience, Subutone, Subulex, Ivory, and White Rain.

Another source is in paper products, and this may be more difficult because it is virtually impossible to know the formaldehyde content of paper without analyzing it.

SUMMARY

1. Read labels and avoid not only formaldehyde itself but also formaldehyde-releasing preservatives (mainly quaternium-15, 2-bromo-2-nitropropane-1,3-diol, imidazolidinyl urea, and diazolidinyl urea), and urea formaldehyde resins.
2. All polyester (but not polyester-cotton blends) and all-cotton fabrics not labeled "durable press, will not shrink more than 4 to 5 percent" or "do not use chlorine bleach" are less likely to contain formaldehyde. Wash clothing and linens several times before their initial use.
3. Ask your dermatologist or physician about performing a test to identify formaldehyde in liquids and textiles about which there is a question.
4. Wear chemically resistant gloves when handling formalin or items containing formaldehyde.
5. Follow instructions for protecting the skin when using nail hardeners. Avoid products labeled as containing sensitizers. Dilute shampoos and hair tonics before using them. Do not use over-the-counter lotions or cosmetics on irritated skin or where you have a rash.
6. Before starting regular use, you can test a product which may or may not contain formaldehyde by applying it to a small tender area of skin daily (such as the neck or where the arm bends) and examine the area each day for several days for eczema.
7. Persons who are exposed occupationally should wear a National Institute for Occupational Safety and Health-approved respirator and chemical-resistant gloves. Direct work with formaldehyde should be done under a hood with ventilation. In any case, avoid contact with eyes, skin, and clothing.

Although most positive patch tests for formaldehyde are relevant provided an intensive search is made for a source, avoidance of eliciting products in the environment remains difficult. For example, 11 formaldehyde-positive Danish contact dermatitis patients were carefully interviewed on their use of all products.[86] Even with identification of the products containing formaldehyde and the substitution of alternative products, two-thirds were not healed 2 to 3 months after initial diagnosis. Some formaldehyde-sensitive patients require intensive investigation and hours of counseling, with uncertain results.

REFERENCES

1. U.S. Pharmaceutical Convention: *United States Pharmacopeia, 20th Revised National Formulary,* 15th ed. Rockville, MD, U.S. Pharmacopeial Convention, 1975.
2. Gerberich HR, Stautzberger AL, Hopkins WC: Formaldehyde, in *Kirk-Othmer Encyclopedia,* vol. 11. New York, Wiley, 1980.
3. Marks JG, De Leo VA: *Contact and Occupational Dermatology.* St. Louis, Mosby Year Book, 1992.
4. *Federal Register* 52.233 Friday Dec. 4, 1987. Occupational exposure to formaldehyde; final rule, p. 46239.
5. National Research Council: *Formaldehyde and Other Aldehydes.* Washington, DC, National Academy of Sciences, 1981.
6. National Institute for Occupational Safety and Health: *Criteria for a Recommended Standard: Occupational Exposure to Formaldehyde.* Washington, DC, U.S. Government Printing Office, 1976, p 176.
7. Balmat JL: *Formaldehyde Institute Methods Manual.* Scarsdale, NY, Formaldehyde Institute, 1983.
8. Kennedy ER, Teass AW, Gagnon VT: Industrial hygiene sampling and analytical methods for formaldehyde, in Turoski V (ed): *Formaldehyde, Analytic Chemistry and Toxicology,* Washington, DC, American Chemical Society, 1985, chap 1.
9. Blohm S: Formaldehyde contact dermatitis: I. A simple method for the determination of small amounts of formaldehyde. *Acta Derm Venereol* 30:450, 1959.
10. American Association of Textile Chemists and Colorists: Test method 112-1968, Determination of formaldehyde in resin-treated fabrics. sealed jar method, in *ATTCC Technical Manual.* Research Triangle Park, NC, American Association of Textile Chemists and Colorists, 1982.
11. Andrews BA, Harper RJ: Formaldehyde release—Are current test methods realistic? *Text Res J* 50:177, 1980.
12. Pizziconi VB: Hazards associated with chemical cleaning and disinfecting agents for reuse, in *Reuse of Disposables, AAMI Tech. Assessment Report.* Arlington, VA, Association for the Advancement of Medical Instrumentation, 1983, pp 163–174.
14. Silberberg I: Apposition of mononuclear cells to Langerhans cells in contact allergic reactions. *Acta Derm Venereol* 53:1, 1973.
15. Shelley WB: Selective uptake of contact allergens by the Langerhans cell. *Arch Dermatol* 113:187, 1977.
16. Marzulli FN, Maibach HI: The use of graded concentrations in studying skin sensitizers: Experimental contact sensitization in man. *Food Cosmet Toxicol* 12:219, 1974.
17. Kligman AM: The identification of contact allergens by human assay: III. The maximization test for screening and rating contact sensitizers. *J Invest Dermatol* 47:393, 1966.
18. Tsuchiya S, Konda M, Okamoto K, Takas Y: Studies on contact sensitivity in the guinea pig. *Contact Dermatology* 88:246, 1982.
19. Jordan WR Jr, Sherman WT, King SE: Threshold responses in formaldehyde sensitive subjects. *J Am Acad Dermatol* 1:44, 1979.
20. Mathias CG, Chappler RR, Maibach HI: Contact urticaria from cinnamic aldehyde. *Arch Dermatol* 116:75, 1980.
21. Cronin E: *Contact Dermatitis.* Edinburgh, Churchill Livingstone, 1980.
22. Fisher AA: Cosmetic dermatitis: II. Reactions to some commonly used preservatives. *Cutis* 26:136, 1980.
23. Frosch PJ, White IR, Rycroft RJ, et al: Contact allergy to Bronopol. *Contact Dermatitis* 22:108, 1990.
24. Storrs FJ, Bell DE: Allergic contact dermatitis to 2-bromo-2-nitropropane-1,3-diol in a hydrophilic ointment. *J Am Acad Dermatol* 8:157, 1983.

25. Jordan WP: Diazolidinyl urea: The antigenic backlash with imidazolidinyl urea. Presented at the 42nd annual meeting of the American Academy of Dermatology, 1983.

26. Mandy SH: Contact dermatitis to substituted imidazolidinyl urea—A common preservative in cosmetics (letter). *Arch Dermatol* 110:463, 1974.

27. Perret CM, Happle R: Contact sensitivity to diazolidinyl urea (Germall 11). *Arch Dermatol Res* 281:57, 1989.

28. Kantor JR, Taylor JS, Ratz JL, Evey PL: Acute allergic dermatitis from diazolidinyl urea (Germall II) in a hair gel. *J Am Acad Dermatol* 13:116, 1985.

29. Hatch KL: Textile dermatitis from formaldehyde, in Feinman SE (ed): *Formaldehyde Sensitivity and Toxicity.* Boca Raton, FL, CRC Press, 1988.

30. Sherertz EF: Clothing dermatitis: Practical aspects for the clinician. *Am J Contact Dermatitis* 3:55, 1992.

31. Mitchell JC: Non-inflammatory onycholysis from formaldehyde-containing nail hardener. *Contact Dermatitis* 7:173, 1981.

32. Kaaber S, Thulin H, Nielsen E: Skin sensitivity to denture base materials in the burning mouth syndrome. *Contact Dermatitis* 5:90, 1979.

33. Zemtsov A, Taylor JS, Evey P, Dijkstra J: Allergic contact dermatitis from formaldehyde in a liquid soap. *Cleve Clin J Med* 57:301, 1990.

34. Bruynzel DP, van Ketel WG, deHaan P: Formaldehyde contact sensitivity and the use of shampoos. *Contact Dermatitis* 10:179, 1984.

35. Cronin E: Formaldehyde is a significant allergen in women with hand eczema. *Contact Dermatitis* 25:276, 1991.

36. Kleinhaus D, Dayss U: Formaldehyde contact allergy (in German). *Derm Beruf Umwelt* 28:101, 1980.

37. Holness DL, Nethercott JR: Dermatitis in hairdressers. *Dermatol Clin* 8:119, 1990.

38. Holness DL, Nethercott JR: Health status of funeral service workers exposed to formaldehyde. *Arch Environ Health* 44:222, 1989.

39. Angelini G, Meneghini CL: Dermatitis in engineers due to synthetic coolants. *Contact Dermatitis* 3:219, 1977.

40. Grattan CE, English JS, Fould IS, Rycroft RJ: Cutting fluid dermatitis. *Contact Dermatitis* 20:372, 1989.

41. Black H: Contact dermatitis from formaldehyde in newsprint. *Contact Dermatitis Newsletter* 10:162, 1972.

42. Romaguera C, Grimat F, Lecha M: Occupational purpuric textile dermatitis from formaldehyde resins. *Contact Dermatitis* 7:152, 1981.

43. Hendrick DJ, Lane DJ: Occupational formaldehyde asthma. *Br J Ind Med* 34:11, 1977.

44. Pirila V, Kilpio O: On dermatitis caused by formaldehyde and its compounds. *Am Med Intern Fenn* 38:38, 1949.

45. von Krogh G, Maibach HI: The contact urticaria syndrome, in Marzulli FN, Maibach HI (eds): *Dermatotoxicology,* 2d ed. New York, Hemisphere, 1983, chap 14.

46. Pisati G, Brini D, Cirla AM: Formaldehyde allergy in a synthetic resins factory (in Italian). *Med Lav* 71:88, 1980.

47. Maurice F, Rivory JP, Larsson PH, et al: Anaphylactic shock caused by formaldehyde in a patient undergoing long term hemodialysis. *J Allergy Clin Immunol* 19:383, 1986.

48. Pardon N, Bompart PV: Some clinical forms of intolerance to phenol-formaldehyde resins (in French). *Med Trav Soc Secur* 20:63, 1959.

49. Rappaport B, Hoffman M: Urticaria due to aliphatic aldehydes: A clinical and experimental study. *JAMA* 116:2656, 1941.

50. Lindskov R: Contact urticaria to formaldehyde. *Contact Dermatitis* 8:333, 1982.

51. Fisher AA: Formaldehyde: Some recent experiences. *Cutis* 17:665, 1976.

52. Helander I: Contact urticaria from leather containing formaldehyde. *Arch Dermatol* 113:1443, 1977.

53. McDaniel W, Marks J: Contact urticaria due to sensitivity of spray starch. *Arch Dermatol* 115:628, 1979.

54. Guyot JD: Report of formaldehyde urticaria. *South Med J* 14:115, 1921.

55. Al-Nashi YG, Al-Rabayi AA: A case of sensitivity to tricresol formaldehyde. *Br Dent J* 142:52, 1977.

56. Kaaber S, Thulin H, Nielsen E: Skin sensitivity to denture base materials in the burning mouth syndrome. *Contact Dermatitis* 5:90, 1979.

57. Ruyter IE: Release of formaldehyde from denture base polymers. *Acta Odontol Scand* 38:17, 1980.

58. North American Contact Dermatitis Group: *Patch Testing in Allergic Contact Dermatitis,* 6th ed. Evanston, IL, American Academy of Dermatology, 1982.

59. Shelley WB: Immediate sunburn-like reaction in a patient with formaldehyde photosensitivity. *Arch Dermatol* 118:117, 1982.

60. Stoors FJ, Rosenthal LE, Adams RM, et al: Prevalence and relevance of allergic reactions in patients patch tested in North America—1984 to 1985. *J Am Acad Dermatol* 20:1038, 1989.

61. Feinman SE: Frequency of allergic contact dermatitis from formaldehyde, in Feinman, SE (ed): *Formaldehyde Sensitivity and Toxicity*. Boca Raton, FL, CRC Press, 1988, ch. 6.

62. Lynde CW, Warshawaky L, Mitchell JC: Screening patch tests in 4190 eczema patients 1972–1981. *Contact Dermatitis* 8:417, 1982.

63. Fregert S, Hjorth N, Magnusson B, et al: Epidemiology of contact dermatitis. *Trans St Johns Hosp Dermatol Soc* 55:17, 1969.

64. Bruckner-Tuderman L, Konig A, Schnyder UW: Patch test results of the Dermatology Clinic Zurich in 1989; personal computer-aided statistical evaluation. *Dermatology* 184:29, 1992.

65. Fan WX, Zhao B: Study on Chinese common allergens of contact dermatitis. *Derm Beruf Umwelt* 38:158, 1990.

66. Hatch KL, Maibach HI: Textile chemical finish dermatitis. *Contact Dermatitis* 14:1, 1986.

67. Bardana EJ Jr, Montanaro A: Formaldehyde: An analysis of its respiratory, cutaneous, and immunologic effects. *Ann Allergy* 66:441, 1991.

68. Patterson R, Pateras V, Grammer LC, Harris KE: Human antibodies against formaldehyde—human serum albumin in individuals exposed to formaldehyde. *Int Arch Allerg Appl Inmmunol* 79:53, 1986.

69. Kramps JA, Peltenburg LTC, Lerklaan PRM, et al: Measurement of specific antibodies in individuals exposed to formaldehyde. *Clin Exp Allergy* 19:509, 1989.

70. Thrasher JD, Madison R, Broughton A, Gard Z: Building-related illness and antibodies to albumin conjugates of formaldehyde, toluene diisocyanate, and trimellitic anhydride. *Am J Indust Med* 15:187, 1991.

71. Howell D, Perkins HA: Anti-N-like antibodies in the sera of patients undergoing chronic hemodialysis. *Vox Sang* 23:291, 1972.

72. Fassbinder W, Frei U, Koch KM: Hemolysis due to formaldehyde-induced anti-N-like antibodies in hemodialysis patients. *Klin Wochenscr* 57:673, 1979.

73. Ebner H, Kraft D: Formaldehyde-induced anaphylaxis after dental treatment? *Contact Dermatitis* 24:307, 1991.

74. Swenberg JA, Kerns WD, Mitchell RJ, et al: Induction of squamous cell carcinomas of the rat nasal cavity by inhalation exposure of formaldehyde vapor. *Cancer Res* 40:3398, 1980.

75. Mashford PM, Jones AR: Formaldehyde metabolism in the rat: A reappraisal. *Xenobiotica* 12:119, 1982.

76. Heck H, Casanova-Schmitz M: Reaction of formaldehyde in the rat nasal mucosa, in Clary J, Gibson JE, Waritz R (eds): *Formaldehyde: Toxicology, Epidemiology, and Mechanisms*. New York, Dekker, 1983, chap 9.

77. *Federal Register* 54.12 Thursday Jan 19, 1989. Rules & Regulations. Limits for Air Contamination, p 2938.

78. American Conference of Governmental Industrial Hygienists (ACGIH): *Threshold Limit Values for Chemical Substances and Physical Agents in the Work Environment with Intended Changes for 1983–4*. ACGIH, Cincinnati, 1983, p 42.

79. Cosmetic Ingredient Review Panel: *Final Report of the Safety Assessment for Formaldehyde*. Cosmetic, Toiletry, and Fragrance Association, Washington DC, 1983.

80. European Economic Community Directive of May 17, 1982 amending the second time directive 761169 on the approximation of the laws of the member states relating to cosmetic products. *Official Journal of the European Community* #L1671, June 15, 1982.

81. *Code of Federal Regulations* 16CFR1500.3(b)(9).

82. 1987 FDA data cited in Feinman SE: Exposure to cosmetics containing formaldehyde, in Feinman SE (ed): *Formaldehyde Sensitivity and Toxicity*. Boca Raton, FL, CRC Press, 1988, chap 7.

83. Adams RA: *Occupational Skin Disease*. New York, Grune & Stratton, 1983.

84. Sudin B: Formaldehyde emission from particleboard and other building material: A study from the Scandinavian countries. Presented at the Particleboard Series Symp. No. 12, Washington State Univ., Pullman, 1978.

85. Mathias CG: Prevention of occupational contact dermatitis. *J Am Acad Dermatol* 23(4 pt 1):742, 1990.

21

ETHYLENEDIAMINE

Jere D. Guin

BACKGROUND

In 1967, in a 4-month period, Provost and Jillson[1] found 13 patients allergic to ethylene-diamine (EDA). The first patient reacted to Mycolog but not to Kenalog, and after a search of the ingredients of Mycolog Cream, ethylenediamine was found to be the cause. This specific ingredient was not on the label, as it was a stabilizer, allowing the use of both mycostatin and neomycin without loss of antimicrobial activity. This report was quickly confirmed by Epstein and Maibach.[2] Following this, many cases were reported, and many more were found which were not reported. While in the original series the allergy seemed to be somewhat monolithic, later reports found numerous concomitant allergies as well as reactions to ethylenediamine in other products and a number of cross-reactions to similar chemicals. Almost a decade earlier, a pharmacist who became allergic when preparing aminophylline suppositories[3] actually represented the first case, according to Hogan.[4] Many medications share the structure of two carbons terminated by one or two amino groups, and a number of human and animal studies have examined what will and will not be tolerated by persons allergic to ethylenediamine.

CHEMISTRY

Ethylenediamine is a two-carbon hydrocarbon bound on each end by an amino group, with the formula $(NH_2\text{-}CH_2\text{-}CH_2\text{-}NH_2)\cdot HCl$.[4] It has been used as a stabilizer in the original Mycolog Cream and its generic equivalents,[4] as a hardener for some epoxy resin systems,[5] and as a buffer to prevent an untoward decrease in the pH of Merthiolate (thimerosal) as well as thimerosal topical solution USP and thimerosal aerosol USP.[6] It is especially suitable for combination with carbon dioxide in air to prevent damage from atmospheric exposure. It is soluble in water and alcohol, and it is a solvent for casein, sulfur, albumin, and shellac. It is also used as an emulsifier. It can be found in latex, antifreeze, and textile lubricants.[7] It has some ability to chelate copper, but in human subjects it is not effective in chelating nickel.[8]

Among the epoxy hardeners studied, ethylenediamine is a potent sensitizer, as is the entire category of aliphatic polyamines.[9] It may also cross-react with diethylenetriamine and triethylenetetramine, which are used as epoxy resin hardeners.[5,8] In fact, there is a very long list of polyamine hardeners, and to make matters worse, the long-term prognosis of some of these epoxy workers is poor.[10]

The prevalence of ethylenediamine allergy depends upon the area reporting. It is 9 percent in Saskatchewan and it reached over 1 percent of *normals* in the San Francisco area,[11] where Mycolog generics and equivalents[12] were commonly prescribed. Allergy to ethylenediamine is also noted in a higher percentage of epoxy-exposed workers in Poland,[5] and 26 percent of Bulgarian petrochemical workers exposed to ethylenediamine are patch-test positive to it.[13] In Belgium the incidence in persons patch tested is >1/2 percent,[14] and in one section of Germany the very light incidence of 0.3% did not warrant keeping it on the screening tray.[15]

WHAT IS THE CLINICAL PICTURE?

The most common presentation in the United States is still the Mycolog-allergic patient, with the caveat that more recently they have been allergic to one of the generics and not Mycolog Cream itself (although EDA seems to have been removed finally from newer supplies of all but one of the generics). In this country the formulation has undergone changes over the years, finally with both ethylenediamine and neomycin being removed from the brand-name product. However, there may be older supplies of several generic preparations[12] which most pharmacists dispensed as Mycolog under the generic substitution laws present in some form in every state of the United States. The rash seen is usually an eczematous spread of the original problem. There are also several more unusual presentations reported, and distributions based on how and where the cream (to which the patient is allergic) is applied.

Most patients reacting to ethylenediamine have an eczema, which worsens despite treatment. This may be anywhere, but it is likely to be where treatment is deliberately applied. For example, Fisher[6] described an early case of spread from the angles of the mouth, where perleche was being treated. It is one of the antigens reported in early infancy[16] and in children. Of two children with widespread nummular eczema, one child had pubic involvement and one had a papulovesicular dermatitis as a secondary eruption.[17]

Hand dermatitis is another presentation. Several workers developed an occupational hand dermatitis from exposure to ethylenediamine in a coolant mixture to which they were exposed at work.[18] A nurse handling aminophylline injections developed hand eczema (and urticaria), which cleared with avoidance.[19] A hand eczema with involvement of the palms and proximal nail folds occurred from exposure to a floor polish remover containing 3% ethylenediamine.[20]

Eczema from epoxy exposure may involve not only the hands but also the face and other areas. This is especially true when the patient is allergic to the hardener.[21] Systemic contact dermatitis can cause an exanthematous eruption[22] or even exfoliative erythroderma.[22,23] It can also progress from an exanthem to exfoliative dermatitis.[22] The latter is not common from drugs, but this is one of those causes. It has been found in persons receiving systemic aminophylline or a cross-reacting medication by several routes, intravenous,[23] oral,[24] and suppository.[22] Ethylenediamine is known to cross-react with piperazine,[25] and one patient became erythrodermic from a cross-reaction with only four tablets of piperazine, which he took for treatment of threadworms.[24]

Several forms of systemic contact dermatitis are known to occur if one considers all reported allergens. The best known is perhaps the flareup of a recent or current contact dermatitis on patch testing or reexposure or the recrudescence of a positive patch test following reexposure. A generalized maculopapular "dermatitis" can occur following intravenous aminophylline.[26] Aminophylline can also do this by suppository[22] or from oral medications.[24]

One cannot accurately predict the allergen from the cutaneous findings, but there are definite patterns which sometimes seem to occur from certain medications. Systemic contact dermatitis from other contact allergens may show itself as a tattoo granuloma, eczema of the elbows, pompholyx, the baboon syndrome (a red rash over the buttocks),[27] or even parapsoriasis. Perhaps the classic systemic contact is the mercury reaction described by Nakayama et al.,[28] with the generalized erythema in its characteristic distribution.

Another presentation of EDA sensitivity is photosensitivity. Photoallergic contact dermatitis of the face has been reported from exposure to cutting oils containing this chemical.[29] Such reactions may be only photoallergic[29] or both contact allergic and photoallergic.[30]

PROGNOSIS

Approximately 25 percent of those allergic will lose their allergy in 10 years. The other side of this is that 75 percent retain it.

WHAT DOES THE POSITIVE PATCH TEST MEAN?

When a patient's allergy comes from exposure to a combination steroid cream (e.g., Mycolog), it may be accompanied by allergy to one or more other ingredients in that cream. This might include especially neomycin, parabens, fragrance ingredients, and triamcinolone. Formerly there were persons allergic to thimerosal, but that was removed from the formula many years ago. Relatively few are seen who are allergic to Mycolog Ointment rather than the cream, as the ointment never contained ethylenediamine.

A person allergic to ethylenediamine from exposure to epoxy hardeners may develop a cross-reaction to a long list of similar chemicals used for the same purpose. There are also medications which may contain this reagent, the most notable being aminophylline, or theophylline ethylenediamine HCl. Many antihistamines also contain this structure as a moiety within the molecule, which may not be available, so there is disagreement as to which medications would not be tolerated in persons allergic to ethylenediamine. Fisher[6] states that tripelennamine (pyrabenzamine) and hydroxyzine may be problems. He also lists Surfadil, which is no longer manufactured. While some suggest that promethazine (Phenergan) might be a problem, this has more recently been denied.[31,32] A few cases of sensitivity have been reported, but the authors did not consider a causal relationship to be prominent or likely.[33]

THE THREE CASES OF NOT-SO-NEUROTIC VULVAR ECZEMA

The fragrance content of Mycolog Cream may also be a source of concomitant allergy,[34] and the pattern seen may be different. The author saw three older women with long-standing vulvar eczema, recalcitrant to treatment.[35] They had been told that this was a form of neurodermatitis which was due to continued stress. Their patch-test data showed reactions to ethylenediamine and to one or more fragrance ingredients found in Mycolog Cream. Following testing, all three were found to be positive to the fragrance materials alpha amylcinnamic alcohol (AACAlc) and alpha amylcinnamic aldehyde (AACAld). The sources of AACAld proved to be laundry detergent in two cases and fabric softener in the third. Two were later reexposed and reacted to clothing laundered with the suspected product, proving a causal relationship. Of 14 persons allergic to either AACAld or AACAlc, only 1 weak responder failed to react to ethylenediamine or another component (at that time) of Mycolog Cream. While AACAld was not listed as an ingredient in the product, it was present by gas liquid chromotography (GLC) analysis, apparently as a contaminant in the commercial-grade AACAlc. Following a change to laundry products free of AACAlc and AACAld, the "neurotic" vulvar eczema cleared completely in all three patients.

WHAT IS THE RELATIONSHIP TO EDTA?

The sodium salt of ethylenediaminetetraacetic acid (EDTA) might be assumed to be a cross-reactor because of the structural similarity, but this is not true. An early publication of three patients with eyelid dermatitis from eyedrops and a positive patch test to EDTA and ethylenediamine was accepted as the rule, but later data changed that as further study failed to show any tendency for EDTA to cause a problem in persons allergic to ethylenediamine.[6] Some persons are allergic to EDTA,[36] but it is apparently not a problem for persons allergic to ethylenediamine.

HOW CAN THIS TYPE OF ALLERGY BE PREVENTED?

There are a number of products containing ethylenediamine which are better avoided, including:

1. Aminophylline, or theophylline ethylenediamine, is used for certain respiratory problems, notably bronchial asthma. It can cause severe reactions by several routes.[22-24] There are products without ethylenediamine which can be substituted, but the generic substitution laws make it necessary for the patient to be alert to possible substitution of theophylline with EDA. The hospital formularies based on bid purchases of generic medications are also a problem, which, however, is not insurmountable. Nevertheless, it represents a perilous pitfall which is constantly present. Hospital personnel who are allergic may react to their patients' medication.
2. Antihistamines which may be a problem include hydroxyzine, antazoline, and mepyramine.[4,37] There is disagreement about promethazine, but most today deny its association. One might be wary of outliers, as there have been anecdotal reports that are

ETHYLENEDIAMINE (EDA)—PATIENT HANDOUT

A patch-test reaction to ethylenediamine (EDA) usually means that the person has been exposed to one of the generic versions of Mycolog Cream or was exposed to Mycolog Cream itself years ago. Mycolog is a combination cortisone-like topical medication with antiyeast activity and formerly with antibiotic activity. It is sometimes thought of as a "shotgun" medication to cover a multitude of problems. The difficulty with it is that to make both the germ killer and antiyeast component work, a stabilizer chemical had to be added, which is where EDA enters the picture. This chemical is a rather potent sensitizer, especially when it is put on a rash and most especially when it is used in the treatment of allergic contact dermatitis without removing the cause. The company marketing the brand-name Mycolog Cream has removed EDA from the formula of the cream, and Mycolog Ointment never had it in the formula. However, because pharmacists can substitute a generic, and because at least one generic formulation still contains it, it remains a common problem.

Another facet to the allergy is that persons allergic to EDA in Mycolog are often allergic to other things in the formula. Neomycin is a chief associated allergy, but this is also in the standard test series, so it is usually discovered. An allergy to an emulsifier may be missed rather easily, and a big problem in some patients is allergy to the perfume which causes allergy to fragrances and flavors found in innumerable places in our environment. A test series to learn whether or not those allergies are present can be helpful. A commonly unrecognized problem is allergy to the cortisone-like active ingredient, which may carry over to other cortisone salves.

There are other sources of EDA which can be troublesome. Persons with asthma and other respiratory problems may receive theophylline EDA or aminophylline, which contains EDA. There are other forms of theophylline which do not, so you should always alert both the physician and pharmacist. Other medications include hydroxyzine (Atarax, Vistaril) where part of the chemical structure is much like that of EDA. This chemical may also be found in tincture of Merthiolate. Early reports that EDA-allergic individuals may be allergic to EDTA, a common preservative (chemically, a salt of EDA tetraacetic acid) are denied by almost all recent data.

An occupational source of the allergy comes from exposure to certain epoxy resin hardeners. Epoxies are plastic polymers used in glues, adhesives, paints, and insulation. They can often be suspected by the presence of two bottles or tubes or packages which have to be mixed. This is not always true, but it usually is. One is the resin and the other is the hardener. The resin is the main sensitizer, but many allergic to it also become allergic to the hardener. Epoxy resin is also in the test kit, and it uncovers about 75 percent of epoxy allergy. Ethylenediamine is also used in the manufacture of rubber and may be in some coolants (used as cutting fluids). Floor polish remover, antifreeze, and animal feed supplements have at times contained EDA.

This information is provided to help persons with contact dermatitis in the understanding of their problem. The contents are subject to change as more information becomes available and are not intended as a substitute for medical treatment.

ETHYLENEDIAMINE (EDA)—PATIENT HANDOUT (*Continued*)

American products considered equivalent to Mycolog Cream include Myco-cream, Mytrex, Tristatin, Myco-Triacet II, and Nystatin-Neomycin-Gramicidin-Triamcinolone Cream.

Brand names of non-U.S. products with similar formulations include Kena-comb, Triacortyl, Halcicomb, Halog TRI Cream, Volog, Alcinon, Dermalog, and Amphocort.

---

worrisome. There are so many alternative medications that it is not worthwhile to take a risk.

3. Tincture of Merthiolate (Lilly) is said to contain EDA.[6] Patch testing to another brand before use might be wise.

4. Industrial exposure to certain epoxy hardeners (aliphatic polyamines) can cause a reaction in some EDA-allergic patients.[5,10,37]

5. Piperazine can cause severe reactions in EDA-allergic persons. This medication is an anthelmintic (worm medicine).[24] That structure is also present in other medications, but the information on cross-sensitivity is lacking.

6. Other sources include animal feed,[38] antifreeze,[7] certain rubber products, and floor polish remover.[20] Obviously the source list is long, but the available information in some areas is meager.

REFERENCES

1. Provost TT, Jillson OF: Ethylenediamine contact dermatitis. *Arch Dermatol* 96:231–234, 1967.
2. Epstein E, Maibach HI: Allergic contact dermatitis. *Arch Dermatol* 98:476–477, 1968.
3. Tass J, Weissberg D: Allergy to aminophylline. *Acta Allerg* 12:39–42, 1958.
4. Hogan DJ: Allergic contact dermatitis to ethylenediamine: A continuing problem. *Dermatol Clin* 8:133–136, 1990.
5. Rudzki E, Krajewska D: Cross-reactions between ethylenediamine, diethylenetriamine and triethylenetetramine. *Contact Dermatitis* 2:311–313, 1976.
6. Fisher AA: Cross reactions between ethylenediamine base in Merthiolate tincture with ethylenediamine HCl. *Contact Dermatitis* 14:181, 1986.
7. *Merck Index,* 9th ed. Rahway, NJ, Merck & Co, 1976, p 499.
8. Burrows D, Rogers S, Beck M, et al: Treatment of nickel dermatitis with Trientine. *Contact Dermatitis* 15:55–57, 1986.
9. Thorgeirsson A: Sensitization capacity of epoxy resin hardeners in the guinea pig. *Acta Derma Venereol* 58:332–336, 1978.
10. Krajewska D, Rudzki E: Sensitivity to epoxy resins and triethylenetetramine. *Contact Dermatitis* 2:135–138, 1976.
11. Prystowsky SD, Allen AM, Smith RW, et al: Allergic contact hypersensitivity to nickel, neomycin, ethylenediamine, and benzocaine: Relationships between age, sex, history of exposure, and reactivity to standard patch tests and use tests in a general population. *Arch Dermatol* 115:959–962, 1979.
12. Fisher AA: The significance of ethylenediamine hydrochloride dermatitis caused by a "generic" nystatin-triamcinolone II cream. *Cutis* 41:241, 1988.
13. Bainova A, Khristeva V, Madzhunov I, Daneva Zh: Dermal exposure to ethylenediamine in the petro-chemical industry. *Problemi Na Khigienata* 12:109–114, 1987.

14. Van Hecke E: Ethylenediamine sensitivity from exposure to epoxy resin hardeners and Mycolog Cream. *Contact Dermatitis* 1:344–348, 1975.
15. Enders F, Przybilla B, Fuchs T, et al: Ethylenediamine contact dermatitis. *Contact Dermatitis* 25:266–267, 1991.
16. Fisher AA: Allergic contact dermatitis in early infancy. *Cutis* 35:315–316, 1985.
17. Caraffini S, Lisi P: Nummular dermatitis-like eruption from ethylenediamine hydrochloride in 2 children. *Contact Dermatitis* 17:313–314, 1987.
18. Crow KD, Peachey RD, Adams JE: Coolant oil dermatitis due to ethylenediamine. *Contact Dermatitis* 4:359–361, 1978.
19. dal Monte A, de Benedictis E, Laffi G: Occupational dermatitis from ethylenediamine hydrochloride. *Contact Dermatitis* 17:254, 1987.
20. English JS, Rycroft RJ: Occupational sensitization to ethylenediamine in a floor polish remover. *Contact Dermatitis* 20:220–221, 1989.
21. Dahlquist I, Fregert S: Allergic contact dermatitis from volatile epoxy hardeners and reactive diluents. *Contact Dermatitis* 5:406–407, 1979.
22. Petrozzi JW, Shore RN: Generalized exfoliative dermatitis from ethylenediamine. *Arch Dermatol* 112:525–526, 1976.
23. Elias JA, Levinson AI: Hypersensitivity reactions to ethylenediamine in aminophylline. *Am Rev Respir Dis* 123:550–552, 1981.
24. Price ML, Hall-Smith SP: Allergy to piperazine in a patient sensitive to ethylenediamine. *Contact Dermatitis* 10:120, 1984.
25. Balato N, Cusano F, Lembo G, Ayala F: Ethylenediamine contact dermatitis. *Contact Dermatitis* 11:112–114, 1984.
26. Berman BA, Ross RN: Ethylenediamine: Systemic eczematous contact-type dermatitis. *Cutis* 31:594–598, 1983.
27. Andersen KE, Hjorth N, Menne T: The baboon syndrome: Systemically induced contact dermatitis. *Contact Dermatitis* 10:97–100, 1984.
28. Nakayama H, Niki F, Shono M, Hada S: Mercury exanthem. *Contact Dermatitis* 9:411–447, 1983.
29. Romaguera C, Grimalt F, Lecha M: Photoallergic dermatitis from ethylenediamine. *Contact Dermatitis* 14:130, 1986.
30. Burry JN: Photocontact dermatitis from ethylenediamine. *Contact Dermatitis* 15:305–306, 1986.
31. Fisher AA: Lack of cross-reaction between promethazine and ethylenediamine (letter). *Contact Dermatitis* 16:236, 1987.
32. King CM, Beck M: Oral promethazine hydrochloride in ethylenediamine-sensitive patients. *Contact Dermatitis* 9:444–447, 1983.
33. White MI: Contact dermatitis from ethylenediamine. *Contact Dermatitis* 4:291–293, 1978.
34. Larsen WG: Allergic contact dermatitis to the perfume in Mycolog Cream. *J Am Acad Dermatol* 1:131–133, 1979.
35. Guin JD, Haffley P: Sensitivity to alpha-amylcinnamic aldehyde and alpha-amylcinnamic alcohol. *J Am Acad Dermatol* 8:76–80, 1983.
36. de Groot AC: Contact allergy to EDTA in a topical corticosteroid preparation. *Contact Dermatitis* 15:250–252, 1986.
37. Balato N, Cusano F, Lembo G, Ayala F: Ethylenediamine dermatitis. *Contact Dermatitis* 15:263–265, 1986.
38. Fisher AA: Allergic contact dermatitis in animal feed handlers. *Cutis* 16:201–202, 1975.

EPOXY PATCH-TEST STANDARD

Jere D. Guin

WHAT IS THE EPOXY RESIN IN THE STANDARD TEST SERIES?

Epoxies are synthetic resins used as adhesives, (hard) surface coatings, electrical insulation materials, coatings for glass fibers, athletic equipment (bows, ski poles, fishing rods, tool handles, prefabrication in construction, paints and varnishes, corrosion inhibitors, aircraft surface protection, and—in combination with an acrylate grouping—dental bonding). Other sources include plastic containers; door handles; ostomy bags; several types of clothing, including shoes and knee pads in jeans; medical equipment such as needles, nasal cannulas, and cardiac pacemakers; printing ink; watch straps; amputation prostheses; and dentures. References for these are given in Chap. 36.

Allergic contact dermatitis to epoxy resins is a leading cause of occupational skin disease, as the *proven and currently relevant* cases constitute almost 8 percent of *all* occupational skin disease in one western country where occupational evaluations are centralized.[1] In this population, only 0.1 to 0.2 percent of the work force is exposed, so the risk of developing occupational sensitivity is relatively high. The actual incidence may well be higher, but epoxy seems to be the third most common cause of occupational allergic contact dermatitis after chromates (cement, leather, electroplating, etc.) and rubber.[1] Most of the occupational allergy would be detected with the standard patch-test allergen, but about 10 percent are allergic to other epoxy structures and a few others are allergic to other components.

SENSITIVITY TO THE COMPONENTS

The reaction to the standard patch-test antigen called *epoxy resin* is a positive test to the most common type of resin. This test will detect about 75 percent or so of reactors, as this is the percentage of the market occupied by this type epoxy resin.[1] This formula is a basic one, comprising two (di) ether-linked hydroxypropane (glycidyl-substituted) phenols (2-*bis*-phenol) bound to acetone which (following binding) is now propane. This gives the formula the chemical name di glycidyl ether of *bis*-phenol acetone or DGEBA. The simplest DGEBA molecule is the one described, which weighs about 340 Da. Larger ones are less sensitizing, although some of the low-molecular-weight monomers can be detected even in the high-molecular-weight resins, so those already allergic will often break out on exposure. Another characteristic is that those allergic to the high-molecular-weight epoxies will usually be detected with the patch test to the DGEBA 340-Da monomer.[2] There is a qualitative (chemical) test for this structure, as described by Fregert and Trulsson[3] which is outlined in Chap. 36.

The total number of commercially available types was 25 by the 1960s. These other epoxy formulas differ in chemical structure and may not be detected by patch testing to the standard DGEBA 340-Da monomer.[4] Most, however, are sold in two separate containers and mixed before using. The second container carries a "hardener," a chemical which cross-links with the epoxy molecule to produce the solid finished product. Allergy to the hardener also develops—this occurred in approximately 24 percent of the cases in one large series.[1] One way one suspects the hardener as part of the picture is that (at least in industrial cases) the face is commonly involved.[5] This does not prove the allergy, but it is sufficiently suggestive to demand a patch test for it.

A third ingredient, called a *reactive diluent,* is usually added to adjust viscosity. The chemical structure is often an aromatic glycidyl ether. These chemicals are potent sensitizers, and they are sometimes, at least, present in the hardened resin. Those allergic to a reactive diluent may or may not be patch-test reactive to the standard antigen.

Because the patch-test material used in the standard series does not detect other epoxy components, it would be useful to test for those in persons who react. The reason is that some of these have other uses or their structure may be similar to another chemical to which one could be exposed. It is much easier to avoid problems if you know what they are and what causes them. Many components other than these are given in Chap. 36.

RECOGNITION

Epoxy resin dermatitis involves the hands and arms in more than 90 percent of cases.[6] The fingers and interdigital web areas are typically affected. The face is involved more than half of the cases, especially when hardener sensitivity is present. While most cases are occupational, glues and dental bonding using ultraviolet-cured epoxy acrylates and other causes can produce (the less common) nonoccupational sensitivity. Typical jobs for reactors are glueing, painting, laminating, and electrical insulating. The highest risk seems to be in those working with epoxies in liquid form.[1] Home use of glue and epoxy paints are the risk factors. One seldom-recognized source of exposure is in dental bonding done with epoxy acrylates which are ultraviolet-cured. Allergy to this material is not common, but those allergic to the epoxy acrylate are often also allergic by the standard epoxy patch-test reagent (DGEBA).

Recognition is often linked to the index of suspicion. One thing to look for is the two-container adhesive. Epoxy resins may occasionally be in "one bag" or one stage, but for the most part the two-container packaging prevails. This one-bag type is more likely to be heat-cured, also, which probably reduces the likelihood of sensitization.

PROTECTION

Gloves must be carefully chosen, as cloth and rubber gloves can make matters worse.[7] Nitrile and nitrile butatoluene gloves are more protective[8] but may be bulky for some jobs.[6] A three-layered lightweight glove (4-H) offers surprising protection to epoxies and is less bulky. These are not inexpensive, however. Lightweight gloves tear more

EPOXY—PATIENT HANDOUT

WHAT DOES A POSITIVE TEST TO EPOXY MEAN?

The positive reaction to epoxy in the standard patch test tray is a reaction to the most commonly used structure of epoxy-resin monomers. Epoxy monomers are chemicals which can be joined to form the polymer, as links are joined to form a chain. Not every epoxy resin has the same structure, but the test material used will find some 75 percent of those allergic to epoxy. However, even when this test is positive, it may or may not point to the cause of your problem, as it could stem from an older, unrelated allergy.

Epoxies are sold as lower-molecular-weight *monomers;* a second chemical used to activate the process is called a *hardener*. The hardener causes the monomer to cross-link into a sort of chain or *polymer*. Products which are *totally* polymerized are not sensitizing, but at room temperature this may, in some resin systems, take months to be complete, so sometimes some of the monomer chemical can be left over. You may be allergic to the resin or to the resin *and* the hardener. The standard test does not test to the hardener, but experience has taught us that almost everyone allergic to the hardeners is also allergic to the monomer. This is why we use the monomer to screen for epoxy allergy. There are also other chemicals in some of these products, but most reports of allergy to them have to do with their industrial use. In occupational exposure, the contents can be uncovered by examining the Material Safety Data Sheet kept at the place of employment.

The positive test means that you should avoid direct contact with epoxy products. These materials are widely used in industry (and at home for that matter) in the following ways:

1. As adhesives and glues. The product may state in the name that it is an epoxy or it may not. Any glue which comes in two tubes is probably an epoxy. There are a few products which are composed of only one component, but this is not the usual case.
2. Paints used for a hard surface or a rustproof primer. Such paints may contain epoxy resins. The paints come in either one or two parts and one has to depend upon the label or the dealer for the information.
3. Electrical insulation materials. Epoxies are often used in these to prevent conduction of electricity. Epoxy products have been widely used on transformers and capacitors for this purpose. This could affect a hobbyist who works with electronic gear. However, this type of exposure is mainly industrial and occupational.

This information is provided to help persons with contact dermatitis in the understanding of their problem. The contents are subject to change as more information becomes available and are not intended as a substitute for medical treatment.

EPOXY—PATIENT HANDOUT (*Continued*)

PREVENTIVE MEASURES

1. Avoidance is the safest approach, but this is not always possible.
2. Epoxies which are larger in molecular weight are less sensitizing. They still contain some of the smaller monomers, but the quantity is lower. Once you are allergic you may react to these, but probably less severely.
3. When one is accidentally exposed, removal of the glue or paint with solvents (acetone, alcohol, or methyl-ethyl ketone) will reduce the exposure. However, routine use of these chemicals is not recommended, as they tend to dry and irritate the skin.
4. Special gloves help to protect the hands, but rubber gloves do not help. Vinyl and neoprene rubber are not totally protective. Nitrile rubber or nitrile butatoluene gloves are protective. For work which requires thin gloves, 4-H gloves, a Danish product, are probably the best solution.
5. A methacrylate (wound) spray (the European product Neobecutane) and to a lesser extent a barrier cream (Kerodex) reportedly help reduce the spread.

---

easily, which can put the patient at increased risk. Use of protection helps but is not absolute. With it, it takes longer on average to develop the allergy[6] and the incidence may be lower. Another practical protective measure is the use of high- rather than low-molecular-weight resins. Complete curing with heat may also help.[9]

The chemistry and clinical findings in epoxy-resin dermatitis are covered in more detail in Chap. 36.

REFERENCES

1. Jolanki R: Occupational skin diseases from epoxy compounds: Epoxy resin compounds, epoxy acrylates and 2,3-epoxypropyl trimethyl ammonium chloride. *Acta Derm Venereol Supple* 159:1–80, 1991.
2. Fregert S. Dahlquist I, Persson K: Sensitizing capacity of substances related to epoxy resin oligomer MW 340, (DGEBA). *Contact Dermatitis* 10:47–48, 1984.
3. Fregert S, Trulsson L: Simple methods for demonstration of epoxy resins of bisphenol A type. *Contact Dermatitis* 4:69–72, 1978.
4. Kanerva L, Jolanki R, Estlander T: Allergic contact dermatitis from non-diglycidyl-ether-of-bisphenol-A epoxy resins. *Contact Dermatitis* 24:293–300, 1984.
5. Dahlquist I, Fregert S: Allergic contact dermatitis from volatile epoxy hardeners and reactive diluents. *Contact Dermatitis* 5:406–407, 1979.
6. Jolanki R, Kanerva L, Estlander T, et al: Occupational dermatoses from epoxy resin compounds. *Contact Dermatitis* 23:172–183, 1990.
7. van Putten PB, Coenraads PJ, Nater JP: Hand dermatoses and contact allergic reactions in construction workers exposed to epoxy resins. *Contact Dermatitis* 10:146–150, 1984.
8. Blanken R, Nater JP, Veenhoff E: Protection against epoxy resins with glove materials. *Contact Dermatitis* 16:46–47, 1987.
9. Holness DL, Nethercott JR: Occupational contact dermatitis due to epoxy resin in a fiberglass binder. *J Occup Med* 31:87–89, 1989.

23

QUATERNIUM-15

Anthony F. Fransway

WHAT IS QUATERNIUM-15?

Quaternium-15 is the dominant member of the family of quaternary ammonium compounds that find use primarily as disinfectants. As the name suggests, the characterizing feature of this class is a methylated nitrogen with four covalent bonds to distinguishing alkyl and aromatic residues. Other prominent members of this family—including alkyl trimethylammonium bromide, benzalkonium chloride, cetrimonium bromide, and benzethonium chloride—are at best rare allergens and are infrequently incorporated into cosmetic and personal care products in comparison with quaternium-15. These will not be further discussed and need not be tested in patients suspected of formaldehyde-releasing biocide sensitivity.

Quaternium-15 is the *cis* isomer of 1-(3-chloroallyl)-3,5,7-triaza-1-azoniaadamantane chloride with a molecular weight of 251.2.[1] This broad-spectrum antimicrobial agent is odorless, colorless, highly water-soluble, insoluble in oils and organic solvents, stable at broad pH and in different ionic formulations, and active against bacteria (particularly *Pseudomonas aeruginosa*), yeasts, and molds. Concentration of use is generally 0.02 to 0.3% by weight in cosmetic formulations. Quaternium-15 as an antimicrobial compares favorably to paraben family members; consequently it is often used as the sole preservative in a cosmetic formulation. Occasionally other preservatives such as the parabens are added to further broaden microbe inhibition.

When a biocide is implicated as the potential cause of allergic contact dermatitis, more than infrequently a generally delicate but occasionally blunt interaction between dermatologists and manufacturers—those who assess epicutaneous allergy and those who use a particular biocide—ensues; quaternium-15 is the most frequent addition to the list of agents undergoing rather intense scrutiny by both groups. The actual importance of finding a "significant" prevalence of allergy in a highly selected population such as those who undergo patch testing has been questioned, particularly in light of the broad application of these products and the millions of consumers who are routinely exposed but experience no difficulty. The issue on its most scientific level balances the importance of numerous factors, including toxicology/toxicity, allergenicity as defined through larger prevalence studies, the quality of the biocide in cosmetic formulations, the price of the biocide, and the investment required to select alternative biocides of equal caliber; at its most practical level it becomes one of perception, with the industry responding and reacting with variable rapidity to the impressions of dermatologists, physicians, and consumers as highlighted in medical and lay publications. The responsiveness of the industry to such perceptions, as well as to the availability of new biocides that may be toxicologically preferable, is highlighted by the frequency of use as voluntarily reported to the FDA and tabulated on a triannual basis.[2] Although representative of only a small proportion of available cosmetic products, quaternium-15 has demonstrated decreasing use over the past 10 years, while other biocides such as imidazolidinyl urea continue to enjoy increasing success.

SOURCES OF EXPOSURE TO QUATERNIUM-15

OCCUPATIONAL

Although quaternium-15 is incorporated into a number of soaps and detergents as a preservative, and despite its frequent use as a cutting-oil biocide, occupational sensitization to quaternium-15 is exceedingly uncommon. As workers are encouraged to wash their hands frequently and remove chemical residues with toxic or allergenic potential, quaternium-15 in detergents and soaps is found to be the occasional source of sensitization. There have been three case reports in the literature of occupational sensitization to quaternium-15, one from exposure to a lotion soap in an individual responsible for the maintenance of machinery in a chicken-processing plant[3] and the other two stemming from rinse-off products in occupations involving hair care.[4] We have also seen one case of occupational sensitization to a quaternium-15–containing hand soap.

COSMETIC AND THERAPEUTIC PRODUCTS

Quaternium-15 is incorporated into a large number of skin and hair care items, particularly rinse-off formulations in which there is a significant proportion of water. The frequency of use of quaternium-15 has declined over the past 9 years, primarily because of the attention directed to this biocide and its identification as a potent formaldehyde donor. Common sources for quaternium-15 include cosmetics, shampoos, conditioners and cream rinses, eyelid makeups, facial moisturizing lotions and creams, shampoos, shaving products, and body powders. In their two landmark studies discussing the causes of allergy to cosmetics, the North American Contact Dermatitis Group found quaternium-15 to be by far the most frequent cause of a preservative allergy, specifically with 6.6 and 9.1 percent of 487 and 713 patients, respectively, found to be allergic to quaternium-15; preservatives were eclipsed only by fragrances as causative of cosmetic reactions.[5,6] Broeckx and colleagues[7] also determined quaternium-15 to be the most frequently reactive preservative in patients suspected of cosmetic allergy, while DeGroot et al.[8] found it second only to methylchloroisothiazolinone/methylisothiazolinone. In tabulating several studies reviewing the frequency of reaction to biocides used in cosmetic products, quaternium-15 was found to be by far the most frequently reactive biocide, with 7.8 percent of 2549 patients from nine individual studies responsive.[5–13] These data are confirmed by White's[14] report of female patients with facial dermatitis, nearly 7 percent of whom were allergic to quaternium-15.

MISCELLANEOUS

Quaternium-15 may also be incorporated into floor waxes and polishes, inks, latex-based paints, laundry starch, paper and pulp products, textile finishing solutions, spinning emulsions, printing pastes, and joint cements. No cases of occupational sensitization have been reported from these particular exposure sources.

CLINICAL PRESENTATIONS OF QUATERNIUM-15 ALLERGY

All cases of occupational sensitization to quaternium-15 to date have involved hand dermatitis, with one case preceded weeks earlier by onycholysis. The use of quaternium-15 in several popular therapeutic moisturizers in the United States accounts for a number of cases presenting with chronic hand eczema. The distribution of dermatitis generally corresponds to the region of moisturizer application. The picture of vivid violaceous dermal erythema without papular dermatitis and with little pruritus but prominent burning sensation is frequently seen with quaternium-15 allergy when this product is applied to facial skin (Fig. 23-1). However, acute and subacute dermatitis presentations and papular and/or vesicular eczema may also be seen (Fig. 23-2).

In the experience of the Mayo Clinic, the most frequent presentation of quaternium-15 allergy is that of positivity in association with formaldehyde and other formaldehyde-releasing biocides.[15] In 181 patients identified to be allergic to quaternium-15 (4.9 percent of all patients tested), less than 30 percent solely reacted to quaternium-15,

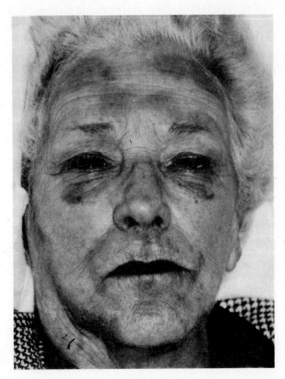

FIG. 23–1. Quaternium-15 cosmetics allergy: the visage of patchy dermal erythema.

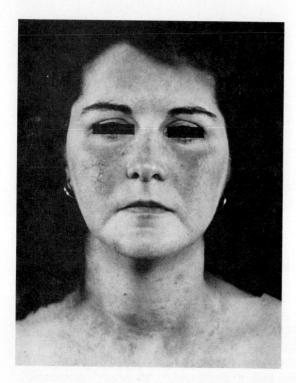

FIG. 23–2. Papular/subacute dermatitis due to quaternium-15 exposure in a popular moisturizing product.

while over 65 percent also responded to formaldehyde and other formaldehyde-releasing biocides. Several patients responded concomitantly only to imidazolidinyl urea or bromonitropropane diol. These data, along with the fact that quaternium-15–positive responses were most often of the same reaction strength or weaker than corresponding formaldehyde responses, suggest that the formaldehyde donor ability of quaternium-15 represents the usual explanation of this reaction. In such situations, it is difficult to identify quaternium-15 specifically as the exposure most proximally related to dermatitis, but one often identifies quaternium-15 as one of many problem antigens in a patient with generalized chronic dermatitis. Many other sources of exposure to formaldehyde and other formaldehyde-donor biocides can often be uncovered. The presentation in this scenario is frequently that of a generalized recalcitrant dermatitis, although one may also see positive patch tests in patients suffering from long-standing atopic dermatitis.

FREQUENCY OF QUATERNIUM-15 POSITIVITY IN SCREENING SERIES

Certain countries—including Italy, the Netherlands, and Canada—have reported very low frequencies of sensitivity to quaternium-15 in screening trays (0.0 to 0.5 percent).[4,16–19] The study of Hogan and colleagues[19] from Canada, exhibiting 4.9 percent positivity in 542 patients, suggests that regional variation within a country may also exist. However, major studies examining quaternium-15 in the western hemisphere

TABLE 23-1. Quaternium-15 Sensitivity in Screening Series

Country	Investigator	Year	Vehicle and Concentration	Number Tested	Percent Positive
USA	NACDG[20]	1970–1976	2% aq.	7000–9000	2.3
USA	NACDG[20]	1978–1979	2% aq.	7001	3.7
USA	NACDG[20]	1979–1982	2% aq.	4193	3.4
UK	Ford and Beck[21]	1983–1984	1% pet.	2298	2.6
USA	NACDG[20]	1984–1985	2% pet. & aq.	4663	6.7, 3.9
USA	Fransway[22]	1990	2% pet.	3415	4.9
USA	Parker and Taylor[24]	1991	2% pet. & aq.	1408	6.3

have suggested that quaternium-15 screening tests are more frequently positive (2.6 to 8.0 percent) (Table 23-1).[20–24] Notable in these data is the North American Contact Dermatitis Group finding of a progressive increase in sensitivity to quaternium-15 over the past 20 years, from 2.3 percent to its present high of over 7 percent. Additional experience is needed to determine whether this figure will diminish with time, as the frequency of quaternium-15 use wanes.

RELEVANCE OF THE POSITIVE RESPONSE TO QUATERNIUM-15

Positive reactions to quaternium-15 are usually relevant, particularly when exuberant or associated with formaldehyde sensitivity. Of Taylor's 89 quaternium-15–allergic patients, the positive reaction was relevant in part or in toto in 56 percent; significance was undetermined in 44 percent, with relevance not excluded.[24] Ford and Beck[21] similarly found 39 of their 59 positive responses (66 percent) to be either probably or possibly relevant. The North American Contact Dermatitis Group has found quaternium-15 to be relevant in the majority of cases exhibiting reactivity (58 percent). This seems to be particularly important in considering the increasing frequency of positive responses in screening series.[23]

NATURE OF THE ALLERGY AND CROSS-REACTING SUBSTANCES

Quaternium-15 positivity is, in the majority of our cases, found in association with and in all probability secondary to formaldehyde sensitivity. Data from other investigators support this concept, all reporting greater than 50 percent of quaternium-15–allergic patients to be also formaldehyde-sensitive. Ford and Beck[21] found 31 of 59 quaternium-15–allergic patients reactive to formaldehyde, with the corresponding figures for Parker and Taylor[24] to be 55 percent (24) and for Fisher[25] to be 86 percent. Cronin[26] experienced a rough concordance rate of 50 percent, while the smaller study by Eiermann and colleagues[5] showed the minority of their quaternium-15 patients (40 percent) to be also formaldehyde-allergic.

Formaldehyde is not the only co-reactive biocide that may be seen on patch testing,

Quaternium-15 is a preservative found in a variety of cosmetics and topical pharmaceutical preparations. By law, all products made in the United States for topical use must have the ingredients listed either on the product package or the box that contains it. To determine whether you are exposed to this preservative to which you have been proven allergic, be sure to check the labeling of ingredients on the package.

Quaternium-15 is most frequently found in hair-care products such as conditioners, rinses, and shampoos as well as several popular moisturizing lotions and a number of cosmetic products. Repeat exposure to a product containing quaternium-15 will probably result in a worsening of your dermatitis. Now that you know you are allergic to this particular ingredient, you must avoid all products that contain it. The following is a detailed but not all-inclusive list of products that may contain quaternium-15:

Cosmetics
Moisturizing creams and lotions
Shampoos
Conditioning agents and cream rinses
Eye makeup
Face makeup
Shaving products
Body powders
Soaps
Disinfectants

Other occupational sources and exposures to quaternium-15 of potential importance include the following:

Adhesives
Floor wax
Floor polish
Water-based inks
Latex paints
Laundry starch
Metal-cutting fluids
Paper pulp
Textile finishing solutions
Spinning emulsions
Printing pastes
Joint cement

Discontinuation of exposure to these products should result in improvement and/or resolution of your dermatitis difficulty.

This information is provided to help persons with contact dermatitis in the understanding of their problem. The contents are subject to change as more information becomes available and are not intended as a substitute for medical treatment.

A number of products may cross-react or co-react with quaternium-15. You should consult with your physician regarding which (if any) of these products need to be avoided as well. The following is, again, a detailed but not all-inclusive list of potential co-reactive substances:

Diazolidinyl urea
Formaldehyde
Imidazolidinyl urea
DMDM hydantoin
Bromonitropropane diol

Quaternium-15 will usually be labeled as such on ingredient packages, but it may go by a number of other names, including the following:

Dowicil 75
Dowicil 100
Dowicil 200
N-(3-chloroallyl) hexaminium chloride
Chloroallyl methenamine chloride
1-(3-chloroallyl)-3,5,7 triaza-1-azoniaadamantane chloride

Should you be exposed to any products with these names on the label, they should be avoided as well.

There are a number of preservatives that are also incorporated into cosmetic products that you may be safely exposed to (assuming you have not shown allergic reaction to these on patch testing as well); such cosmetic products should be selected. Acceptable preservatives include methylparaben, ethylparaben, propylparaben, butylparaben, benzylparaben, methylchloroisothiazolinone/methylisothiazolinone, methyldibromoglutaronitrile/phenoxyethanol, sorbic acid, and propylene glycol.

If you are concerned about a particular cosmetic product and its safety for application to your skin, a use test is advised. In this self-administered test, a small amount of the cosmetic product (particularly moisturizers, lotions, and cosmetics) is applied to an area on the inside of the elbow or over the upper arm twice a day for 1 week. If no redness or itching develops in the area, the same procedure is repeated over a small area in front of the ear on one of your cheeks. If still no response is noted, the product is probably safe for you to use, although you should continue to use caution regarding widespread use until you are certain it is well tolerated. *Note:* The use test is not acceptable for detergents, soaps, hair care products such as shampoos and conditioners, and mascaras or eyeliners. Again, consult your physician regarding which of these products, if any, would be safe for you to use.

as in our series of 181 patients with quaternium-15 allergy, 18 percent responded also to imidazolidinyl urea and 15 percent bromonitropropane diol.[15] Diazolidinyl urea, DMDM hydantoin, and, more rarely, other formaldehyde-releasing biocides may also be concomitantly positive.

Obviously, then, quaternium-15 is most frequently positive on the basis of its formaldehyde release, although fewer than 50 percent of cases may be sensitized sui generis. The fact that quaternium-15 is the biocide with the greatest potential for formaldehyde release (100 ppm at 0.1% concentration) would support this conclusion.[27] Flexibility in determining the importance of the positive response, particularly while considering other positive formaldehyde-releasing biocides, is necessary in determining relevance of response.[27]

PATCH-TEST CONSIDERATIONS

Quaternium-15 is generally tested at 2% concentration in petrolatum. Irritant responses are exceedingly infrequent at this concentration. In patients believed to have preservative sensitivity, it is important to test not only the biocides in the standard tray (formaldehyde and imidazolidinyl urea) but also other formaldehyde-releasing biocides including DMDM hydantoin, diazolidinyl urea, and bromonitropropane diol to determine as precisely as possible the spectrum, severity, and extent of sensitivity. Studies reporting testing to quaternium-15 in water as well as petrolatum have found petrolatum to be a more sensitive delivery system. Only three of Parker and Taylor's[24] patients who reacted to the antigen in an aqueous vehicle and not to petrolatum were identified, whereas the converse of petrolatum-positive, aqueous-negative was found in 35 patients.

PREVENTION AND MANAGEMENT

SOLE REACTIVITY OF QUATERNIUM-15

In the setting where only quaternium-15 is positive, this specific biocide may be avoided. In the case of occupational sensitization, soaps and cutting oils that do not contain quaternium-15 may be selected; for the patient sensitized to cosmetic and hair products, alternative products without quaternium-15 should be substituted. The allergic person should scan ingredient labels religiously to confirm the absence of quaternium-15. There are no data to show that quaternium-15 allergy wanes with time; therefore the patient should avoid this biocide indefinitely. Other formaldehyde-releasing biocides, most notably imidazolidinyl urea, should be safe for use.

THE CONCOMITANT QUATERNIUM-15 AND ALTERNATIVE FORMALDEHYE-RELEASING BIOCIDE SENSITIVITY

One must individualize the approach to the patient who is allergic to quaternium-15 as well as formaldehyde or other formaldehyde-releasing biocides. Should the sole co-reactive antigen be formaldehyde, agents of this class with a very low potential to release formaldehyde may be quite well tolerated by the patient (again, most notably imidazolidinyl urea). Prior to widespread application of any such product, a use test should be done. The issue is less clear if the patient also responds to bromonitropropane diol or DMDM hydantoin, which, although more potent formaldehyde donors than imidazolidinyl urea, suggest a decreased threshold of formaldehyde sensitivity. A recommended general rule is that *if the patient has positive response to three or more formaldehyde-releasing biocides, he or she should endeavor to avoid all members of the class.* If that is not possible, a use test of an imidazolidinyl urea–containing product seems a prudent approach, again assuming imidazolidinyl urea is negative on patch testing.

The patient with broad-spectrum formaldehyde-releasing biocide sensitivity, including imidazolidinyl urea, should select cosmetic products that do not contain any members of the family. Acceptable alternatives include sorbic acid, propylene glycol, members of the paraben family, methylchloroisothiazolinone/methylisothiazolinone, methyldibromoglutaronitrile/phenoxyethanol, and benzyl alcohol. In such patients, testing a specific biocide to ascertain negativity and provocative use testing of any product prior to widespread use on the skin is advisable.

Quaternium-15 at 2% concentration in petrolatum is not believed to be an irritant, so any positive reaction should be assumed to be of potential relevance, and the patient should avoid the substance. If the strength of reaction is in question, repeat patch testing is warranted.[28]

REFERENCES

1. Marouchoc SR: Dowicil 200 preservative, in Kabara JJ (ed): *Cosmetic and Drug Preservation: Principles and Practice.* New York, Dekker, 1984, pp 143–164.
2. Frequency of preservative use in cosmetic formulations as disclosed to FDA—1990. *J Cosmet Toilet* 105:45, 1990.
3. Marren P, DeBerker D, Dawber RPR, et al: Occupational contact dermatitis due to quaternium-15 presenting as nail dystrophy. *Contact Dermatitis* 25:253, 1991.
4. Tosti A, Piraccini BM, Bardazzi F: Occupational contact dermatitis to quaternium-15. *Contact Dermatitis* 23:41, 1990.
5. Eiermann JH, Larsen W, Maibach HI, et al: Prospective study of cosmetic reactions 1977–1980. *J Am Acad Dermatol* 6:909, 1982.
6. Adams RM, Maibach I, Clendenning WE, et al: A five-year study of cosmetic reactions. *J Am Acad Dermatol* 13:1062, 1985.
7. Broeckx W, Blondeel A, Dooms-Goossens A, et al: Cosmetic intolerance. *Contact Dermatitis* 16:189, 1987.
8. DeGroot AC, Beverdam EGA, Ayong CT, et al: The role of contact allergy in the spectrum of adverse effects caused by cosmetics and toiletries. *Contact Dermatitis* 19:195, 1988.
9. Fransway AF: The problem of preservation in the 1990s: I. Statement of the problem, solution(s) of the industry, and the current use of formaldehyde and formaldehyde-releasing biocides. *Am J Contact Dermatitis* 2:6, 1991.
10. Emmons WW, Marks JG: Immediate and delayed reactions to cosmetic ingredients. *Contact Dermatitis* 13:258, 1985.
11. Romaguera C, Camarasa JMG, Alomar A, et al: Patch tests with allergens related to cosmetics. *Contact Dermatitis* 6:167, 1983.
12. DeGroot AC, Liem DH, Nater JP, et al: Patch tests with fragrance materials and preservatives. *Contact Dermatitis* 12:87, 1985.

13. Dooms-Goosens A, Deboulle K, Dooms M, et al: Imidazolidinyl urea dermatitis. *Contact Dermatitis* 14:322, 1986.
14. White IR: Prevalence of sensitivity to quaternium-15. Presentation at 8th International Symposium on Contact Dermatitis, Cambridge, March 20–22, 1986.
15. Fransway AF, Schmitz NA: The problem of preservation in the 1990s: II. Formaldehyde and formaldehyde-releasing biocides: Incidence of cross-reactivity and the significance of the positive response to formaldehyde. *Am J Contact Dermatitis* 2:78, 1991.
16. DeGroot AC, Weyand JW, Bos JD, et al: Contact allergy to preservatives (I). *Contact Dermatitis* 14:120, 1986.
17. DeGroot AC, Bos JD, Jagtman BA, et al: Contact allergy to preservation (II). *Contact Dermatitis* 15:218, 1986.
18. DeGroot AC: Contact allergy to cosmetics: Causative ingredients. *Contact Dermatitis* 17:26, 1987.
19. Hogan DJ, Hill M, Lane PR: Results of routine patch tests of 542 patients in Saskatoon, Canada. *Contact Dermatitis* 19:120, 1988.
20. NACDG data, as published in Feinman SE: *Formaldehyde Sensitivity and Toxicity.* Boca Raton, FL, CRC Press, 1988, pp 73, 85.
21. Ford GP, Beck MH: Reactions to quaternium-15, bronopol, and Germall 115 in a standard series. *Contact Dermatitis* 14:271, 1986.
22. Fransway AF: Isothiazolinone sensitivity. *Lancet* 1:990, 1989.
23. Storrs FJ, Rosenthal LE, Adams RM, et al: Prevalence and relevance of allergic-reactions in patients patch tested in North America—1984–1985. *J Am Acad Dermatol* 20:1038, 1989.
24. Parker LV, Taylor JS: A five-year study of contact allergy to quaternium-15. *Am J Contact Dermatitis* 2:231, 1991.
25. Fisher AA: Cosmetic dermatitis. Part II: Reactions to some commonly used preservatives. *Cutis* 26:136, 1980.
26. Cronin E: *Contact Dermatitis.* New York, Churchill Livingstone, 1980, pp 788–797.
27. Jordan WP, Sherman WJ, King SE: Threshold responses in formaldehyde-sensitive subjects. *J Am Acad Dermatol* 1:44, 1979.
28. Beyer KH, Bergfeld WF, Bernot WO, et al: Final report on the safety assessment of quaternium-15. *J Am Coll Toxicol* 5:61, 1986.

24

p-tert-BUTYLPHENOL FORMALDEHYDE RESIN

Jere D. Guin

HOW WOULD ONE SUSPECT ALLERGY TO p-tert-BUTYLPHENOL FORMALDEHYDE RESIN?

This antigen is part of the standard test series, and positive tests are often obtained on routine screening. It also is part of many shoe series, so one is likely to discover the allergy on screening patients with contact dermatitis. There is often an opportunity to look for relevance when a positive test is present.

Suspecting p-tert-butylphenol formaldehyde resin (PTBPFR) from the rash is some-times possible, as many patients who react primarily to this antigen have plantar dermatitis from the chloroprene rubber (neoprene) cement in the sponge rubber insoles of shoes,[1] especially athletic shoes. One may also see hand eczema.[2] In one series, 67 percent were women, and many patients were atopic.[3] However, the most interesting statistic is that 13 percent of the children who were patch tested reacted to PTBPFR.[4] The reason for this may well be related to the wearing of this type of footwear.

The adhesive effect of PTBPFR seems to be ideal for chloroprene rubber. The macromolecular end product fills in gaps and crevices on both surfaces, and with its natural tackiness, it becomes an excellent adhesive for the purpose. Allergy to PTBPFR has induced a number of cases of shoe dermatitis where PTBPFR is widely used with chloroprene adhesives.

HOW CAN A FINISHED RESIN BE ALLERGENIC?

Malten and Seutter[5] questioned why the finished product would be allergenic, as the polymer is too large for easy absorption and the chemistry suggests that relatively little of the original ingredients remain in the finished product.

The resin PTBPFR is manufactured as a condensation product of formaldehyde and p-tert-butylphenol (PTBP) at 60°C.[5] In a fresh sample of the finished resin, a trace of PTBP is still around, but fewer than 20 percent of those sensitive to PTBPFR are allergic to PTBP, the original chemical before formaldehyde and polymerization. There are products in the older resins after aging and environmental challenge. Malten and

Seutter postulate that there may be some deterioration of the resin in the long-term presence of acid and water, which may be why many patients seem to break out more to old shoes than new shoes.

A typical nail-bed reaction has also been produced by PTBPFR. The eruption was almost identical to those seen with allergy to acrylic nail preparations and cyanoacrylate adhesives.[6]

One may see allergy to PTBPFR as either an occupational or a consumer-type problem. An occupational association can be found in cobblers[7] (which seems to be an anachronism), automobile workers working with weather stripping, from paper,[8] and, of course, where the chemical is manufactured. According to Marks and DeLeo,[9] dentists and dental technicians are also at risk. Consumers may react to a prosthesis,[10] an adhesive for watchbands,[11] and leather objects as well as athletic tape,[12,13] adhesive labels,[14] ink and paper, film developer, motor oil, plywood, boxes, disinfectants and insecticides, and products used in woodworking and ceramics.[2,9] Materials such as do-it-yourself glues, masonry sealants, and "glass wool" may contain PTBPFR.[3]

PATCH-TESTING RESULTS

Sensitivity to PTBPFR has been assumed by some to be caused by allergy to the PTBP component, but this does not explain the patch-test results to components. Prevalence in persons who were patch tested was about 1.5 percent in one European series, which matches other published data. Of 30 persons reacting to PTBPFR, only 1 was allergic to PTBP and 3 were allergic to phenol formaldehyde resin.[3] Allergy to PTBPFR is somewhat more commonly reported than PTBP allergy, but this may be because we do not include a test for the latter as part of the standard series. Where PTBPFR and phenol formaldehyde resins are seen concomitantly, allergy to leather objects (e.g., watchbands) might be suspected.[3]

The PTBPFR patch-test antigen used is a polymer and not the PTBP monomer used to produce the resin. The monomer is also used as an antioxidant, as a germicide, and for a variety of other uses. Most patch-test reactors to PTBPFR are not formaldehyde-allergic, according to Malten.[5] In Bruze's series, the incidence of formaldehyde allergy was higher in those allergic to two different (non-PTBPFR) PFRs[15] but only in 1 of 12 who were PTBPFR-allergic. This may be related to the concentration present, as there is a significant quantity of free formaldehyde in many commercial PTBPFR resins.[16–18] There is also the possibility of variation from one batch to the next,[19] so testing to the one used on the job could show this.

Should a patient be positive to one of the two components used in the manufacture of PTBPFR, formaldehyde sources are given in Chap. 20. The other component, *p-tert*-butylphenol, is widely used as an antioxidant, an antiseptic, a plasticizer for plastics, a pour-point depressant and emulsion breaker for petroleum, a plasticizer for cellulose acetate, in deodorants as a germicide, as a fumigant, and so on.[20] Malten et al.[21] say that it is also used in manufacture of varnish and lacquer resins and as a soap antioxidant.

About 30 or 40 years ago, all persons allergic to PTBPFR were considered to be allergic to PTBP. However there appeared on the scene persons who did not fit what was accepted dogma; they were allergic to the resin *without* allergy to PTBP. Production of PTBPFR is now done mostly without excess PTBP,[4] so that this primary chemical

p-tert-BUTYLPHENOL FORMALDEHYDE RESIN—PATIENT HANDOUT

WHAT IS p-tert-BUTYLPHENOL FORMALDEHYDE RESIN (PTBPFR)?

This chemical is a "plastic" material used mostly as an adhesive especially for leather and water-resistant rubber products. The resin used for patch testing is a polymer (a chainlike connection of the monomer(s) which would be links in the chain) made from formaldehyde and tertiary-butylphenol. There is very little of the original components left in the finished resin, but moisture may gradually reverse the process, forming breakdown chemicals which can cause allergy. PTBPFR is ideally suited for use as an adhesive, since it contracts as it fills in microscopic cracks and crevices on opposing surfaces producing a very tight bonding. It is an ideal adhesive for certain materials because it has a tackiness for the surfaces of leather and rubber, and it binds cloth to leather.

WHERE DOES ONE GET EXPOSED TO THIS MATERIAL?

In 1958 a report appeared of sensitivity in shoe repairmen. At the time there was an excess amount of phenol (carbolic acid) following synthesis, but this was corrected. Today, exposure is probably principally from adhesives. This varies in its source—from adhesive labels, which would be uncommon, to the insoles of athletic shoes, the most common source. There the rubber insoles are likely to contain p-tert-butylphenol formaldehyde resin used as an adhesive. This may be why PTBPFR patch-test material gives positive reactions more often in children than one might anticipate from its frequency of response in routine testing.

Products containing rubber or leather may also be sources. Reactions to clothing include leather items such as a watch strap, a belt or a hatband, a raincoat fabric finish, handbags, and shoes, especially sponge rubber insoles in athletic shoes. Medical items which have caused a problem include a hearing aid, a prosthesis, a brace, and athletic tape.

Occupational exposures include those working with fiberglass products, plywood, masonry sealant, automobile manufacture, foundry work, inks and glues, as well as in shoe repair, although the last source does not occur so often today.

WHAT CAUSES THE ALLERGY?

While the precise cause(s) are not known with certainty, some patients sensitive to PTBPFR seem to be allergic to several breakdown products (called *hydroxymethyl derivatives*), but others do not. These chemicals are assumed to be breakdown products of PTBPFR caused by adding water (from sweat, etc.) and reversing the chemical process which formed the resin in the first place. PTBPFR is very similar to phenol formaldehyde resins (such as Bakelite), but phenol formaldehyde resins usually do not cause a reaction in persons allergic to PTBPFR.

This information is provided to help persons with contact dermatitis in the understanding of their problem. The contents are subject to change as more information becomes available and are not intended as a substitute for medical treatment.

would not be left in significant quantity in the final product, and today that concomitant allergy to the primary chemical is not so common.[17] The PTBPFR test is not adequate to detect other phenol formaldehyde resins; more closely related antigens are required for that purpose.[18]

Because formaldehyde is such a prominent sensitizer, one might assume that it is the problem in these systems. However, the data do not bear this out,[18] at least not in some studies. We frequently see concomitant formaldehyde sensitivity in persons who react mildly to PTBPFR, as our PTBPFR antigen contains detectable levels of free formaldehyde on testing. According to published reports, formaldehyde may[13,16] or may not[5] be found in the PTBPFR used.

REFERENCES

1. Angelini G, Vena GA, Meneghini CL: Shoe contact dermatitis. *Contact Dermatitis* 6:279, 1980.
2. Adams RM: "Spontaneous flare" to *p-tert*-butylphenol formaldehyde resin. *Contact Dermatitis* 1:321, 1975.
3. Geldof BA, Roesyanto ID, van Joost T: Clinical aspects of *para*-tertiary-butylphenolformaldehyde resin (PTBP-FR) allergy. *Contact Dermatitis* 21:312, 1989.
4. Barros MA, Baptista A, Correia TM, Azevedo F: Patch testing in children: A study of 562 schoolchildren. *Contact Dermatitis* 25:156, 1991.
5. Malten KE, Seutter E: Allergenic degradation products of *para*-tertiary butylphenolformaldehyde plastic. *Contact Dermatitis* 12:222, 1985.
6. Rycroft RJ, Wilkinson JD, Holmes R, Hay RJ: Contact sensitization to *p*-tertiary butylphenol (PTBP) resin in plastic nail adhesive. *Clin Exp Dermatol* 5:441, 1980.
7. Malten KE: Occupational eczema due to *p*-tertiary butylphenol in a shoe adhesive. *Dermatologica* 117:103, 1958.
8. Malten KE, Seutter E: Phenolformaldehyde resin in paper. *Contact Dermatitis* 11:127, 1984.
9. Marks JG, DeLeo VA: Exposure list: *para-tert*-butylphenol formaldehyde resin, in *Contact and Occupational Dermatology*. St. Louis, Mosby, 1992, p 96.
10. Romaguera C, Grimalt F, Vilaplana J: Paratertiary butylphenol formaldehyde resin in prosthesis. *Contact Dermatitis* 12:174, 1985.
11. Foussereau J, Petitjean J, Barre JG: Eczema due to wristwatch bands induced by allergy to formol-p.t. butylphenol resins of leather glue (resins of the C.K.R. 1634 type) [Fre] *Bull Soc Fr Dermatol Syphilol* 75:630, 1968.
12. Foussereau J, Petitjean J, Barre JG: Eczema due to wristwatch bands induced by allergy to formol-p.t. butylphenol resins of leather glue (resins of the C.K.R. 1634 type)[Fre]. *Bull Soc Fr Dermatol Syphilol* 75:630, 1968.
13. Foussereau J, Cavelier C, Selig D: Occupational eczema from *para*-tertiary-butylphenol formaldehyde resins: A review of the sensitizing resins. *Contact Dermatitis* 2:254, 1976.
14. Dahlquist I: Contact allergy to paratertiary butylphenol formaldehyde resin in an adhesive label. *Contact Dermatitis* 10:54, 1984.
15. Bruze M: Simultaneous reactions to phenol-formaldehyde resins colophony/hydroabietyl alcohol and balsam of Peru/perfume mixture. *Contact Dermatitis* 14:119, 1986.
16. Bruze M: Sensitizers in PTBP-formaldehyde resins (letter). *Contact Dermatitis* 14:132, 1986.
17. Foussereau J, Cavelier C, Selig D: Occupational eczema from *para*-tertiary-butylphenol formaldehyde resins: A review of the sensitizing resins. *Contact Dermatitis* 2:254, 1976.
18. Bruze M, Fregert S, Zimerson E: Contact allergy to phenol-formaldehyde resins. *Contact Dermatitis* 12:81, 1985.
19. Fregert S: Batch-consciousness in dermatologic management. *Acta Derm Venereol* 59 Suppl 85:63, 1979.
20. Kahn G: Depigmentation caused by phenolic detergent germicides. *Arch Dermatol* 102:177, 1970.
21. Malten KE, Seutter E, Hara I, Nakajima T: Occupational vitiligo due to paratertiary butylphenol and homologues. *Trans St John's Hosp Dermatol Soc* 57:115, 1971.

25

MERCAPTO MIX

Jere D. Guin

WHAT IS MERCAPTO MIX?

This is a mixture of chemicals which are often used in rubber products. Mixtures of related materials are frequently used in allergy testing in order to save time and money and because of the limited number of tests which can be applied. There are many problems with using a mixture rather than testing with each reagent in optimal concentration, but as a practical matter mixtures are very useful. This particular mixture comprises three different but chemically related rubber "accelerators," which are used in the curing of rubber. The chemicals apparently become available on exposure and are liberated and absorbed through the skin. One study of rubber chemicals in gloves found the level of some chemicals to be equal to the test concentrations used for patch testing.

Manufacturing methodology varies so much and there are so many rubber chemicals available that one cannot know with certainty what is contained in a product. Even when the manufacturer furnishes information on the contents, there may be chemicals in a product which are unknown to the manufacturer. The reasons for this are many. Commercial-grade chemicals are seldom pure, and oxidation, heat, and so on may change those originally there. Many products are assembled from manufactured components, such as shoes, and the methodology and composition may not be under the supervision of the final manufacturer. Also, in the case of rubber, chemicals may be added to the latex gathered from the tree, which would not be known unless an analysis were made of each lot of the raw material. Therefore, it is often less important to know what specific chemical caused the allergy than where it is likely to be found. In such an environment, use of mixtures provides the physician with more individual chemicals in his or her test series than would be available if individual reagents were used.

The mercapto mix formerly comprised four rather than three rubber accelerators, as 2-mercaptobenzothiazole (MBT) was included. This was removed, as MBT is used so widely that it deserves separate status, since that allows it to be tested in optimal concentration. The patch testing results with the mixture have been compared with those using individual chemicals, and about 20 percent fewer positives are found. Is this acceptable? That depends upon each case. Certainly it is useful as a screening series. However if this test is negative in a person who strongly suggests rubber sensitivity, retesting with individual reagents is suggested.

The differences created by testing with mixes rather than single chemicals are many, as Mitchell[1] pointed out many years ago. The concentration is generally lower in mixes,

237

which could lead to false negatives. Indeed, this may be a problem with the mercapto mix, as the mix concentration proved to be too low and MBT has now been separated for testing as a single antigen. Mitchell was also concerned about the stability of the chemicals, and using four at once may add to the problem. One form of interaction which he considered was quenching, which might occur in a mixture. This is the suppressive influence of one substance on the sensitizing ability of another—for example, the effect of eugenol on sensitization by cinnamic aldehyde.[2] Basically there are false-negatives because the concentration is lower, but the dose may sometimes be reinforcing if the behavior of each single chemical is influenced by others in the mixture. Quenching has been shown to occur in sensitization[2] and in nonimmunologic contact urticaria[3] but not in elicitation of subjects already allergic.[4]

Another concern is the occurrence of both false-positive reactions from irritation and false-negative results ostensibly from dilution of the active chemical.[5] The reverse is at least theoretically possible, as weaker allergens used together may elicit a reaction in subthreshold concentration, according to McClelland and Shuster,[6] who showed an additive effect on elicitation responses. The mercapto mix will pick up an occasional positive response which would have been missed by testing to MBT,[7] but this is the exception rather than the rule. With a mix comprising 0.25% of each of four antigens, only 14/169 allergic to either or both were mix-positive and MBT negative.[8] Even when the concentration was raised to 0.33% each, of 73 allergic to MBT and/or the mix, only 8 were MBT-negative and mix-positive.

The composition of the mercapto mix is 0.33% each of N-cyclohexyl-2-benzothiazolesulfenamide; 2,2'-benzothiazyl disulfide; and 4-morpholinyl-2-benzothiazyl disulfide. These are sometimes abbreviated as CBS, MBTS (which unfortunately does not match any chemical name) or DBTD for dibenzothiazyl disulfide, and MMBT. According to Cronin,[9] the order of positive responses is MMBT> CBS> MBTS. All of these are closely related to MBT in structure, with the 2-thiol component necessary for cross-reactivity.[10]

In one series of 145 rubber-allergic patients, the most commonly positive reagent was the mercapto mix.[11] One should be aware of the differences in the European data from those from the United States, as the mix there comprises four chemicals (MBT is included) each at 0.5% concentration (it is 0.33% each in the mix used in the United States). The level of sensitivity to the mercapto mix in the United States is about 2.1 percent; it is somewhat lower in Europe.[12] Of some 200 persons tested to multiple individual rubber accelerators, 11 of 16 positive to any reacted to more than one. This is not surprising, as many are closely related chemically and they are often found in the same product. In another European series, however, the percentage of mercapto mix patients was less than one-fourth that of the thiuram mix,[11] but this included many with occupational dermatitis caused by latex gloves, which is commonly associated with thiuram sensitivity. Rubber gloves (and probably other products as well) which are ostensibly free of a rubber chemical may actually have it present on analysis,[13] so one would be wise to test patients to the item itself before declaring it safe.

N-CYCLOHEXYL-2-BENZOTHIAZOLESULFENAMIDE

This chemical, also known as CBS, is a benzothiazole accelerator which is sometimes used in manufacture of tires of natural and synthetic rubber or to substitute for MBTS/DPG systems in other applications. The basic structure is that of MBT linked to the cyclohexyl structure through an amine linkage. The technical aspects are not important to the physician, but one can see the benzothiazole component in the structure, so one would expect it sometimes to cross-react with other benzothiazole accelerators.

2,2'-BENZOTHIAZYL DISULFIDE

This substance, or MBTS, is another benzothiazole which is closely related to MBT. It is used as such for both natural and synthetic rubber, but the latter may be combined with a secondary accelerator. It may be in both white and colored materials. In products to be in repeated contact with food, its content is limited to 1.5% maximum, according to 21 CFR section 177.26. This chemical is formed from MBT by heat and oxidation and may be a sensitizer in some shoes. One recent publication suggests that MBT is converted by oxidation into this compound, which then is the actual cause of allergic contact dermatitis to MBT. It has been isolated along with MBT from athletic shoes causing insole dermatitis, but it was not possible to know whether it was in the original formula of the rubber content or formed from oxidative change. It may also be found in chloroprene rubber as a plasticizer.

4-MORPHOLINYL-2-BENZOTHIAZYL DISULFIDE

Industrially, this product is used where extended processing safety is a worry, as for thick treads or extrusions, in products with a high furnace black loading, and products to be stored for extended periods.

PATCH TESTING

There is obviously considerable overlap between the mercapto mix and MBT. In one study 9/10 reacted to MBT, 2 to the mix and MBT and 1 only to the mix. It is known that MBT may be converted easily into DBTD at a pH of 6.5 and that all three components of the mercapto mix will form MBT in the presence of glutathione.[14] The tendency to sensitize to the morpholinyl-substituted benzothiazole was shown in one study to be greater, with 80 percent of the animals sensitized to MMBT reacting to MBT but only 50 percent of those MBT-sensitized responding to MMBT on elicitation.[15] This was thought to have been from the affinity the morpholinyl moiety had for S-H and amine groups of amino acid moieties of protein.[16]

WHAT IS THE BEST WAY TO PREVENT CONTACT WITH ONE OF THESE CHEMICALS?

Most studies do not list the objects to which patients broke out except that rubber gloves are a common sensitizer, especially for thiuram-positive patients. Shoes are a leading cause of MBT sensitivity, and these patients frequently overlap with those who are sensitive to the mercapto mix. Insole dermatitis may also occur to DBTD (MBTS).[17] For shoe sensitivity, avoidance of sponge rubber insoles is advised and advance patch testing to shoes is advised. For glove-allergic patients, Elastyren gloves are usually tolerated, but these contain a low level of carbamate, so testing should be done to determine whether or not the patient will tolerate them. Tactylon is very hypoallergenic, and these gloves can be used in persons allergic to both rubber and vinyl. Vinyl is

MERCAPTO MIX AND 2-MERCAPTOBENZOTHIAZOLE—PATIENT HANDOUT

WHAT ARE 2-MERCAPTOBENZOTHIAZOLE (MBT) AND MERCAPTO MIX (MBT MIX)?

These chemicals are "rubber chemicals", as they are largely used in curing both natural rubber and certain synthetic rubbers. Natural rubber comes from the sap or latex of a tree *Hevea braziliensis*. In its natural state, untreated natural rubber is not suitable for many uses. To improve stability and physical properties, natural rubber is heated and chemically treated to produce cross-linkages. Chemicals used in the latter process are called *accelerators*. An important category of accelerators is the benzothiazoles. This includes MBT and the chemicals in MBT mix. Some synthetic rubber such as styrene-butadiene requires an even greater amount of MBT than other sulfur donors.

HOW COMMON IS THIS ALLERGY?

The prevalence of allergy to MBT varies with the geographic region. In North America in 1985–1989, the prevalance of reactions to 1% MBT was 2.1 percent and to MBT mix was 2.5 percent of persons suspected to have contact dermatitis. So many of these rubber chemicals are similar in chemical structure that we do not always know which one caused the original allergy. However, those who are allergic should avoid articles likely to contain related rubber chemicals.

WHAT PRODUCTS CAUSE THE ALLERGIC CONTACT DERMATITIS IN SOMEONE ALLERGIC TO MBT OR MBT MIX?

Mercaptobenzothiazole is the most common cause of allergy to the insoles in shoes. This causes a rash on the bottom of the feet, sparing the arch and the toes where they are attached, but worse where there is pressure. At least one of the rubber chemicals in MBT mix can also do this.

When spandex (a synthetic elastic material, e.g., Lycra) was newly released, MBT was found in some of those products, but it is not in them today. However, one can see MBT in a variety of rubber products such as brassiere cups, rubber bands, finger cots, rubber banknote counters, rubber swim caps, face masks, and gas masks. MBT may also be in rubber products used in food preparation such as hoses, gloves, or spatulas.

MBT is sometimes found in rubber gloves, although that allergy is usually caused by another rubber chemical. Other health care products which may contain MBT include catheters, veterinary medications, elastic bandages, rubber stoppers in medical syringes, and (as a contaminant in) the injectable solution of a medication called *digoxin*, to name a few. MBT is sometimes found in hot water bottles and baby bottle nipples. It occasionally causes allergy in condoms. There can be MBT in items of clothing where it is incorporated into the threads of the material, elastic waistbands, girdles, suspenders, and protective aprons as well as gloves, boots, and shoes.

MERCAPTO MIX AND 2-MERCAPTOBENZOTHIAZOLE— PATIENT HANDOUT (*Continued*)

There are also a number of unsuspected sources of exposure which are either not rubber or do not seem to be rubber. MBT has also been used in an anticorrosive agent, in an antifreeze mixture, in insecticides, fungicides, and laboratory reagents. It has been reported to be in photographic film, tools (especially the grip), handlebar grips, cleansers and detergents, cushions, sponges, paints, tubing, rubber sponges, and cement tubes.

WHAT SHOULD BE DONE TO PREVENT EXPOSURE TO THESE CHEMICALS?

Be wary of any rubber product, especially shoes made with rubber (as athletic shoes) or padded with foam rubber. One would do well to test the lining before wearing any pair purchased as a substitute. All-leather shoes may be safe, but many persons fail to identify the sponge rubber insole when present and pay for their indiscretion by breaking out. In addition to selecting a safe pair of shoes, you must not wear any socks or stockings which have been worn in the shoes to which you are allergic. Furthermore, elasticized stockings are suspect. Some persons allergic to MBT will break out on the elbows from rubber in upholstered furniture. For those who must wear elastic (support) hose, a product free of rubber can be purchased from Jobst, Inc., PO Box 653, Toledo, Ohio 43694 [Tel. (800) 221-7570]. Avoid going barefoot on rubber-backed carpet and cover the padded arms of upholstered furniture with a towel.

Glove allergy is a bit easier, as lists are available for gloves free of MBT. However, before wearing any of the "safe" brands, test yourself to be certain there are no other chemicals in the gloves to which you might be allergic. Wearing vinyl gloves is another alternative, but again test yourself to be certain, as a number of individuals are allergic to both. Should you be allergic to both rubber and vinyl gloves, polyethylene or Tactylon gloves should be satisfactory. The latter are available (sterile and nonsterile) from SmartPractice, 3400 McDowell, Phoenix, Arizona 85008-7899.

Handling rubber objects can cause a problem where your hands touch your skin, so try to avoid direct contact when you have to touch rubber objects until you are clear. A polyethylene glove can be used to apply cosmetics. Sponges used to apply cosmetics often contain rubber chemicals, so avoid using them.

often substituted by hospital personnel as a practical solution, and it is frequently a satisfactory solution. Testing the patient to be certain is advised, as allergy to vinyl is far from rare. Two publications have given charts on the chemical content in latex examination and surgical gloves,[18,19] but chemicals unrecognized by the manufacturer may be present anyway,[13] so testing the patient to a piece of the glove is advised. This should usually be done on the outer upper arm as it is a good area for transdermal absorption and it is convenient for solid objects.

Reports of allergy to a facial mask,[20] to an amputation prosthesis,[21] and many other such contactants have appeared. Plantar pustulosis may also occur in persons allergic to chemicals in the mercapto mix.[22]

One can do single tests to find the causative one of the three antigens included in the mix. Most who react will also react with MBT, and avoidance of that is covered in the section on that (single) chemical. The handout for MBT is probably in order for those allergic to the mercapto mix, although usage of these chemicals does not always overlap.

In interpreting the results, consider a positive test as evidence of the group, as there is a great tendency for cross-reactions, and MBT is positive in most.

REFERENCES

1. Mitchell JC: Patch testing with mixes. *Contact Dermatitis* 7:98–104, 1981.
2. Opdyke DLJ: Inhibition of sensitization reactions induced by certain aldehydes. *Food Cosmet Toxicol* 14:197–198, 1976.
3. Guin JD, Meyer BN, Drake RD, Haffley P: The effect of quenching agents on contact urticaria by cinnamic aldehyde. *J Am Acad Dermatol* 10:45–51, 1984.
4. Basketter DA, Allenby CF: Studies of the quenching phenomenon in delayed contact hypersensitivity reactions. *Contact Dermatitis* 25:160–171, 1991.
5. Epstein E: Simplified patch test screening with mixtures. *Arch Dermatol* 95:269–274, 1967.
6. McLelland J, Shuster S: Contact dermatitis with negative patch tests: The additive effect of allergens in combination. *Br J Dermatol* 122:623–630, 1990.
7. Mitchell JC, Clendenning WE, Cronin E, et al: Patch testing with mercaptobenzothiazole and mercapto mix. *Contact Dermatitis* 2:123–124, 1976.
8. Lynde CW, Mitchell JC, Adams RM, et al: Patch testing with mercaptobenzothiazole and mercapto mixes. *Contact Dermatitis* 8:273–274, 1982.
9. Cronin E: *Contact Dermatitis.* Edinburgh, Churchill Livingstone, 1980, p 730.
10. Fregert S: Cross sensitivity pattern of 2-mercaptobenzothiazole (MBT). *Acta Derm Venereol* 49:45–50, 1962.
11. von Hintzenstern J, Heese A, Koch HU, et al: Frequency, spectrum and occupational relevance of type IV allergies to rubber chemicals. *Contact Dermatitis* 24:244–252, 1991.
12. Nethercott JR, Holness DL, Adams RM, et al. Patch testing with a routine screening tray in North America, 1985 through 1989: Frequency of response. *Am J Contact Dermatitis* 2:122–129, 1991.
13. Knudsen BB, Larsen E, Egsgaard H, Menne T: Release of thiurams and carbamates from rubber gloves. *Contact Dermatitis* 28:63–69, 1993.
14. Hansson C, Agrup G: Stability of the mercaptobenzothiazole compounds. *Contact Dermatitis* 28:29–34, 1993.
15. Wang XS, Suskind RR: Comparative studies of the sensitization potential of morpholine, 2-mercaptobenzothiazole and 2 of their derivatives in guinea pigs. *Contact Dermatitis* 19:11–15, 1988.
16. Wang XS, Tabor MW: Studies of the reactivity of morpholine, 2-mercaptobenzothiazole and 2 of their derivatives with selected amino acids. *Contact Dermatitis.* 19:16–21, 1988.
17. Jung JH, McLaughlin JL, Stannard J, Guin JD: Isolation, via activity-directed fractionation, of mercaptobenzothiazole and dibenzothiazyl disulfide as 2 allergens responsible for tennis shoe dermatitis. *Contact Dermatitis* 19:254–259, 1988.
18. Heese A, van Hintzenstern J, Peters KP, et al: Allergic and irritant reactions to rubber gloves in medical health services: Spectrum, diagnostic approach, and therapy. (Published erratum appears in *J Am Acad Dermatol* 26:403, 1992.) *J Am Acad Dermatol* 25:831–839, 1991.
19. Rich P, Belozer ML, Norris P, Storrs FJ: Allergic contact dermatitis to two antioxidants in latex gloves: 4,4′-thiobis(6-tert-butyl-meta-cresol) (Lowinox 44S36) and butylhydroxyanisole: Allergen alternatives for glove-allergic patients. (Published erratum appears in *J Am Acad Dermatol* 26:144, 1992.) *J Am Acad Dermatol* 24:37–43, 1991.
20. Fowler JF Jr, Callen JP: Facial dermatitis from a neoprene rubber mask. *Contact Dermatitis* 18:310–311, 1988.
21. Baptista A, Barros MA, Azenha A: Allergic contact dermatitis on an amputation stump. *Contact Dermatitis* 26:140–141, 1992.
22. Pecegueiro M, Brandao M: Contact plantar pustulosis. *Contact Dermatitis* 11:126–127, 1984.

26

BLACK RUBBER MIX

Jere D. Guin

WHAT IS BLACK RUBBER MIX?

This is a mixture of certain chemicals used in the processing of rubber to make the product more resistant to breakdown, cracking, and crumbling in the air. Rubber would not weather well if it did not contain antidegradants to help prevent damage from oxygen and ozone and to provide protection from flex cracking and heat aging. An excellent group of such chemicals is the one comprising the derivatives of p-phenylaminediamine (PPD). Three of these are in the test material: N-phenyl-N'-isopropyl-p-phenylenediamine (IPPD) in a concentration of 0.1% and N-phenyl-N'-cyclohexyl-p-phenylenediamine (CPPD) and N, N'-diphenyl-p-phenylenediamine (DPPD) each in a 0.25% concentration. While there are nonstaining antioxidants, the black rubber products provide good protection at the cost of their staining qualities. Typical applications would be in tires, radiator hoses, and so on. In the United States, IPPD is seldom used as such today, but it is commonly present in European products.[1] Most individuals allergic to IPPD will also break out to N(1,3-dimethylbutyl)-N'-phenyl-p-phenylenediamine (DMPPD), the chemical usually substituted, so the test material used is still relevant.

WHY USE A MIX?

This is covered in the section on the mercapto mix, but essentially the mix allows one to test to three or four chemicals at one time, saving time, trouble, and money. In addition, it may uncover some sensitive patients that one would not find using a single such chemical. Of course, the problem with mixes is that the optimum concentration is often not possible, and irritation can easily occur unless the mixture is standardized.

HOW DO PPD-RELATED CHEMICALS DIFFER FROM OTHER RUBBER CHEMICALS

The structure of chemicals within this group is based on N,N' substitution of the basic paraphenylenediamine molecule. There are many categories of rubber chemicals grouped according to use or structure. Categorization of use is often done according to the dominant activity, as there may be more than one use of a single rubber chemical or family of rubber chemicals. Some of these chemicals accelerate the process of cross-linkage or curing, some act as retarders, some are inert "fillers," some are used for foams or "blowers," some act as mould lubricants, and some prevent degradation. In the last category, which comprises largely antioxidants and antiozonants, one of the best chemical groups for this purpose is the one structurally related to PPD. These chemicals also stain the rubber, so this mixture of such agents is called the black rubber mix. The PPD-related rubber chemicals are used in both natural and synthetic products. While the greatest use has been in tires, these antioxidants are found in a wide variety of products, usually recognizable by the color of the product.

HOW IS ALLERGY TO BLACK RUBBER MIX RECOGNIZED?

One can often get a clue from a patient presenting with contact dermatitis who has a history or signs of rubber allergy. The percentage of those allergic to other rubber chemicals—such as thiurams, benzothiazoles, or carbamates—who are also allergic to PPD mix varies with the population. The PPD-related chemicals are more often associated with occupationally induced allergy.[2] In some series of industrial cases,[2] it is the leading sensitizer, with a reported prevalence rate of 37 per thousand.[2]

Of 158 persons allergic to rubber, PPD mix produced a positive patch test in 40. It was third in order of frequency after thiurams and carbamates.[3] In countries where IPPD is still used, it may be the leading rubber allergen in workers in tire manufacturing. In one European study, 42 of 56 IPPD-allergic persons acquired sensitivity to IPPD from occupational exposure. Of these, 17 were in tire manufacture, 9 were automobile mechanics, 9 were drivers, and 7 had other industrial exposure.[4]

The location of the eruption depends upon the source, but hand dermatitis is typical. The eruption is often a fissured dermatitis of the hands with a lichenified dermatitis of the wrists and forearms[5] in persons handling tires,[6] because the antigen frequently contaminates the surface[7] and the eruption may spread to other areas, such as the chest and axillae.[8] One reason for this may be the tendency for IPPD, CPPD, and DPPD to concentrate on the surface of the black rubber objects. This predisposes the patient to hand contact and hand transfer. In one large series, 47 percent had hand involvement. This often is caused by handling black rubber tires, hoses, and so on, but unusual contact can occur. One person reacted after holding a policeman's rubber-covered billy club (truncheon or blackjack); the eruption cleared when the rubber was replaced by leather.[9] Another person reacted after holding the black rubber "wishbone" of a wind-surfer; the cure was to switch to an equivalent aluminum component.[10] One report of dermatitis from rubber finger stalls in postal sorters found IPPD in the product when the manufacturer ostensibly did not know it was there.[11] Perhaps another reason one sees surface transfer is that IPPD is a potent sensitizer—at such low levels that it is tested at 0.1% concentration.[12]

With hand transfer, the face may be involved as well, and direct transfer also can be less obvious. Shaw and Wilkinson[60] had a patient with localized eczema of the leg, following an injury, who proved to be aggravating the condition by rubbing it with the tip of her walking stick. The tip was made of black rubber and she was, of course, allergic to black rubber mix.

The eruption can also be seen from clothing (e.g., socks where an eczema was circumferentially distributed on the calf[13]). There are also reports of contact to the eyelids from an eyelash curler[14] and a radarscope,[15] on the face where a rubber mask was worn,[16] and on the body where underclothing was worn,[17] but this must be somewhat unusual.

Shoe (or boot)[18] dermatitis may stem from PPD-related chemicals or from PPD dyes. Some do not feel that shoe dyes are likely to be PPD-related,[19] but Lynde et al.[20] found that 5 of 32 shoe-allergic persons were sensitive to PPD and not to isopropyl-phenyl-o-phenylenediamine on standard testing to shoe chemicals.[20] Certainly an eruption can be present on the feet from black rubber chemicals.[21,21a] Persons with allergy to both PPD and black rubber mix are probably rubber-, rather than dye-sensitive, although reactions to dye reportedly still occur.[22] A black watch strap can cause a band of contact dermatitis on the wrist,[23,24] and specific areas of the face may be involved from contact with unsuspected objects such as swim goggles[25] or eyeglass straps[26] or where a spectacle chain was attached by a black rubber piece.[27]

There are also unusual presentations that one might never suspect without knowing of the entity. For example, purpuric contact dermatitis can occur from these chemicals.[20,28,29] Erythema multiform can also occur from contact allergy.[30] Another clinically atypical picture is that of palmoplantar pustulosis.[31] Photodermatitis has been reported from PPD, but the data in that report does not include a positive test to black rubber mix.[32]

Perhaps the most sherlockian case history was reported by Dooms-Goossens et al.,[33] who had a patient with a dermatitis of the hands and the perioral area of the face and allergy to black rubber mix. This person, a chemist, carefully watched his contact in his laboratory, but he broke out on attending monthly meetings of the European Economic Community in Brussels, where he regularly gave a report. The rash appeared on the day after his meetings and improved steadily afterward until the next meeting. He painstakingly avoided contact with black rubber, even protecting the hands from contact by wearing cotton gloves. He also looked diligently but unsuccessfully for the source. The authors watched his behavior when in the EEC building and discovered that he rode an escalator and grasped the black rubber railing without realizing it was made of black rubber. Avoidance solved the problem. Perhaps the most unusual part of this case is the location on the face as well as the hands, as the allergen was apparently transferred from the hands. Dooms-Goossens remembered a case published by Goh[34] of a patient exposed to the handle grips on his motorcycle.

I had a similar case of a patient with *Candida* cheilitis who was given an ointment to treat the condition. She came in with a contact dermatitis of the lips and circumoral area and—as it proved—she was not allergic to the ointment. However, she was positive on patch testing to black rubber mix in the standard screening series. Apparently the oil-based ointment tended to degrade some rubber object she had touched. She then picked up the antigen and transferred it to her face every time she applied an ointment to her lips. On watching her own behavior she discovered the culprits: they were the black rubber pads on the undersurface of her stapler, which she used every weekend in publishing her church bulletin. Again, recognition and avoidance solved the problem.

CROSS-REACTIVITY

Since PPD is already in the standard patch-test series, why add three chemically related substances? The reason is that PPD testing does not reliably find allergy to these chemicals. Certainly it may, but the rate of responses to PPD- in IPPD-sensitized subjects is only about 37.5 percent.[2] There is species specificity between IPPD and PPD in the ability of each to induce allergy, with PPD being a more potent sensitizer in the guinea pig[35] and IPPD causing more allergy in human beings.[36] IPPD is a strong sensitizer in human subjects,[36] with concentrations as low as 0.01% being adequate to produce sensitivity.[37]

Chemicals in the black rubber mix (IPPD, CPPD, and DPPD) tend to cross-react with PPD, but this is far from universal. In Poland, over half of PPD-allergic persons are allergic to IPPD as well.[38] In recent years, many rubber manufacturers in western countries have substituted N-(1,3-dimethylbutyl)-N'-phenyl-p-phenylenediamine (DMPPD) for IPPD because it is less sensitizing. It may cross-react, however, as patch-test data shows that chemical to regularly cause responses in IPPD-allergic persons.[39] All three chemicals in the black rubber mix are sensitizers in clinical reports, and there is cross-reactivity in guinea-pig data.[39] The basic molecular structural characteristics contributing to sensitization seem to be the primary amino group with the aromatic ring, the basic nature caused by substitution on the ring, and the presence of components which are electron donors rather than electron acceptors.[40]

PATCH TESTING

Suppliers of patch-testing materials sell antigens containing the individual chemicals, but most testing is done with the mixture of three chemicals: IPPD 0.1% plus CPPD and DPPD, each in a 0.25% concentration in petrolatum. Years ago some investigators used higher concentrations of black rubber chemicals, but because of active sensitization from the testing, the concentration was reduced from 2% to 0.25%,[41] and in this country IPPD is tested at 0.1% both in the mix and individually. The other two, CPPD and DPPD, are individually tested at a concentration of 1%. These are commercial-grade chemicals, so there may be some contamination as well as cross-reactivity with other chemicals in the group. There is seldom a reason to go to great lengths to determine the specific PPD-substituted chemical(s) to which the patient is allergic, as the patient will not be able to determine which black rubber product contains which chemical anyway. The rank order for reactivity in the group is IPPD>CPPD>DPPD. Testing to IPPD alone rather than the mix would miss 10%.[42]

In Poland, the incidence of sensitivity to black rubber has been reported to be 8.7 percent of persons patch tested in one series, but these patients had not complained of rubber sensitivity. Whether this was caused by a hidden source, cross-reactivity, or a false-positive response is not clear.[38] When patients in that series reacted to other rubber chemicals, there was obvious relevance, which is surprising in view of the widespread use of IPPD in Poland.

In European centers, about 0.6 to 0.7 percent of those tested react to the black rubber mix,[42] while in the United States screening examinations turn up a response in about 2.1% of those tested.[43] The incidence may be much higher, however, in those allergic to rubber from sources other than gloves, although it is not nearly as common as thiuram sensitivity even in this group.[44]

There may be a genetic basis for susceptibility, as in one series there was an increased incidence in persons positive for HLA-B40, and there was a negative correlation for HLA-A10.[45]

SOURCES

Sources of contact with black rubber are largely determinable by a commonsense approach: If a rubber object is black, it *very* likely contains these chemicals and should be avoided. The list would be incredibly long. Many of the published case reports are given in Table 26-1.

OCCUPATION

In occupational dermatitis to rubber, the PPD-related aromatic amines are commonly the cause of rubber allergy. In one series, of a total of 56 persons with allergic contact dermatitis to IPPD, 42 cases were considered to have been caused by occupational contacts, 17 cases were found among workers in tire manufacture, 9 in car mechanics, 9 in drivers, and 7 in various industrial occupations.[4] When one thinks of industrial exposure from the manufacture of rubber chemicals, jobs related to tire manufacture are typical. Less obvious may be those workers who assemble boots and shoes, cushions, insulation on electrical wiring, floor mats, and even the rubber pads under tabletop appliances or office equipment.

Anyone who handles automotive parts, such as hoses, is probably going to be exposed. Mechanics and body shop employees, salvage workers, automobile sales-

TABLE 26–1. Sources of Black Rubber Exposure

Acrylates[47]	Hoses[47]
Automatic milking machines[47]	Orthopedic bandage[55]
Automobile tires[2,51]	Patch testing[56]
Banknote counter (rubber bands)[52]	Radarscope[15]
Belts[51]	Rubber repair cement[50]
Blackjack tabletop[9]	Scuba mask[16]
Bootee[36]	Shoe sole[36]
Boots[20]	Shoes[22]
Cables[51]	Spectacle strap[27]
Camera eyepiece[53]	Squash ball[57]
Cloth shoes[21]	Stapler foot
Cushion[36]	Stockings[58,59]
Escalator rail[33]	Truck cushions[50]
Eyelash curler[26]	Tubing[47]
Finger stall[11]	Underclothing[17]
Flower bouquet band[54]	Walking stick[60]
Gasoline[50]	Watch strap[23,24]
Gloves[51]	Windsurfer "wishbone"[10]
Handlebar grip[34]	

WHAT IS THE BLACK RUBBER MIX?

This is a mixture of three rubber chemicals which sometimes cause contact allergy. The mixture is used to test for sensitivity to three potential causes of rubber allergy with one test. As with other mixtures, using a mixture rather than a separate test in the optimum concentration is very practical, but it is a compromise. These chemicals are added to certain types of rubber to protect the product from the harmful effects of exposure to oxygen and ozone, which can damage rubber. They impart a black color to the rubber, so they are "black rubber" chemicals, and the mixture is a mixture of black rubber chemicals or "black rubber mix."

WHAT DOES A POSITIVE TEST MEAN?

Not every positive test is accurate, but usually a positive test indicates allergy to one of the chemicals normally found in black rubber products and that you may possibly react to such products. The sources are often so subtle that one would not even consider the exposure. For example, it may mean you will break out to an appliance's electrical cord, which is usually covered with black rubber. One unusual case involved someone who broke out on the face after holding a black rubber railing on an escalator! The tiny amount of the chemicals from the black rubber railing were enough to cause the allergy when the hands transferred them to the face. Hand transfer of these chemicals from handling rubber products is a very real possibility in persons with a positive patch test to black rubber mix.

HOW DO I KNOW THAT THIS CAUSED THE PROBLEM?

This can be difficult to prove, but it is not hard to suspect. The important thing is to recognize the potential sources and avoid touching them without protection. A patch test to the material will tell you whether or not you are allergic to it, and your doctor can show you how to do this. The rash may be where your skin contacts the object, as under a black rubber watch strap, but a rash on the eyelids or lips may come from your handling the object with the hands and then touching these areas.

WHERE WOULD I LIKELY COME INTO CONTACT WITH BLACK RUBBER?

The sources are incredibly numerous. Some examples have already been mentioned. Perhaps the principal exposure occurs in industry, where workers are

---

This information is provided to help persons with contact dermatitis in the understanding of their problem. The contents are subject to change as more information becomes available and are not intended as a substitute for medical treatment.

exposed to tires, radiator hoses, or weatherstripping for automobile windows or where they may handle the chemicals or the rubber to be used for such purposes. Clothing sources in the United States are not especially common, but elastic in socks, a brassiere, or underwear has contained these chemicals and caused allergy. Rubber handlebars can cause hand eczema, and a black rubber cushion around an eyepiece can cause a poison ivy–like rash around the eye of an allergic person. Persons have been exposed to black rubber on a sailboat, in an eyelash curler, and even in a medicine dropper. Because these chemicals have a structure similar to that of the dye used on hair, persons who dye their hair and their barbers and beauticians are also at risk to become allergic to the dye if they are allergic to black rubber mix.

Occupational exposure can result in epidemics among workers in industry. Unusual sources sometimes become obvious when many persons become allergic. A good example of the latter is in the case of dairy farmers who became allergic to the black rubber used on milking machines.

A seldom recognized problem is the tendency of oily substances such as hand lotions, moisturizers, and prescription ointments to damage rubber. This means that the object touched may release more of the chemicals when it is degraded. Some patients have even unknowingly picked up the chemical by having the prescription ointment on their hands; they have then transferred the allergy to the eyelids, lips, and other areas.

HOW CAN I KNOW WHETHER OR NOT AN OBJECT CONTAINS THE SUBSTANCE THAT CAUSES MY ALLERGY

The best way to suspect that you may be allergic is to check the color. If it looks like it is made of rubber and it is black, it probably will be a problem. If you are in regular contact and you want to be certain, you can test yourself by putting shavings of the rubber on your skin under a piece of paper tape. Sometimes a small square of Saran wrap is used to cover the rubber scrapings so that a square shape is formed. You should limit the size of the Saran to just larger than the pieces of rubber and fold it back to make a square. Tack it down on the outer (upper) arm and leave it for 2 days. Mark the skin when you take the bandage off and look for redness and itching. Pressure under the bandage can cause irritation and may make you think you are allergic when you are not. Don't test yourself to just any object either, as some things are irritating when tested in this manner. If you are in doubt, have your doctor help you with it.

WHAT ARE SOME EXAMPLES?

Black rubber tires (both natural and synthetic), cables, belting, hoses, cushions in trucks, rubber cement, scuba masks, oxygen masks, shoe soles, tips of walking

(Continued)

BLACK RUBBER (PPD) MIX—PATIENT HANDOUT *(Continued)*

sticks and the feet of appliances, electric cords, sandals, "cloth" slippers, squash balls, black rubber gloves, eyepiece covers, eyeglass straps, gasoline, finger stalls, rubber bands, boots and shoes, sports equipment, the rubber pads under staplers, and even a police billy club covered with rubber. The list is so much longer that it is impossible to name everything, but you should understand by now. The rest is common sense and taking the time to be careful.

Now look around you and find a black rubber object. Now find another. If you can't, look at your feet. Are the heels on your shoes rubber? Look at the floor mats on the stairs or in your car. Look under the items on your desk. Is there a rubber pad on the undersurface? Is it black? Look at the electrical outlets in the room. Is there a cord plugged into one of them? Is it black? Practice this and you'll find many sources. Watch what you touch with your hands and look for the source(s) any time you break out.

persons, automotive parts clerks, tire fitters, tire salespersons, and so on are all at risk. Service station, garage, and parking attendants as well as car washers, drivers, and truckers are also exposed. Persons retreading tires would handle material containing these chemicals on a regular basis.

Some occupations are more difficult to suspect. These would include military personnel operating a radarscope, scuba divers, motorcycle riders including police personnel, hospital employees,[46] electrical workers (who handle insulated wire and cable), and repairpersons. Bank tellers, postal workers, and florists all use elastic bands which sometimes contain these chemicals. Dairy farmers may break out to the black rubber components of automatic milking machines.[47,48] More examples include painters, engineers, machine operators, boiler maintenance workers, aircraft fitters, and plant hire contractors.[49]

Sometimes it calls for real detective work to uncover the occupational association. The church secretary who reacted to the rubber feet (pads) on her stapler and Dooms-Goosens' patient who broke out to an escalator railing were both "at work." One is occupationally exposed when mowing lawns (the grips on the handles of the mower) or when repairing boots and shoes. A photographer may touch black rubber (the eyepiece, the lens, or case of the camera). The list is endless, and the average patient needs considerable counseling when the patch test to black rubber mix is read as positive. A handout is included but is not a substitute for explanation in person.

REFERENCES

1. Herve-Bazin B, Gradiski D, Duprat P, et al: Occupational eczema from *N*-isopropyl-*N'*-phenylparaphenylenediamine (IPPD) and *N*-dimethyl-1,3 butyl-*N'*-phenylparaphenylenediamine (DMPPD) in tires. *Contact Dermatitis* 3:1–15, 1977.

2. Kilpikari I: Occupational contact dermatitis among rubber workers. *Contact Dermatitis* 8:359–362, 1982.
3. Lammintausta K, Kalimo K: Sensitivity to rubber: Study with rubber mixes and individual rubber chemicals. *Derm Beruf Umwelt* 33:204–208, 1985.
4. Foussereau J, Cavelier C: Has *N*-isopropyl-*N'*-phenylparaphenylenediamine a place among standard allergens? Importance of this allergen in rubber intolerance. *Dermatologica* 155:164–167, 1977.
5. Calnan CD: Lichenoid dermatitis from isopropylaminodiphenylamine. *Contact Dermatitis Newsletter* 10:237, 1971.
6. Jordan WP: Contact dermatitis from *N*-isopropyl-*N'*-phenylparaphenylenediamine. *Arch Dermatol* 103:85–87, 1971.
7. Fregert S: Relapse of hand dermatitis after short contact with tires. *Contact Dermatitis Newsletter* 13:351, 1973.
8. Ancona A, Monroy F, Fernandez-Diez J: Occupational dermatitis from IPPD in tires. *Contact Dermatitis* 8:91–94, 1982.
9. Brandao FM: Occupational contact dermatitis from rubber antioxidants. *Contact Dermatitis* 4:246, 1978.
10. Tennstedt D, Lachapelle JM: Windsurfer dermatitis from black rubber components. *Contact Dermatitis* 7:160–161, 1981.
11. Roed-Petersen J, Hjorth N, Jordan WP, Bourlas M: Postsorters' rubber fingerstall dermatitis. *Contact Dermatitis* 3:143–147, 1977.
12. Wilkinson DS: Sensitivity to *N*-isopropyl-*N'*-phenyl-*p*-phenylenediamine. *Contact Dermatitis Newsletter* 3:37, 1968.
13. Fisher AA: Nonoccupational dermatitis due to "black" paraphenylenediamine rubber chemicals: Part I. *Cutis* 49:163–164, 1992.
14. Vestey JP, Buxton PK, Savin JA: Eyelash curler dermatitis. *Contact Dermatitis* 13:274–275, 1985.
15. Hamada T, Horiguchi S: Chronic melanodermatitis due to the rubber peephole of a ship radarscope. *Contact Dermatitis* 4:245–246, 1978.
16. Maibach HI: Scuba diver facial dermatitis: Allergic contact dermatitis to *N*-isopropyl-*N'*-phenylparaphenylenediamine. *Contact Dermatitis* 1:330, 1975.
17. Batschvarov B, Minkov DM: Dermatitis and purpura from rubber in clothing. *Trans St. Johns Hosp Dermatol Assoc* 54:178–182, 1968.
18. Ho VC, Mitchell JC: Allergic contact dermatitis from rubber boots. *Contact Dermatitis* 12:110–111, 1985.
19. Storrs FJ: Dermatitis from clothing and shoes, in Fisher AA (ed): *Contact Dermatitis,* 3d ed. Philadelphia, Lea & Febiger, 1986, p 323.
20. Lynde CW, Washawski L, Mitchell JC: Patch test results with a shoewear screening tray in 119 patients, 1977–80. *Contact Dermatitis* 8:423–425, 1982.
21. Leppard BJ, Parhizgar B: Contact dermatitis to PPD rubber in Maleki shoes. *Contact Dermatitis* 3:91–93, 1977.
21a. Romaguera C, Grimalt F, Vilaplana J: Eczematous and purpuric allergic contact dermatitis from boots. *Contact Dermatitis* 21:269, 1989.
22. Romaguera C, Grimalt F, Vilaplana J: Shoe contact dermatitis. *Contact Dermatitis* 18:178, 1988.
23. Romaguera C, Aguirre A, Diaz Perez JL, Grimalt F: Watch strap dermatitis. *Contact Dermatitis* 14:260–261, 1986.
24. Foussereau J, Cavelier C, Protois JC: A case of allergic isopropyl-*p*-phenylenediamine (IPPD) dermatitis from a watch strap. *Contact Dermatitis* 18:253, 1988.
25. Romaguera C, Grimalt F, Vilaplana J: Contact dermatitis from swimming goggles. *Contact Dermatitis* 18:178–179, 1988.
26. McKenna KE, McMillan C: Facial contact dermatitis due to black rubber. *Contact Dermatitis* 26:270–271, 1992.
27. Conde-Salazar L, Guimaraens D, Romero LV, Gonzalez MA: Unusual allergic contact dermatitis to aromatic amines. *Contact Dermatitis* 17:42–44, 1987.
28. Shmunes E: Purpuric allergic contact dermatitis to paraphenylenediamine. *Contact Dermatitis* 4:225–229, 1978.
29. Roed-Petersen J, Clemmensen OJ, Menne T, Larsen E: Purpuric contact dermatitis from black rubber chemicals. *Contact Dermatitis* 18:166–168, 1988.
30. Foussereau J, Cavelier C, Protois JC, et al: A case of erythema multiforme with allergy to isopropyl-*p*-phenylenediamine of rubber. *Contact Dermatitis* 18:183, 1988.

31. Schoel J, Frosch PJ: Allergic contact eczema caused by rubber-containing substances simulating pustulosis palmaris. *Derm Beruf Umwelt* 38:178–180, 1990.

32. LeVine MJ: Idiopathic photodermatitis with a positive paraphenylenediamine photopatch test. *Arch Dermatol* 120:1488–1490, 1984.

33. Dooms-Goossens A, Degreef H, de Veylder H, Maselis T: Unusual sensitization to black rubber. *Contact Dermatitis* 17:47–48, 1987.

34. Goh CL: Hand dermatitis from a rubber motorcycle handle. *Contact Dermatitis* 16:40–41, 1987.

35. Kligman AM, Magnusson B: *Allergic Contact Dermatitis in the Guinea Pig.* Springfield, Ill, Charles C Thomas, 1970.

36. Cronin E: *Contact Dermatitis.* Edinburgh, Churchill Livingstone, 1980.

37. Roed-Petersen J, Hjorth N, Jordan WP, Bourlas M: Postsorters' rubber fingerstall dermatitis. *Contact Dermatitis* 3:143–147, 1977.

38. Rudzki E, Ostaszewski K, Grzywa Z, Kozlowska A: Sensitivity to some rubber additives. *Contact Dermatitis* 2:24–27, 1976.

39. Benezra C, Sigman CS, Bagheri D, et al: A systematic search for structure-activity relationships of skin sensitizers: II. *Para*-phenylenediamine. *Semin Dermatol* 8:88–93, 1989.

40. Malkowski J, Klenieswka D, Maibach H: Relationship between chemical structure and allergenicity: Aromatic amines. *Derm Beruf Umwelt* 31:48–50, 1983.

41. Rudzki E, Napiorkowska I: Active sensitization to IPPD. *Contact Dermatitis* 10:126–127, 1984.

42. Menne T, White IR, Bruynzeel DP, Dooms-Goossens A: Patch test reactivity to the PPD-black-rubber-mix (industrial rubber chemicals) and individual ingredients. *Contact Dermatitis* 26:354, 1992.

43. Nethercott JR, Holness DL, Adams RM, et al: Patch testing with a routine screening tray in North America, 1985 through 1989: I. Frequency of response. *Am J Contact Dermatitis* 2:122–129, 1991.

44. von Hintzenstern J, Heese A, Koch HU, et al: Frequency, spectrum and occupational relevance of type IV allergies to rubber chemicals. *Contact Dermatitis* 24:244–252, 1991.

45. Hegyl E, Busova B, Niks M: HLA-A and -B antigens in IPPD-sensitive persons. *Contact Dermatitis* 22:228–229, 1990.

46. Carlsen L, Andersen KE, Egsgaard H: IPPD contact allergy from an orthopedic bandage. *Contact Dermatitis* 17:119–121, 1987.

47. Nater JP: Hypersensitivity to rubber. *Berufs-Dermatosen* 23:161–168, 1975.

48. Lintum JC, Nater JP: Allergic contact dermatitis caused by rubber chemicals in dairy workers. *Dermatologica* 148:42–44, 1974.

49. Alfonzo C: Allergic contact dermatitis to isopropylaminodiphenylamine (IPPD). *Contact Dermatitis* 5:145–147, 1979.

50. Fineman SE: Sensitivity to rubber chemicals. *J Toxicol Cutan Ocul Toxicol* 6:117–153, 1987.

51. Riboldi A, Lobaccaro M: Occupational contact dermatitis from rubber. *Clin Dermatol* 10:149–155, 1992.

52. Erikssen G, Ostlund E: Rubber band note counters as a cause of eczema among employees at a Swedish post office. *Acta Derm Venereol* 48:212–214, 1968.

53. Soto Giro J, Vazquez FJ, Leache YA, Quintanilla E: Contact dermatitis by sensitization to amine-type antioxidants. *Allergol Immunopathol* 17:263–265, 1989.

54. Foussereau J, Cavelier C, Protois JC, et al: A case of erythema multiforme with allergy to isopropyl-*p*-phenylenediamine of rubber. *Contact Dermatitis* 18:183, 1988.

55. Carlsen L, Andersen KE, Egsgaard H: IPPD contact allergy from an orthopedic bandage. *Contact Dermatitis* 17:119–121, 1987.

56. Rudzki E, Napiorkowska I: Active sensitization to IPPD. *Contact Dermatitis* 10:126–127, 1984.

57. Cronin E: Squash ball dermatitis. *Contact Dermatitis Newsletter* 13:365, 1973.

58. Fisher AA: Nonoccupational dermatitis to "black" rubber mix: Part II. *Cutis* 49:229–230, 1992.

59. Vollum DI, Marten RH: Contact dermatitis from 4-isopropylaminodiphenylamine. *Trans St. Johns Hosp Assoc Dermatol Assoc* 54:73–74, 1968.

60. Shaw S, Wilkinson DS: Unexpected cause of IPPD sensitivity. *Contact Dermatitis* 11:258, 1984.

27

POTASSIUM DICHROMATE

Jere D. Guin

WHAT ARE CHROMATES?

Chromium is a common metal making up a significant part of the earth's crust (200 ppm average)[1] and seawater (1 to 2.5 ppb),[1] 4×10^{-5} to 4.6×10^{-4} ppm), most of which is in the insoluble form. It is important biologically, being involved in the metabolism of carbohydrates and lipids. Commercially, it is obtained from an ore in which it is combined with iron. It is used in many ways in industry, especially in stainless and other types of steel, in making pigments and corrosion inhibitors, in tanning leather, in photoengraving and photography, in certain tattoo pigments, in colored inks for lithography, in mordants for dyeing, and in many other applications. The greatest source of contact dermatitis is from exposure to cement and mortar, where chrome is a contaminant in rather low concentration. Sensitization is to chromium salts, or chromates.

HOW IS CONTACT DERMATITIS TO CHROMATES RECOGNIZED?

Most cases of contact dermatitis from chromates are on the hands and fingers, with a few, perhaps as many as 15 percent, becoming widespread. Occasionally the eruption is localized to the feet. The face is less often involved, but a few patients develop a generalized eruption which mimics photodermatitis, as it is located in exposed sites. The diagnosis is made after patch testing confirms what is seen and after a relevant history is obtained. Traditionally, most cases have been in men and were occupationally induced, but this is changing in nations where ferrous sulfate has been added to cement.[2] The ratio of women to men has been increasing, with a resultant decline in the construction industry. Potassium dichromate is a commonly positive patch-test reaction in the pediatric population, and the opportunity for exposure seems to determine the prevalence. Hexavalent chromium is a potent allergen and the incidence of new sensitivities is high where there is a high degree of exposure, as where ore is smelted.[3]

WHAT OCCUPATIONS ARE LIKELY TO BE ASSOCIATED WITH ALLERGY TO CHROMATES?

The list of occupations in which allergy to chromium may arise is very long, starting with mining and smelting. The most common association, however, is with cement, mortar, and plaster in the construction trades. Cement workers are especially at risk, as are bricklayers.

In a prefabrication plant in Singapore, the prevalence of chromate allergy was 8.5 percent, although one-third of these individuals were not symptomatic.[4] Outside the United States, many persons with (Portland) cement dermatitis are also allergic to cobalt; according to Adams,[5] however, this is not true within the United States. The reason is not known, but it may have to do with concomitant sensitization. Almost all persons allergic to cobalt are also allergic to chromate, but perhaps only one-third of those sensitive to chromate are cobalt-allergic.[6] The chromate content of cement varies widely by report. Adams[5] gives the content of soluble chromium (the sensitizing component) as 1 to 30 ppm in the United States, but it is low by any standard. The important factor is the water-soluble chromate content,[6] and alkalinity also apparently contributes to sensitizing capacity. The original method of Portland cement manufacture did not involve oxidation; today, however, air is blown into rotating drums where the chromium content is changed in valence by oxidation. While it may be possible to use ingredients low in chromium content, the gypsum that is added would still be a problem.[6] The sensitizing potential of chromium in cement depends upon the valence (Cr^{vi}), solubility (potassium, sodium, calcium, and ammonium salts are soluble), pH (chromates occur at an acid pH, while dichromates occur at an alkaline pH), quantity (5 ppm is adequate), and the presence of reducing material (the addition of ferrous sulfate changes Cr^{vi} to Cr^{iii}).[6]

Painting and paint manufacture can be associated, as can metal (rustproofing) primers containing zinc chromates. Zinc potassium chromate comprises both zinc chromate and potassium dichromate. The latter is in a concentration higher than the one used for patch testing and thus is a potential sensitizer.[7] Those vulnerable to exposure from painting would include artists as well as house painters and others working with pigments.

Glazers in the pottery industry are commonly known to develop irritant hand eczema, but they also may develop allergy to chromates. Metalworkers may become sensitive to any of several metals, including chrome. This can happen in workers with sheet metal who are already allergic following contact with the metal[8] and from additives to soluble oils.[9] An unusual source of coolant dermatitis was the coolant used in pressing phonograph records.[10]

Persons in other occupations involving chromate exposure include turners, tailors, truck and locomotive drivers, rubber and plastics workers, printers and lithographers,[11] gas workers, and chemists. Chromates are also used in foundry bricks and the linings of boilers. Added risk exists in electroplating,[12] blueprint developing, the tanning of leather, etc., and in many areas of construction, although the preponderance of cases in industry is in cement workers, masons, plasterers, and so on. Many metalworkers are exposed, especially where chrome is used as a corrosion inhibitor for zinc-coated (galvanized) metals. Table 27-1 gives a longer list of known sources of occupational exposure.

TABLE 27–1. Occupations Associated with Chromate Allergy— Partial List

Cement working[20]	Archiving[26]
Bricklaying	Glazing and pottery[48]
Plastering[20]	Engineering[11]
Chromium plating[12]	Blueprinting[5]
Cooking[20]	Explosive and gunpowder manufacture[5]
Dye making[5]	Fireworks manufacture[5]
Dyeing[3]	Candlemaking[5]
Engraving[5]	Tanning[5]
Fitting[20]	Tile laying[20]
Printing and lithography[11]	Boiler scaling[5]
Photography[5]	Biology[5]
Rubber[20]	Furniture polishing[5]
Plastics[11]	Glass working[5]
Gas workers	Histology[5]
Chemists[5]	Match manufacture[5]
Workers handling antirust agents	Linoleum working[5]
Wood preservation and staining[5]	Paper waterproofing[5]
Defatting solvent application[45]	Pencil manufacture[5]
Food laboratory[46]	Locomotive operation[5]
Painting (including artists)[47]	Refractory brickmaking[5]
Machinists[5]	Soap manufacture[5]
Metalworkers	Graphics[11]
Manufacturing (assembly)[20]	Radio and TV[11]
Grinding (paint)[26]	Farming[11]
Welding[5,20]	Foods[11]
Scaffolding[20]	Textiles[11]
Stainless steel manufacture[5]	Cleaning[11]
Battery manufacture[5]	Household work[11]
Oil and gas drilling[5]	Turners[11]
Roofing and shingle manufacture[5]	Physicians (surgeons)
Tattooing[26]	

EXPOSURE TO ARTICLES OF CLOTHING

Clothing dermatitis is not an area where one might normally suspect chromate allergy, but shoe dermatitis may stem from chrome-tanned leather[13] and certain textiles may contain chromates.[14] Most laundry products apparently do not contain enough chrome to be a practical problem in the United States,[15] but a chromate dye in a European bleach was said to possibly cause allergy in housewives.[16] Hatters working in the dyeing room with chromate mordants can, if allergic, have a problem.[13]

SYSTEMIC CONTACT DERMATITIS

Ingestion of chromium can cause systemic contact dermatitis,[17,18] which not infrequently accompanies pompholyx. Lesions may also be seen on the elbows.[19] Some dietary sources are given in Table 27-2. However, how this happens is a good question, as trivalent chromium is not absorbed, and the acid concentration of the stomach converts

TABLE 27–2. Dietary Sources of Chromium[a]

Foods with higher concentrations
  Thyme, 10.00 μg/g
  Black pepper, 3.3 μg/g
  Cloves, 1.50 μg/g
Foods with minute quantities
  Drinking water, 0 to 0.112 ppm
  Dairy products, mean 0.10 μg/g
  Meat and fish, mean 0.11 μg/g
  Vegetables, mean 0.03 μg/g
  Fruit, mean 0.02 μg/g
  Grain, mean 0.04 μg/g
Animal diets contain higher amounts
  Dog food pellets, 4.24 μg/g
Other vegetation unlikely to be eaten, such as
  Wild cherry leaves, 0.57 μg/g
  Pasture grass, 1.30 μg/g
  Cigarettes, 0.39 μg/g

[a]Total human body content is about 6 mg of chromium; there is a higher concentration in infants, and animals generally have very much higher concentrations. There are three reasons for the low concentration in the human body: (1) Most chromium in earth is in the insoluble chromite form; (2) vegetation consumed by humans tends to be that with the lowest concentration; (3) any hexavalent chromium which is absorbed is changed in the acid media of the stomach to the trivalent form, which is not absorbed.[44] Therefore one may question whether or not dietary chromium is relevant.
Source: From Burrows.[20]

hexavalent chromium to the trivalent form. One authority[20] observed that these individuals must be achlorhydric! Experimentally, higher oral doses can also cause nonresponsiveness.[21]

Exposure can come from orthopedic metals,[22] pacemaker wires,[17] drugs,[17] acupuncture needles,[23] or even ingested food or water.[24] Spontaneous flares occur where persons previously had contact dermatitis, or a positive patch test may be seen. Tattoo reactions are said to occur, but they must be rare, as none were found in a very large series.[25]

ARE ALL FORMS OF CHROMIUM CAUSES OF ALLERGY?

For many years there was a controversy over the valence of the sensitizing form of chrome. Trivalent chromium is not absorbed well percutaneously, so it is not suitable for patch testing.[26] Essentially, both trivalent and hexavalent salts will produce a reaction when injected intradermally,[27] but only the hexavalent will do so when applied topically, as trivalent chromium is not absorbed percutaneously in sufficient quantity. Either, when absorbed, can be a problem in sensitive individuals.

PATCH TESTING FOR CHROMATE SENSITIVITY

Patch testing to 0.5% potassium dichromate is a routine part of the standard patch-test series. The concentration to be used for this purpose has been evaluated many times, as the usual concentration is a marginal irritant, causing false-positive reactions in many persons tested. Patch testing with too high a concentration can be irritating. Another complication is keloid formation.[28]

A positive patch-test reaction to 0.5% potassium dichromate may be caused not only by a true allergy but also by a (false-positive) irritant reaction. Of 108 reactions in one series, 44 were regarded as irritant and 15 were doubtful.[29] Tests to 0.375% potassium dichromate in petrolatum are seldom irritant, but this concentration does not find all of those who are allergic.[30] In doubtful cases, one can use the lower concentration and it probably indicates allergy if positive.

The time of application can be as short as 24 h and still provide over 90 percent of the total absorption expected.[31] Reading of the test should be done twice, with the first reading at 3 or 4 days, as day 4 gives a somewhat higher yield than day 2.[32] This is one of the antigens which produces delayed responses, so an additional delayed reading at day 7 is recommended.[33]

The vehicle used is usually petrolatum, but an aqueous solution can also be used (some have even claimed it is superior at 48 h).[34] However, the pH influences absorption. At a pH above 12, the mean threshold for sensitive subjects is at a concentration of 0.08%, while it is 0.15% for petrolatum and 0.27% in distilled water. The increased absorption at an alkaline pH helps explain sensitization from the incredibly low levels in cement, which is very alkaline when wet.

Storage of the antigen at room temperature can also influence the result, as potassium dichromate loses homogeneity compared with the same antigen stored at 4°C (39.2°F).[35] The patient should also be asked about systemic or local corticosteroid use, as this may interfere with the results.[36]

WHEN IS A POSITIVE PATCH-TEST REACTION RELEVANT?

Where the patient presents with what seems to be contact dermatitis and there is a clear history of exposure, relevance seems clear. Assuming there is a putative contact eczema as a reason for patch testing, one would do well to look thoroughly for a source. Table 27-3 lists some published sources of exposure. Of course, should a spontaneous flareup occur, then an association with a single positive patch test is strongly suggested. If multiple prominently positive patch-test responses are present, repeating the test with isolated antigens may be informative. Suspected sources could be checked for presence of chrome, using the diphenylcarbazine spot test.

In one series, about 70 percent of those with what was interpreted as a positive reaction were considered relevant. Burrows[20] feels that this will increase as we learn better how to find hidden sources of contact. Some workers with a positive patch test have never had any form of contact dermatitis, but they are apparently at risk if adequately exposed.[37]

TABLE 27–3. Some Sources of Exposure to Chromates

Oil from metal working[49]	Ashes[25]
Postage stamps[50]	Cigarettes[25]
Batteries[5]	Surgical (chromic) gut suture[25]
Coolant oils[51]	Jeweler's enamel[25]
Offset printing[52]	Laboratory reagent[46]
Green baize tabletops for blackjack[53]	Newspaper[25]
Milk testers[46,54,55]	Rubber gloves[62]
TV screens[56]	Orthopedic pins or screws[17,22]
Shoes[57]	Pacemaker[62]
Quicklime[58]	Paint[47]
Magnetic tapes[59]	Solvent[45]
Detergents and bleaches[60]	Tattoo dye[25]
Boiler linings[61]	Test reagent (laboratory)[63]
Refractory materials	Military uniforms[14]
Matches[25]	Defatting solvent[45]
Leather[25]	Homeopathic drug[17]

Source: Refs. 5 and 20.

WHAT ABOUT REACTIONS WHICH ARE NOT ALLERGIC?

Irritant reactions are common in many situations, especially where there is exposure to higher concentrations or to chromic acid. Chrome ulcers occur on broken or eczematous skin. This also occurs on the moist nasal septum, especially where ventilation is inadequate and the worker does not wear an approved respirator. Inhalation causes lung problems and can lead to an increased risk for lung cancer as well.

PREVENTION

Prevention of the irritant reactions may call for more than is required by the criteria laid down by many governmental regulations. In a review published in 1978, the following steps were routine in Great Britain, but even these may not have been adequate for many situations[20]:

1. Tests every 14 days to ensure that levels do not exceed
   a. 0.5 mg Cr/m^3 air of soluble chromous salt
   b. 0.1 mg Cr/m^3 air of chromates, dichromates, or chromic acid
   c. 1.0 mg Cr/m^3 air of chromium metal and insoluble salts (not hexavalent)

2. Monthly medical examinations
3. Regular inspection of the hands and forearms
4. Preventive measures (e.g., gloves, washing facilities, and a 25% lanolin in petrolatum cream)

Certainly the better the ventilation, the better the chance of reducing the incidence of respiratory problems. The wearing of an approved respirator is also necessary for some jobs where exposure is high. Samitz[37A] used 10% aqueous ascorbic acid as a

POTASSIUM DICHROMATE ALLERGY—PATIENT HANDOUT

WHAT IS CHROMATE ALLERGY?

A positive patch test to potassium dichromate is evidence that one will break out to materials containing chromium salts. While one normally might think that a metal object is at fault, it is more likely to be an ingredient of cement, mortar, pigments, leather, photographic or blueprint materials, or radiator coolant. This is one of the more common causes of an allergic eczema, which can be very slow to respond to treatment.

IN WHOM IS SUCH ALLERGY USUALLY SEEN?

Allergy to chromates is more common in men than women, and most cases are occupational. It is also one of the more common allergies encountered in children.

WHERE IS CHROMIUM FOUND?

Chromium is found in some types of soil, but this is not a problem with regard to allergy. Sources of exposure which may cause allergy include cement, leather, pigments (in cosmetics, paints, inks, and tattoos), pottery, matches, radiator fluid and coolant, certain gut surgical suture material, and products used in engraving and electroplating. According to some, metallic chromium plating is not a problem, but according to others, it *is*. Reaction to acupuncture needles containing chromium has been reported. By far the most important source of exposure is cement and mortar, as these are the most common sources as original causes. Chromium in cement and mortar is in very low concentration but the alkaline nature of the wet material probably increases the potential for causing allergy. Exposure to most leather as well as certain colored inks and other pigments can cause chromate dermatitis.

WHICH OCCUPATIONS ARE MOST AT RISK?

The occupation most commonly associated with contact allergy to chromate is construction work, where contact with mortar, cement, or plaster is common. The dust may be a problem, as the distribution of rash is frequently in exposed or open areas, such as the face, neck, hands, and arms.

Chromates are used to tan leather, dye textiles and furs, process blueprints and photographs, and make pigments used in inks, paints, tattoos, and cosmetics. They are also used for rust protection in boilers, radiators, and coolants. Persons

This information is provided to help persons with contact dermatitis in the understanding of their problem. The contents are subject to change as more information becomes available and are not intended as a substitute for medical treatment.

working in the smelting of chrome from iron chrome have, in years past, been especially at risk. Metalworkers and welders sometimes react as well. Electroplating workers may develop ulcers (which are burns and not allergic reactions) or sensitization dermatitis. Workers exposed to unusual occupational sources include milk testers, lithographers, potters, and diesel locomotive mechanics, but the list is long. Some cases are not occupational; for example, some patients have broken out to household bleach or radiator cleaner, and some can react to chrome pigments in a tattoo. Some individuals with mouth eruptions and chromate allergy can be allergic to the metal components of a denture.

CAN ONE HAVE A PROBLEM WITHOUT BEING ALLERGIC?

Wet cement is very irritating to normal skin; severe blistering and burns can occur if one is exposed directly without wearing protective boots or if the wet cement gets inside one's gloves. However, this is due to the cement and not its chromate content. Workers in electroplating can develop ulcers on the skin from chromic acid burns, and those who do not wear respirators may develop ulcers in the nose, which can flatten the nose. Lung problems can also occur from inhaling fumes.

HOW LONG DOES THE ALLERGY LAST?

About two-thirds of those sensitive to chromates will still be allergic when tested several years later. Looking at it another way, most of those who develop the sensitivity at work still break out even though they change to jobs where they are no longer exposed. The reason for this is not known, but experimental studies suggest that the chromate in the skin is very slow to leave.

WHAT CAN BE DONE TO PREVENT THE PROBLEM IN PERSONS ALREADY ALLERGIC?

Avoidance is important, but it may not be adequate. Cement and mortar can be treated with 0.35% iron sulfate (or when the chromate content is <5μg/g cement, 0.20% is sufficient) to change the chrome content chemically and make it hard to absorb through the skin. A barrier cream can be made from ascorbic acid (vitamin C) and EDTA (a chemical which binds metals), which helps some people.

There is also some evidence that water and foods containing chrome can flare the eruption and make it more difficult to manage. This has prompted some to

(Continued)

---

recommend dietary avoidance, but others deny a benefit, as stomach acids make dietary chromates difficult to absorb.

HOW DO I KNOW WHAT OBJECTS CONTAIN CHROMATE?

If you have access to a chemistry laboratory, you may be able to test certain materials for chrome. The test has to be done where acids can be used, as dilute acids are added to the object in hot water. One adds a 1% alcoholic solution of diphenyl carbazide and looks for a red color.

---

reducing agent to change the valence of chromium from hexavalent to trivalent. A similar barrier product has been evaluated, using added tartaric acid, glycine, and/or EDTA, for which benefit has been claimed.[38]

Concomitant reactions may occur to other metals, perhaps due to opportunity for exposure. Persons allergic to potassium dichromate 0.5% probably should be tested to other antigens as well, since three-fourths of persons allergic to potassium dichromate react to other antigens, especially nickel, cobalt, and rubber.[20] This is especially true for persons working with metals or (for Europeans) cement. A cross-reaction with zirconium has been reported.[39]

PROGNOSIS

Chromate dermatitis tends to be persistent, with 79 percent of those positive 4 to 7 years previously still having a positive patch test and 76 percent still having difficulty with the rash.[40] Approximately 69 or 70 percent have a persistent rash despite treatment,[16] especially when the initial diagnosis is delayed[41], and the condition persists in more than half even when a job change has been made to remove the individual from exposure.[42] Reactivity, however, may change in either direction with time.[43]

REFERENCES

1. Love AHG: Chromium—Biological and analytical considerations, in Burrows D (ed): *Chromium Metabolism and Toxicity*. Boca Raton, FL, CRC Press, 1983.
2. Farm G: Changing patterns in chromate allergy. *Contact Dermatitis* 5:298–299, 1986.
3. Schwartz L, Tulipan L, Birmingham DJ: *Occupational Diseases of the Skin*. Philadelphia, Lea & Febiger, 1957, pp 294–299, 829–834.
4. Goh CL, Gan SL, Ngui SJ: Occupational dermatitis in a prefabrication construction factory. *Contact Dermatitis* 15:235–240, 1986.

5. Adams RM: *Occupational Skin Disease*. New York, Grune & Stratton, 1983, pp 397–399.
6. Fregert S: Chromium valencies and cement dermatitis. *Br J Dermatol* 105(suppl 21):7–9, 1981.
7. Adams RM, Fregert S, Gruvberger B, Maibach HI: Water solubility of zinc chromate primer paints used as antirust agents. *Contact Dermatitis* 2:357–358, 1976.
8. Rycroft RJ, Calnan CD: Relapse of chromate dermatitis from sheet metal. *Contact Dermatitis* 3:177–180, 1977.
9. Calnan CD: Chromate dermatitis from soluble oil. *Contact Dermatitis* 4:378, 1978.
10. Calnan CD: Chromate in coolant water of gramophone record presses. *Contact Dermatitis* 4:346–347, 1978.
11. Peltonen L, Fraki J: Prevalence of dichromate sensitivity. *Contact Dermatitis* 9:190–194, 1983.
12. Lee HS, Goh CL: Occupational dermatosis among chrome platers. *Contact Dermatitis* 18:89–93, 1988.
13. Bajaj AK, Gupta SC, Chatterjee AK, Singh KG: Shoe dermatitis in India. *Contact Dermatitis* 19:372–375, 1988.
14. Fregert S, Gruvberger B, Foransson K, Norman S: Allergic contact dermatitis from chromate in military textiles. *Contact Dermatitis* 4:223–224, 1978.
15. Hostynek JJ, Maibach HI: Chromium in U.S. household bleach. *Contact Dermatitis* 18:206–209, 1988.
16. Dooms-Goossens A, Ceuterick A, Vanmaele N, Degreef H: Follow-up study of patients with contact dermatitis caused by chromates, nickel, and cobalt. *Dermatologica* 160:249–260, 1980.
17. van Ulsen J, Stolz E, van Joost T: Chromate dermatitis from a homeopathic drug. *Contact Dermatitis* 18:56–57, 1988.
18. Schleiff P: Provokation of the Chromatekzems zu Testzwecken durch interne Chrom Zufuhr. *Hautarzt* 19:209–210, 1968.
19. Kaaber K, Sjlin KE, Menne T: Elbow eruptions in nickel and chromate dermatitis. *Contact Dermatitis* 9:213–216, 1983.
20. Burrows D: Chromium and the skin. *Br J Dermatol* 99:587–595, 1978.
21. Christensen OB, Christensen MB, Maibach HI: Flare-up reactions and desensitization from oral dosing in chromate-sensitive guinea pigs. *Contact Dermatitis* 10:277–279, 1984.
22. Munro-Ashman D, Miller AJ: Rejection of metal to metal prosthesis and skin sensitivity to cobalt. *Contact Dermatitis* 2:65–67, 1976.
23. Tanii T, Kono T, Katoh J, et al: A case of prurigo pigmentosa considered to be contact allergy to chromium in an acupuncture needle. *Acta Derm Venereol* 71:66–67, 1991.
24. Kaaber K, Veien NK: The significance of chromate ingestion in patients allergic to chromate. *Acta Derm Venereol* 57:321–323, 1977.
25. Rudzki E, Kozlowska A: Causes of chromate dermatitis in Poland. *Contact Dermatitis* 6:191–196, 1980.
26. Samitz MH, Katz S: A study of the chemical reaction between chromium and skin. *J Invest Dermatol* 43:35–43, 1964.
27. Fregert S, Rorsman H: Allergy to trivalent chromium. *Arch Dermatol* 90:4–6, 1964.
28. Calnan CD: Keloid formation after patch tests. *Contact Dermatitis* 7:279–280, 1981.
29. Storrs FJ, Rosenthal LE, Adams RM, et al: Prevalence and relevance of allergic reactions in patients patch tested in North America—1984 to 1985. *J Am Acad Dermatol* 20:1038–1045, 1989.
30. Burrows D, Andersen KE, Camarasa JG, et al: Trial of 0.5% versus 0.375% potassium dichromate: European Environmental and Contact Dermatitis Research Group (EECDRG). *Contact Dermatitis* 21:351, 1989.
31. Rudzki E, Zakrzewski Z, Prokopczyk G, Kozowska A: Patch tests with potassium dichromate removed after 24 and 48 hours. *Contact Dermatitis* 2:309–310, 1976.
32. Shehade SA, Beck MH, Hillier VF: Epidemiological survey of standard series patch test results and observations on day 2 and day 4 readings. *Contact Dermatitis* 24:119–122, 1991.
33. Macfarlane AW, Curley RK, Graham RM, et al: Delayed patch test reactions at days 7 and 9. *Contact Dermatitis* 20:127–132, 1989.
34. Samsoen M, Stampf JL, Lelievre G, Foussereau J: Patch testing with hexavalent chromium salts in different vehicles and with nickel and cobalt in petrolatum. *Derm Beruf Umwelt* 30:181–184, 1982.
35. Goh CL, Kwok SF: The influence of temperature on the concentration homogeneity of patch test materials. *Contact Dermatitis* 15:231–234, 1986.
36. Sukanto H, Nater JP, Bleumink E: Influence of topically applied corticosteroids on patch test reactions. *Contact Dermatitis* 7:180–185, 1981.
37. Burrows D, Calnan CD: Cement dermatitis: II. Clinical aspects. *Trans St. Johns Hosp Derm Soc* 51:27–39, 1965.

37a. Samitz MH, Shrager J: Prevention of dermatitis in the printing and lithography industries. *Arch Dermatol* 94:307–309, 1966.

38. Romaguera C, Vilaplana J, Grimalt F, et al: Prophylaxis of patients with sensitization to chrome and nickel using a cosmetic preparation for topical use. *Med Cutan Ibero-Latino-Americana* 11:139–146, 1983.

39. Turk JL, Parker D: Sensitization with Cr, Ni and Zr salts and allergic type granuloma formation in the guinea pig. *J Invest Dermatol* 68:341–345, 1977.

40. Thormann J, Jespersen NB, Joensen HD: Persistence of contact allergy to chromium. *Contact Dermatitis* 5:261–264, 1979.

41. Halbert AR, Gebauer KA, Wall LM: Prognosis of occupational chromate dermatitis. *Contact Dermatitis* 27:214–219, 1992.

42. Halbert AR, Gebauer KA, Wall LM: Prognosis of occupational chromate dermatitis. *Contact Dermatitis* 27:214–219, 1992.

43. Lisi P, Simonetti S: Contact sensitivity in children and adults with atopic dermatitis—A chronological study. *Dermatologica* 171:1–7, 1985.

44. Donaldson RM, Barreras RF: Intestinal absorption of trace elements of chromium. *J Lab Clin Med* 68:484–493, 1966.

45. Ros AM, Bang-Pedersen NB: Chromate in defatting solvent. *Contact Dermatitis* 3:105, 1977.

46. Rudzki E, Czerwinska-Dihnz C: Sensitivity to dichromate in milk testers. *Contact Dermatitis* 3:1057–1058, 1977.

47. van Ketel WG: Low incidence of occupational dermatitis from chromate. *Contact Dermatitis* 10:249, 1984.

48. Wilkinson SM, Heagerty AHM, English JSC: Hand dermatitis in the pottery industry. *Contact Dermatitis* 26:91–94, 1992.

49. Alomar A, Conde-Salazar L, Romaguera C: Occupational dermatoses from cutting oils. *Contact Dermatitis* 12:129–138, 1985.

50. Fregert S, Gruvberger B, Mitchell JC: Contact dermatitis to postage stamps. *Contact Dermatitis* 1:328, 1975.

51. Einarsson O, Kylin B, Lindstedt G, Wahlberg JE: Chromium, cobalt and nickel in used cutting fluids. *Contact Dermatitis,* 1:182, 1975.

52. Malten KE: Cobalt and chromium in offset printing. *Contact Dermatitis,* 1:120, 1975.

53. Fisher A: Blackjack disease and other chromate puzzles. *Cutis* 18:21, 1976.

54. Huriez CL, Maetin P, Lefebvre M: Sensitivity to dichromate in a milk analysis laboratory. *Contact Dermatitis* 1:247, 1975.

55. Rogers S, Burrows D: Contact dermatitis to chrome in milk testers. *Contact Dermatitis* 1:387, 1975.

56. Stevenson CJ: Fluorescence as a clue to contamination in TV workers. *Contact Dermatitis* 1:242, 1975.

57. Varelzides A, Katsambas A, Georgala S, et al: Shoe dermatitis in Greece. *Dermatologica* 149:236, 1974.

58. Weiler K-J, Rüssel HA: Das Chromekzem durch Branntkalk. *Berufsdermatosen* 22:116, 1974.

59. Krook G, Fregert S, Gruvberger B: Chromate and cobalt eczema due to magnetic tapes. *Contact Dermatitis* 3:60, 1977.

60. Garcia-Perez A, Martin-Pascual A, Sanchez-Misiego A: Chrome content in bleaches and detergents: Its relationship to hand dermatitis in women. *Acta Derm Venereol* 53:353, 1973.

61. Rycroft RJR, Calnan CD: Chromate dermatitis from a boiler lining. *Contact Dermatitis* 3:198, 1977.

62. Conde-Salazar L, Marto Castano A, Arroyo Vicente M: Determination of chrome in rubber gloves. *Contact Dermatitis* 6:237–238, 1980.

63. Pedersen NB: Chromate in a food laboratory. *Contact Dermatitis* 3:105, 1977.

28

BALSAM OF PERU

Jere D. Guin

Balsam of Peru is a fragrance material derived from a species of tree native to El Salvador in Central America. Botanically it is *Myroxolon balsamum*,[1] a member of the pea family (Leguminosae or Fabaceae). At maturity it may reach some 20 to 30 m (98 ft) in height. Trees are productive after they are about 5 years old, although trees younger than 25 years give a poorer quality of balsam.[2] It is called *balsam of Peru* because El Salvador once was a Peruvian colony, and it was under the seal of the viceroy of Peru that the commodity was shipped from Central America in the early days.[1,2] The term *balsam* is used for a viscous, colored, aromatic plant product, soluble in alcohol but not in water and obtained by spontaneous or artificially induced flow from an incision through the bark.[3] The term *balm* is sometimes used the same way. These plant materials have an ancient tradition of medicinal use. Indeed, balsam of Peru has some activity against bacteria, fungus, lice, and scabies,[1] and it has been used as an expectorant.[2]

Balsam of Peru in ointment form has been used in Europe on burns,[2] but it is much less used medicinally[1] in the United States. It is also a natural fragrance material, but its use is now restricted to those products treated to reduce allergy.[3,4] In Hjorth's[1] series, men became allergic mostly through medicinal use, while most women were sensitized through exposure to use of fragrance materials. In the United States, balsam of Peru can be found in some popular hemorrhoidal suppositories, but most allergies seem to be related to perfume sensitivity. This plant balsam is a complex resinous mixture, the dominant content being coniferyl benzoate and cinnamyl cinnamate. The principal sensitizers are found in the resinous residue, which is ether-soluble and precipitated by petroleum ether.[1] Hjorth found that further characterization is difficult because of the tendency for this material to oxidize and polymerize.

The most sensitizing portion of balsam of Peru is in the ether-soluble resinous portion, comprising only some 3.9 percent of the total. To approach this from the other end, persons reactive to balsam of Peru today are less likely to react to the resin, probably because they were sensitized by fragrance exposure rather than by balsam of Peru.[5] Mitchell[6] found that 57 of 142 persons allergic to balsam of Peru did not break out to the "components," a battery of specific perfume-related antigens. The cinnamates and eugenol gave more reactions, but 57 were negative despite allergy to balsam of Peru. Testing with fragrance ingredients known to be present in balsam of Peru showed that cinnamic alcohol and acid were more likely to cause a reaction than was cinnamic aldehyde. The failure of 57 of the 142 to react to any known ingredient confirms that a significant number who react are allergic to something other than the fragrance components. In Hjorth's series of persons highly allergic to the whole material, only 5 of 16 reacted to "claire de Perou," which is essentially the fragrance material with the resinous portion removed. For persons who were primarily sensitized by exposure to fragrance material rather than to balsam of Peru itself, this may not hold true. Balsam of Peru is also helpful in uncovering sensitivity to soap perfume.[1,7]

WHAT IS SEEN CLINICALLY?

In the United States, the pattern of the eruption in persons who patch test positive to balsam of Peru is essentially the same as that for perfume or fragrance allergy. In Hjorth's[1] (Danish) series, more than two-thirds of those allergic to balsam of Peru were women. However some 60 percent of those patch tested were women. Some 25 years later, the incidence in Denmark was equal between men and women, about 4 percent of each having positive reactions, but more than twice as many women were patch tested.[8] The incidence is higher in older persons and lower below age 30.[8] In the United States, the incidence is 3.8 percent of those tested under age 40 and 6.7 percent over age 40.[9]

The location of the eruption depends upon exposure, but in Hjorth's series[1] eczema of the hands was most common, followed by the legs, face, feet, arms, and neck in that order. A computer analysis of location showed balsam of Peru sensitivity to be associated with dermatitis of the forehead, cheeks, and (lower) legs.[10] In China, those facial eczemas caused by cosmetics were associated with balsam of Peru sensitivity.[11]

In Rystedt's[12] series of hand eczema from atopic dermatitis, balsam of Peru and fragrance mix were the two antigens significantly associated. In other series reactions to these same two antigens, colophony, nickel, and cobalt are often present.[13,14] Colophony (rosin) is also related to sensitivity to perfumes and spices but not to balsam of Peru.[2] Sensitivity to nickel is felt by some to be related to atopy. Even though such allergy is increased, irritant dermatitis remains extremely important.[13]

Allergy to balsam of Peru also is associated with leg ulcers and stasis eczema.[15,16] In one series with a large group with lower leg dermatitis, about 19 percent reacted to balsam of Peru and many reacted to cetearyl products (Lanettes) as well suggesting cosmetic product sensitization.[17]

For those ingesting the antigen, one might expect a flareup at a previous site; pompholyx; symmetrical maculopapulovesicular or urticarial eruptions of eyelids, axillae, antecubital areas, and neck; erythema multiforme; exfoliative dermatitis[18]; or an eruption of the face with "secondary" vasculitis-like lesions on the legs with purpura from topical treatment.[19]

Balsam of Peru also gives a higher response rate than many other antigens in the pediatric population,[20] where reportedly it is second only to nickel.[21]

BALSAM OF PERU—PATIENT HANDOUT

WHAT IS BALSAM OF PERU?

Balsam of Peru is an aromatic resinous plant material obtained by wounding the bark of a particular tree in El Salvador. Balsam is an alcohol-soluble resinous secretion and Peru comes from El Salvador's being a Peruvian colony when the material was named. It has been used as a "healing" salve because it feels and smells good and has antibacterial, antifungal, and antiparasitic activity.

Today, however, a positive patch test to balsam of Peru is usually associated with perfume sensitivity. It also warns of problems from flavoring, both artificial and natural, as perfumes and flavors are often the same substances. The opportunity for exposure to balsam of Peru is higher in some European countries, where it has been used as a salve for burns. In Europe, men may become allergic from using the salve (perhaps on a burn), while most women become allergic from perfumes. In the United States, balsam of Peru is found in some hemorrhoidal suppositories and surgical dressings, but otherwise it is a marker or indicator for allergy to perfumes acquired from other exposure.

WHAT PROBLEMS ARE ASSOCIATED WITH ALLERGY TO BALSAM OF PERU?

Several problems can be related. Persons with hand eczema are especially at risk to develop perfume allergy where balsam of Peru is a marker. It is also an indicator for allergy to perfumes and spices, especially cinnamon, cloves, nutmeg, and paprika for those allergic to spices or flavors. Oral exposure to these can cause sore mouth (tongue), a rash of the lips or angles of the mouth, or a flare elsewhere, such as tiny watery bumps on the hands.

Some persons react to perfumes, colognes, or fragrances added to cosmetics, after-shaves, deodorants, or other cosmetics. A common cause of allergy to fragrances comes from their presence in lotions applied to the skin around a leg ulcer or to a rash associated with swelling of the ankle. One must be extremely careful about what is used on that type skin as it is very easy to become allergic.

Balsam of Peru can also be positive in children, and the causes would be similar to those in adults.

ARE THERE OTHER SOURCES OF EXPOSURE?

Yes, sometimes, eating foods containing related chemicals will cause a previous rash to flare or may create a new problem. This does not always happen, but it

---

This information is provided to help persons with contact dermatitis in the understanding of their problem. The contents are subject to change as more information becomes available and are not intended as a substitute for medical treatment.

is best to avoid it. Avoid the following foods and medicines until you can prove (with medical supervision) that you are not allergic:

Citrus peel: oranges, lemon, grapefruit, tangerines, etc.
Artificially flavored baked goods, gum, candy
Perfumed tea, tobacco, coffee, etc.
Cough medicine and lozenges
Eugenol (in a dentist's office, it causes the clovelike odor)
Ice cream, colas
Spices: cinnamon, cloves, nutmeg, paprika, chili sauce, chutney, pickled herring, pickled vegetables, paté, liver pastes, vermouth, bitters, spiced beverages

HOW CAN ONE AVOID EXPOSURE?

Fortunately, fragrance-free products are much more available than they were only a few years ago:

1. Fragrance-free laundry detergents include Cheer Free (the regular one has perfume) and Tide Fragrance Free (the regular one is scented).
2. Bounce is available in a fragrance-free form.
3. Paper products available without fragrance include Kleenex (the Softique may contain fragrance, but the regular form does not), Northern Tissue, and Charmin Free as well as others.
4. Toilet soaps without perfume include Basis Soap and unscented forms of Neutrogena and Purpose.
5. Shampoo is a problem, as all shampoos contain fragrance. Ivory has an unscented shampoo which has a masking fragrance. Some can use fragrance-free soap with soft or mineral-free water. Some persons allergic to cinnamates (including balsam of Peru and cinnamic aldehyde) will tolerate a herbal-scented shampoo. This has the odor of green leaves rather than flowers and is called a *green note*. Allergy to that scent is not uncommon, and sensitivity to perfume ingredients can be broad, so such tolerance is by no means universal.
6. Fragrance-free cosmetic lines are widely available.

If you are suspicious, a usage test will help, in that you apply or use the product twice daily for a week. You can apply creams to a quarter-sized area in front of the elbow or the neck. If there is no reaction after a week, you will probably tolerate the product. When using a shampoo, watch the areas adjacent to the scalp (e.g., the forehead and ears).

Be careful not to use irritant cosmetics in a usage test except as they are normally used. Shampoos, soaps, and cleansers can cause a rash which is not allergic if they are covered or overused on tender areas.

HOW DOES ONE AVOID CONTACT WITH BALSAM OF PERU?

In the United States, avoiding balsam of Peru is relatively easy, but avoiding cross-reacting allergens is anything but easy. Fundamental to avoidance is elimination of exposure to fragrance materials. Some things have to be omitted and fragrance-free products are advised. According to Hjorth,[1] Englehardt found that things containing benzoic acid and benzyl benzoate may also cause a reaction in persons allergic to balsam of Peru.

For balsam of Peru–allergic persons with hand eczema, an often unsuspected source of contact is spices used in cooking.[15,22] In one series of 50 persons who were allergic to spices, 48, or 96 percent, were allergic to balsam of Peru.[23] The spices more often causing a reaction include cloves, Jamaican pepper, and cinnamon.[22] Those allergic to indicator tests (balsam of Peru fragrance mix, colophony, and wood tars) are much more likely to be sensitive to spices than the general population of persons being patch tested, especially to cloves, nutmeg, and paprika.[24] (In another series which added galanga, curry, ginger, garlic, and onion, none of the patients was allergic to balsam of Peru but many reacted to fragrance mix.[25])

Another often unrecognized source of contact is with flavors and foods. Several lists of foods have been published, but the worst items may be citrus peel, colas, vermouth, and artificial flavors.[26] A diet low in potential reactors has been proposed.[27] Oral challenge can produce pompholyx,[22] or it may aggravate the problem. However, some aggravation occurs in persons not allergic to balsam of Peru. This may be nonspecific.[28]

Rare sources of exposure would be other balsams, benzyl benzoate, or plastics with a positive test to resorcinol monobenzoate.

FOODS AND MEDICATIONS THAT MAY CAUSE REACTIONS IN INDIVIDUALS ALLERGIC TO BALSAM OF PERU INCLUDE THE FOLLOWING[27]:

Citrus peel: oranges, lemon, grapefruit, bitter orange, tangerine, mandarin oranges, etc.

Essence-flavored products: baked goods, candy, gum

Wine, scented teas, tobacco, etc.

Cough medications and lozenges

Eugenol

Ice cream

Colas and other soft drinks

Spices: Cinnamon, cloves, vanilla, curry (products from these include: ketchup, chili sauce, chutney, pickled herring, pickled vegetables such as beets and cucumbers, baked goods, paté, liver paste, vermouth, bitters, spiced beverages)

Fruit

Wine

ASSOCIATED ALLERGENS

Not only is balsam of Peru valuable in uncovering persons allergic to spices and fragrances, but it also cross-reacts with other balsams, benzyl benzoate, and benzoic acid. Sensitivities to colophony and balsam of Peru are linked, as is propolis.[29]

REFERENCES

1. Hjorth N: *Eczematous Allergy to Balsams, Applied Perfumes and Flavoring Agents.* Copenhagen, Munksgaard, 1961.
2. Walter GT: Balsam of Peru. *Perfumes Essential Oils Rev* 705–707, 1968.
3. Guin JD: History, manufacture, and cutaneous reactions to perfumes, in Frost P, Horwitz SN (eds): *Principles of Cosmetics for the Dermatologist.* St. Louis, Mosby, 1982, pp 111–129.
4. International Fragrance Association Code of Practice (IFRA). Amended 1991.
5. Matthies C, Dooms-Goossens A, Lachapelle JM, et al: Patch testing with fractionated balsam of Peru. *Contact Dermatitis* 19:384–385, 1988.
6. Mitchell JC: Contact hypersensitivity to some perfume materials. *Contact Dermatitis* 1:196–199, 1975.
7. Burry JN: Environmental dermatitis: Contact dermatitis from perfumes in soap. *Med J Austr* 145:160–162, 1986.
8. Christophersen J, Menne T, Tanghj P, et al: Clinical patch test data evaluated by multivariate analysis: Danish Contact Dermatitis Group. *Contact Dermatitis* 21:291–299, 1989.
9. Nethercott JR, Holness DL, Adams RM, et al: Patch testing with a routine screening tray in North America: 1983 through 1989: III. Age and response. *Am J Contact Dermatitis* 2:198–201, 1991.
10. Edman B: Sites of contact dermatitis in relationship to particular allergens. *Contact Dermatitis* 13:129–135, 1985.
11. Zhao B, Fan WX: Facial contact dermatitis: Pathogenetic factors in China. *Int J Dermatol* 30:485–486, 1991.
12. Rystedt I: Hand eczema and long-term prognosis in atopic dermatitis. *Acta Derm Venereol Suppl* 117:1–59, 1985.
13. Meding B: Epidemiology of hand eczema in an industrial city. *Acta Derm Venereol Suppl* 153:1–43, 1990.
14. Nilsson E: Contact sensitivity and urticaria in "wet" work. *Contact Dermatitis* 13:321–328, 1985.
15. Frenzel U, Gutekunst A: Allergic phenomena in the treatment of leg ulcer. *Phlebologie* 38:389–394, 1985.
16. Lembo G, Balato N, Giordano C, Ayala F: Contact sensitization in stasis dermatitis and chronic leg ulcers: Study of 112 patients. *Min Med* 75:1133–1135, 1984.
17. Lindemayr H, Drobil M: Eczema of the lower leg and contact allergy. *Hautarzt* 36:227–231, 1985.
18. Dooms-Goossens A, Dubelloy R, Degreef H: Contact and systemic contact-type dermatitis to spices. *Dermatol Clin* 8:89–93, 1990.
19. Bruynzeel DP, van den Hoogenband HM, Koedijk F: Purpuric vasculitis-like eruption in a patient sensitive to balsam of Peru. *Contact Dermatitis* 11:207–209, 1984.
20. Rademaker M, Forsyth A: Contact dermatitis in children. *Contact Dermatitis* 20:104–107, 1989.
21. Kuiters GR, Smitt JH, Cohen EB, Bos JD: Allergic contact dermatitis in children and young adults. *Arch Dermatol* 125:1531–1533, 1989.
22. Niinimaki A: Scratch-chamber tests in food handler dermatitis. *Contact Dermatitis* 16:11–20, 1987.
23. Niinimaki A: Delayed-type allergy to spices. *Contact Dermatitis* 11:34–40, 1984.
24. van den Akker TW, Roesyanto-Mahadi ID, van Toorenenbergen AW, van Joost T: Contact allergy to spices. *Contact Dermatitis* 22:267–272, 1990.
25. Bruynzeel DP, Prevoo RLMA: Patch tests with some spices. *Dermatol Clin* 8:85–87, 1990.
26. Larsen WG: How to instruct patients sensitive to fragrances. *J Am Acad Dermatol* 21(4 pt 2):880–884, 1989.
27. Veien NK, Hattel T, Justesen O, Nrholm A: Reduction of intake of balsams in patients sensitive to balsam of Peru. *Contact Dermatitis* 12:270–273, 1985.
28. Veien NK, Hattel T, Justesen O, Nrholm N: Oral challenge with balsam of Peru. *Contact Dermatitis* 12:104–107, 1985.
29. Machackova J: The incidence of allergy to propolis in 605 consecutive patients patch tested in Prague. *Contact Dermatitis* 18:210–212, 1988.

29

NICKEL SULFATE

Jere D. Guin

WHAT IS THE MEANING OF NICKEL ALLERGY?

Nickel sensitivity is extremely common and a problem of consequence, especially to women who may have allergy to jewelry and snaps on clothing. The problem is not limited to that group, however, as hand dermatitis is commonly associated with nickel sensitivity, although it may not be causally related.

The prevalence varies from one country to another, perhaps because of differences in behavior of the populations. Nickel dermatitis is by any measurement common. In the United States about 10.5 percent of those patch tested were allergic to nickel sulfate 5% in petrolatum,[1] but even in the general population prevalence is on the general order of 10 percent in this country.[2] However, it is higher in women than in men.[3] In Canada, the prevalence of persons patch tested was 17.4 percent. In another study, it was 5.1 percent in men and 16.7 percent in women.

In most countries the incidence among those patch tested for suspected contact dermatitis ranges from 6.4 to 16 percent, but some studies have found that from 16.7 percent to over 30 percent of those patch tested were positive.[4-10] The experience in Europe parallels that in America. Overall, the percentage of reactors among persons patch tested for possible contact dermatitis to nickel between 1967 and 1990 ranged from 0.4 to 8.5 percent in men and 0.5 to 43.7 percent in women.[11]

The greater prevalence in women may be prominent and age-related.[12] Nickel allergy often begins early, as schoolgirls with pierced ears had a 13 percent prevalence, while in those without pierced ears it was only 1 percent.[13] Nickel sensitivity overall is ten times as common in women as it is in men.[2] Ear piercing seems to induce nickel sensitivity. Although the prevalence is lower in women who do not have pierced ears, it is still higher than in men when age-matched groups are compared.[14] Women tend to become allergic at a younger age and to be sensitized by jewelry. Both men and women have a tendency toward an association with hand eczema, and that association is more common in men.[15] Prevalence is also higher in persons with photodermatitis.[16]

Nickel is also a common sensitizer in the pediatric population,[17-23] and infants can be sensitized.[24] Rudzki et al.[25] found that about one in five children aged 6 to 15 were allergic to nickel, and the prevalence of allergy was equal in boys and girls. However girls above age 15 were much more likely to be allergic than boys of that age group.[25]

ARE THESE TESTS RELEVANT?

Many persons with positive patch tests to nickel do not present with nickel dermatitis,[26] but more than 90 percent will have a history which probably correlates.[4]

Also, occupations where exposure to metals is routine are not necessarily the cause of the sensitivity, as 25 of 79 persons aged 15 to 19 were nickel-allergic on preemployment tests.[27] Even among metalworkers who were nickel-allergic, most had a prior history of jewelry dermatitis.[28]

HOW DOES ONE RECOGNIZE CONTACT DERMATITIS TO NICKEL?

Easily the most consistent picture in nickel allergy is that of an eczematous eruption or scar where the ears have been pierced to accommodate earrings. Cheap earrings are the source of contact allergy in a high percentage of patients,[29] but most of those who develop sensitivity from earrings do not present with that picture but rather have a positive history when the patch test to nickel is positive.[30] Some may present with hypertrophic scars or keloids. The reason earrings are a problem may be related to both the metallurgy and the efficiency of plasma in releasing nickel from metal objects.[31]

An eczema where other jewelry is worn is also suspect, but other diseases must be ruled out. For example, tinea under a watch may look eczematous but can be confirmed with a KOH preparation.[32] In a person known to be nickel-sensitive, the dimethylglyoxime test for free nickel in the jewelry is extremely useful.

In years past, most cases were associated with the metal clasps on garter belts or stocking supports. In the United Kingdom they were called suspenders, but the change from stockings to pantyhose solved that.

An abdominal eruption in an adolescent girl makes one think of exposure to the metal snaps in blue jeans (Fig. 29-1), which may be accompanied by hand eczema as

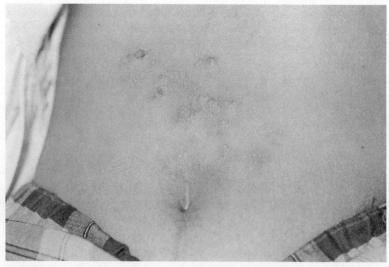

FIG. 29-1. Jean snap dermatitis in a nickel-allergic adolescent.

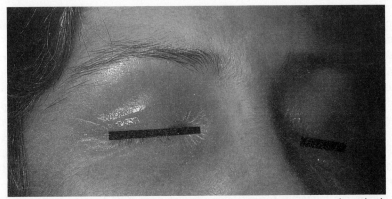

FIG. 29–2. Hand transfer contact dermatitis of the eyelids. the source was the patient's metal nail file.

well.[33] A postoperative nickel dermatitis of the abdomen and inner thigh can also be caused by use of a nonstainless retractor during surgery.[34] Stainless steel clips sensitized one patient after thyroid surgery, causing a severe eruption in the wound site after 3 weeks.[35]

Eyelid dermatitis may occur from nickel-contaminated cosmetics[36] or a nail file (Fig. 29-2), but persons with eyelid dermatitis are nickel-allergic less often than expected.[37]

Another person developed an osteomyelitis-like reaction around stainless steel wires used to treat a mandibular fracture,[38] and stomatitis and the sore mouth syndrome may be associated with sensitivity to dental metals,[39–41] but exposure to nickel in a dental alloy will not always cause a detectable reaction.[42]

The incidence of systemic contact dermatitis from nickel (Fig. 29-3) is not easily obtained. An eruption over the knee, elbow, mouth, and face may be associated with an orthopedic implant or dental prosthesis.[43–47] The former seems unusual, as no patients with metal to plastic arthroplasty implants showed cutaneous effects despite patch-test conversion in a few.[48] A dermatitis of the arms, periorbital edema, and eczema under jean snaps developed from orthodontic bands without stomatitis.[49] Some develop sensi-

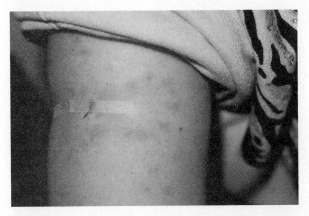

FIG. 29–3. Systemic contact dermatitis following nickel exposure. The histology was that of a fixed erythema.

tivity after arthroplasty, but loosening did not accompany allergy in one series.[50] Noneczematous eruptions may occur from pocket change (Figs. 29-4 and 29-5) or even systemic exposure.[51]

Possible airborne contact has been reported from metal spraying (as an alternative to plating) with nickel and chromium in the vapor.[52] I have seen airborne contact from a vapor with high nickel content.

A controversial subject is the development of endogenous eczema or pompholyx following nickel exposure. Many nickel-sensitive persons have recurrent episodes of pompholyx.[53] Burrows[54] says that the "apron pattern," which is sometimes regarded as nickel sensitivity, is considered by Cronin and others to be a constitutional eczema. The idea that pompholyx is induced by dietary nickel has two principal flaws. One is that it takes 5 mg or more of oral nickel, which is much too high ever to be physiologic. The other is the tendency for systemic contact dermatitis to produce more changes than pompholyx.[54] Roduner et al.[55] found no difference in the effect of oral nickel on pompholyx and "non-pompholyx" eczema.

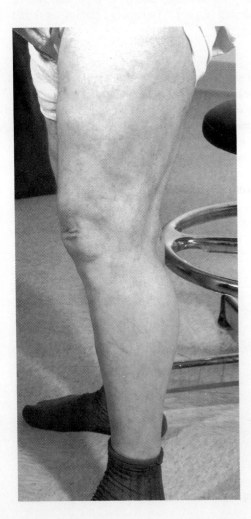

FIG. 29–4. Dermal (noneczematous) contact from nickel.

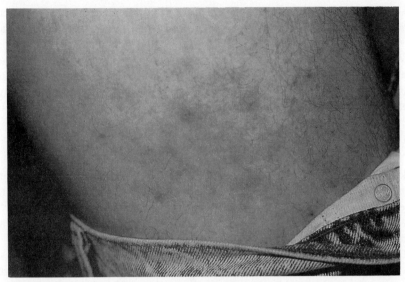

FIG. 29–5. Contact allergy on the thigh from change carried in the pocket.

Möller,[55a] however, feels that nickel is a cause but not the only cause of pompholyx. The association with hand eczema is undeniable, and this is especially true for pompholyx. The cutaneous reaction from nickel is dose-dependent, with a high provocation at 2.5 to 5.6 mg and less at 0.5 mg. He also noted the benefit with diet and disulfiram (which is used to chelate the metal) and the aggravation with challenge.

Systemic contact may produce pompholyx with elbow dermatitis (which runs a course parallel to hand dermatitis)[56] or dermatitis in the axillae with spread over the inner thighs (as part of the baboon syndrome).[57] Sensitization from systemic exposure has also been reported, and a widespread eruption can be seen from orthopedic implants or a pacemaker,[58] even one made of stainless steel. The eruption sometimes starts where metal exposure occurred.[59]

Unusual presentations attributed to nickel allergy include circular excoriations of the back, where biopsy showed superficial vasculitis,[60] erythema multiforme,[61,62] a lichen striatus–like eruption from bookbinding glue,[63] lichenoid dermatitis,[64] granuloma annulare,[65] and an eruption from a razor mimicking sycosis barbae.[66] Fransway and Winkelmann[67] had four patients who developed cutaneous T-cell lymphoma ostensibly from chronic antigenic stimulation, and one of these was nickel-allergic. Allergic contact urticaria, rhinitis, and asthma may occur from nickel,[68] as may joint or muscle stiffness.[69]

Finally, many persons with a history of metal sensitivity are patch-test negative to nickel. Of 28 with a positive history, 13 were negative on testing, and 8 of 23 with positive tests lacked a history of a problem.[70]

PATCH TESTING

Patch testing to nickel has been done for so long that one might logically assume that all of the technical problems have been solved. Unfortunately this is far from true. Even experts do not agree on many points, some of which seem quite important. There are differences in the salt to use, the vehicle, the method of occlusion, and the need for intradermal testing, to name a few. The standard test reagent is 5% nickel sulfate in petrolatum, and we have more experience with that reagent than any other, although I have used many comparing the two sides and often trying to define whether a unilateral response was an irritant or a false negative test on the other side. With all of the problems, testing to nickel and indeed to other metals is important, as it often provides valuable confirmation and sometimes an unsuspected response which is relevant.

THE ANTIGEN

Nickel chloride produces more positive responses than nickel sulfate,[71,72] but it is more likely to produce an irritant response.[73] Irritation may be reduced by using a petrolatum rather than an aqueous vehicle for nickel chloride. Lammintausta and Maibach[74] feel that the tendency for irritation by nickel chloride has limited its usefulness as an allergen, and my experience has been the same.

Nickel alloys which release adequate amounts may also be used for patch testing. An old-time favorite is a nickel (U.S.) coin, which is not of World War II vintage. To be safe, one can test the coin with dimethylglyoxime before applying it, but this test would only prove presence of 10 μg, which is the limit of detection.

THE CONCENTRATION

A concentration of 5% has been selected as perhaps the best, as a 2.5% concentration will miss about 20%.[75] However, some suggest the 2.5% concentration for infants,[18] and the atopic patient.[76]

In reading the test results, weak and moderately strong positive patch-test reactions to metal salts may be irritant and some recommend the results be checked with serial dilution tests or at least that retesting be done.[62]

Rarely, there may be some use for testing with a higher concentration of nickel sulfate in persons with a strongly positive history and a negative patch test to a 5% concentration. Dooms-Goossens found two patients who had strong histories but failed to react to 5% nickel sulfate in either petrolatum or water and even 1:10,000 on intradermal testing, but had + + responses with 10% nickel sulfate in petrolatum.[77] Möller concluded that those with a positive history but negative tests are probably atopics,[78] but persons with a positive history and negative patch testing also can be evaluated further by using nickel chloride rather than nickel sulfate[79,80] or using DMSO as the vehicle.[81] Another method is oral provocation (although this may be positive without allergy).

Sometimes open testing elicits a response within a few hours. It has been recommended as a possible screening test, although it detects about 93 percent of reactors by 48 h.[82] Intradermal testing sometimes reveals positive tests not found on patch testing,[83] and it will detect a few reactors who do not have positive patch tests but do have a history suggesting nickel allergy.[83] There are three indications for intradermal testing:

1. Interpretation of the patch test is difficult.
2. A patch test is negative despite a strong history.
3. It is necessary to confirm or refute a previous diagnosis.

The method used by Möller[84] was 0.016% nickel sulfate in a tuberculin syringe (with a stainless steel needle). It took 0.1 mL to produce the desired 4-mm wheal on the volar forearm. A 4-mm or greater reaction at 72 h was interpreted as positive.

Homogeneity can also be a problem. This is worse when the antigen is not refrigerated.[85] Many (14 to 16 out of 25) persons allergic to 5% nickel sulfate in petrolatum (11,200 ppm) react to 112 ppm, and 1 of 25 reacted to 1.12 ppm.[86] The amount of nickel in the standard patch test varies sixfold because while 12 to 18 μL is the desired amount, the actual content is 9 to 50 μL.[87] The amount added to a Finn chamber is 12 to 18 μL (although studies show that a range of 9 to 50 μL can be seen in current use). The range of concentrations of nickel in 5% nickel sulfate in 25 samples was 0.7 to 1.1%.[88]

THE VEHICLE

The vehicle is a bit more controversial. Some prefer the aqueous form,[75,89] as provocation is higher.[31] Reactivity varies with the vehicle in the following order: DMSO>PG>water>cetromacrogol>petrolatum.[90] Softisan produced stronger reactions than petrolatum in 19 of 23 patients.[91]

TIME OF OCCLUSION

Time of occlusion is traditionally 48 h, but Bruze[92] found that 5-h occlusion was possible provided that higher concentrations were used.

TIME FOR READING

When reading times of 24 and 48 h are compared, they are the same in 74 percent, positive at 48 h only in 17 percent, and positive at 24 h only in 8.5 percent.[71] Reading on day 4 detected 14 percent of 873 nickel reactors who were negative on day 2.[93]

IRRITANT REACTIONS

Pustular reactions are produced in persons with atopic dermatitis when patches are placed on follicular papules, erythema, lichenification, or areas of trauma.[94] *Corynebacterium acnes* sufficient to produce small pustules will lead to a pustular response from nickel patch tests in all cases, and any inflammatory can cause this in 5 percent of cases.[95] Even rabbits show this at injection sites.[96] Fischer and Rystedt[97] found the 6.5 percent of follicular and irritant reactions could be separated from the allergic by serial dilution from 5% to 0.0025% in both petrolatum and water. They found more nonallergic reactions when petrolatum was the vehicle, despite using Finn chambers. Wahlberg[76] also concluded that this reaction is more likely with a petrolatum vehicle and it is both concentration- and vehicle-dependent, as one sees it only with the highest concentration.

OTHER TECHNICAL PROBLEMS

Use of aluminum chambers with nickel solutions may cause etching of the aluminum and a reduction of nickel content in saline solutions. This is explained by the fact that aluminum has a greater affinity for electrons than cobalt or nickel, causing an electron exchange.[98] In the chapter on patch testing, Bruze discusses irritancy from nonpetrolatum vehicles. Applying the metal alloys themselves will give a positive response if 1 μg/cm^2/week or more of nickel is released, and a weak reaction if release is below 0.5 μg/cm^2/week.[99]

According to McClelland et al.,[100] "The response to both allergen and irritant was greater than to either alone. Doses of allergen, which did not produce a response when applied alone, produced a response when an irritant was added. Irritants therefore increase the allergic contact dermatitis response and may explain the presence of contact dermatitis in patients with negative patch tests." There are, of course, other probable causes.

In some women there is also a tendency for lower threshold and greater sensitivity premenstrually.[101] Estradiol enhances nickel-induced blast formation of lymphocytes.[102]

Retesting in the same area is accentuated, but retesting after 3 to 6 weeks may be accompanied by downregulation.[103]

TESTING ON THE ORAL MUCOSA

Mucosal evaluation has been done with metallic plates with high nickel content under a maxillary acrylic plate. This was left on 48 h and read 24 h later.[104]

RELATIONSHIP TO SENSITIVITY TO OTHER METALS

In 5.8 percent of one patch-tested population, both nickel and cobalt were positive. Almost half of these persons had hand eczema. Those with a strongly positive patch test to nickel are 50 times more likely to have a strong cobalt allergy than a control population.[105]

Walton found that all of the copper reactors were also nickel-sensitive, but the reasons are currently not clear.

Commercial sources of copper, chromium, cobalt, and palladium patch-test materials may contain nickel contamination, which is generally not enough to cause a positive response in most subjects but may do so in highly sensitive persons.[106,107] Camarasa et al.[108] studied seven persons highly allergic to both nickel and palladium and found the palladium patch-test material free of nickel. Possible explanations include the following[109]:

False-positive reaction.
Reactions are concomitant due to both metals being used together.
Both metals are in Group VII in the periodic table.
Contamination of the test material.

Burrows found that all palladium reactors on testing to PdC$_2$ were negative to the pure metal foil,[109] but in another study, 3 of 29 persons with reactions to both metals reacted to a palladium disk.[110] A summary of results at multiple centers found that 3 of 42 reactors were not nickel-allergic. There were 39 who reacted to palladium and nickel and 15 who reacted to palladium, nickel, and cobalt.[111] Since cobalt reagents seem to contain more contaminant nickel than palladium materials, these results are probably not due to contaminant nickel in palladium test material.

The association of nickel and cobalt sensitivity may be caused by concomitant sensitization, as most persons in that category are women with hand eczema; that is, the sensitivity may be a phenomenon secondary to preexisting hand eczema.[112] According to Eedy et al.,[107] the content of nickel in the various metals used as patch-testing reagent sources was as follows:

Nickel: 9360 to 19,400 ppm
Cobalt: 0900 to 3180 ppm
Chromium: 0040 to 4280 ppm
Palladium: 10 to 100 ppm
Copper: 20 to 170 ppm

Lammintausta[113] found, in an animal study, that both nickel and cobalt sensitization had an enhancing effect of reactivity to the other metal, but in human subjects sensitivity may be specific.[114]

NICKEL ALLERGY AND HAND ECZEMA

The association of nickel allergy with hand eczema has attracted much attention. According to Möller,[9] the hand eczema typically follows nickel sensitivity by a number of years, and it seems to be independent of exposure to nickel. It is certainly endogenous and can flare even with avoidance, although challenge by ingestion can induce a flare. The reduction of nickel in the diet is reportedly beneficial in many. About 60 percent of persons who started on a low-nickel diet continued after 5 years, and almost all of these thought it was beneficial.[115]

Hyposensitization by oral administration of nickel has also been attempted. Some success reportedly was achieved with 5 mg but not 0.5 mg once weekly for 6 weeks as measured by patch testing before and after.[116] The urine and serum levels were not elevated, however. Perhaps this is because they are increased earlier than 7 days. Sudden challenge with higher amounts is less well tolerated.[117]

Hand eczema in housewives is commonly (78 percent) caused by contact dermatitis, with one large study finding a similar incidence of irritant (45 percent) and allergic (43 percent) contact[118] and another finding that 38 percent were caused by allergy.[119] Nickel allergy is very common in persons with hand eczema.[120–122] In the general population there is a 19 percent prevalence of hand dermatitis, but this rises to 43 percent in nickel-allergic women. In a prospective study, nickel sensitivity predisposed to hand eczema[123]; in another, it was associated with more relapses.[124] The influence on hand eczema is not genetic, as the prevalence of hand eczema was the same in nickel-sensitive monozygotic and dizygotic twins, and this was comparable with the prevalence in the general population.[125]

Patch tests are positive in some persons without a history of skin disease. Of 274 such orthopedic patients undergoing surgery, 22 percent had at least one reaction in the standard series, with a prevalence of 7 percent to nickel.[26]

SOURCES

The sources of contact are often obvious, but there are persons with a positive patch-test reaction who have no history of a contact problem.[26,75] The most common source may be earrings, but one seldom sees a patient who presents with earlobe dermatitis as the principal complaint. More often this is the source of sensitivity, but other sources cause the presenting picture. It may be an object as obvious as a metal snap on clothing or one as cryptic as clothing contaminated from an iron or from pocket change. One should also think not only of external sources but, on occasion, of internal sources as well. Systemic contact may come from a patch test, a prosthesis, and even perhaps from the diet.

Some of the reported sources can be found in Table 29-1. This comes from published reports. However, through the years, I have seen nickel allergy caused by a wide variety of objects, ranging from a metal edge on a desk at school to a spray from a hopper containing metal bolts. Common sense, the pattern and location, a positive patch test, and diligence will usually unravel the puzzle.

Another clinical problem is occupationally induced nickel sensitivity. Several occupations have been reported to be at higher risk, although sensitivity in these may not necessarily be causally related to work. The increase in the frequency of nickel sensitivity in women with pierced ears as opposed to those with unpierced ears is highly significant ($p < .001$), and it is more likely to be the underlying cause than the occupation. In men, nickel sensitivity is much less common,[126] and occupational factors are more often implicated.

Among 66 hairdressers, 18 were allergic to nickel [less than p-phenylenediamine (PPD)].[127] One reason is that nickel is released from metal objects used with thioglycolate solutions.[128,129] However, another possible scenario is the tendency for persons in this occupation to have pierced ears. When *apprentice* hairdressers were compared with student nurses, nickel allergy was twice as common among the former, and this was perhaps due not only to the slightly higher prevalence of pierced ears among hairdressers but also to their having had it done at a younger age.[130] Occupations associated in women include hairdressers, chefs, and cleaning women. Men engaged in engineering, building, and mining are at increased risk,[15] but electroplating[131] and electroforming[72] also provide a high level of exposure.

TREATMENT

The most obvious approach to the treatment of nickel sensitivity is to prevent exposure in some manner. This can be done by recognizing the sources and avoiding contact, by (antigen) substitution of materials which are safe, and by using barriers to contact or absorption. Avoidance of systemic exposure reportedly helps, and deliberate exposure can also be used to advantage.

ANTIGEN SUBSTITUTION

For many nickel-allergic patients, the most useful substitution is perhaps that of earrings made from "safe" alloys. Hypoallergenic earrings release 0.005 μg of nickel, while

TABLE 29–1. Sources of Exposure to Nickel

Accupuncture needles[172-174]	Hooks and garter	Paper clips[174]
Ballpoint pens (rare)[8]	supports[174,199]	Pens[74]
Belt buckles[8,174]	Hydrogenated fat[200]	Pencils[174]
Bicycle handlebars[174]	ID tags[174,178a]	Plated cutlery[8]
Blackboard chalk[175,176]	Intravenous infusion needles[201]	Pocket knives[8]
Blow-dry hairbrush[177]	Jeans rivets and snaps[199]	Powder paint[214]
Bobby pins[174]	Jewelry: necklace, earrings[174,194]	Prams[8]
Bracelet[178a]	Key rings[8]	Purse[8]
Brassiere wire supports[174]	Keys[8,174,178a,202]	Razors[174]
Buttons on blue jeans[174]	Kitchen equipment[8,174]	Safety pins[178a]
Carriages[174]	Kitchen handles[8]	Sanitary goods[194]
Case[178a]	Kitchen utensils[194]	Sanitary napkin pins[174]
Chrome platers[179]	Knitting needles (not now in	Scissors[8,174,202]
Cigarette lighter[174]	U.K.)[8]	Sewing machines[8,174]
Clips, safety pins[8]	Letter opener[8,202]	Shoelace tips[178a]
Coins[8,174,178a]	Lighters[8]	Shoe buckles[174]
Coin (swallowing)[180]	Lipstick, powder cases[8,174]	Snaps on undergarments[174]
Contact lens cleaning solution[181]	Magnets[178]	Spectacle frames[178a,215,216]
Curlers[174]	Mascara[203]	Stainless-steel sinks, pans[8]
Dermo-jet[174,182-184]	Medallion[174,178]	Steel wool—Grade "O"[174]
Door handles[8,174]	Metal arch supports[174]	Steel wool[210] and soap pads[217]
Doorknob[178a]	Metal chairs[174]	Stethoscope[218]
Drawer handles[174]	Metal chair arm rests[174]	Surgical retractors[34]
Earrings[174]	Metal connector on catheter[204]	Table edge[202]
EKG electrodes[185]	Metal gates[205]	Tailoring tools[194]
Electrocautery plate[186]	Metal machinery, pipes,	Taps[8]
Epilating needles[174]	handles[8]	Telephone dials[8,174]
Eye pencil[187]	Metal pins held in the mouth[174]	Telephone[202]
Eyeglass frames[174]	Metal plating[206]	Television dial[8,202]
Eyelash curler[174,188,189]	Metal sinks[174]	Thimbles[174]
Eyelets on shoes[174]	Metal thimbles[8]	Tin openers[8]
Eyeshadow[190,191]	Metal toys[178a]	Transcutaneous electrical
Fertilizers[192]	Metal working fluids[207]	nerve stimulation[219]
Fingernails (higher than toenails)[193]	Metallic threads (shawl)[208]	Typewriter parts[174]
Food	Molded bricks used in	Umbrellas[174]
Furniture frames[8]	construction[209]	Vacuum cleaners[174]
Galvanic baths[194]	Multiple injector syringe[210]	Watch straps[174,178a,194]
Garter snaps[174]	Necklaces[174]	Wheelchair frame[202]
Guitar strings[195]	Needles[174]	White gold or cheap metal rings[8]
Hairdressing tools[194]	Objects handled[194]	White gold crowns[174]
Hairpins[174]	Orthodontic headgear (metal	Window catches[8]
Handbag, case handles[8,174]	buckle)[211]	Wristband to dissipate static
Heart valves[174,196]	Orthodontic wires and	electricity[220]
Hemodialysis equipment[197]	bands[212]	Zipper[8,174,178a,194,199]
Hip prostheses[198]	Palladium[213]	

[a]Pediatric patients.

unused posts and earrings release 0.005 to 25 μg. Those causing a problem released up to 442 μg, and it took <0.05 μg to break out.[132] According to Fisher,[133] stainless steel ear-piercing kits are available from H & A Enterprises (143-19 25th Street, Whitestone, NY 11357). Hypoallergenic jewelry is widely available, but it is a good idea for patients to learn to test items for free nickel before exposure. This can be done with the dimethylglyoxime stick test[134] as follows:

1. Two reagents are used in the test: 1% dimethylglyoxime in alcohol and 10% ammonia water.
2. A few drops of each reagent are placed on a cotton-tipped applicator so that it is moist. Two or so is usually enough.
3. The metal surface is rubbed with the applicator and observed for a red color.
4. A color change to red indicates the presence of free nickel.

The test is extremely useful and is commonly prescribed for nickel-allergic patients at our institution. The nickel spot test detects free nickel down to 10 ppm,[54,135] and the sensitivity threshold of most patients is above 11.2 ppm. While there are persons who react strongly to levels well below 10 ppm on patch testing on normal skin,[86] earrings that cause dermatitis usually release more than the threshold level,[132] so the test is very practical. However, it also has limitations. Some alloys are not as easily detected as others,[99,136] but alloys releasing more than 1 μg/cm^2/week give positive reactions, while those releasing less than 0.5 μg/cm^2/week give weak responses.[99] However, some patients will react to white gold, which contains some 0.5 ppm and has a negative dimethylglyoxime test.[135,137]

The presence of free nickel will also be influenced by environmental factors. Sweat will leach 0.6 to 99 ppm from stainless steel, physiological saline 0.5 to 9.8 ppm, and blood 2.6 to 17.4 ppm from stainless steel objects. In tissue, nickel levels of up to 34 to 53 ppm can be found immediately adjacent to a vitallium implant, but the metal is not detectable 1 cm away.[138] Fisher criticized this study because, although both vitallium and stainless steel contain nickel in the alloys, a study with vitallium cannot be used to represent what might happen with stainless steel.[89]

In Denmark, regulations have been adopted to reduce the nickel content of fasteners, ornaments, jewelry, and the like by using the dimethylglyoxime test, which ostensibly demonstrates a release of at least 0.5 μg/cm^2/week.[139] Most but not all nickel-allergic persons will tolerate other metals, such as copper, brass, bronze, palladium, and gold.[140] Therefore after testing to a new alloy it may be possible to substitute it if the test is negative.

BARRIERS AND COATINGS

Polyurethane coating of metal objects containing nickel may retard reactions (8 of 11 patients) provided that the material is intact, while a fabric flap may help prevent nickel dermatitis from clothing.[141] Rubber gloves are not adequate, as nickel will penetrate them.[142]

Chelating agents with disulfiram (Antabuse) or trientene have undergone trials, but the results are inconclusive.[15,53,135,143-148] Disulfiram is closely related to many of the rubber chemicals in structure, and it splits into two molecules of diethyldithiocarbamate

HANDOUT FOR NICKEL-ALLERGIC PERSONS

HOW DOES ONE BECOME ALLERGIC TO NICKEL?

Nickel sensitivity is something that some of us acquire after we are born. It is usually from exposure where there is some inflammation, but by far the most common underlying event is ear piercing. Women who have had their ears pierced are more than ten times as likely to become nickel-sensitive as those who have not. Occupational allergy is more likely in men than in women in the United States.

WILL I BE ALLERGIC FOR LIFE?

Perhaps, but this is not certain. Nickel-allergic persons who have obvious dermatitis may have persistent problems, but those who are positive on patch testing but do not have a rash tend to do much better. Children who are patch-test-positive to nickel are often no longer allergic after three years.

WHAT USUALLY CAUSES THE RASH TO APPEAR?

Sweat leaches nickel out of many types of metal, especially steel. The "free" nickel is then absorbed into the skin, where it causes the rash. Tissue fluids are even more likely to dissolve nickel in jewelry, so the open wound from ear piercing can be a difficult problem.

HOW DO I KNOW WHICH ITEMS CONTAIN FREE NICKEL?

Steel which is not stainless steel is suspect, and even stainless occasionally can cause a problem. However, you can test jewelry and metal objects for free nickel with a "nickel spot test." Nickel spot test kits are marketed by Allerderm Laboratories, but if your local physician or pharmacy does not carry it, you can obtain one from the Skin and Allergy Shop, 310 East Broadway, Louisville, KY 40202 or (800) 366-6483.

Directions are as follows:

1. Two reagents are used in the test: 1% dimethylglyoxime in alcohol and 10% ammonia water.
2. A few drops of each reagent are placed on a cotton-tipped applicator so that it is moist. One or two is usually enough.
3. The metal surface is rubbed with the applicator and observed for a red color.
4. The color change to red indicates presence of free nickel.

This information is provided to help persons with contact dermatitis in the understanding of their problem. The contents are subject to change as more information becomes available and are not intended as a substitute for medical treatment.

This very simple test will detect relatively low levels of free nickel, but some very sensitive persons may occasionally break out to metal objects that test negative. "Hypoallergenic jewelry" often does not have enough free nickel to cause a rash, but testing an object first is advised, as some articles which are said to be safe may not be.

HOW DO I AVOID CONTACT WITH NICKEL?

Substituting nickel-free jewelry is advised. There should be a layer of cloth between the skin and hooks and snaps on clothing. Coins and key rings can be kept in a plastic coin purse, and highly allergic persons should avoid inadvertent transfer of nickel on the hands or fingernails. Plastic or stainless steel objects can often be substituted. For example, eyeglass frames of plastic can be used rather than those of metal. Coating objects with polyurethane or nail polish can be of temporary benefit if one is not allergic to those materials. Cloth, cellophane, and other types of tape or cloth may be used to prevent direct contact with the skin, but such things are only helpful temporarily, as sooner or later you will probably become exposed. Rubber gloves do not adequately protect, but plastic gloves help, especially the thicker ones.

Sometimes a dental prosthesis (false teeth or a bridge) may contain free nickel. Metal clips used in surgery may also become a problem if corroded. Whether orthopedic implants cause a significant problem is controversial, but most authorities believe that modern implants are seldom a problem. Levels of nickel can be found around some types of implant, but there was no problem in healing in a fairly large series of nickel-allergic persons who underwent such surgery.

WHAT ABOUT NICKEL IN THE DIET?

This is also controversial. Some types of hand eczema are much more common in persons who are nickel-allergic, but it is difficult to show that one causes the other. A diet list is available showing which foods are high in nickel. Water from the tap in some localities may contain more nickel in the early morning, ostensibly because it picks up nickel from metal pipes overnight. An iron skillet might be a problem, but Teflon-coated and aluminum cookware should ordinarily not release nickel. Stainless steel cookware contains nickel, but not free nickel unless one uses it to cook or heat acid foods. Again, the nickel spot test can be helpful in establishing which objects are probably safe.

AM I LIKELY TO BECOME ALLERGIC TO OTHER METALS?

Allergy to copper and cobalt is more common in those who are nickel-allergic than in those who are not. To be safe, you can ask to be tested to these metals. Palladium sensitivity is also associated with allergy to nickel, but persons who react to palladium on patch test often do not break out to metallic palladium (found in jewelry and certain dental metals).

TABLE 29-2. Diet Instruction for the Reduction of Nickel Intake

It is not necessary to restrict intake of the following:

All kinds of meat and poultry, fish, and eggs. Milk, unflavored yogurt, butter, margarine, cheese, and yeast.

Vegetables: asparagus, red beets, broccoli, Brussels sprout, white cabbage, cauliflower, champignons, Chinese cabbage, corn, cucumber, dill, eggplant, garlic (in moderation), mushrooms, onions (in moderation), parsley, green and red peppers, and potatoes

Grain products: finely milled rye and wheat flour, whole grain rye and wheat bread (in moderation), white rice and breakfast foods made of rice, cornflakes, cornmeal, cornstarch, macaroni, popcorn, rice, spaghetti, wheat flour, whole grain rye and wheat bread (in moderation)

Fruits: peaches, pears, raisins, rhubarb and all berries *except* raspberries

Drinks: coffee and tea (not too strong, and in moderation), soft drinks, alcoholic beverages (distilled products and drinks made from these)

Miscellaneous items, including spaghetti and yeast

The following foods have a high nickel content, and intake should be restricted: Shellfish like shrimp, crawfish, prawns, and mussels.

Vegetables: beans (green, brown, white), kale, leeks, lentils, lettuce, soy protein powder, spinach, peas, and sprouts made from beans and lucerne.

The grain products, buckwheat, millet, oatmeal, wheat bran (i.e., bran and fiber products), including muesli, unpolished rice, rye bran, bran biscuits, and fiber tablets and multigrain breads

Fruits: dates, figs, pineapple, prunes, and raspberries

Drinks: chocolate and cocoa drinks, and tea from drink dispensers

Miscellaneous items including almonds, baking powder (in large amounts), linseed, hazelnuts and other nuts, peanuts, soya-containing foods such as meat with soya additives, sesame seeds, sunflower seeds, sweets containing chocolate, marzipan, nuts, strong licorice, and vitamins containing nickel

The first liter of water taken from the tap in the morning should not be used in food preparation, as nickel may be released from the tap during the night. Nickel-plated kitchen utensils, such as eggbeaters and teaballs, should be replaced.

Acid foods such as stewed fruits and rhubarb cooked in stainless steel utensils should be avoided. The acids in the foods can cause nickel to be released from the utensils. Tinned foods should be eaten only in moderation.

You will judge the value of the diet by the results. Therefore do not start when you are likely to cheat, as when starting a vacation or planning to attend holiday parties. Follow the diet for at least 1 to 2 months. It can be difficult to change eating habits for a long period of time. So adhere to the instructions as closely as possible when eating at home. The greatest problem is eating out. When eating away from home, the diet may have to be modified, but use discretion.

Source: Adapted from Veien and Andersen,[162] by permission.

after absorption.[149] Sometimes a flare is seen after start of treatment and before improvement is noted.[150] In one patient, improvement was noted repeatedly following courses of treatment with both diethyldithiocarbamate and tetraethylthiuram disulfide.[151]

Epidermal levels are apparently best reduced by NaEDTA,[152] which reportedly can be used with some success in a barrier cream.[153] A barrier using diethyldithiocarbamate was not effective.[154]

DIET

The benefit of a "low-nickel" diet is controversial. Oral challenge with five times the normal nickel content of the diet tends to exacerbate hand eczema in many nickel-sensitive patients,[155] but similar levels may exacerbate hand eczema even in persons who are not patch-test positive to nickel.[156,157]

It takes about 2.5 mg or more to cause a flare, while the normal dietary intake is closer to 0.5 mg.[135] Twenty times the average daily intake caused a flare in 9 of 12 persons after about 1 to 20 h.[157a] Seventeen of 28 became worse after 2.5 mg and 9 of 17 improved following 6 weeks of reduced dietary nickel with an accompanying suppression of urinary levels. Seven of the nine experienced exacerbations after resuming normal intake.[158] In another study, 0.5 and 2.5 mg did not cause a flare, but 5.0 mg increased the severity of pompholyx. The serum levels at the higher dose were 2 1/2 times normal.[159] However, some studies deny that dietary nickel or metal hip prostheses perpetuate nickel dermatitis.[144] Urinary levels are increased over the 2 or 3 days after oral challenge,[160] but one study found little correlation between flares of dermatitis and urinary levels.[161] Perhaps a sudden increase in dietary levels is the determining factor,[117] or it may be necessary to deplete body stores of nickel to determine the role of dietary nickel in hand eczema.[143]

Dietary sources have been detailed by Veien[162] and others, and tap water seems to contain much higher nickel levels in the early morning when first drawn, with 250 μg in 250 mL. Hot water contained more than cold. Flushing for only 5 min eliminated the higher values.[163] Overall, water from the water works before transmission had very low levels of nickel, and most samples from suburban locations was below 1 μg/L. The higher levels occur apparently from the delivery system.[164] Nickel may come from canned foods and acid foods (those with oxalic acid especially) may release nickel from stainless steel cookware.[165] The dimethylglyoxime test may not be adequate to detect levels which will cause a problem in some people.[142,166] None was released from aluminum, enamel, or Teflon cookware.[167] There may be increased absorption with indomethacin therapy.[168]

Vegetables grown with nickel supplementation of the soil may develop higher levels.[169] Underground water was the suspected contact source in one patient, as concentrated samples elicited a positive test in a nickel-sensitive patient with chronic facial dermatitis.[170] A diet with reduced nickel content as proposed by Veien is found in Table 29-2. Another possible way to reduce absorption is to take oral disodium chromoglycate.[171]

REFERENCES

1. Nethercott JR, Holness DL, Adams RM, et al: Patch testing with a routine screening tray in North America through 1989: I. Frequency of response. *Am J Contact Dermatitis* 2:122, 1991.
2. Prystowsky SD, Allen AM, Smith RW, et al: Allergic contact hypersensitivity to nickel, neomycin, ethylenediamine and benzocaine: Relationship between age, sex, history of exposure and reactivity to standard patch tests and use tests in a general population. *Arch Dermatol* 115:959, 1979.
3. Nethercott JR, Holness DL, Adams RM, et al: Patch testing with a routine screening tray in North America through 1989: II. Gender and response. *Am J Contact Dermatitis* 2:130, 1991.
4. Nethercott JR, Holness DL: Cutaneous nickel sensitivity in Toronto, Canada. *J Am Acad Dermatol* 22:756, 1990.
5. Hogan DJ, Hill M, Lane PR: Results of routine patch testing of 542 patients in Saskatoon, Canada. *Contact Dermatitis* 19:120, 1988.
6. Sertoli A, Gola M, Martinelli M, et al: Epidemiology of contact dermatitis. *Semin Dermatol* 8:120, 1989.
7. Zhang XM, Niklasson B, Li SY: Patch testing in cases of eczema and dermatitis in Beijing, China. *Contact Dermatitis* 25:224, 1991.

8. Wilkinson DS, Wilkinson JD: Nickel allergy and hand eczema, in Maibach HI, Menne T (eds): *Nickel and the Skin: Immunology and Toxicology.* Boca Raton, FL, CRC Press, 1989, p 133.
9. Moller H: Nickel dermatitis: Problems solved and unsolved. *Contact Dermatitis* 23:217, 1990.
10. Lunder M: Variable incidence of nickel dermatitis. *Contact Dermatitis* 18:287, 1988.
11. Basketter DA, Briatico-Vangosa G, Kaestner W, et al: Nickel, cobalt and chromium in consumer products: A role in allergic contact dermatitis? *Contact Dermatitis* 28:15, 1993.
12. Menne T, Christophersen J, Green A: Epidemiology of nickel dermatitis, in Maibach HI, Menne T (eds): *Nickel and the Skin: Immunology and Toxicology.* Boca Raton, FL, CRC Press, 1989, pp 112–113.
13. Larsson-Stymne B, Widstrom L: Ear piercing—A cause of nickel allergy in schoolgirls? *Contact Dermatitis* 13:289, 1985.
14. McDonagh AJ, Wright AL, Cork MJ, Gawkrodger DJ: Nickel sensitivity: The influence of ear piercing and atopy. *Br J Dermatol* 126:16, 1992.
15. Gawkrodger DJ, Vestey JP, Wong WK, Buxton PK: Contact clinic survey of nickel-sensitive subjects. *Contact Dermatitis* 14:165, 1986.
16. Barber KA, Cronin E: Patch and photopatch testing in chronic actinic dermatitis. *Contact Dermatitis* 10:69, 1984.
17. Weston WL, Weston JA: Allergic contact dermatitis in children. *Am J Dis Child* 138:932, 1984.
18. Hjorth N: Contact dermatitis in children. *Acta Derm Venereol Supple* 95:36, 1981.
19. Pevny I, Brennenstuhl M, Razinskas G: Patch testing in children: II. Results and case reports. *Contact Dermatitis* 11:302, 1984.
20. Veien NK, Hattel T, Justesen O, Norholm A: Contact dermatitis in children. *Contact Dermatitis* 8:373, 1982.
21. Brandao FM, Faria A, Marques MS, et al: Allergic contact dermatitis in children: A multicenter study of the Portuguese Contact Dermatitis Group (GPEDC). *Contact Dermatitis* 26:112, 1992.
22. Kuiters GR, Smitt JH, Cohen EB, Bos JD: Allergic contact dermatitis in children and young adults. *Arch Dermatol* 125:1531, 1989.
23. Weston WL, Weston JA, Kinoshita J, et al: Prevalence of positive epicutaneous tests among infants, children, and adolescents. *Pediatrics* 78:1070, 1986.
24. Ho VC, Johnston MM: Nickel dermatitis in infants. *Contact Dermatitis* 15:270, 1986.
25. Rudzki E, Grzywa Z, Rebandel P: Patch testing in children. *Contact Dermatitis* 17:117, 1987.
26. Magnusson B, Moller H: Contact allergy without skin disease. *Acta Derm Venereol* 59 (Suppl 89):113, 1979.
27. Kraus SM, Muselinovic NZ: Pre-employment screening for contact dermatitis among the pupils of a metal industry school. *Contact Dermatitis* 24:342, 1991.
28. Rystedt I, Fischer T: Relationship between nickel and cobalt sensitization in hard metal workers. *Contact Dermatitis* 9:195, 1983.
29. Santucci B, Ferrari PV, Cristaudo A, et al: Nickel dermatitis from cheap earrings. *Contact Dermatitis* 21:245, 1989.
30. Cronin E: Contact dermatitis: 8. The significance of nickel sensitivity in women. *Br J Dermatol* 84:96, 1971.
31. Emmett EA, Risby TH, Jiang L, et al: Allergic contact dermatitis to nickel: Bioavailability from consumer products and provocation threshold. *J Am Acad Dermatol* 19:314, 1988.
32. Ayres S Jr, Mihan R: Wristwatch ringworm. *Arch Dermatol* 102:235, 1970.
33. Brandrup F, Larsen FS: Nickel dermatitis provoked by buttons in blue jeans. *Contact Dermatitis* 5:148, 1979.
34. Kvorning SA: Post-operative dermatitis following non-epidermal nickel contact. *Contact Dermatitis* 1:327, 1975.
35. Nurse DS: Nickel sensitivity induced by skin clips. *Contact Dermatitis* 6:497, 1980.
36. van Ketel WG, Liem DH: Eyelid dermatitis from nickel contaminated cosmetics. *Contact Dermatitis* 7:217, 1981.
37. Nethercott JR, Nield G, Holness DL: A review of 79 cases of eyelid dermatitis. *J Am Acad Dermatol* 21:223, 1989.
38. Roed-Petersen B, Roed-Petersen J, Jorgensen KD: Nickel allergy and osteomyelitis in a patient with metal osteosynthesis of a jaw fracture. *Contact Dermatitis* 5:108, 1979.
39. Kaaber S, Thulin H, Nielsen E: Skin sensitivity to denture base materials in the burning mouth syndrome. *Contact Dermatitis* 5:90, 1979.

40. van Loon LA, van Elsas PW, van Joost T, Davidson CL: Contact stomatitis and dermatitis to nickel and palladium. *Contact Dermatitis* 11:294, 1984.

41. Romaguera C, Vilaplana J, Grimalt F: Contact stomatitis from a dental prosthesis. *Contact Dermatitis* 21:204, 1989.

42. Spiechowicz E, Glantz PO, Axell T, Chmielewski W: Oral exposure to a nickel-containing dental alloy of persons with hypersensitive skin reactions to nickel. *Contact Dermatitis* 10:206, 1984.

43. Munro-Ashman D, Miller AJ: Rejection of metal to metal prosthesis and skin sensitivity to cobalt. *Contact Dermatitis* 2:65, 1976.

44. Grimalt F, Romaguera C: Acute nickel dermatitis from a metal implant. *Contact Dermatitis* 6:441, 1980.

45. Olveti E: Contact dermatitis from an acrylic-metal dental prosthesis. *Contact Dermatitis* 24:57, 1991.

46. Fernandez JP, Veron C, Hildebrand HF, Martin P: Nickel allergy to dental prostheses. *Contact Dermatitis* 14:312, 1986.

47. Temesvari E, Racz I: Nickel sensitivity from dental prosthesis. *Contact Dermatitis* 18:50, 1988.

48. Nater JP, Brain RG, Deutman R, Mulder TJ: The development of metal hypersensitivity in patients with metal-to-plastic hip arthroplasties. *Contact Dermatitis* 2:259, 1976.

49. Wilson AG, Gould DJ: Nickel dermatitis from a dental prosthesis without buccal involvement. *Contact Dermatitis* 21:53, 1989.

50. Waterman AH, Schrik JJ: Allergy in hip arthroplasty. *Contact Dermatitis* 13:294, 1985.

51. Veien NK, Christiansen AH, Svejgaard E, Kaaber K: Antibodies against nickel-albumin in rabbits and man. *Contact Dermatitis* 5:378, 1979.

52. Handfield-Jones S, Boyle J, Harman RR: Contact allergy caused by metal sprays. *Contact Dermatitis* 16:44, 1987.

53. Christensen OB, Moller H: Nickel allergy and hand eczema. *Contact Dermatitis* 1:129, 1975.

54. Burrows D: Is systemic nickel important (editorial)? *J Am Acad Dermatol* 26:632, 1992.

55. Roduner J, Haudenschild-Falb E, Kunz E, et al: Peroral nickel provocation in nondyshidrosiform and dyshidrosiform nickel eczema. *Hautarzt* 38:262, 1987.

55a. Möller H: Yes, systemic nickel is probably important. *J Am Acad Dermatol* 28:511, 1993.

56. Kaaber K, Sjolin KE, Menne T: Elbow eruptions in nickel and chromate dermatitis. *Contact Dermatitis* 9:213, 1983.

57. Andersen KE, Hjorth N, Menne T: The baboon syndrome: Systemically-induced allergic contact dermatitis. *Contact Dermatitis* 10:97, 1984.

58. Landwehr AJ, van Ketal WG: Pompholyx after implantation of a nickel-containing pacemaker in a nickel-allergic patient. *Contact Dermatitis* 9:147, 1983.

59. Tilsley DA, Rotstein H: Sensitivity caused by internal exposure to nickel, chrome and cobalt. *Contact Dermatitis* 6:175, 1980.

60. Hjorth N: Nickel vasculitis. *Contact Dermatitis* 2:356, 1976.

61. Cook LJ: Associated nickel and cobalt contact dermatitis presenting as erythema multiforme. *Contact Dermatitis* 8:280, 1982.

62. Fischer T, Rystedt I: False-positive, follicular and irritant patch test reactions to metal salts. *Contact Dermatitis* 12:93, 1985.

63. Schena D, Nigro MA: Allergic contact dermatitis from nickel with unusual localization. *Contact Dermatitis* 27:330, 1992.

64. Lombardi P, Campolmi P, Sertoli A: Lichenoid dermatitis caused by nickel salts? *Contact Dermatitis* 9:520, 1983.

65. Stransky L: Contact granuloma annulare. *Contact Dermatitis* 16:106, 1987.

66. Goh CL, Ng SK: Nickel dermatitis mimicking sycosis barbae. *Contact Dermatitis* 16:42, 1987.

67. Fransway AF, Winkelmann RK: Chronic dermatitis evolving to mycosis fungoides: Report of four cases and review of the literature. *Cutis* 41:330, 1988.

68. Estlander T, Kanerva L, Tupasela O, et al: Immediate and delayed allergy to nickel with contact urticaria, rhinitis, asthma and contact dermatitis. *Clin Exp Allergy* 23:306, 1993.

69. Theermann R, Wirth CJ: Shoulder stiffness and metal allergy—A possible link? A single case report (Ger). *Zeitschrift fur Orthopadie und Ihre Grenzgebiete* 127:65, 1989.

70. Kieffer M: Nickel sensitivity: Relationship between history and patch test reaction. *Contact Dermatitis* 5:398, 1979.

71. Kalimo K, Lammintausta K: 24 and 48 h allergen exposure in patch testing. Comparative study with 11 common contact allergens and NiCl$_2$. *Contact Dermatitis* 10:25, 1984.

72. Wall LM, Calnan CD: Occupational nickel dermatitis in the electroforming industry. *Contact Dermatitis* 6:414, 1980.
73. Vendenburg JJ, Epstein WL: Experimental nickel contact sensitization in man. *J Invest Dermatol* 41:413, 1963.
74. Lammintausta K, Maibach HI: Clinical concepts in nickel testing, in Maibach HI, Menne T (eds): *Nickel and the Skin: Immunology and Toxicology,* Boca Raton, FL, CRC Press, 1989, p 93.
75. Fisher AA: Problems attending patch testing for nickel sensitivity. *Cutis* 29:148, 157, 186, 1982.
76. Wahlberg JE: Immunoglobulin E, atopy, and nickel allergy. *Cutis* 18:715, 720, 1976.
77. Dooms-Goossens A, Naert C, Crispeels MT, Degreef H: Is a 5% nickel sulphate patch test concentration adequate? *Contact Dermatitis* 6:232, 1980.
78. Moller H, Svensson A: Metal sensitivity: Positive history but negative test indicates atopy. *Contact Dermatitis* 14:57, 1986.
79. Menne T: Nickel allergy reliability of patch test evaluated in female twins. *Dermatosen* 29:156, 1981.
80. Cronin E: *Contact S Dermatitis.* Edinburgh, Churchill Livingstone, 1980.
81. van Ketal WG: Patch testing with nickel sulfate in DMSO (letter). *Contact Dermatitis* 4:167, 1978.
82. Christensen OB, Wall LM: Open, closed and intradermal testing in nickel allergy. *Contact Dermatitis* 16:21, 1987.
83. Meneghini C, Angelini G: Intradermal test in contact allergy to metals. *Acta Derm Venereol Suppl* 59:123, 1979.
84. Moller H: Intradermal testing in doubtful cases of contact allergy to metals. *Contact Dermatitis* 20:120, 1989.
85. Goh CL, Kwok SF: The influence of temperature on the concentration homogeneity of patch test materials. *Contact Dermatitis* 15:231, 1986.
86. Allenby CF, Goodwin BF: Influence of detergent washing powders on minimal elicited patch test concentrations of nickel and chromium. *Contact Dermatitis* 9:491, 1983.
87. Fischer T, Maibach H: Recovery of nickel sulphate from a standard patch test. *Contact Dermatitis* 11:134, 1984.
88. Fischer T, Maibach H: Amount of nickel applied with a standard patch test. *Contact Dermatitis* 11:285, 1984.
89. Fisher AA: Metal dermatitis—Some questions and answers. *Cutis* 19:156, 164, 169, 1977.
90. Mendelow AY, Forsyth A, Florence AT, Baillie AJ: Patch testing for nickel allergy: The influence of the vehicle on the response rate to topical nickel sulphate. *Contact Dermatitis* 13:29, 1985.
91. Väänänen A, Hannuksela M: Softisan—A new vehicle for patch testing. *Contact Dermatitis* 14:215, 1986.
92. Bruze M: Patch testing with nickel sulphate under occlusion for five hours. *Acta Derm Venereol* 68:361, 1988.
93. Shehade SA, Beck MH, Hillier VF: Epidemiological survey of standard series patch test results and observations on day 2 and day 4 readings. *Contact Dermatitis* 24:119, 1991.
94. Uehara M, Takahashi C, Ofuji S: Pustular patch test reactions in atopic dermatitis. *Arch Dermatol* 111:1154, 1975.
95. Stone OJ, Johnson DA: Pustular patch test—experimentally induced. *Arch Dermatol* 95:618, 1967.
96. Wahlberg JE, Maibach HI: Sterile cutaneous pustules: A manifestation of primary irritancy? Identification of contact pustulogens. *J Invest Dermatol* 76:381, 1981.
97. Fischer T, Rystedt I: False-positive, follicular and irritant patch test reactions to metal salts. *Contact Dermatitis* 12:93, 1985.
98. Fischer T, Maibach H: Aluminium in Finn chambers reacts with cobalt and nickel salts in patch test materials. *Contact Dermatitis* 12:200, 1985.
99. Menne T, Brandup F, Thestrup-Pedersen K, et al: Patch test reactivity to nickel alloys. *Contact Dermatitis* 16:255, 1987.
100. McLelland J, Shuster S, Matthews JN: "Irritants" increase the response to an allergen in allergic contact dermatitis. *Arch Dermatol* 127:1016, 1991.
101. McLelland J, Lawrence CM: Premenstrual exacerbation of nickel allergy (letter). *Br J Dermatol* 125:83, 1991.
102. Silvennoinen-Kassinen S, Isotalo H, Jakkula H: Estradiol enhances nickel-induced blast transformation. *Contact Dermatitis* 11:260, 1984.
103. Hindsen M, Christensen OB: Delayed hypersensitivity reactions following allergic and irritant inflammation. *Acta Derm Venereol* 72:220, 1992.

104. Axell T, Spiechowicz E, Glantz PO, et al: A new method for intraoral patch testing. *Contact Dermatitis* 15:58, 1986.
105. van Joost T, van Everdingen JJ: Sensitization to cobalt associated with nickel allergy: Clinical and statistical studies. *Acta Derm Venereol* 62:525, 1982.
106. Karlberg AT, Boman A, Wahlberg JE: Copper—A rare sensitizer. *Contact Dermatitis* 9:134, 1983.
107. Eedy DJ, Burrows D, McMaster D: The nickel content of certain commercially available metallic patch test materials and its relevance in nickel-sensitive subjects. *Contact Dermatitis* 24:11, 1991.
108. Camarasa JG, Serra-Baldrich E, Lluch M, et al: Recent unexplained patch test reactions to palladium. *Contact Dermatitis* 20:388, 1989.
109. Todd DJ, Burrows D: Patch testing with pure palladium metal in patients with sensitivity to palladium chloride. *Contact Dermatitis* 26:327, 1992.
110. de Fine Olivarius F, Menne T: Contact dermatitis from metallic palladium in patients reacting to palladium chloride. *Contact Dermatitis* 27:71, 1992.
111. Camarasa JG, Burrows D, Menne T, et al: Palladium contact sensitivity. *Contact Dermatitis* 24:370, 1991.
112. Menne T: Relationship between cobalt and nickel sensitization in females. *Contact Dermatitis* 6:337, 1980.
113. Lammintausta K, Pitknen OP, Kalimo K, Jansen CT: Interrelationship of nickel and cobalt contact sensitization. *Contact Dermatitis* 13:148, 1985.
114. Cavelier C, Foussereau J, Gille P, Zissu D: Allergy to nickel or cobalt: Tolerance to nickel and cobalt samples in man and in the guinea pig allergic or sensitized to these metals. *Contact Dermatitis* 21:72, 1989.
115. Veien NK, Hattel T, Justesen O, Nørholm A: Dietary treatment of nickel dermatitis. *Acta Derm Venereol* 65:138, 1985.
116. Sjovall P, Christensen OB, Moller H: Oral hyposensitization in nickel allergy. *J Am Acad Dermatol* 17:774, 1987.
117. Santucci B, Cristaudo A, Cannistraci C, Picardo M: Nickel sensitivity: Effects of prolonged oral intake of the element. *Contact Dermatitis* 19:202, 1988.
118. Calnan CD, Bandmann HJ, Cronin E, et al: Hand dermatitis in housewives. *Br J Dermatol* 82:543, 1970.
119. Agrup G: Hand eczema. *Acta Derm Venereol* 49, *Suppl* 61, 1969.
120. Meding B: Epidemiology of hand eczema in an industrial city. *Acta Derm Venereol Suppl* 153:1, 1990.
121. Peltonen L: Nickel sensitivity in the general population. *Contact Dermatitis* 5:27, 1979.
122. Lantinga H, Nater JP, Coenraads PJ: Prevalence, incidence and course of eczema on the hands and forearms in a sample of the general population. *Contact Dermatitis* 10:135, 1984.
123. Menne T, Borgan O, Green A: Nickel allergy and hand dermatitis in a stratified sample of the Danish female population: An epidemiological study including a statistic appendix. *Acta Derm Venereol* 62:35, 1982.
124. Lammintausta K, Kalimo K, Aantaa S: Course of hand dermatitis in hospital workers. *Contact Dermatitis* 8:327, 1982.
125. Menne T, Holm NV: Hand eczema in nickel-sensitive female twins: Genetic predisposition and environmental factors. *Contact Dermatitis* 9:289, 1983.
126. McDonagh AJ, Wright AL, Cork MJ, Gawkrodger DJ: Nickel sensitivity: The influence of ear piercing and atopy. *Br J Dermatol* 126:16, 1992.
127. Lynde CW, Mitchell JC: Patch test results in 66 hairdressers 1973–81. *Contact Dermatitis* 8:302, 1982.
128. Dahlquist I, Fregert S, Gruvberger B: Release of nickel from plated utensils in permanent wave liquids. *Contact Dermatitis* 5:52, 1979.
129. Brandao FM: Release of nickel by permanent wave liquids, shown by the dimethylglyoxime test. *Contact Dermatitis* 5:406, 1979.
130. van der Burg CK, Bruynzeel DP, Vreeburg KJ, et al: Hand eczema in hairdressers and nurses: A prospective study. I. Evaluation of atopy and nickel hypersensitivity at the start of apprenticeship. *Contact Dermatitis* 14:275, 1986.
131. Fischer T: Occupational nickel dermatitis, in Maibach HI, Menne T (eds): *Nickel and the Skin: Immunology and Toxicology.* Boca Raton, FL, CRC Press, 1989, pp 117–132.
132. Fischer T, Fregert S, Gruvberger B, Rystedt I: Nickel release from ear piercing kits and earrings. *Contact Dermatitis* 10:39, 1984.
133. Fisher AA: Ear piercing and sensitivity to nickel and gold (letter). *J Am Acad Dermatol* 17:853, 1987.

134. Shore RN, Binnick S: Dimethylglyoxime stick test for easier detection of nickel. *Arch Dermatol* 113:1734, 1977.
135. Burrows D: The Prosser White oration 1988. Mischievous metals—chromate, cobalt, nickel and mercury. *Clin Exp Dermatol* 14:266, 1989.
136. Menne T, Andersen KE, Kaaber K, et al: Evaluation of dimethylglyoxime stick tests for detection of nickel. *Derm Beruf Umwelt* 35:128, 1987.
137. Fischer T, Fregert S, Gruvberger B, Rystedt I: Contact sensitivity to nickel in white gold. *Contact Dermatitis* 10:23, 1984.
138. Samitz MH, Katz SA: Nickel dermatitis hazards from prostheses: In vivo and in vitro solubilization studies. *Br J Dermatol* 92:287, 1975.
139. Menne T, Rasmussen K: Regulation of nickel exposure in Denmark. *Contact Dermatitis* 23:57, 1990.
140. Romaguera C, Grimalt F, Vilaplana J: Contact dermatitis from nickel: An investigation of its sources. *Contact Dermatitis* 19:52, 1988.
141. Moseley JC, Allen HJ Jr: Polyurethane coating in the prevention of nickel dermatitis. *Arch Dermatol* 103:58, 1971.
142. Wall LM: Nickel penetration through rubber gloves. *Contact Dermatitis* 6:461, 1980.
143. Jordan WP Jr, King SE: Nickel feeding in nickel-sensitive patients with hand eczema. *J Am Acad Dermatol* 1:506, 1979.
144. Burrows D, Creswell S, Merrett JD: Nickel, hands and hip prostheses. *Br J Dermatol* 105:437, 1981.
145. Veien NK, Hattel T, Justesen O, Norholm A: Oral challenge with nickel and cobalt in patients with positive patch tests to nickel and/or cobalt. *Acta Derm Venereol* 67:321, 1987.
146. Kaaber K, Menne T, Veien N, Hougaard P: Treatment of nickel dermatitis with Antabuse: a double blind study. *Contact Dermatitis* 9:297, 1983.
147. Christensen JD: Disulfiram treatment of three patients with nickel dermatitis. *Contact Dermatitis* 8:105, 1982.
148. Burrows D, Rogers S, Beck M, et al: Treatment of nickel dermatitis with Trientine. *Contact Dermatitis* 15:55, 1986.
149. Klein LR, Fowler JF Jr: Nickel dermatitis recall during disulfiram therapy for alcohol abuse. *J Am Acad Dermatol* 26:645, 1992.
150. Kaaber K, Menne T, Tjell JC, Veien N: Antabuse treatment of nickel dermatitis: Chelation—a new principle in the treatment of nickel dermatitis. *Contact Dermatitis* 5:221, 1979.
151. Menne T, Kaaber K: Treatment of pompholyx due to nickel allergy with chelating agents. *Contact Dermatitis* 4:289, 1978.
152. Fullerton A, Hoelgaard A: Binding of nickel to human epidermis in vitro. *Br J Dermatol* 119:675, 1988.
153. van Ketel WG, Bruynzeel DP: Chelating effect of EDTA on nickel. *Contact Dermatitis* 11:311, 1984.
154. van Ketel WG, Bruynzeel DP: The possible chelating effect of sodium diethyldithiocarbamate (DDC) in nickel allergic patients: Patch test procedures, with nickel on DDC pretreated skin. *Derm Beruf Umwelt* 30:198, 1982.
155. Nielsen GD, Jepsen LV, Jorgensen PJ, et al: Nickel-sensitive patients with vesicular hand eczema: Oral challenge with a diet naturally high in nickel. *Br J Dermatol* 122:299, 1990.
156. Veien NK, Kaaber K: Nickel, cobalt and chromium sensitivity in patients with pompholyx (dyshidrotic eczema). *Contact Dermatitis* 5:371, 1979.
157. Veien NK, Hattel T, Justesen O, Norholm A: Oral challenge with metal salts: I. Vesicular patch-test-negative hand eczema. *Contact Dermatitis* 9:402, 1983.
157a. Christensen OB, Moller H: External and internal exposure to the antigen in the hand eczema of nickel allergy. *Contact Dermatitis* 1:136, 1975.
158. Kaaber K, Veien NK, Tjell JC: Low nickel diet in the treatment of patients with chronic nickel dermatitis. *Br J Dermatol* 98:197, 1978.
159. Gawkrodger DJ, Cook SW, Fell GS, Hunter JA: Nickel dermatitis: The reaction to oral nickel challenge. *Br J Dermatol* 115:33, 1986.
160. Menne T, Mikkelsen HI, Solgaard P: Nickel excretion in urine after oral administration. *Contact Dermatitis* 4:106, 1978.
161. de Jongh GJ, Spruit D: Factors influencing nickel dermatitis, II. *Contact Dermatitis* 4:149, 1978.
162. Veien NK, Andersen MR: Nickel and Danish food. *Acta Derm Venereol* 66:502, 1986.
163. Andersen KE, Nielsen GD, Flyvholm MA, et al: Nickel in tap water. *Contact Dermatitis* 9:140, 1983.
164. Gammelgaard B, Andersen JR: Nickel in tap water. *Contact Dermatitis* 12:123, 1985.

165. Brun R, Nickel in food: the role of stainless-steel utensils. *Contact Dermatitis* 5:43, 1979.

166. Katz SA, Samitz MH: Leaching of nickel from stainless steel consumer commodities. *Acta Derm Venereol* 55:113, 1975.

167. Christensen OB, Moller H: Release of nickel from cooking utensils. *Contact Dermatitis* 4:343, 1978.

168. Spruit D: Increased nickel absorption following indomethacin therapy. *Contact Dermatitis* 5:62, 1979.

169. Christensen OB: Effect on growth and nickel content of cabbage plants watered with nickel solutions. *Contact Dermatitis* 5:239, 1979.

170. Lee AY, Lee YS: A case of allergic contact dermatitis due to nickel in underground water. *Contact Dermatitis* 22:141, 1990.

171. Pigatto PD, Gibelli E, Fumagalli M, et al: Disodium cromoglycate versus diet in the treatment and prevention of nickel-positive pompholyx (see comments). *Contact Dermatitis* 22:27, 1990.

172. Romaguera C, Grimalt F: Nickel dermatitis from acupuncture needles. *Contact Dermatitis* 5:195, 1979.

173. Romaguera C, Grimalt F: Contact dermatitis from a permanent acupuncture needle. *Contact Dermatitis* 7:156, 1981.

174. Fisher AA: Nickel—the ubiquitous contact allergen, in Fisher AA (ed): *Contact Dermatitis*. Philadelphia, Lea & Febiger, 1986, pp 745–761.

175. Zanca A, Nigro M, Luciani P, et al: The release of nickel from blackboard chalk may cause contact dermatitis. *Contact Dermatitis* 19:143, 1988.

176. Raith L, Jaeger K: The nickel content of chalk—cause of contact dermatitis? *Contact Dermatitis* 14:61, 1986.

177. Dahlquist I: "Nickel itch" from a blow-dry hair brush. *Contact Dermatitis* 8:217, 1982.

178. Fisher AA: Nickel dermatitis in children. *Cutis* 47:19, 1991.

179. Lee HS, Goh CL: Occupational dermatosis among chrome platers. *Contact Dermatitis* 18:89, 1988.

180. Lacroix J, Morin CL, Colin PP: Nickel dermatitis from a foreign body in the stomach. *J Pediatr* 95:428, 1979.

181. Vilaplana J, Romaguera C, Grimalt F: Contact dermatitis from nickel and cobalt in a contact lens cleaning solution. *Contact Dermatitis* 24:232, 1991.

182. Lachapelle JM, Tennstedt D: An anatomo-clinical study of delayed skin allergic reactions to nickel following intradermal injections of lidocaine with a Dermo-jet. *Contact Dermatitis* 8:193, 1982.

183. Fernandez de Corres L, Garrastazu MT, Soloeta R, Escayol P: Nickel contact dermatitis in a blood bank. *Contact Dermatitis* 8:32, 1982.

184. Lachapelle JM, Tennstedt D, Lauwerys R, et al: Release of nickel into fluid stored in the reservoir of Dermo-Jets. *Contact Dermatitis* 8:122, 1982.

185. Fisher AA: Dermatologic hazards of electrocardiography. *Cutis* 20:686, 1977.

186. Trevisan G, Kokelj F: Allergic contact dermatitis from nickel in an electrocautery plate. *Contact Dermatitis* 26:267, 1992.

187. Zemba C, Romaguera C, Vilaplana J: Allergic contact dermatitis from nickel in an eye pencil. *Contact Dermatitis* 27:116, 1992.

188. Romaguera C, Grimalt F: Dermatitis from nickel eyelash curler. *Contact Dermatitis* 12:174, 1985.

189. Drandrup F: Nickel eyelid dermatitis from an eyelash curler. *Contact Dermatitis* 25:77, 1991.

190. Goh CL, Ng SK, Kwok SF: Allergic contact dermatitis from nickel in eyeshadow. *Contact Dermatitis* 20:380, 1989.

191. van Ketel WG: Occupational contact with coins in nickel-allergic patients. *Contact Dermatitis* 12:108, 1985.

192. Pecegueiro M: Contact dermatitis due to nickel in fertilizers. *Contact Dermatitis* 22:114, 1990.

193. Gammelgaard B, Veien NK: Nickel in nails, hair and plasma from nickel-hypersensitive women. *Acta Derm Venereol* 70:417, 1990.

194. Nebenfuhrer L, Kohanka V, Vincze E, et al: Sources of nickel allergy in Budapest. *Contact Dermatitis* 10:116, 1984.

195. Marshman G, Kennedy CT: Guitar-string dermatitis. *Contact Dermatitis* 26:134, 1992.

196. Krushell JS, Burnett JW: Nickel dermatitis. *Cutis* 45:87, 1990.

197. Olerud JE, Lee MY, Uvelli DA, et al: Presumptive nickel dermatitis from hemodialysis. *Arch Dermatol* 120:1066, 1984.

198. Carlsson A, Moller H: Implantation of orthopaedic devices in patients with metal allergy. *Acta Derm Venereol* 69:62, 1989.

199. Cavelier C, Foussereau J, Massin M: Nickel allergy: Analysis of metal clothing objects and patch testing to metal samples. *Contact Dermatitis* 12:65, 1985.

200. Mitchell JC: The skin and chemical additives to foods. *Arch Dermatol* 104:329, 1971.
201. Romaguera C, Grimalt F, Vilaplana J: Nickel dermatitis from an infusion needle. *Contact Dermatitis* 12:181, 1985.
202. Fisher AA:P The dimethylglyoxime test in the prevention and management of nickel dermatitis. *Cutis* 46:467, 1990.
203. Karlberg AT, Liden C, Ehrin E: Colophony in mascara as a cause of eyelid dermatitis: Chemical analyses and patch testing. *Acta Derm Venereol* 71:445, 1991.
204. Vrignaud S, Gross GB, Wiesel M: Contact dermatitis caused by a peripheral intravenous catheter with metallic connector. *Ann Fr Anesth Reanim* 10:475, 1991.
205. Olumide Y: Contact dermatitis in Nigeria: I. Hand dermatitis in women. *Contact Dermatitis* 17:85, 1987.
206. Mathur AK: Occupational dermatitis and absorption in a metal plater. *Contact Dermatitis* 9:530, 1983.
207. Samitz MH, Katz SA: Skin hazards from nickel and chromium salts in association with cutting oil operations. *Contact Dermatitis* 1:158, 1975.
208. Hegyi E, Gasparik J: The nickel content of metallic threads in an Indian shawl. *Contact Dermatitis* 21:107, 1989.
209. Hegyi E, Gasparik J: The nickel content of moulded bricks as building material. *Contact Dermatitis* 21:63, 1989.
210. Fernandez de Corres L, Bernaola G, Munoz D, et al: The innumerable sources of nickel. *Contact Dermatitis* 19:386, 1988.
211. Burden DJ, Eedy DJ: Orthodontic headgear related to allergic contact dermatitis: A case report. *Br Dent J* 170:447, 1991.
212. Bass JK, Fine H, Cisneros GJ: Nickel hypersensitivity in the orthodontic patient. *Am J Orthodont Dentofac Orthop* 103:280, 1993.
213. Wahlberg JE, Boman AS: Cross-reactivity to palladium and nickel studied in the guinea pig. *Acta Derm Venereol* 72:95, 1992.
214. Bannar-Martin BR, Rycroft RJ: Nickel dermatitis from a powder paint. *Contact Dermatitis* 22:50, 1990.
215. Grimalt F, Romaguera C: Nickel allergy and spectacle frame contact acne. *Contact Dermatitis* 4:377, 1978.
216. Sun CC: Allergic contact dermatitis of the face from contact with nickel and ammoniated mercury in spectacle frames and skin-lightening creams. *Contact Dermatitis* 17:306, 1987.
217. Dawber R, Sonnex T: Nickel dermatitis due to steel fibre and soap cleaning pads. *Contact Dermatitis* 8:342, 1982.
218. Bischof RO: Stethoscope dermatitis: An unusual presentation. *Cutis* 51:244, 1993.
219. Fisher AA: Dermatitis associated with transcutaneous electrical nerve stimulation. *Cutis* 21:24, 33, 47, 1978.
220. Widstrom L, Bergstrom B, Wennerholm C: Nickel allergy and wrist strap to dissipate static electricity. *Contact Dermatitis* 15:299, 1986.
221. Veien NK, Hattel T, Laurberg G: Low nickel diet: An open, prospective trial. *J Am Acad Dermatol* 29:1002, 1993.

SPECIAL CATEGORIES
IN CONTACT DERMATITIS
AND ECZEMA

30

CLOTHING

Tuula Estlander
Riitta Jolanki
Lasse Kanerva

Clothing is an essential part of everyday life. Clothes also reflect something about their wearer—for instance, the wearer's age, occupation, and attitude to fashion. Clothing includes, in addition to the different garments, also shoes, boots, and accessories such as stockings, gloves, hats, and belts. Innumerable materials are used in the manufacture of wearing apparel, but the most important of these are textiles, leather, rubber, plastic, and fur. Additional materials such as metals and wood may be used in zippers, buttons, and decorations.

Although most people are able to use their wearing apparel without any problems, skin disorders are connected with almost every material used. Apart from the materials themselves, chemical contamination of the materials may also be responsible for the symptoms attributed to the clothing.

An estimation of the actual frequency of clothing dermatitis among the general population is a difficult task. No epidemiologic data are available to allow determination of the proportion of this type of dermatoses. Nevertheless, skin disorders caused by wearing apparel can be considered to be relatively rare when the vast production of clothing is borne in mind. Most reports on dermatoses due to clothing usually describe sporadic cases or minor epidemics only.[1-8]

Recent reports[7-10] and everyday clinical practice, however, suggest that the occurrence of clothing-induced dermatoses might be underestimated and that the possibility of this type of dermatitis should be kept in mind.

TYPES OF SKIN DISORDERS AND THEIR MECHANISMS OF DEVELOPMENT

Clothing can evoke both skin sensitization and irritation which may appear as contact dermatoses, commonly as contact dermatitis (eczema), seldom as contact urticaria.[1,4] Irritant dermatoses are probably more common than allergic ones. Allergic disorders are, however, more important. Allergy, once developed, is a permanent state of the organism, and dermatitis recurs when the contact with the specific sensitizer is renewed. Special types of contact dermatoses such as pigmented, pigmented purpuric, or purpuric eruptions[11–17] and phototoxic dermatitis[18] may also occur, but they are rarities.

Allergic contact eczema develops as a result of an immunologic delayed (type IV) allergic reaction to different materials, usually to chemicals which have come into contact with the skin (Figs. 30-1 to 30-9). Skin patch testing is the specific method by which the causative agent of allergic contact eczema can most reliably be detected (Fig. 30-10) and thus distinguished from irritant contact eczema.[1,19–23]

Contact urticaria may also be developed by immunologic and nonimmunologic mechanisms.[23,24] Allergic contact urticaria is a result of an immediate (type I) allergic reaction. The symptoms appear quickly, generally within 5 to 30 min after the skin has come into contact with the causative agents—usually plant or animal proteins, sometimes chemical compounds. The causative agent can be found by using skin tests developed to detect type I allergy, usually prick or scratch tests and blood investigations,in order to show specific immunoglobulin E (IgE) antibodies to the suspected agents.[23–28] Sometimes skin challenges are done with the suspected agents—e.g., with natural rubber latex (NRL) gloves[25,27,27a,28]—as well as use tests with suspected garments.[7]

CAUSATIVE AGENTS OF DERMATOSES

Unfinished and undyed natural or synthetic textile, leather, and fur materials do not in practice induce contact sensitization (type IV allergy),[1,4,29] but allergic contact urticaria (type I allergy) caused by NRL[25] and some other natural materials is well known.[1,4,29] Delayed-type allergic skin sensitization is usually caused by textiles, leather, and fur, treated both chemically and mechanically,[1–10,30] and ready-made rubber[1,4,23,27,31–38] and sometimes plastic articles.[1,4,23,33,37]

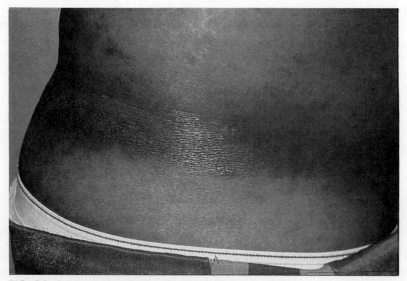

FIG. 30–1. Waistband dermatitis from the waistband of underwear.

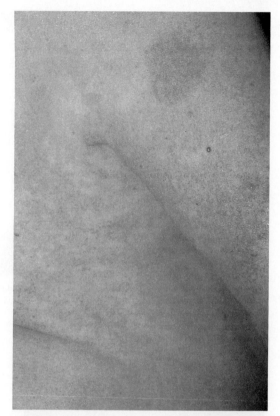

FIG. 30-2. Contact dermatitis to clothing contaminated with nitrogen mustard ointment. Prominent contact dermatitis can be seen over a treated plaque of cutaneous T-cell lymphoma (CTCL) as well as where contaminated clothing came into contact with the skin.

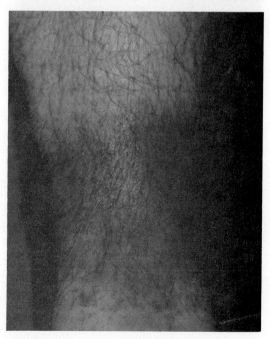

FIG. 30-3. Contact dermatitis to a sock. Patch test was positive to the area of the sock matching the eczema.

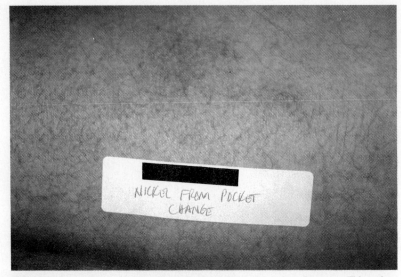

FIG. 30–4. Contact dermatitis to nickel contaminating the pocket of trousers. This patient also reacted to his shirt collar, which was contaminated with nickel from his steam iron.

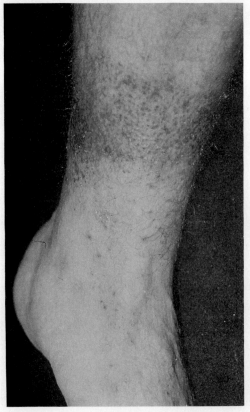

FIG. 30–5. Thiourea allergy from diethylthiourea in a wet suit. This patient tolerated a wet suit free of thioureas.

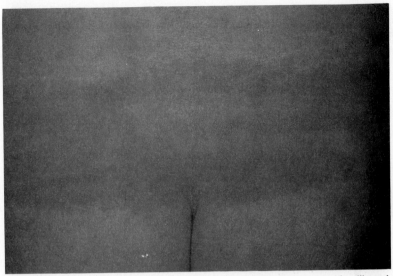

FIG. 30–6. Bleached rubber syndrome. All rubber tests were negative except zinc dibenzyl-dithiocarbamate treated with a chlorine bleach.

PREDISPOSING FACTORS AND THE SITES OF THE DERMATOSES

All factors which promote the release of chemicals from clothing into the skin—as well as factors which are able to damage the skin, making it more vulnerable to external contactants—also promote the development of clothing dermatitis. These factors include sweating, friction, pressure, shaving of armpits, use of depilatory agents and deodorants,[1,4] and wet, tight, poorly fitting clothes, gloves, and shoes.

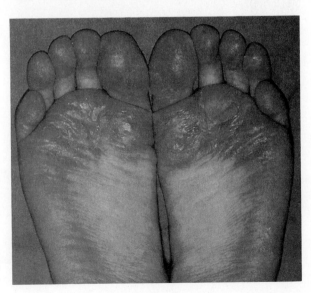

FIG. 30–7. Contact to the insoles of athletic shoes.

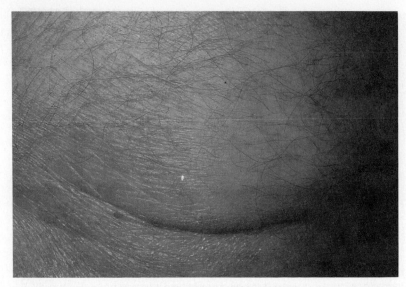

FIG. 30–8. Reaction to a formaldehyde-releasing textile finish in a formaldehyde-allergic patient. The area involved has more pressure from clothing than nearby uninvolved skin.

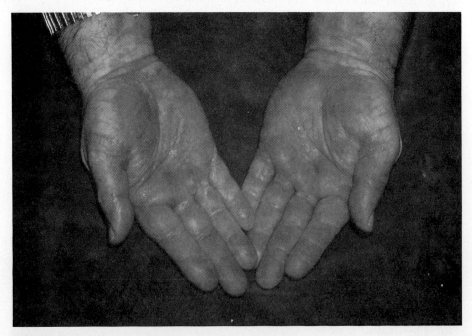

FIG. 30–9. Allergic contact dermatitis to work gloves.

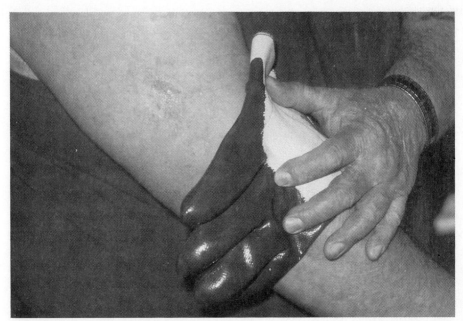

FIG. 30–10. Causative gloves and positive patch test.

Clothing dermatitis is usually distributed over the skin surface where the offending garment is in close contact with the skin; e.g., axillary borders, neck, and antecubital fossae and waist. Hands and arms are the sites of glove dermatitis, and the dorsa of the feet and legs are the sites of shoe and boot dermatitis as well as the sites of dermatitis caused by stockings and socks. Popliteal fossae, as well as inner and dorsal aspects of thighs, are sites of the dermatitis caused by pantyhose or tights. The hands and face are often affected in all types of clothing dermatoses. They are the most common sites of occupationally induced textile dermatitis. The dermatitis may also have been distributed in a less striking manner over different parts of the body, mimicking endogenous dermatoses such as seborrheic dermatitis, atopic dermatitis, or neurodermatitis.[1,4,7]

The outer appearance of the dermatitis may also differ from that of typical eczematous eruptions and appear as persistent erythematous wheal-type or transient urticarial lesions or an eruption resembling erythema multiforme.[9] Sometimes diffuse itching of the affected skin areas is the only sign of a textile-dependent skin disorder.[1,9]

CAUSES OF ALLERGIC CONTACT ECZEMA

TEXTILES

The chief sensitizers in textiles are colorants and their intermediates, sometimes mordants; chemical finishes, especially durable-press finishes; and sometimes flame retardants.[1–10,27,39–41] Formaldehyde is an important allergen in durable-press finishes and flame retardants.[1,3,4,7,27,40,41] Formaldehyde can also be present in some resin binders[42,43] used in the pigment printing of fabrics and in fabric softeners.[4,44] Colophony (rosin) and lanolin alcohols, used in the finishing of some materials, and antistatic agents may also sensitize.[4,10,39] The other potential causes include rubber in some elastic parts of garments (underwear, swimwear, bandages), phenolformaldehyde and *p-tert*-butylphenolformaldehyde resins used in the waterproofing of some materials, antimicrobials, spot removers,[1,4,7,10,39] and epoxy resin in some glues[4] and in the print of textile labels.[45] Nickel in zippers and decorations may also be the cause of textile dermatitis.[9,10,38]

DYES

Most of the dyes and pigments produced in the world are used for the dyeing of textiles, leather, and furs. The dyes and pigments can be classified in many ways. For example, a colorant may take its name from the method by which it is applied to the fibers (e.g., disperse, reactive, acid, vat, azoic, or oxidation base dyes) or a colorant may be named according to its chemical structure (e.g., azo and anthraquinone dyes). Disperse and reactive dyes belong to the most widely used textile dyes. Disperse dyes have been in use since 1920. Reactive dyes are among the newest ones. The first reactive dyes were developed in the late 1950s. Azoic (naphthol) dyes are among the oldest dyes. They have been used since the late 1800s but are not much used today, at least in industrialized countries.[46-51]

Usually the dyeing of textiles is carried out in water solutions, and the dye molecules attach themselves to the fibers by adsorption, but reactive dyes react with the textile fibers, forming permanent covalent bonds with the fibers. Pigments must be fixed in the fibers with a resin binder. They are used in the printing of textiles. Also other dyes (e.g., disperse dyes and reactive dyes) can be used in the printing of textiles.[1,4,42,43,46,52]

The dyes (the methods of application) are chosen according to the types of fibers used. Dyes of different composition are required to color materials made of different fibers. Disperse dyes are used to dye synthetic or semisynthetic materials. They are water-insoluble dyes which, during the dyeing process, are dissolved in the fibers from a water solution containing a dispersing agent. Vat dyes are water-soluble dyes and are used to color natural fibers. They are applied to the fiber in colorless form, and the final color is produced by oxidation of the dye. Acid dyes and reactive dyes are suitable for dyeing both synthetic and natural fibers. They can also be used to dye leather. In accordance with their names, acid dyes are normally applied from dye solutions containing some acid (e.g., sulfuric, formic, or acetic). Oxidation-base dyes and azoic dyes belong to developed dyes, which means that the final color is produced ("developed") often in two stages in the fiber. Oxidation-base dyes are used to dye mainly furs and for the permanent dyeing of hair. Each of these dye groups may contain dyes of different chemical constitution. For instance disperse dyes may contain azo, anthraquinone, nitro, methine, and quinoline dyes.[1,2,4,5,30,43,46]

The dyes manufactured for commercial use are classified according to their type of application (e.g., Disperse Orange 3, Disperse Blue 124), and they have various trade names.[39,46,47] They usually contain one or more dye compounds, by-products, impurities, and auxiliary substances.[48-52] When a certain commercial dye is in question, the best information on its properties is usually obtained from *The Colour Index,* a large reference book published by the American Association of Textile Chemists and Colorists and the British Society of Dyers and Colourists. The *Index* lists, for example, the colour index (CI) name, chemical class, colour index constitution number (CI no.) if the chemical structure of the dye has been given to the Index, commercial names, and hue of the dye. Unfortunately all textile dyes are not given in the *Index,* and some of the dyes included are no longer in commercial use.

A dyed fabric contains about 2 percent dyes, but the color of a dyed fabric does not give much information about the dyes used. For instance in a blue fabric, the sensitizing dye may be yellow or brown. The development of sensitization depends partly on the method of the dye application and partly on the chemical structure of the dye to be applied to the fiber. A dyed fabric may provoke sensitization when the surplus dye or a starting compound of the dye is retained in the fabric, when a dye is not completely fixed in the fiber, or when the fabric contains a strong sensitizer. Sensitization is in practice caused by organic synthetic dyes which are directly attached to the fibers. Pigments which have no affinity to the fibers are only occasional sensitizers.[1,2,4,5,30]

Most cases of allergic clothing dye dermatitis have been elicited by wearing stockings and other dyed garments.[1,2,4,5,7-10] Occupational cases occur only sporadically and are due to the handling of dyed textiles or the wearing of dyed work or protective clothing without undergarments.[1,4,9,10,30,53]

Disperse dyes of azo and anthraquinone dye classes are the most common sensitizers:

Disperse Blue 35. CAS number 12222–75–2

anthraquinone dye

Disperse Orange 3. CAS number 730–40–5

azo dye

Disperse dyes used to color synthetic or semisynthetic fibers are not always fast fixable in the fibers.[1,2,5,30] Thus sensitizing garments often bleed during sweating and the washing of the garment.

Azoic or naphthol dyes:

Naphthol AS. CAS number 92–77–3

azoic or naphthol dye

have also induced some cases of clothing dermatitis. They are used in the dyeing of cotton. The method is used especially in the developing countries. The dyeing process takes place in two stages by which the desired color is developed in the fiber using two dye components, a diazonium compound and a naphthol coupling compound. Both of these can sensitize, but the reported cases have been due to naphthol compounds.[12,14,16,30,53] The colorfastness of the dyes (dyed materials neither stain the skin nor easily bleed during washings) is rather good, but residual free dye has been demonstrated in the sensitizing dyed fabrics.[53]

Sensitizers may also be present in other dye groups used to dye textiles (e.g., fabrics dyed with vat dyes and acid dyes have caused allergic contact eczema).[30,54] Some new nondisperse dyes taken into use in the textile industry have also been shown to be sensitizers.[55]

Reactive dyes are an exception where dyed textiles are concerned. Allergic (type IV) sensitization has occurred only in the dyeing of textiles when the dyes have been handled as such.[30,43,52,56] Fabrics dyed with reactive dyes are probably safe to the consumer as far as causing allergy. Because reactive dyes form covalent bonds with cellulose, protein, or synthetic fibers, the dyes are fixed firmly in the fibers assuming that the dyeing process is not faulty and the fibers are of good quality.[30,52]

Among workers in textile dyeing plants and dye factories, however, severe type I allergy symptoms (asthma, rhinitis, urticaria, contact urticaria) connected with the exposure to reactive dyes are even more important than type IV allergic contact eczema.[57-61] Even a lethal case of asthma has been reported from occupational exposure to reactive dyes.[58] Those sensitized to reactive dyes often have both respiratory and skin symptoms.[52,56-61]

It should also be remembered that sometimes a dye is transformed into a sensitizer as a result of finishing processes. Phosgene (2,5-dichlorophenyl)hydrazones, new sensitizers among textile dyes, were found to be formed only when a fabric dyed with certain azoic dyes had been bleached with sodium hypochlorite solution.[62,63] Another example is a disperse stocking dye which caused an allergic skin reaction only after the stocking had been handled with a special finish which is a lanolin emulsion, the emulsifying agent being a cationic substance.[64]

In addition to dyes themselves, chromium, which can be a constituent in some metal complex dyes or used to fix the dye in the fiber or used as a mordant before dyeing, has been described as the cause of dermatitis evoked by dyed textiles.[10,65-67]

FINISHES

The finishing agents of textiles are other sources of allergy due to clothing. Most cases of allergic eczema have been elicited by formaldehyde-based finishing resins (Fig. 30-8), but acrylates are also among potential allergens, as well as flame retardants, amtimicrobials, and antistatic agents.[1,3,4,7,40,41,68,69]

The purpose of durable-press finishes is to make textiles crease-resistant, unshrinkable, colorfast, water-repellent, and/or flame retardant. The finishing resins based on formaldehyde are formed in the interstices of textile fibers when formaldehyde reacts with substances such as ureas, melamines, methylol carbamates, and triazons.[3] Free unreacted formaldehyde, or formaldehyde formed when a resin has decomposed due to hydrolysis, or the resin or reactant itself, have been responsible for dermatoses.[1,3,4,7,27,40,41,68,69]

Between the 1950s and the 1970s, urea and melamine formaldehyde resins were the most common causes of dermatoses due to resin-finished textiles; mostly formaldehyde has been the actual sensitizer.[1,4] Dermatitis has been evoked by garments made of cotton or cotton blends worn every day and also by sheets.[1,3,4,40,41,69,70] Occasional occupational sensitization has occurred due to the wearing of work clothes and sewing or cutting of finished fabrics.[27]

The amount of free formaldehyde in the causative textiles has been as much as 12,000 mg/kg. By the beginning of the 1980s, the development of better N-methylol compounds led to a decrease in the release of formaldehyde from textiles. When dimethyloldihydroxyethyleneurea (DMDHEU) is used, the amount of formaldehyde is between 1500 and 2000 mg/kg; when methylated DMDHEU is used, the amount is 250 to 500 mg/kg.[3] It has also been estimated that 750 mg/kg or more[71] is required before sensitization develops, but those already sensitized to formaldehyde may get skin symptoms even when the amount is less than 750 mg/kg. A reduction in the formaldehyde content has also been suggested to cause a reduction in the allergy to formaldehyde.[72]

The release of formaldehyde from textiles decreases with the number of home launderings, usually with alkaline washing agents. But in some cases formaldehyde release can be even greater from washed than from unwashed finished textiles. Changes in the fabric pH during laundering are suggested to be a reason for the increase in the release of formaldehyde. Other factors affecting the increased release of formaldehyde include elevated temperature and high relative humidity. On the other hand, the use of washing agents containing chlorine bleaches can prevent the release of formaldehyde. Then the content of formaldehyde in the textiles does not decrease as compared with washings with chlorine-free washing agents.[3]

Formaldehyde may also be a sensitizer in resin binders necessary in the printing of textiles with dyes and pigments.[42,43] It can also be contained as a preservative in fabric softeners used as after-wash products.[4,44] Flame retardants are other sources of formaldehyde and formaldehyde resins.[4] For instance, Pyrovatex CP and Propan, both durable flame retardants, may also release formaldehyde.

Dicyandiamid is a new potential sensitizer among flame retardants. A case of allergic dermatitis from the chemical has been described in the factory manufacturing flame retardants.[73]

LEATHER AND FURS

Dermatitis caused by leather and furs is far less common than dermatitis due to textile materials. Chromium compounds used in the tanning process, shoe and leather glues, and dyes are the most important contact allergens. The causative articles include leather shoes and boots, gloves, garments used without underwear, belts and watch straps, as well as furs and fur products. Occupational sensitization caused by chromium or occasionally by colorants usually occurs due to the wearing of chrome tanned or dyed leather gloves. Experiments done with materials of leather gloves, using synthetic[74] and human sweat, have shown that chromium is released into sweat in amounts sufficient

TABLE 30-1. Chromium Content of Industrial Leather Gloves Determined by Atomic Absorption Spectrophotometry

Number of glove samples	Total Cr, μg/g	Cr measured sweat, μg/g	Percent of total Cr
8[a]	11,000–18,000	250–1,800, human, pH 6.5	2–13
7[b]	11,000–36,000	100–1,300, synthetic, pH 6.5	

[a]Jolanki R, Institute of Occupational Health, Helsinki, Finland, 1982 (unpublished).
[b]Fregert S, Gruvberger B: *Contact Dermatitis* 5:189, 1979.

to induce sensitization (Table 30-1). Chromium compounds, glues, and dyes present in military boots, safety boots, and shoes may also be the cause of occupationally induced sensitization.[1,4,30,38,75–81]

SHOE LEATHER

Chromium compounds are most commonly used in tanning (95 percent), but formaldehyde and glutaraldehyde are also used in tanning processes and may be sensitizers in the corresponding materials. Other alternative tanning processes include vegetable tanning with plant or fruit extracts and synthetic tanning using many chemical agents. After tanning, the leather is processed with fat liquoring (e.g., using sulfonated or cod liver oil or synthetic fish oil), then dyed, and finally handled with a leather finish. Fat liquoring and finishing chemicals contain antimicrobials (e.g., *N*-octyl-4-isothiazolin-3-one, 1,2-benzisothiazolin-3-one, and 2-thiocyanomethyl benzothiazole). Shoe insoles may be made of vegetable-tanned leather, rubber, or polyurethane. In addition, insoles can be prepared of wood or leather fibers suspended in emulsions of different rubber resins, which also contain antimicrobials. Shoe uppers, especially in athletic shoes,[81] can also be made of textile materials containing rubber and polyurethane (see also Chaps. 17 and 31).

SHOE ADHESIVES

Shoe adhesives include hot melted materials (e.g., polymers of ethyl vinyl acetate, polyamides, polyesters), urethane, neoprene, and NRL. They may contain many allergenic additives including synthetic resins such as *p*-tertiary butylphenolformaldehyde resins, phenolformaldehyde resins, epoxy resins, acrylic resins, and rubber additives (e.g., dodecyl mercaptane, thiurams, and mercaptobenzothiazole), and antimicrobials. Heel and toe counters made of polyester or cotton materials may also be impregnated with synthetic resins.[81]

DYES

Dye dermatitis induced by leather and fur dyes is fairly uncommon. Only a few reports have been published. Information available on the constitution of sensitizing leather dyes is scarce. Only in one case caused by safety boots[82] has the actual sensitizer, an azo dye, been determined, but it is probable that azo dyes more generally are responsible for leather dye dermatitis.[27] Dermatitis due to fur dyes has been reported from black-dyed furs, namely mink and fox furs. p-Phenylenediamine, a black dye also used as a permanent hair dye, has been the sensitizer. Both occupational cases due to the making of fur products and nonoccupational cases due to the wearing of dyed furs have been published.[1,4,30] Rhinitis and asthma have also been connected with the handling of dyed furs by fur workers.[1,30]

RUBBER

Rubber products are prepared from natural rubber latex (NRL) or synthetic rubber polymers to which many chemicals are added during the manufacturing process.[1,25,27,32] Rubber can cause allergic contact eczema (type IV allergy) both during the manufacturing process and in the form of completely cured (vulcanized) products. Simultaneous immediate (type I) allergy may occur with delayed allergy to rubber (see discussion of contact urticaria below). Additives, especially accelerators and antioxidants, are the chief allergens (type IV allergy) found in rubber materials. These additives do not become structural components of the rubber substance and can be present in a relatively free state in the material. The thiuram group, the mercaptobenzothiazole group, the carbamates, the guanidine group, and the thioureas contain the most important allergenic accelerators.[1,23,31–37,84,85] The first three groups of accelerators contain the most common allergens for those who have become sensitized from the use of rubber gloves.[31–37] Sensitization to thioureas has been reported from contact with insoles of athletic shoes (ethylbutyl thiourea)[85] and wet suits (diethylthiourea)[86] (Fig. 30-5), as well as from the use of neoprene gloves (diphenylthiourea).[87] Amines, which are p-phenylenediamine derivatives are examples of sensitizing antioxidants.[1,23,32] Other antioxidants [e.g., 4,4'-thiobis(6-*tert*-butyl-*meta*-cresol)] and butylhydroxyanisole have also been shown to be sensitizers in rubber gloves.[88] Nonallergenic additives may also become sensitizers after having been transformed by chemicals which have come into contact with rubber.[32]

Rubber gloves have long been an important cause of allergic contact eczema (type IV allergy) caused by rubber. They are also the most important cause of occupationally derived rubber eczema.[27,31,34–37] For instance, in Finland, about 60 percent of all occupationally derived cases of rubber eczema are induced by protective gloves made of rubber.[27] Dermatitis from rubberized gloves is shown in Fig. 30-9.

Recently some compounds in glove dusting powder, such as antimicrobials, have been suggested as potential causes of rubber glove dermatitis.[34,35]

Rubber boots are another source of both occupational and nonoccupational rubber eczema.[32,79] Rubber soles and stiffeners in shoes and boots made of materials other than rubber may also be responsible for allergic rubber eczema (see also Chaps. 31 and 34). Wet suits worn by divers and wind-surfers as well as rubber bands and other elastic parts containing rubber in undergarments (Figs. 30-1 and 30-6) and swimming suits can also evoke allergy to rubber. Rubber shoulder pads and dress shields can also be sources of rubber allergy.[4,32,38,79,81,84–86]

PLASTICS

Completely cured plastic materials are not generally considered to be sensitizers. Plasticizers, stabilizers, UV absorbers, antimicrobials, flame retardants, and colorants are additives and potential contact allergens in plastics.[1,23] The reported cases are scarce and for the most part due to the wearing of gloves and boots made of polyvinyl chloride (PVC). The actual sensitizer has usually remained undetermined, but a specific colorant[89] and some plasticizers[90] have been responsible for the reported cases caused by protective gloves and plastic fabrics.[1,4,37,91] Footwear can also be considered a potential cause of allergic contact dermatitis due to plastic materials. A case induced by bisphenol A in the plastic material of footwear has been reported.[83] Diaminodiphenylmethane may also be a potential allergen in shoe uppers containing polyurethane foam.[1,81]

NICKEL

Nickel can sensitize both in metal form and as a soluble compound. It is the most common cause of delayed-type allergy among women. At least 10 percent of women are allergic to nickel.[92,93] Nickel-plated metal objects and metal parts containing nickel used in clothing and accessories can induce allergy to nickel and cause eczema in sensitized individuals. Dermatitis typically occurs at the sites of contact with buttons, zippers, clips, clasps, jeans studs, and buckles.[1,4,38] Metal objects carried in the pockets of trousers may also be the cause of nickel dermatitis. Jeans buttons used in overalls, removable buttons with metal fasteners used in some work clothes, and buckles in "health" sandals may be responsible for occupational dermatitis due to nickel.

CAUSES OF IRRITANT CONTACT ECZEMA

Irritation is another mechanism by which clothing dermatitis can develop. Coarse wool and synthetic fibers are often responsible, especially when the skin is dry (aging and atopic skin).[38] The handling of coarse-textured textile materials may also be the cause of occupational dermatitis.[94] Buckles, buttons, boot tops, coarse seams, brassieres, and tight belts may cause friction and pressure against the skin and thus irritate the skin, leading to eczematous eruptions. These may sometimes be pigmented or purpuric.[38] Airtight synthetic materials such as textiles, rubbers, and plastics may cause irritation and softening of the skin due to sweating in warm conditions—for instance, at work-places. Remnants of washing agents—e.g., in cases where the rinsing of the washing machine is not sufficient (disturbances in the program)—and solvents (e.g., perchlore-thylene)[95] used in the cleaning of clothes may also be responsible for irritation due to clothing as well as contamination from materials (e.g., glass and mineral fibers)[38,95a] and chemicals (e.g., tributyltin oxide)[96] handled at work and in hobbies.[97]

CONTACT URTICARIA

Contact urticaria evoked by clothing is rare compared with contact eczema. Most cases have resulted from wearing gloves made of natural rubber latex (NRL). Similar symptoms have also resulted from contact with other rubber products made of NRL (e.g., balloons, condoms, condom urinals, medical adhesives, and dental coffer-dams).[98–103] The phenomenon has been known for only some 10 years. In 1988 in

Finland, an academic dissertation concerning type I rubber glove allergy was published.[25] All symptoms of the hospital workers using surgical gloves made of NRL on a daily basis were analyzed in the dissertation. About 3 percent of these workers had allergy to NRL, and 7 percent of the doctors and nurses in the surgical unit had allergy to NRL based on prick test results. When industrial workers regularly using NRL gloves were examined, 4 percent of them were found to be allergic to NRL.[102] It has also been estimated that 1 percent of the entire population, at least in Finland, has allergy to NRL. Asthma and occupational asthma caused by latex in household gloves and by latex in plant manufacturing surgical gloves have also been described.[104,105]

Surgical gloves are made of NRL, which is polyisoprene but which contains about 2 percent protein.[105] Proteins of 10,000 to 70,000 Da molecular mass in NRL are considered to be the most important responsible allergens causing the urticarial reaction.[106] Additives, such as accelerators, are other potential allergens. Recently, an increasing number of cases of rubber contact urticaria from rubber additives has been reported.[34,35,107,108]

Contact urticaria due to glove dusting powder has also been reported as a complication arising from the use of powdered surgical gloves. It is less common than contact urticaria caused by NRL, and only occasional cases have been reported.[34,35,110–112] The cause of the reaction is also suspected to be proteinaceous materials, such as protein impurities in glove donning powder made of corn (maize) starch.[110] However, glove powder can be contaminated with latex allergens. Airborne contaminated powder may cause symptoms of rhinitis and conjunctivitis in sensitized persons (e.g., among medical personnel).[113]

It is important to diagnose persons who have type I allergy to NRL, glove powders, or rubber additives correctly, since their local urticarial reactions may be followed by other, more troublesome or serious symptoms including eye irritation, rhinitis, asthma, and even life-threatening anaphylaxis.[25] Several serious cases of anaphylaxis or anaphylactoid reactions in both adults and children from exposure to gloves and other rubber materials during various surgical operations (cesarean sections, spina bifida operations, nasal surgery),[114–117] medical examinations (rectal and gynecologic)[100,108,109,118,119] and dental examinations and treatments[100,120] as well as from contact with materials other than those used in medical or dental operations (e.g., rubber balloons, condoms[99,100,108,109]) have been reported. Anaphylaxis due to NRL leading to a patient's death has also been described.[109] Atopic persons are more susceptible than nonatopics to get type I contact urticaria reactions, and their distant symptoms from other organs; e.g., nose and lungs, seem to be more common and severe.[25,100] However, the contact urticarial reaction may attack nonatopics as well.[25,100] Surgeons, gynecologists, pediatricians, dentists, and other doctors or nurses performing operations on a patient who is allergic to NRL must wear gloves made of synthetic rubber or plastic. No rubber objects should be used during such operations.

Apart from NRL, glove powder, and rubber additives, only occasional cases of allergic contact urticaria due to natural silk and wool have been described.[29] Recently a textile finish described as a cationic condensation product of dicyandiamide, formaldehyde, ammonium chloride, and ethylenediamine was reported to induce a contact urticarial reaction leading to the collapse of the patient.[121] Formaldehyde, both in textiles and leather, has also been responsible for contact urticaria as well as urticarial reactions, probably with nonimmunologic mechanisms.[27,69,122,123] In addition, laryngitis, pneumonitis, and asthma from formaldehyde have been described.[123] Cases of formaldehyde asthma caused by the steam-ironing of fabrics finished with formaldehyde-based resins have also been reported.[124]

INVESTIGATIONS

LOCALIZATION OF DERMATITIS

The typical localization and appearance of the dermatitis (see also Chaps. 3 and 4, on allergic contact dermatitis and its recognition) and a positive anamnesis consistent with suspected wearing apparel, accessories, or metal objects in garments or shoes will confirm a suspicion of clothing-induced dermatitis. In cases where the patient is not convinced about the existence of clothing dermatitis or cannot give any clue as to what garment might be the cause of the skin problems, all wearing apparel used at home or at work should be included in the list of possible causative agents. Apart from wearing apparel, other textile products which may come into contact with the skin should also be remembered as possible causes of textile dermatitis. These include bed linen, carpeting, upholstery fabrics, and other items such as wigs, purses, sleeping bags, and backpacks.[7,125,126]

PATCH TESTING WITH COMMERCIAL DYE AND TEXTILE FINISH ALLERGENS

In cases where textile, leather, or fur items are the suspects, patch testing should include a standard series[23] (e.g., European, commercially available from Chemotechnique Diagnostics, Edvard Olsv. 2, P.O. Box 80, 230 42 Tygelsjö, Malmö, Sweden), see Table 30-2.[127] Detailed information about the standard series is given in Ref. 23. Patch testing with extra series (Tables 30-3 and 30-4; Chemotechnique),[127] according to the suspected materials or sites of dermatitis, is almost always necessary. Positive reactions to standard series paraphenylenediamine (PPDA) and formaldehyde may point to clothing allergy. PPDA is used to dye furs (e.g., mink and fox) and for the permanent dyeing of hair[1,30] but not of textiles.[2] A positive reaction to PPDA may also refer to azo dye allergy, because cross-allergy between PPDA and azo dyes (e.g., used to dye textiles, leather, and furs) occurs to some extent.[1,2,4,5,7,30] Formaldehyde gives a positive patch-test reaction in many but not all cases of allergic dermatitis caused by formaldehyde-based textile finishes.[1,4,7,40,68] Patch testing with formaldehyde may also be problematic,[4,27] but the use of a dilution series (e.g., 2, 1, and 0.5% in water) makes the interpretation of test results easier.[27] Therefore patch testing with specific textile colors and finish series (e.g., Chemotechnique, Table 30-3)[127,131,132] and with some extra allergens relevant to textile, leather, and fur dyes of the azo group (p-aminoazobenzene, o-nitro-paraphenylenediamine, Chemotechnique) is needed and will further help to diagnose allergic contact dermatitis due to wearing apparel.[30] p-Aminoazobenzene (4-aminoazobenzene) can also be found in the shoe series (Chemotechnique, Table 30-4) and o-nitro-paraphenylenediamine (2-nitro-4-phenylenediamine) in the hairdressing series (Chemotechnique).[127] If the complete series of textile colors and finishes is not available for use,

TABLE 30–2. European Standard Patch-Test Series[a]

Compound	Conc. % (W/W)	Vehicle
Potassium dichromate	0.5	pet
4-Phenylenediamine base	1.0	pet
Thiuram mix	0.25	pet
Neomycin sulfate	20.0	pet
Cobalt chloride	1.0	pet
Benzocaine	5.0	pet
Nickel sulfate	5.0	pet
Quinolone mix	6.0	pet
Colophony	20.0	pet
Parabens	12.0	pet
Black rubber mix	0.6	pet
Wool alcohols	30.0	pet
Mercapto mix	2.0	pet
Epoxy resin	1.0	pet
Balsam of Peru	25.0	pet
4-*tert*-Butylphenol formaldehyde resin	1.0	pet
Mercaptobenzothiazole	2.0	pet
Formaldehyde	1.0	aq
Fragrance mix	8.0	pet
Sesquiterpene lactone mix	0.1	pet
Quaternium 15 (Dowicil 200)	1.0	pet
Primin	0.01	pet
Cl + Me-isothiazolinone (Kathon CG, 100 ppm)	0.67	aq

[a] Commercially available from Chemotechnique Diagnostics, Edvard Olsv. 2, P.O. Box 80, 230 42 Tygelsjö, Malmö, Sweden.[127]

TABLE 30–3. Textile Colors and Finish Series[a]

Compound	Conc. % (W/W)	Vehicle
Disperse Yellow 3	1.0	pet
Disperse Orange 3	1.0	pet
Disperse Red 1	1.0	pet
Disperse Red 17	1.0	pet
Disperse Blue 153	1.0	pet
Disperse Blue 3	1.0	pet
Disperse Blue 35	1.0	pet
Dimethylol dihydroxyethyleneurea (Fix.CPN)	4.5	aq
Dimethylol propyleneurea (Fix.PH)	5.0	aq
Tetramethylol acetylenediurea (Fix.140)	5.0	aq
Disperse Blue 106	1.0	pet
Ethyleneurea, melamineformaldehyde (Fix.Ac)	5.0	pet
Urea formaldehyde (Kaurit S)	10.0	pet
Melamine formaldehyde (Kaurit M70)	7.0	pet
Disperse Blue 85	1.0	pet
Disperse Orange 1	1.0	pet
Disperse Orange 13	1.0	pet
Disperse Brown 1	1.0	pet
Disperse Yellow 9	1.0	pet
Disperse Blue 124	1.0	pet
Basic Red 46	1.0	pet

[a] Commercially available from Chemotechnique Diagnostics, Edvard Olsv. 2, P.O. Box 80, 230 42 Tygelsjö, Malmö, Sweden.[127]

TABLE 30–4. Shoe Series[a]

Compound	Conc. % (w/w)	Vehicle
N-Isopropyl-N-phenyl-4-phenylenediamine[b]	0.1	pet
Glutaraldehyde	0.2	aq
Disperse Orange 3[c]	1.0	pet
Acid Yellow 36	1.0	pet
Hydroquinone monobenzylether	1.0	pet
Thiuram mix[d]	1.0	pet
Potassium dichromate[d]	0.5	pet
4-tert-Butylphenol formaldehyde resin[d]	1.0	pet
4-Phenylenediamine base[d]	1.0	pet
Nickel sulfate[d]	5.0	pet
Colophony[d]	20.0	pet
Formaldehyde[d]	1.0	aq
Diphenylthiourea[b]	1.0	pet
2-Mercaptobenzothiazole[b]	2.0	pet
Diethylthiourea[b]	1.0	pet
Diphenylguanidine[b]	1.0	pet
Dibutylthiourea[b]	1.0	pet
Epoxy resin[d]	1.0	pet
Dodecylmercaptan[b]	0.1	pet
Cl + Me-isothiazolinone (kathon CG, 200 ppm)[d]	1.34	aq
4-Aminobenzene	0.25	pet
2-n-Octyl-4-isothiazolin-3-one	0.1	pet

[a]Commercially available from Chemotechnique Diagnostics, Edvard Olsv. 2, P.O. Box 80, 230 42 Tygelsjö, Malmö, Sweden.[127]
[b]Included in the rubber additive series, Table 30-5.
[c]Included in the textile colors series, Table 30-3.
[d]Included in the standard series, Table 30-2.

testing with urea formaldehyde resin (ureaformaldehyde, Table 30-3) and four disperse dyes—Disperse Blue 124, Disperse Red 1, Disperse Yellow 3, and Disperse Orange 3 (Table 30-3)—will be useful and give more information than testing with a standard series alone in identifying patients allergic to textile finishes and dyes.[7–9,27,40,68]

PATCH TESTING WITH ACTUAL DYES USED IN SUSPECTED TEXTILE, LEATHER, AND FUR ITEMS

In cases where dyed textile, leather, and furs are the suspects, the best results are, of course, obtained by performing patch tests with the actual dyes and finishes used in the materials. At least in some countries, information on the chemicals used may be obtained from the manufacturers of textiles, as well as samples for testings. Further information about commercially used colorants can be found in *The Colour Index*. When the chemicals themselves are not available for testing, it would be useful if at least some information concerning the types of fibers, dyes, or finishes could be obtained from the distributors or manufacturers of the products or fabrics, giving a hint of the dye groups used.[30]

PATCH TESTING WITH SUSPECTED TEXTILE, LEATHER, OR FUR MATERIALS

Patch testing with pieces of moistened fabric, leather, or fur skins as such can be performed.[23,30] For these tests, an application time of 2 or sometimes 3 days is usually enough. The pieces of fabric can also be soaked in water for 10 to 15 min before the application of the patch tests where there is suspicion of allergy to finishes and for 30 to 60 min in acetone or ethanol where dye allergy is suspected.[2,7,23] Apart from soaking pieces of fabric in water and solvents, extracts can be made for testing by boiling pieces of suspected textile materials in water or in ethanol.[128] If the dyes are the causative agents, the tests with the dyed materials usually give positive results; whereas in cases where the finishes (e.g., durable-press finishes) are the causes, the test will probably give negative results.[1,4]

IDENTIFICATION OF THE CAUSATIVE AGENT IN THE MATERIAL

Where allergy to formaldehyde is concerned, formaldehyde can be detected in the suspected products using the chromotropic acid method[129] and a more specific complementary method (lutidine method)[23] using acetylacetone as a reagent.[130] Also, the Schiff reagent method is suitable for detecting formaldehyde in textiles. For details on how to perform tests using the chromotropic acid, see Appendix A; for that and Schiff's reagent methods, see Ref. 4; for the lutidine method, see Refs. 23, 130, or Appendix A.

When a dyed material gives only a positive patch-test reaction, it is important to confirm the reaction by retesting to exclude an irritant reaction. The recognition of the causative allergen will need time-consuming chemical analyses and cooperation between an expert chemist and the manufacturer of the material. Even when commercial dyes are used for testing, it may be difficult to determine the actual allergen. Again, analyses of the dyes (thin-layer chromatography, high performance liquid chromatography, atomic absorption spectrometry, gas chromatography, mass spectrometry)[133] and cooperation of the manufacturer of the dye are important in determining the sensitizer.

PATCH TESTING WHEN SHOE ALLERGY IS SUSPECTED

When shoes are the suspects, scrapings or pieces of the lining and other materials inside the shoe[75] can be used for patch testing. If large, thin pieces with smooth surfaces and regular edges are used, interpretation of the test results may be easier.[81] Patch testing with a standard series, however, will detect the most common causes of allergic shoe dermatitis.[81] The use of a specific shoe series (Table 30-4),[127] sometimes also a rubber additive series (Table 30-5), and a plastics and glues series (Table 30-6) might be necessary in some cases (see Chaps. 24, 31, 34, 36). Apart from allergens included in the shoe series (Table 30-4), several other allergenic compounds can be used in the manufacture of shoes.[81] Further investigations to identify the actual allergen in the shoe materials are needed when a material sample gives only a positive patch-test reaction (see above).

TABLE 30–5. Rubber Additives Series[a]

Compound	Conc. % (w/w)	Vehicle
Tetramethylthiuram disulfide	1.0	pet
Tetramethylthiuram monosulfide	1.0	pet
Tetraethylthiuram disulfide	1.0	pet
Dipentamethylenethiuram disulfide	1.0	pet
N-Cyclohexyl-N-phenyl-4-phenylenediamine	1.0	pet
N,N-Diphenyl-4-phenylenediamine	1.0	pet
N-Isopropyl-N-phenyl-4-phenylenediamine	1.0	pet
2-Mercaptobenzothiazole	1.0	pet
N-Cyclohexylbenzothiazyl sulphenamide	1.0	pet
Dibenzothiazyl disulfide	1.0	pet
Morpholinylmercaptobenzothiazole	1.0	pet
Diphenylguanidine	1.0	pet
Zinc diethyldithiocarbamate	1.0	pet
Zinc dibutyldithiocarbamate	1.0	pet
N,N-Di-beta-naphthyl-4-phenylenediamine	1.0	pet
N-Phenyl-2-naphthylamine	1.0	pet
Hexamethylenetetramine	2.0	pet
Diaminodiphenylmethane	0.5	pet
Dibutylthiourea	1.0	pet
Zinc dimethyldithiocarbamate	1.0	pet
2,2,4-Trimethyl-1,2-dihydroquinoline	1.0	pet
Diethylthiourea	1.0	pet
Dibultylthiourea	1.0	pet
Dodecylmercaptan	0.1	pet

[a]Commercially available from Chemotechnique Diagnostics, Edvard Olsv. 2, P.O. Box 80, 230 42 Tygelsjö, Malmö, Sweden.[127]

PATCH TESTING WHEN RUBBER AND PLASTIC ALLERGY IS SUSPECTED

When rubber and plastic materials are suspected of causing type IV allergic contact eczema, tests with pieces of the materials[27] should always be performed, because only a restricted number of potential allergens are commercially available. The standard series (Table 30-2), which contains three rubber mixes[23,127] and mercaptobenzothiazole, probably recognizes most cases of rubber allergy.[1,31–37] Other additives not included in the standard series (e.g., thiourea compounds—see Chap. 17) may also be the causes of rubber allergy. Therefore a vast rubber series (Table 30-5) is often necessary. The possibility of type I allergy should also be remembered, especially in cases of glove-induced dermatitis (see also Chap. 34).

When allergy to a plastic material is suspected, the use of the plastics and glues series may be useful (Table 30-6). In cases where the material only gives a positive patch-test reaction, attempts (see above) should be made to confirm the type of reaction and to identify the allergen.

INVESTIGATIONS IN CONTACT URTICARIA

In cases where allergic contact urticaria is suspected and also in uncertain cases where the results of skin tests and IgE determinations are not quite clear, skin tests and

TABLE 30–6. Plastics and Glues Series*a*

Compound	Conc. % (w/w)	Vehicle
Hydroquinone	1.0	pet
Dibutyl phthalate	5.0	pet
Phenyl salicylate	1.0	pet
Diethylhexylphthalate (Dioctylphthalate)	2.0	pet
2,6-Ditert-butyl-cresol (BHT)	2.0	pet
2 (2-Hydroxy-5-methylphenol)-benzotriazol	1.0	pet
Benzoyl peroxide	1.0	pet
4-*tert*-Butylcatechol (PTBC)	0.5	pet
Azodiisobutyrodinitrile	1.0	pet
Bisphenol A	1.0	pet
Tricresyl phosphate	5.0	pet
Phenol formaldehyde resin (P-F-R-2)	1.0	pet
p-*tert*-Butylphenol formaldehyde resin*b*	1.0	pet
Triphenyl phosphate	5.0	pet
Toluenesulfonamide formaldehyde resin	10.1	pet
Resorcinol monobenzoate	1.0	pet
2-Phenylindole	2.0	pet
2-*tert*-Butyl-4-methoxyphenol (BHA)	2.0	pet
Abitol	10.0	pet
4-*tert*-Butylphenol	1.0	pet
2-Monomethylol phenol	1.0	pet
Diphenylthiourea*c*	1.0	pet
2-n-Octyl-4-isothiazolin-3-one	0.1	pet
Cyclohexanone resin	1.0	pet
Triglycidyl isocyanurate	0.5	pet

*a*Commercially available from Chemotechnique Diagnostics, Edvard Olsv. 2, P.O. Box 80, 230 42 Tygelsjö, Malmö, Sweden.[127]
*b*Included in the standard series, Table 30-2.
*c*Included in the rubber additives series, Table 30-5.

specific IgE determinations (RASTs) showing immediate allergy[23,28] and appropriate challenges should be performed.[25–28,134] When challenges are done, the risk of anaphylactic reactions should be kept in mind.[25,52,61]

TREATMENT AND PRINCIPLES OF THE PREVENTION OF SKIN DISORDERS DUE TO CLOTHING

The most important aspect in the treatment of dermatoses due to clothing is to recognize the causative agent or agents and to avoid contact with them. In addition, most patients also need symptomatic local medication before the skin symptoms disappear.

When the definite cause is known, it may be quite easy to give detailed advice to the patient; but when the cause remains unknown, only rough advice can be given, and the patient may again come into contact with new garments evoking skin problems. In some cases patients who have multiple sensitivities to undetermined (disperse) azo dyes have been able to wear only undyed white garments. Washing of the dyed materials does not solve the dermatitis problem of a patient allergic to textile dye.[7] Garments made of cotton, rayon, silk, and wool can be recommended for patients sensitized to disperse dyes.[1,4,7] For patients who have multiple dye allergies, garments made of fabrics dyed with reactive dyes may be other alternatives.[52] Patients who have been sensitized to durable-press finishes should avoid garments made of cotton or cotton blends and also any other fabrics made of blends of synthetic and natural fibers.[1,4,7] Textile labels may possibly give some information as to finishes. However, it would be safer not to rely on the markings in the labels but to wash new textile garments before use. In problematic cases, it would be worthwhile to test for formaldehyde content in all garments to be used (see Chap. 20 and Appendix C).

Even more problems are encountered in cases of shoe allergy, especially in cases of allergy to shoe glues. Apart from avoiding contact with allergens of footwear, it is also important to control hyperhidrosis and possible friction caused by the materials. Alternatives to those sensitized to leather are usually using all nonleather materials (e.g., athletic shoes which contain textile materials and polyurethane or rubber). In cases of allergy to chromates, shoes containing vegetable-tanned soles, linings, and insoles can be used. Many cases of shoe allergy, however, remain unsolved and must be managed according to the patch-test results and actual symptoms, often empirically. Plastic shoes or boots and wooden shoes with vegetable-tanned uppers not glued in the place can be recommended.[81,135]

Textile footwear might also be feasible in some cases, at least at home, in offices, and during the summer. In a cold climate, thick socks or inner shoes made of textile materials used in relatively loose shoes or boots often prevent allergens from coming into contact with the skin and thus also prevent the development of dermatitis.

In cases of type I or IV allergy to household and industrial rubber gloves, gloves made of polyvinyl chloride (PVC) or other plastic materials[96,136] are probably the safest alternatives to rubber gloves. In cases of type IV allergy to surgical and examination gloves, there is more information about alternatives available. NRL gloves or synthetic rubber gloves can be selected, in most cases, according to patch-test results with rubber additive series, avoiding gloves containing the specific allergen. In cases of type I allergy to NRL, apart from PVC gloves, some synthetic rubber gloves can be recommended. If "hypoallergenic" NRL gloves are selected, it is safest first to apply tests before using the gloves.[25–28,134] Lists of recommended alternatives of surgical and examination gloves for rubber glove–allergic patients can be found in Refs. 34, 35, and 88. For persons allergic to both latex and vinyl gloves, Tactylon gloves may be tried after patch testing.

Although reported cases of dermatoses due to protective and work clothing are even less common than those caused by everyday clothes, it is important to pay attention to the materials and garment patterns of all clothes, shoes, or boots used at work as well as the materials worn closest to the skin. Perspiration and mechanical friction caused by poorly fitting tight clothes increase the risk of skin irritation and sensitization to dyes and finishing agents. Therefore only good-quality textile materials should be used. Whenever possible, the materials should be breathable to prevent irritation caused by sweating. Dyes or colorants in textiles and leather must be well fixed to the materials so that they are not released by perspiration. The garments should be well fitted, especially the sleeves should be loose and the seams smooth enough not to irritate the skin. When finishing resins are used, they should be of high quality and should not release formaldehyde in amounts sufficient to sensitize. Metal objects in the clothing and in other articles should not contain releasable nickel. Clothes contaminated with hazardous chemicals should be discarded. For details concerning the use of protective gloves, see also Refs. 97 and 137.

REFERENCES

1. Cronin E: *Contact Dermatitis.* Edinburgh, Churchill Livingstone, 1980.
2. Hatch KL, Maibach HI: Textile dye dermatitis: A review. *J Am Acad Dermatol* 12:1079–1092, 1985.
3. Hatch KL, Maibach HI: Textile chemical finish dermatitis: A review. *Contact Dermatitis* 14:1–13, 1986.
4. Stoors FJ: Dermatitis from clothing and shoes, in Fisher AA (ed): *Contact Dermatitis,* 3d ed. Philadelphia, Lea & Febiger, 1986, pp 283–337.
5. Feinman SE, Doyle EA: Sensitization to dyes in textiles and other consumer products. *J Toxicol–Cut Ocular Toxicol* 3:195–222, 1988.
6. Estlander T: Skin disorders caused by clothing, in *Proceedings: Quality and Usage of Protective Clothing.* Kittilä, Finland, NOKOBETEFF IV, February 5-7, 1992, pp 130–136.
7. Sherertz EF: Clothing dermatitis: Practical aspects for the clinician. *Am J Contact Dermatitis* 3:55–64, 1992.
8. Balato N, Lembo G, Patruno C, Ayla F: Prevalence of textile dye contact sensitization. *Contact Dermatitis* 23:111–126, 1990.
9. Seidenari S, Manzini BM, Danese P: Contact sensitization to textile dyes: Description of 100 cases. *Contact Dermatitis* 24:253–258, 1991.
10. Gasperini M, Farli M, Lombardi P, Sertoli A: Contact dermatitis in the textile and garment industry, in Frosch PJ, Dooms-Goossens A, Lachapelle J-M, et al (eds): *Current Topics in Contact Dermatitis.* Berlin, Springer Verlag, 1989, pp 326–329.
11. Batschvarov B, Minkov DM: Dermatitis and purpura from rubber in clothing. *Trans St John's Dermatol Soc* 59:178–182, 1968.
12. Ancona-Alayón A, Escobar-Márques R, Gonzáles-Mendoza A, et al: Occupational pigmented contact dermatitis from Naphthol AS. *Contact Dermatitis* 2:129–134, 1976.
13. Shmunes E: Purpuric allergic contact dermatitis to paraphenylenediamine. *Contact Dermatitis* 4:225–229, 1978.
14. Kieć-Świerczyńska M: Occupational contact dermatitis in the workers employed in production of Texas textiles. *Dermatosen* 30:41–43, 1982.
15. Fisher AA: Purpuric contact dermatitis. *Cutis* 33:346–351, 1984.
16. Hayakawa R, Matsunaga K, Kojima S, et al: Naphthol AS as a cause of pigmented contact dermatitis. *Contact Dermatitis* 13:20–25, 1985.
17. van der Ween JPW, Neering H, de Haan P, Bruynzeel DP: Pigmented purpuric clothing dermatitis due to Disperse Blue 85. *Contact Dermatitis* 19:222–223, 1988.
18. Hjorth N, Möller H: Phototoxic textile dermatitis ("bikini dermatitis"). *Arch Dermatol* 112:1445–1447, 1976.
19. Pirilä V: Chamber test versus patch test for epicutaneous testing. *Contact Dermatitis* 1:48–52, 1975.
20. Hannuksela M: Epicutaneous testing. *Allergy* 34:5–10, 1979.
21. Adams RM: Patch testing: A recapitulation. *J Am Acad Derm* 5:629–642, 1981.
22. Fischer T, Maibach HI: Improved, but not perfect, patch testing. *Am J Contact Dermatitis* 1:73–90, 1990.
23. Rycroft RJG, Menné T, Frosch PJ, Benezra (eds): *Textbook of Contact Dermatitis.* Berlin, Heidelberg, Springer-Verlag, 1992.
24. Lahti A, Maibach HI: Immediate contact reactions, in Menné T, Maibach HI (eds): *Exogenous Dermatoses: Environmental Dermatitis.* Boca Raton, FL, CRC Press, 1991, pp 21–35.
25. Turjanmaa K: Latex glove contact urticaria (thesis). University of Tampere, Finland, 1988.
26. Wass U: Studies on IgE antibodies induced by low-molecular-weight chemicals (thesis). Göteborg, Sweden, 1989.
27. Estlander T: Occupational skin disease in Finland. Observations made during 1974u–1988 at the Institute of Occupational Health, Helsinki (thesis). *Acta Derm Venereol* (suppl 115), 1–85, 1990.
27a. Turjanmaa K: Contact urticoria from latex gloves, in Mellström G, Wahlberg JE, Maibach HI (eds): *Protective Gloves for Occupational Use.* Series in Clinical and Research Dermatology. Boca Raton, FL, CRC Press, 1994, pp 241–254.
28. Kanerva L, Estlander T, Jolanki R: Skin testing for immediate hypersensitivity in occupational allergology, in Menné T, Maibach HI (eds): *Exogenous dermatoses: Environmental dermatitis.* Boca Raton, FL, CRC Press, 1991, pp 103–126.

29. Hatch KL, Maibach HI: Textile fiber dermatitis. *Contact Dermatitis* 12:1–11, 1985.
30. Estlander T, Kanerva L, Jolanki R: Occupational allergic dermatoses from textile, leather, and fur dyes. *Am J Contact Dermatitis* 1:13–20, 1990.
31. Lammintausta K, Kalimo K: Sensitivity to rubber: Study with rubber mixes and individual rubber chemicals. *Dermatosen* 33:204–208, 1985.
32. Taylor JS: Rubber, in Fisher AA (ed): *Contact Dermatitis,* 3d ed. Philadelphia, Lea & Febiger, 1986, pp 603–643.
33. Estlander T, Kanerva L, Jolanki R: Dermatitis and urticaria from rubber and plastic gloves. *Contact Dermatitis* 14:20–25, 1986.
34. Heese A, v Hintzenstern J, Peters K-P, Koch HU: Typ-IV Allergien gegen Gummihandschuhe— Inzidenz, Allergene, Diagnostik und Therapie (Allergies of delayed type against rubber gloves— incidence, allergens, diagnostic approach, therapy). *Z Hautk* 66:25–32, 1991.
35. Heese A, v Hintzenstern J, Peters K-P, et al: Allergic and irritant reactions to rubber gloves in medical health services. *J Am Acad Dermatol* 25:831–839, 1991.
36. von Hintzenstern J, Heese A, Koch HU, et al: Frequency, spectrum and occupational relevance of type IV allergies to rubber chemicals. *Contact Dermatitis* 24:244–252, 1991.
37. Frosch PJ, Born CM, Schütz R: Kontaktallergien auf Gummi-, Operations- und Vinylhandschuhe. *Hautarzt* 38:210–217, 1987.
38. Adams RM: Dermatitis due to clothing. *Cutis* 5:577–582, 1972.
39. Foussereau J, Benezra C, Maibach HI: Textile industry, in *Occupational Contact Dermatitis: Clinical and Chemical Aspects,* 1st ed. Copenhagen, Munksgaard, 1982, pp 260–266.
40. Andersen K, Hamann K: Cost benefit of patch testing with textile finish resins. *Contact Dermatitis* 8:64–67, 1982.
41. Hatch KL: Textile dermatitis from formaldehyde, in Feinman SE (ed): *Formaldehyde Sensitivity and Toxicity.* Boca Raton, FL, CRC Press, 1988, pp 91–103.
42. Herve-Bazin B, Foussereau J, Cavelier C: L'eczéma allergique au support de pigments textiles. *Berufsdermatosen* 25:113–118, 1977.
43. Estlander T, Jolanki R, Kanerva L, Plosila M: An artist's allergy to reactive dyes and formaldehyde. *Contact Dermatitis* 23:303–304, 1990.
44. Kofoed ML: Contact dermatitis to formaldehyde in fabric softeners. *Contact Dermatitis* 11:254, 1984.
45. Fregert S, Orsmark K: Allergic contact dermatitis due to epoxy resin in textile labels. *Contact Dermatitis* 11:131–132, 1984.
46. Abrahart EN: *Dyes and Their Intermediates.* London, Arnold, 1977.
47. Jenkins CL: Dye hazards report. *Dangerous Properties of Industrial Materials Report,* July/August:5, 1981.
48. Horning RH: The contribution of dyes to the metal content of textile mill effluents. *Textile Chemist Colorist* 12:275–277, 1972.
49. Fregert S, Trulsson L: Difficulties in tracing sensitizing textile dyes. *Contact Dermatitis* 4:174, 1978.
50. Brandle I, Stampf JL, Foussereau J: Thin-layer chromatography of organic dye allergens. *Contact Dermatitis* 10:254–255, 1984.
51. Foussereau J, Dallara JM: Purity of standardized textile dye allergens: A thin layer chromatography study. *Contact Dermatitis* 14:303–306, 1986.
52. Estlander T: Allergic dermatoses and respiratory diseases from reactive dyes. *Contact Dermatitis* 18:290–297, 1988.
53. Roed-Petersen J, Batsberg W, Larsen E: Contact dermatitis from Naphthol AS. *Contact Dermatitis* 22:161–163, 1990.
54. Wilson HTH, Cronin E: Dermatitis from dyed uniform. *Br J Derm* 85:67–69, 1971.
55. Manzini BM, Seidenari S, Danese P, Motolese A: Contact sensitization to newly patch tested nondisperse textile dyes. *Contact Dermatitis* 25:331–332, 1991.
56. Thoren K, Meding B, Nordlinger R, Belin L: Contact dermatitis and asthma from reactive dyes. *Contact Dermatitis* 15:186, 1986.
57. Alanko K, Keskinen H, Björksten F, Ojanen S: Immediate-type hypersensitivity to reactive dyes. *Clin Allergy* 8:25–31, 1978.
58. Docker A, Wattie JM, Topping MD, et al: Clinical and immunological investigations of respiratory disease in workers using reactive dyes. *Br J Ind Med* 44:534–541, 1987.
59. Park HS, Kim YJ, Lee MK, Hong C-S: Occupational asthma and IgE antibodies to reactive dyes. *Yonsei Med J* 30:298–304, 1989.

60. Park HS, Hong C-S: The significance of specific IgG and IgG4 antibodies to a reactive dye in exposed workers. *Clin Exp Allergy* 21:357–362, 1991.
61. Romano C, Sulotto F, Pavan I, et al: A new case of occupational asthma from reactive dyes with severe anaphylactic response to the specific challenge. *Am J Ind Med* 21:209–216, 1992.
62. Kojima S, Momma J: Phosgene(2,5-dichlorophenyl)hydrazone, a new strong sensitizer. *Contact Dermatitis* 20:235–236, 1989.
63. Kojima S, Momma J, Kaniwa M, et al: Phosgene (chlorophenyl)hydrazones, strong sensitizers found in yellow sweaters bleached with sodium hypochlorite, defined as causative allergens for contact dermatitis by an experimental screening method in animals. *Contact Dermatitis* 23:129–141, 1990.
64. Imbeau SA, Reed CE: Nylon Stockings dermatitis: An unusual example. *Contact Dermatitis* 5:163–164, 1979.
65. Dorn H: Chronische Ekzeme durch Kleiderfarben und Textilhilfsprodukte. *Archs Klin Exp Derm* 211:291–297, 1960.
66. Ebner H: Chromatkontaktallergie als Ursache von Bekleidungsekzemen. *Dermatologica* 135:355–361, 1967.
67. Fregert S, Gruvberger B, Göransson K, Normark S: Allergic contact dermatitis from chromate in military textiles. *Contact Dermatitis* 4:223–224, 1978.
68. Malten KE: Textile finish contact hypersensitivity. *Arch Dermatol* 89:215–221, 1964.
69. Andersen KE, Maibach HI: Multiple application delayed onset urticaria: possible relation to certain unusual formalin and textile reactions? *Contact Dermatitis* 10:227–234, 1984.
70. Tegner E: Sheet dermatitis. *Acta Derm Venereol* 65:254–257, 1985.
71. Fisher AA, Kanof NB, Biondi EM: Free formaldehyde in textiles and paper. *Arch Dermatol* 86:753–756, 1962.
72. Sugai T, Yamamoto S: Decrease in the incidence of contact sensitivity to formaldehyde. *Contact Dermatitis* 2,154, 1980.
73. Senff H, Kuhlwein A, Hausen BM: Allergisches Kontaktekzem auf Dicyandiamid. *Dermatosen* 36:99–101, 1988.
74. Fregert S, Gruvberger B: Chromium in industrial leather gloves. *Contact Dermatitis* 5:189, 1979.
75. Grimalt F, Romaguera C: New resin allergens in shoe contact dermatitis. *Contact Dermatitis* 1:169–174, 1975.
76. Angelini G, Vena A, Meneghini CL: Shoe contact dermatitis. *Contact Dermatitis* 6:279–283, 1980.
77. Oumeish OY, Rushaidat QM: Contact dermatitis to military boots in Jordan. *Contact Dermatitis* 6:498, 1980.
78. Malten KE, Rath R, Pastors PHM: p-tert.-Butylphenol formaldehyde and other causes of shoe dermatitis. *Dermatosen* 31:149–153, 1983.
79. Foussereau J, Tomb R, Cavelier C: Allergic contact dermatitis from safety clothes and individual protective devices. *Dermatol Clin* 8:127–132, 1990.
80. Sharma SC, Handa S, Sharma VK, Kaur S: Footwear dermatitis in northern India. *Contact Dermatitis* 25:57–58, 1991.
81. Podmore P: Shoes, in Rycroft RJG, Ménne T, Frosch PJ, Benezra (eds): *Textbook of Contact Dermatitis*. Berlin, Springer-Verlag, 1992, pp 515–526.
82. Ancona A, Seviere L, Trejo A, Monroy F: Dermatitis from an azo-dye in industrial leather protective shoes. *Contact Dermatitis* 8:220–221, 1982.
83. Srivas CR, Devadiga R, Aroor AR: Footwear dermatitis due to bisphenol A. *Contact Dermatitis* 20:150–151, 1989.
84. Jung JH, McLaughlin JL, Stannard J, Guin JD: Isolation, via activity-directed fractionation, of mercaptobenzothiazole and dibenzothiazyl disulfide as 2 allergens responsible for tennis shoe dermatitis. *Contact Dermatitis* 19:254–259, 1988.
85. Roberts JI, Hanifin JM: Athletic shoe dermatitis, contact allergy to ethybutyl thiourea. *JAMA* 241:275–276, 1979.
86. Adams RM: Contact allergic dermatitis due to diethylthiourea in a wetsuit. *Contact Dermatitis* 8:277–278, 1982.
87. Masmoudi ML, Lachapelle J-M: Occupational dermatitis to dihydroxydiphenyl and diphenylthiourea in neoprene gloves. *Contact Dermatitis* 16:290–291, 1987.
88. Rich P, Belozer ML, Norris P, Storrs FJ: Allergic contact dermatitis to two antioxidants in latex gloves: 4,4'-thiobis(6-tert-butyl-meta-cresol) (Lowinox 44S36) and butylhydroxyanisole—Allergen alternatives for glove-allergic patients. *J Am Acad Dermatol* 24:37–43, 1991.

89. Jolanki R, Kanerva L, Estlander T: Organic pigments in plastics can cause allergic contact dermatitis. *Acta Derm Venereol (Suppl)* 134:95–97, 1987.

90. Fregert S, Rorsman H: Allergens in epoxy resins. *Acta Allergol* 19:296–199, 1964.

91. Kanerva L, Jolanki R, Estlander T: Organic pigment as a cause of plastic glove dermatitis. *Contact Dermatitis* 13:41–43, 1985.

92. Christensen OB: Nickel dermatitis: An update. *Dermatol Clin* 8:37–40, 1990.

93. Fowler JF: Allergic contact dermatitis to metals. *Am J Contact Dermatitis* 1:212–223, 1990.

94. Launis L, Laine A: Toxic dermatitis in a Finnish textile factory. *Contact Dermatitis* 6:51, 1980.

95. Redmond SF, Schappert KR: Occupational dermatitis associated with garment. *J Occup Med* 29:243–244, 1987.

95a. Tarvainen K, Jolanki R, Forsman-Grönholm L: Reinforced plastics industry: Exposure, skin diseases and skin protection, in *Proceedings: Quality and Usage of Protective Clothing*. Kittilä, Finland, NOKOBETEFF IV, February 5-7, 1992, pp 147–150.

96. Grace CT, Ng SK, Cheong LL: Recurrent irritant contact dermatitis due to tributyltin oxide on work clothes. *Contact Dermatitis* 25:250–251, 1991.

97. Estlander T, Jolanki R: How to protect the hands. *Derm Clin* 6:105–114, 1988.

98. Bransbury AJ: Allergy to rubber condom urinals and medical adhesives in male spinal injury patient. *Contact Dermatitis* 5:317–323, 1979.

99. Axelsson IGK, Eriksson M, Wrangsjö K: Anaphylaxis and angioedema due to rubber allergy in children. *Acta Paediatr Scand* 77:314–316, 1988.

100. Wrangsjö K, Wahlberg JE, Axelsson IGK: IgE-mediated allergy to natural rubber in 30 patients with contact urticaria. *Contact Dermatitis* 19:264–271, 1988.

101. Turjanmaa K, Reunala T: Condoms as a source of latex allergen and cause of contact urticaria. *Contact Dermatitis* 20:360–364, 1989.

102. Taylor J, Evey P, Helm T, Wagner W: Contact urticaria and anaphylaxis from latex. *Contact Dermatitis* 23:277–278, 1990.

103. Hamann CP: Natural rubber latex protein sensitivity in review. *Am J Contact Dermatitis* 4:4–21, 1993.

104. Seifert HU, Seifert B, Wahl R, et al: Immunoglobulin E-vermittelte Kontakturtikaria bzw. Asthma bronchiale durch Latex-enthaltende Haushaltsgummihandschuhe: Drei Fallberichte. *Dermatosen* 35:137–139, 1987.

105. Tarlo SM, Wong L, Roos J, Booth N: Occupational asthma caused by latex in a surgical glove manufacturing plant. *J Allergy Clin Immunol* 85:626–631, 1990.

106. Alenius H, Turjanmaa K, Palosuo T, et al: Surgical latex glove allergy: Characterization of rubber protein allergens by immunoblotting. *Int Arch Allergy Appl Immunol* 96:376–380, 1991.

107. Helander I, Mäkelä A: Contact urticaria to zinc diethyldithiocarbamate (ZDC). *Contact Dermatitis* 9:327–328, 1983.

108. Belsito DV: Contact urticaria caused by rubber: Analysis of seven cases. *Dermatologic Clinics* 8:61–66, 1990.

109. Ownby DR, Tomlanovich M, Sammons N, McCullough J: Anaphylaxis associated with latex allergy during barium enema examinations. *AJR* 156:903–908, 1991.

110. van der Meeren HLM, van Erp PEJ: Life-threatening contact urticaria from glove powder. *Contact Dermatitis* 13:190–191, 1986.

111. Fisher AA: Contact urticaria due to corn starch surgical glove powder. *Cutis* 38:307–308, 1986.

112. Fisher AA: Contact urticaria and anaphylactoid reaction to corn starch surgical glove powder. *Contact Dermatitis* 16:224–225, 1987.

113. Turjanmaa K, Reunala T, Alenius H, Brummer-Korvenkontio H, Palosuo T: Allergens in latex surgical gloves and glove powder. *Lancet* 29:1588, 1990.

114. Turjanmaa K, Reunala T, Tuimala R, Kärkkäinen T: Allergy to latex gloves: Unusual complication during delivery. *Br Med J* 297:1029, 1988.

115. Morales C, Basomba A, Carreira J, Sastre A: Anaphylaxis produced rubber glove contact: Case reports and immunological identification of the antigens involved. *Clin Exp Allergy* 19:425–430, 1989.

116. Slater JE: Rubber anaphylaxis. *N Engl J Med* 320:1126–1130, 1989.

117. Zenarola P: Rubber latex allergy: Unusual complication during surgery. *Contact Dermatitis* 21:197–198, 1989.

118. Fabro L, Mülethaler K, Wüthrich B: Anaphylaktische Reaktion auf Latex, ein Soforttypallergen von zunehmender Bedeutung. *Hautarzt* 40:208–211, 1989.

119. Taylor JS, Cassettari DO, Wagner W, Helm T: Contact urticaria and anaphylaxis to latex. *J Am Acad Dermatol* 21:874–877, 1989.
120. Grattan CEH, Kennedy CTC: Angioedema during dental treatment. *Contact Dermatitis* 13:333–349, 1985.
121. de Groot AC, Gerkens F: Contact urticaria from a chemical textile finish. *Contact Dermatitis* 20:63–64, 1989.
122. Helander I: Contact urticaria from leather containing formaldehyde. *Arch Dermatol* 113:1443, 1977.
123. Feinman SE: *Formaldehyde Sensitivity and Toxicity.* Boca Raton, Fla, CRC Press, 1988.
124. Nordman H, Keskinen H, Tuppurainen M: Formaldehyde asthma—rare or overlooked? *J Allergy Clin Immunol* 75:91–99, 1985.
125. Brown R: Allergy to dyes in permanent-press linen. *Contact Dermatitis* 22:303–304, 1990.
126. Shehade SA, Beck MH: Contact Dermatitis from disperse dyes in synthetic wigs. *Contact Dermatitis* 23:124–125, 1990.
127. Patch Test Allergens. Chemotechnique Diagnostics, Malmö, Sweden. *Product Catalogue* 1992/93.
128. Fregert S: Extraction of allergens for patch testing. *Acta Derm Venereol* 44:107–109, 1964.
129. Blohm S-G: Formaldehyde contact dermatitis. *Acta Derm Venereol* 39:450–453, 1959.
130. Fregert S, Dahlquist I, Gruvberger B: A simple method for detection of formaldehyde. *Contact Dermatitis* 10:132–134, 1984.
131. Menezes Brandâo F, Altermatt C, Pecegueiro M, et al: Contact dermatitis to Disperse Blue 106. *Contact Dermatitis* 13:80–84, 1985.
132. Menezes-Brandâo F, Hausen BM: Cross reaction between Disperse Blues 106 and 124. *Contact Dermatitis* 16:289–190, 1987.
133. Fregert S: Physicochemical methods for detection of contact allergens. *Dermatol Clin* 6:97–104, 1988.
134. Lahti A, Turjanmaa K: Prick and use tests with 6 glove brands in patients with immediate allergy to rubber proteins. *Contact Dermatitis* 26:259–262, 1992.
135. Mathias CGT, Maibach HI: Polyvinyl chloride boots in the management of shoe dermatitis in industrial workers. *Contact Dermatitis* 5:249–250, 1979.
136. Chemical Protection List, 4 H Safety A/S Lyngby, Denmark, 1/1992.
137. Hellström GA, Wahlberg JE, Maibach HI (eds): *Protective Gloves for Occupational Use.* Boca Raton, FL, CRC Press, 1994.

31

SHOES

Patricia Podmore

Contact dermatitis on the feet is a common and difficult problem. The difficulty arises in that feet are constantly exposed to a wide variety of possible allergens, some of which are known and regularly tested to in today's patch-testing kit but a larger majority of which are as yet unknown and therefore not contained in routine patch-test series.[1] This problem has arisen particularly in recent years as a result of the rapidly changing world of footwear manufacture. Shoes, particularly athletic shoes, are manufactured all over the world. The ingredients used in their manufacture are therefore not always readily available, tend to be rapidly changing, and tend to vary widely from country to country. A further problem is that footwear may be manufactured in many different sites, with different portions of the shoe being made in different countries, making collation of a comprehensive patch-testing kit an extremely difficult task.

The diagnosis of footwear-allergic contact dermatitis, as in any case of contact dermatitis, is based on the patient's history and the distribution of the dermatitic rash. Careful inquiry should be made as to whether or not the onset of the rash bears any relationship to purchase of a new pair of shoes. Patch testing as well as a battery of the chemical ingredients of manufacture should include small portions of the shoes, particularly those portions which are in close contact with the dermatitic area.[2] It is important to ensure that these clippings from the shoe be not large enough or so shaped as to cause a spurious friction reaction. The distribution of the rash is particularly important, as the architecture of the average pair of modern shoes is quite complex and each portion of the shoe may contain a widely different group of allergens (Fig. 31-1). It is therefore important for the investigator to have a mental picture of the structure of the average shoe as well as a working knowledge of the types of allergens likely to be included in the suspect component. This task can be made more difficult by a time delay before the clinician sees the rash, as there may have been blurring of the more specific distribution of the dermatitis. It is well worth the time and effort necessary to exclude underlying constitutional eczema as being the explanation for foot eczema or foot dermatitis prior to embarking on what is often a difficult journey of identification of the causative allergens in a case of allergic contact dermatitis to footwear. Similarly, a fungal infection should be excluded by carrying out microscopy with scrapings of the affected area of the foot and culture of the scrapings.

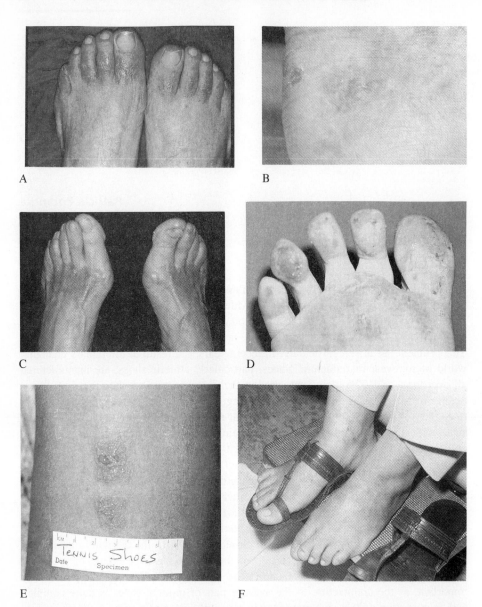

FIG. 31–1. *A.* Eczema of the dorsum of the toes but sparing the plantar surfaces is typical of rubber-box-toe dermatitis. This was formerly a common form of shoe allergy. (See color Plate 8*A.*)   *B.* Heel dermatitis in a patient allergic to black rubber. This patient also reacted to a black watchband.   *C.* Allergic contact dermatitis to elastic in stretch loafers. (See color Plate 8*B.*)   *D.* Insole dermatitis in a rubber-allergic patient. (See color Plate 8*C.*)   *E.* Positive patch test to shoes in the patient illustrated in *D.   F.* Contact to Indian buffalo-hide sandal straps. This is thought to be a reaction to vegetable-tanned leather.   *G.* Thiuram sensitivity in a patient with allergy to rubber gloves. *H.* Reaction to *p-tert* butylphenol formaldehyde resin, a component of the adhesive often used with sponge rubber insoles.

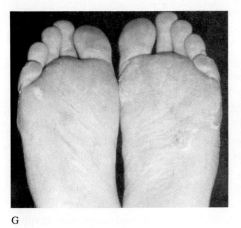 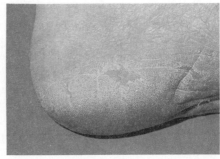

G   H

FIG. 31–1. (*Continued*)

The average shoe consists of the following components:

1. Shoe uppers
2. Shoe sole
3. Shoe insoles
4. Heel and toe counters

These components are all bound together by various types of adhesive chemicals.

SHOE UPPERS

Shoe uppers, particularly in the last few years, have undergone a dramatic metamorphosis in that prior to the advent of athletic footwear, virtually all shoes contained leather uppers, either of a vegetable-tanned nature or, alternatively, of a chromate-tanned nature. However, nowadays shoe uppers can contain a vast range of synthetic materials, including polyurethane and neoprene foam. It is important to have a working knowledge of the types of chemicals contained in each different type of upper.

Leather is tanned by a two-stage process.[3] Chrome tanning is the most common tanning process in use. However, an upper which is chrome-tanned is also retanned and may be retanned by one of the other methods which include vegetable tanning, synthetic tanning, alum tanning, and formaldehyde tanning. Vegetable tanning has become less common nowadays, but it does have a role in footwear manufacture. It tends to yield a highly resilient and water-resistant leather but also a leather which is harder, less malleable and therefore more difficult to work with than either chrome-tanned leather or synthetic-tanned leather. The vegetable tannins are all plant or fruit extracts; the particular ones in use today are quebracho, wattle, myrobolans, and chestnut extracts. These are wood extracts which are approximately 60 percent tannins. Vegetable-tanned leather tends to be found particularly in shoe soles rather than shoe uppers nowadays. It is also less used for economic reasons in that vegetable tanning is a long slow process taking approximately 3 weeks, compared with other methods of tanning which would take only a matter of hours or up to 2 days. Chrome tanning, which is the most common type, exposes the wearer to the allergen potassium dichromate. Formaldehyde or alum tanning is carried out using formaldehyde or glutaraldehyde, and this yields a shoe which is particularly water-resistant. Synthetic tanning is usually used as a final or secondary tannage, and this tends to utilize chemicals such as naphthalene sulfonic acid and phenol resins, dimethylol urea, dicyandiamide, and melamine formaldehyde resin. Tanning is the initial process in leather manufacture and is followed by a series of steps to yield a malleable, resilient material which will conform to modern wishes of appearance of the leather upper in terms of the finishing that nowadays leather has to undergo in order to compete in the high-fashion stakes.

Tanning is followed by an oiling process, using oils such as cod liver oil, synthetic moellon oil, and sulfonated neatsfoot oil. Dyeing is the next process, followed by finishing. The finish combines several steps which are mainly designed to produce the final appearance of the leather with a variety of agents such as metal stains, acrylic resins, nitrocellulose finishes, and water-repellent coats. All these steps may involve chemicals that can cause sensitization and footwear dermatitis.

Leather uppers have been largely replaced in recent years, particularly in our young population, by the foam uppers of athletic footwear. These foams tend to be either polyurethane or neoprene. Polyurethane is a relatively inert substance. A wide range of chemicals is used in its manufacture. A majority of these are totally polymerized or are absent at the time of wearing. However, it is possible that some of the catalysts involved in the polyurethane reaction persist as possible allergens. Common catalysts in use at present in the polyurethane chemical industry are the tertiary or quaternary amines. Another common foam material is neoprene. Neoprene foam is actually rubber foam, as neoprene is a synthetic rubber agent.[4] Table 31-1 lists the various different chemicals and their titles which are used in rubber manufacture. Table 31-2 lists the actual ingredients of neoprene itself. These, therefore, are the chemicals which should be used when testing usually a patient who has presented with a dorsal foot dermatitis and who continually wears athletic type footwear.[5-8] At the time of patch testing, it is important also to test portions of the sponge removed from the upper. Frequently, unfortunately, a positive reaction may be obtained to the sponge with totally negative reactions to the specific allergens leading to great difficulty in identifying the causative allergen.

TABLE 31–1. Chemicals Used in Rubber Manufacture

Vulcanizers	Diorthotolyl guanidine
	Dicumyl peroxide
Accelerators	Ethylene thiourea
Antioxidants	Octylated diphenylamines
	2,2,4-Trimethyl-1,2-dihydroquinoline
	Butylated hydroxytoluene
	Diphenylamines
Pigment	Titanium dioxide
Resins	Coumarone indene resins
	Terpene phenolic resins
	p-tert-Butylphenol formaldehyde resin
Blowing agents	Azodicarbonamide
	4,4-Oxybis (benzenesulfonylhydrazide)

TABLE 31–2. Neoprene Formulation

Chlorinated rubber (neoprene)
Phenolic resin (*p-tert*-butylphenol formaldehyde resin
  or terpene phenolic resin)
Magnesium oxide
Zinc oxide
Ethylene thiourea
Dioctyl-4-phenylenediamine
Fillers: sodium/calcium silicate
Tetramethylthiuram disulfide
Diorthotolyl guanidine
Sodium dibutyldithiocarbamate

SHOE SOLES

Most of the substances used in shoe uppers can also be used in shoe soles (i.e., either chrome- or vegetable-tanned leather or alternatively neoprene or polyurethane in the solid form). Therefore the various chemicals used for testing the shoe uppers will be relevant also to the soles. Other types of rubber may also be used in shoe sole manufacture. There are many different types of rubbers, which tend to have different properties which are used to advantage by the manufacturer.[8] The most commonly used types for shoe soles are natural rubber or polybutadiene rubber.

SHOE INSOLES

Shoe insoles are an extremely important part of the shoe in allergic contact dermatitis. It is important, however, to make a differential diagnosis at this stage in that there are a lot of constitutional causes of plantar dermatosis. If the distribution of the rash is in the sole of the foot with sparing of the toe creases, a diagnosis of allergic contact dermatitis to the shoe insole should not be ignored. Shoe insoles, once again, can be made of leather—chrome- or vegetable-tanned—or of polyurethane or neoprene foam. Another material in use in cheaper shoes particularly is a fiberboard material. This is a composite material usually made of paper fibers or occasionally wood or even leather fibers which are solidified in a glue matrix. Fiberboard, therefore, tends to open a wide range of possibilities of allergens causing plantar foot dermatitis, including leather chemicals, rubber chemicals, adhesive chemicals, and biocides.[9-13]

ADHESIVES

Adhesives used in footwear include the following:

1. Hot metal adhesives
2. Latex adhesives
3. Urethane adhesives
4. Neoprene adhesives

Hot metal adhesives are high-molecular-weight polymers of no importance as causative agents of allergic contact dermatitis. Latex adhesives are natural rubber in solution and are therefore found in all the rubber chemicals. Neoprene and urethane adhesives similarly implicate chemicals used in neoprene and urethane manufacture. The adhesives are used throughout the shoe and therefore can cause dermatitis in any distribution on the foot, dorsal or plantar.

HEEL AND TOE COUNTERS

If a shoe is to retain its shape, it is necessary to stiffen it at the toe and heel; this leads to the addition of what are known as heel and toe counters. These can vary from very complex structures right down to a simple layer of hot-melt adhesive in the inside of the toe or heel of the shoe. Chemicals that can be used to make heel and toe counters include, again, mainly the adhesive chemicals and also substances such as phenol formaldehyde resin, melamine formaldehyde, and urea formaldehyde resin.

MANAGEMENT OF FOOTWEAR-ALLERGIC DERMATITIS

As mentioned at the start of this chapter, a diagnosis of footwear-allergic contact dermatitis is made based on the patient's history, the onset of the rash in relation to a particular type of footwear, and the distribution of the rash. It is particularly helpful if the patient is presenting early on in the disease, prior to the development of a more widespread eczematization. Having made a working diagnosis, it is important then for the clinician to take a careful history from the patient about his or her footwear and preferably, if possible, have the patient bring all the types of footwear used to the clinic for examination and possible patch testing. Any troublesome pair should be identified by the patient and be particularly selected for testing of small portions of the areas of shoe corresponding to the areas of dermatitis, taking care again, as mentioned above, to apply thin slivers of the material in question to the back in order to prevent a spurious frictional reaction. Patch testing should then be carried out. It is also important to patch test these patients to the standard battery as—despite all the problems mentioned above of the changing world of shoe manufacture and our ignorance in terms of the specific chemicals involved in footwear—a reasonable percentage of cases of footwear-allergic contact dermatitis may be diagnosed using the standard tray. That series contains potassium dichromate, covering leather allergy; mercaptobenzothiazole, thiuram, and other rubber antigens; and particularly butyl phenol formaldehyde.[14–17] Any of these can be culprits in footwear-allergic contact dermatitis. The standard battery also contains some biocides that may be encountered in footwear.[9–13] If there has been a positive reaction to any portion of the patient's own shoes, the manufacturer of these should be contacted and consulted about the exact ingredients of the portion of the shoes that caused a positive reaction. More extensive patch testing can be carried out to the chemicals listed in Table 31-3. These chemicals are not yet readily available and can even be difficult to obtain and difficult to maintain in the correct concentrations. A list of the areas in which they are found is included in Table 31-3. This provides advice which can be given to the patient on what type of footwear to avoid. However in the absence of a positive diagnosis of the causative allergen, it is still important to try to help the patient identify the specific types of footwear that may be causing problems so that they can be avoided. Sources of specialty shoes are given in Table 34-6 (Chap. 34).

TABLE 31–3. Extended Shoe Chemical Tray

Toluene sulfonamide formaldehyde resin	10% pet.
4,4'-Diaminodiphenylmethane	0.5% pet
2,2,4-Trimethyl-1,2-dihydroquinoline	1% pet.
1H-Benzotriazole	1% pet.
4,4'-Dithiomorpholine	1% pet.
Coumarone indene resin	20% pet.
Terpene phenolic resin	20% pet.
Tetramethyl butanediamine	1% pet.
N-Octyl-4-isothiazolin-3-one 8% in propylene glycol 92% (Kathon LP)	0.1% pet.
Bismuth neodecanoate	1% pet.
N,N-Diethyl thiourea	1% pet.
Ethylbutyl thiourea	1% pet.
N,N-Dibutyl thiourea	1% pet.
3-Methyl thiazolidine 2-thion (Vulcacit CRU)	1% pet.
Ethylene thiourea	1% pet.
Disperse orange 3	1% pet.
Disperse yellow 3	1% pet.
Copper 8-quinolinolate	1% pet.
Diorthotolyl guanidine	1% pet.
Dioctyl phthalate	5% pet.
N-Dodecyl mercaptan	0.1% pet.
Glutaraldehyde	1% aq.
Urea-formaldehyde resin	10% pet.
Dicyandiamide	0.1% aq.
Toluene sulphonhydrazide	0.5% alc.
Dimethylaminoethyl ether (Niax1)	1% pet.
Azodicarbonamide (Azobisformamide)	0.5% pet.

JUVENILE PLANTAR DERMATOSIS

Juvenile plantar dermatosis is a fascinating condition found more commonly in young boys than young girls, the age ranging between 5 and 12. It is occasionally seasonal in nature but follows a very specific clinical pattern.[18] The children affected all have involvement of the plantar surfaces of their feet in a contact distribution, with sparing of the toe creases and of the insteps. The skin becomes atrophic and shiny and easily hacked. There can be severe blistering, which tends virtually always to be accompanied by extreme discomfort, leading to the child having difficulty even in walking. To date no specific allergic cause has been found, although the morphological appearance certainly fits with an allergic contact dermatitis. It is a condition which is more common in children who either have themselves a history of atopy or, alternatively, have a family history of atopy. It is a condition that does tend to disappear with time, and no specific causative allergen has been identified as yet. It may be possible that these children are reacting to a chemical which we have not yet identified in the footwear or alternatively to a combination of chemicals. Certainly the warm, humid environment of the shoe is a major contributing factor, as improvement can be obtained in these children by recommending the wearing of leather-lined shoes with leather uppers (preferably with the leather lining stitched and not glued in place), shoes slightly larger than necessary for the feet, leather insoles with leather soles, and the avoidance of dyed nylon socks. It is also thought that the common use of underfloor central heating in schools contributes to the problem.

CONCLUSION

In conclusion allergic contact dermatitis to footwear is a common and a difficult problem. Successful management requires careful history taking from and examination of the patient. Patch testing to the standard battery may be sufficient to yield a diagnosis of the causative allergen. However, further extensive patch testing may also be carried out. Unfortunately, the list of allergens used for testing at present is by no means complete, so the absence of a positive reaction should not be taken as excluding a diagnosis of allergic contact dermatitis. Juvenile plantar dermatosis is a specific entity which tends to affect young boys in particular; it may be seasonal in incidence and tends to be found in families with a higher incidence of atopy. Clinically, it is a condition which would suggest allergic contact dermatitis, but to date no specific causative allergen has been found.

REFERENCES

1. Storrs F: Dermatitis from clothing and shoes, in Fisher AA (ed): *Contact Dermatitis,* 3d ed. Philadelphia, Lea & Febiger, 1980, p 283.
2. Cronin E: *Contact Dermatitis.* Edinburgh, Churchill Livingstone, 1980.
3. Thorstensen TC: *Practical Leather Technology,* 3d ed. Melbourne, FL, Krieger Publishing Co., 1985.
4. Rabbit RO: *The Vanderbilt Rubber Handbook.* Norwalk, CT, Vanderbilt, 1978.
5. Roberts JL, Hanifin JM: Athletic shoe dermatitis, contact allergy to ethylbutyl thiourea. *JAMA* 241:275, 1979.
6. Roberts JL, Hanifin JM: Contact allergy and cross reactivity to substituted thiourea compounds. *Contact Dermatitis* 6:138, 1980.
7. Bruze M, Fregert S: Allergic contact dermatitis from ethylene thiourea. *Contact Dermatitis* 9:208, 1983.
8. Camarsqa JE, Romaguera C, Conde Salazar L, et al: Thiourea reactivity in Spain. *Contact Dermatitis* 12:220, 1985.
9. Bang Pedersen N: Occupational allergy from 1,2-benziothiazolin-3-one and other preservatives in plastic emulsions. *Contact Dermatitis* 2:340, 1976.
10. Thormann J: Contact dermatitis to a new fungicide, 2-n-octyl-4-isothiazolin-3-one. *Contact Dermatitis* 8:204, 1982.
11. Mathias TCG, Andersen KE, Hamann K: Allergic contact dermatitis from 2-n-octyl-4-isothiazolin-3-one, a paint mildewicide. *Contact Dermatitis* 9:507, 1983.
12. Anderson KE, Veien N: Biocide patch tests. *Contact Dermatitis* 12:99, 1985.
13. Pilger C, Nethercott JR, Weksberg F: Allergic contact dermatitis due to a biocide containing 5-chloro-2-methyl-4-isothizolin-3-one. *Contact Dermatitis* 14:201, 1986.
14. Malten K, Seutter E: Allergenic degradation products of paratertiary butyl phenol formaldehyde plastic. *Contact Dermatitis* 12:222, 1985.
15. Malten KE, Rath R, Pasters HM: Paratertiary butyl phenol formaldehyde and other causes of shoe dermatitis. *Dermatosen* 31:149, 1983.
16. Malten KE: Contact sensitisations caused by para-tertiary butyl phenol and certain phenol formaldehyde-containing glues. *Dermatologica* 135:541, 1967.
17. Foussereau J, Cavalier C, Selig D: Occupational eczema from paratertiary butylphenol formaldehyde resins: A review of the sensitising resins. *Contact Dermatitis* 2:254, 1976.
18. Rook, Wilkinson, Ebling: in Champion RH, Burton JL, Ebling FJG (eds): *Textbook of Dermatology,* 5th ed. London, Blackwell Scientific, 1992.

32

COSMETICS

Anton C. de Groot

WHAT ARE COSMETICS?

According to U.S. regulations, the Federal Food, Drug, and Cosmetic (FD&C) Act defines cosmetics as *articles intended to be applied to the human body for cleansing, beautifying, promoting attractiveness, or altering the appearance without affecting the body's structure or functions.* Included in this definition are products such as skin creams, lotions, perfumes, lipsticks, fingernail polishes, eye and facial makeup preparations, shampoos, permanent waves, hair colors, toothpastes, and deodorants. Cosmetics marketed in the United States, whether manufactured here or imported from abroad, must be in compliance with the provisions of the FD&C Act, the Fair Packaging and Labeling Act, and the regulations published under the authority of these laws.

Products that are cosmetics but are also intended to treat or prevent disease or affect the structure or function of the human body are also considered drugs. Examples are anticaries toothpastes (e.g., fluoride toothpastes), sunscreen preparations intended to protect against sunburn, antiperspirants that are also deodorants, and antidandruff shampoos. These products must comply with both the drug and cosmetic provisions of the law.[1]

FREQUENCY AND NATURE OF ADVERSE REACTIONS TO COSMETICS

Cosmetic products are used by nearly everyone. Although serious adverse reactions are rare, side effects do occur. Adverse reactions include the following[2]: irritation (subjective and/or objective), contact allergy, photosensitivity, immediate contact reactions (contact urticaria), acne/folliculitis, (unintentional) color changes of the skin and appendages, and (rarely) systemic side effects. In an epidemiologic study among 1609 individuals of the general population in the Netherlands, it was found that over 12 percent (men, 9 percent; women, 16 percent) had experienced side effects that were attributed to cosmetic products in the preceding 5 years.[3] In clients of beauticians, this percentage was 25.[4] Most reactions were caused by irritation, notably from personal cleanliness products such as soaps, shampoos, bath foams, and deodorants. Contact allergy was estimated to have been the cause of the reaction in approximately 10 percent of all cases.[4]

In dermatologic practice, allergy to cosmetic products has been diagnosed in 0.6 percent of all referrals and in 5 to 10 percent of all patients suspected of having allergic contact dermatitis.[5,6] The percentage of the general population that is allergic to cosmetics or cosmetic ingredients has been roughly estimated at 2 to 3 percent of adults.[6]

In this chapter, only contact allergic dermatitis as a side effect of cosmetics is discussed.

CLINICAL PICTURE OF ALLERGIC COSMETIC DERMATITIS

The clinical picture of allergic cosmetic dermatitis depends on the type of products used (and, consequently, the sites of application) and the degree of the patient's sensitivity. Usually, cosmetics and their ingredients are weak allergens and the dermatitis resulting from cosmetic allergy is mild: erythema, mild edema, desquamation, and papules. Weeping vesicular dermatitis rarely occurs, although some products, especially the permanent hair dyes, may cause fierce reactions. Allergic reactions to the permanent dyes are usually most prominent on the face and ears rather than on the scalp (Figs. 32-1 and 32-2).

Contact allergic dermatitis from cosmetic products can sometimes be recognized easily. Examples include reactions to deodorant, eyeshadow, perfume, and lipstick (Figs. 32-3 and 32-4). In more than half of all cases, however, the diagnosis of cosmetic allergy is suspected neither by the patient nor the physician.[5,7] The typical patient suffering from allergic cosmetic dermatitis is a woman aged 20 to 45 with mild erythema, edema, and scaling of the eyelids (Fig. 32-5). The face itself is also frequently

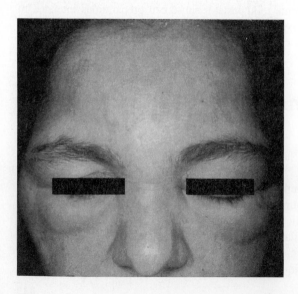

FIG. 32–1. Allergic cosmetic dermatitis of the face with strong periorbital edema due to hair-dye allergy. (See color Plate 9.)

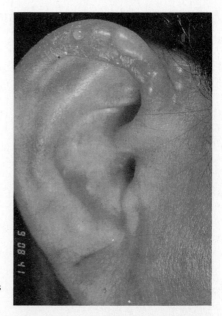

FIG. 32-2. Bullous cosmetic dermatitis on the ears due to hair-dye allergy. (See color Plate 10.)

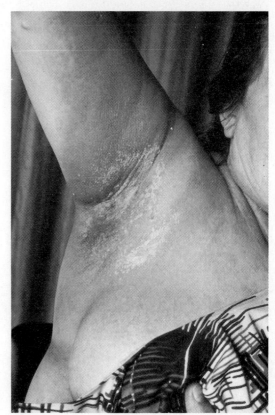

FIG. 32-3. Allergic contact dermatitis from a deodorant. (See color Plate 11.)

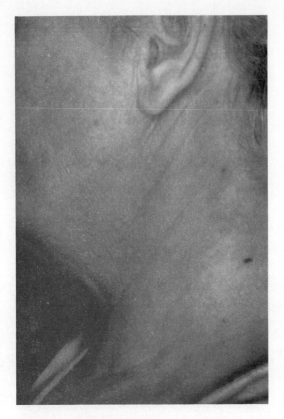

FIG. 32–4. Allergic contact dermatitis from perfume. (See color Plate 12.)

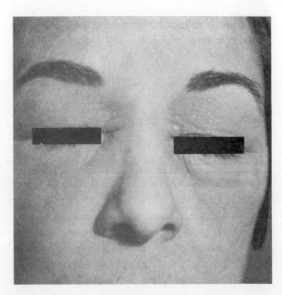

FIG. 32–5. Allergic cosmetic dermatitis: typical example of mild involvement of the eyelids. (See color Plate 13.)

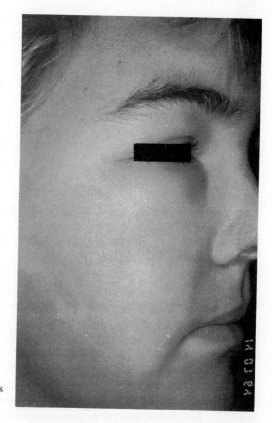

FIG. 32–6. Allergic cosmetic dermatitis involving the face. (See color Plate 14.)

involved (Fig. 32-6); often the dermatitis is limited to the face and/or eyelids. Other common sites for cosmetic dermatitis are the neck, arms, and hands. However, all parts of the body may be involved. Most often, the cosmetics have been applied to previously healthy skin (especially on the face), nails, or hair. However, allergic cosmetic dermatitis may also be caused by products used on previously damaged skin, notably irritant contact dermatitis (hands) and atopic dermatitis (hands, arms, and legs).[5]

PRODUCTS CAUSING ALLERGIC COSMETIC DERMATITIS

In general, most reactions are caused by "stay-on" or "leave-on" products (i.e., cosmetics which remain on the skin after application). Cosmetic products of the "rinse-off" variety such as shampoo, soap, bath and shower foam, and toothpaste infrequently cause allergic reactions. This applies to both sensitization to such products and to elicitation of contact dermatitis in sensitized subjects. This may conveniently be explained by the low concentration of possible allergens by dilution of the products under normal circumstances of use and by the relatively short contact time with the skin.

Several studies performed in various countries such as the United States,[7,8] the Netherlands,[5] Sweden,[9] Spain,[10] and France[11] have investigated the cosmetic products responsible for allergic cosmetic dermatitis. The results have varied considerably, probably reflecting different patterns of cosmetic usage and the sample size; for a summary, see Ref. 2. In the study performed by the members of the North American Contact Dermatitis Group (NACDG),[7] 578 patients were allergic to 600 products. Most reactions were caused by skin-care products, followed by hair cosmetics, facial makeup products, nail cosmetics (lacquers and hardeners), fragrance products, shaving preparations, and eye makeup products (Table 32-1). Of course, trends in cosmetic usage (e.g., the growing cosmetic market for men and the development of new products such as "kiddy cosmetics" and hair gel) may influence the situation.

ALLERGENS

Only two studies[5,7] have systematically investigated the allergens in cosmetic products by patch testing patients with proven cosmetic-related allergic contact dermatitis with some or all of the ingredients of the responsible products. In both studies, fragrances and preservatives were the most common allergens. During 64 months (1977 to 1983), the members of the NACDG studied 578 patients with proven cosmetic allergy.[7] To identify the causative ingredients, 403 patients (70 percent) were patch tested with some (273 patients) or all (130 patients) the ingredients. This resulted in the identification of 87 ingredients or classes of ingredients that had caused allergic cosmetic dermatitis (Tables 32-2 and 32-3).

Of the functional classes of cosmetic ingredients, fragrances caused most reactions, followed by preservatives and antioxidants, hair colors, nail lacquer resins and acrylates, lanolin and its derivatives, permanent waving agents, and sunscreens (Table 32-2). Of the individual ingredients identified as allergens, most were unspecified fragrances, followed by quaternium-15, p-phenylenediamine, glyceryl thioglycolate, propylene glycol, toluenesulfonamide/formaldehyde resin, imidazolidinyl urea, parabens, cinnamic alcohol, 2-bromo-2-nitropropane-1,3-diol, formaldehyde, and lanolin (Table 32-3). More recently, attention has focused on the preservative methylisothiazolinone/methylchloroisothiazolinone (Kathon CG) as an important contact allergen.[12-14] In some

TABLE 32–1. Products Responsible for Allergic Cosmetic Dermatitis in 578 U.S. Patients

Products, $N = 600$	Number and Percentage[a] of Reactions	
Skin care products	175	(29)
Hair cosmetics	143	(24)
Facial makeup	61	(10)
Nail cosmetics	53	(9)
Fragrances	43	(7)
Shaving preparations	21	(4)
Eye makeup	18	(3)
Other products	86	(14)

[a]Percentages in parentheses.
Source: Adams and Maibach.[7]

TABLE 32–2. Ingredients Responsible for Cosmetic Allergy in 578 U.S. Patients

Class		Number of Reactions
Fragrances		162
Fragrance, unspecified	67	
Cinnamic alcohol	17	
Hydroxycitronellal	11	
Musk ambrette	11	
Isoeugenol	10	
Geraniol	8	
Cinnamic aldehyde	6	
Others (4 or less)	32	
Preservatives and antioxidants		161
Quaternium-15	65	
Imidazolidinyl urea	21	
Parabens, unspecified	19	
2-Bromo-2-nitropropane-1,3-diol	16	
Formaldehyde	16	
Sorbic acid	6	
Others (3 or less)	18	
Hair Colors		45
p-Phenylenediamine	41	
Resorcinol	3	
2-Nitro-p-phenylenediamine	1	
Nail lacquer resins and acrylates		32
Toluenesulfonamide/formaldehyde resin	23	
Ethyl methacrylate	5	
Other (meth)acrylates	4	
Lanolin (derivates)		31
Lanolin	15	
Lanolin alcohol	12	
Lanolin oil	2	
Others	2	
Permanent waving agents		26
Glyceryl thioglycolate	25	
Thioglycolate (unspecified)	1	
Sunscreens		21
Glyceryl PABA	5	
Octyl dimethyl PABA	5	
PABA	3	
Others (2 or less)	8	
Miscellaneous		28

Source: Adams and Maibach.[7]

European countries, this preservative became one of the most important contact allergens and the most frequent cause of allergic cosmetic dermatitis[5,12–14]; but it is now also becoming an important contact allergen in the United States.[15–17] Other "new" cosmetic sensitizers include diazolidinyl urea,[18,19] methyldibromoglutaronitrile,[20,21] the dibenzoylmethanes,[22,23] and cocamidopropyl betaine.[24]

TABLE 32-3. Most Frequent Causative Ingredients in 578 U.S. Patients with Cosmetic Allergy

Ingredient	Function	Number of Reactions
Fragrance (unspecified)	Fragrance	67
Quaternium-15	Preservative	65
p-Phenylenediamine	Hair color	41
Glyceryl thioglycolate	Permanent-waving agent	25
Propylene glycol	Humectant/moisturizer	25
Toluenesulfonamide/formaldehyde resin	Nail lacquer resin	23
Imidazolidinyl urea	Preservative	21
Parabens	Preservatives	19
Cinnamic alcohol	Fragrance	17
2-Bromo-2-nitropropane-1,3-diol	Preservative	16
Formaldehyde	Preservative	16
Lanolin	Moisturizer/emulsifier	15
Lanolin alcohol	Moisturizer/emulsifier	12
Hydroxycitronellal	Fragrance	11
Musk ambrette	Fragrance	11
Isoeugenol	Fragrance	10

Source: Adams and Maibach.[7]

FRAGRANCES

Fragrances are the most frequent cause of cosmetic allergy, both from products primarily used for their scent (perfumes, colognes, eaux de toilette, aftershave, deodorants) and from other scented products. Occasionally, patients allergic to fragrances experience flares of their dermatitis caused by ingestion of these chemicals as flavorings in foods and beverages.[25] Perfumes contain 12 to 20 percent of the perfume compound, colognes 2 to 5 percent, perfume lotions and perfume de toilette 5 to 8 percent, and other cosmetics 0.2 to 1 percent. A fragrance may consist of 10 to 300 fragrance components. The exact allergen is usually not identified, but when it is, most reactions are caused by isoeugenol, eugenol, oak moss absolute, cinnamic alcohol, cinnamic aldehyde, and hydroxycitronellal. Musk ambrette, used as a fragrance fixative, has been responsible for many cases of contact allergy and especially photocontact allergy[26] (see also Chap. 33).

PRESERVATIVES

Preservatives[27-29] (see also Chap. 40) are added to water-containing cosmetics to inhibit the growth of nonpathogenic and pathogenic microorganisms, which may cause degradation of the product or endanger the health of the consumer.

Formaldehyde

Formaldehyde is a frequent sensitizer and a ubiquitous allergen. Routine testing in patients with suspected allergic contact dermatitis yields prevalence rates of sensitization of over 6 percent in the United States,[30] but most cases are from noncosmetic sources.

The cosmetic industry uses free formaldehyde almost exclusively in rinse-off products, which rarely gives rise to cosmetic allergy. This antigen is discussed in Chap. 20, and Fransway has reviewed formaldehyde-related preservative allergy.[27,28]

Formaldehyde Donors

Formaldehyde donors are preservatives that, in the presence of water, release formaldehyde. Therefore, cosmetics preserved with such chemicals will contain free formaldehyde, the amount depending on the preservative used, its concentration, and the amount of water present in the product. Formaldehyde donors used in cosmetics and toiletries include quaternium-15, imidazolidinyl urea, diazolidinyl urea, 2-bromo-2-nitropropane-1,3-diol, and DMDM hydantoin. Quaternium-15 releases the most and imidazolidinyl urea the least free formaldehyde.[31] Contact allergy to formaldehyde donors may be due to the preservative itself or to formaldehyde sensitivity. For a review, see Refs. 27 and 28. The formaldehyde donors appear to be gaining in popularity as preservatives in cosmetics. Formaldehyde, however, has largely been replaced by other chemicals, because it is suspected (when inhaled as a gas) of being a possible human carcinogen.[32]

QUATERNIUM-15 (DOWICIL 200). Quaternium-15 is the most frequent preservative sensitizer in cosmetic products.[7] Routine testing by the NACDG yielded a prevalence rate of 6.2 percent in patients suspected of allergic contact dermatitis.[30] Half of these reactions may be caused by formaldehyde sensitivity.[33] At the commonly used concentration of 0.1%, quaternium-15 releases about 100 ppm free formaldehyde, which in many formaldehyde-sensitive patients is sufficient to cause allergic cosmetic dermatitis.

IMIDAZOLIDINYL UREA (GERMALL 115). Imidazolidinyl urea releases little formaldehyde and consequently poses little threat to formaldehyde-sensitive subjects. In the United States, the prevalence rate of contact allergy to imidazolidinyl urea is 2 percent.[30] Cross-reactions to and from the related preservative diazolidinyl urea may be observed.[18]

DIAZOLIDINYL UREA (GERMALL II). Diazolidinyl urea is chemically related to imidazolidinyl urea.[18] It has been in use only since 1982 and is the most active preservative of the imidazolidinyl urea group. Routine testing by the NACDG resulted in a prevalence rate of sensitization of 2.4 percent in patients suspected of having allergic contact dermatitis.[30] Diazolidinyl urea appears to be a stronger sensitizer than imidazolidinyl urea.[34] Patients allergic to this preservative may or may not react to formaldehyde.[18]

2-BROMO-2-NITROPROPANE-1,3-DIOL (BRONOPOL). Bronopol has been responsible for so many cases of allergic cosmetic dermatitis from Eucerin cream in the United States that the manufacturer decided to replace it.[35,36] Another concern is that its interaction with amines and amides can result in the formation of nitrosamines and nitrosamides, which are suspected to be carcinogens. In Europe, Bronopol is an infrequent sensitizer.[37]

DMDM HYDANTOIN. DMDM hydantoin (dimethylol dimethyl hydantoin, Glydant) has so far not been implicated as causing cosmetic allergy. However, it has been demonstrated that some patients allergic to formaldehyde may react upon patch testing to DMDM hydantoin.[38] In addition, provocation tests with a cream containing 0.25% w/w

DMDM hydantoin in formaldehyde-sensitive subjects elicited a positive response in some of them, indicating that patients who are allergic to formaldehyde may be at risk of developing allergic cosmetic dermatitis from products preserved with DMDM hydantoin.[38]

Parabens

The paraben esters (benzyl, butyl, ethyl, methyl, propyl) are the most widely used preservatives in cosmetic products and may be considered very safe from an allergologic point of view,[39] especially in the low concentrations used in cosmetics. In Europe, routine testing with the parabens yields low rates of sensitization (less than 1 percent),[40] and in the United States they are not tested in the NACDG routine series.[30] Most cases of sensitization to parabens are caused from the use of topical pharmaceutical preparations on eczematous skin or leg ulcers. For a review of paraben sensitivity, see Ref. 29.

Methyl(Chloro)Isothiazolinone (MI/MCI, Kathon CG)

MI/MCI is a preservative system containing, as active ingredients, a mixture of methylchloroisothiazolinone and methylisothiazolinone. The most widely used commercial product is Kathon CG (where CG denotes cosmetic grade), which contains 1.5 percent active ingredients. In recent years, this highly effective preservative has become a major cause of cosmetic allergy in most European countries.[5] The subject has been reviewed.[12–14] In the United States, prevalence rates of 1.7 to 1.9 percent (NACDG[15,17]) and 3.6 percent (Mayo Clinic[16]) have been observed. The use concentration of MI/MCI is mostly between 3 to 15 ppm, which is usually far below the threshold for detection of allergy with patch tests, indicating that most allergic patients will not react to the product upon patch testing. Therefore, MCI/MI always has to be tested separately (100 ppm water) whenever cosmetic allergy is suspected.

HAIR COLORS

Hair colors may be temporary, semipermanent, or permanent. Most cases of cosmetic allergy from hair dyes are caused by the (permanent) oxidation dyes of the para- type (p-phenylenediamine and related dyes). In recent years, the incidence of dermatitis due to hair dyes containing p-phenylenediamine (derivatives) appears to have decreased. This is attributed to the provision of cautionary notices on the product, awareness of the risk, patch testing of the product by future users, improvements in the technical quality of the cosmetic product, and improvements in the technique of application of these dyes. Nevertheless, p-phenylenediamine remains an important cause of cosmetic allergy,[7] since 6.4 percent of all patients routinely tested by the NACDG reacted to it.[30] These oxidation dyes are also an occupational hazard for hairdressers and beauticians.[41] The chemistry of and adverse reactions to oxidation coloring agents have been reviewed[42] (see also Chap. 13).

GLYCERYL THIOGLYCOLATE

Glyceryl thioglycolate, a waving agent used in acid permanent-waving products, may sensitize consumers,[7,43] but it is usually an occupational hazard for the hairdresser.[41,44] Patients allergic to glyceryl thioglycolate infrequently react to ammonium thioglycolate, the chemical traditionally used in permanent wave procedures.

PROPYLENE GLYCOL

Propylene glycol (1,2-propanediol) is widely used as a vehicle for pharmaceutical preparations. In cosmetics, it acts as humectant (or moisturizer), as it is capable of retaining moisture over a wide range of relative humidity. The literature on irritant and allergic reactions to propylene glycol has been reviewed.[29,45] A major problem with testing for possible allergy is the optimal test concentration and the differentiation between irritant and allergic test responses. The NACDG currently recommends a 10 percent aqueous propylene glycol solution for patch testing. Allergic contact sensitization may be confirmed by repeated patch testing, usage tests, or oral provocation in selected cases. Given the nearly universal presence of propylene glycol in topical preparations and cosmetics, it may be very hard for allergic persons to avoid.

TOLUENESULFONAMIDE/FORMALDEHYDE RESIN AND ACRYLATES

Toluenesulfonamide/formaldehyde resin (TSFR) is the usual resin in the majority of nail varnishes (lacquers and nail hardeners). It is used in preference to the less allergenic polyester resins because it is resistant to chipping. It is a common cause of cosmetic allergy.[5,7,46] Contact allergy to the resin manifests itself as patchy dermatitis in the neck or on the eyelids (resembling seborrheic dermatitis), or on the upper chest, the external auditory meatus, the vulva, and the anus. Although the user avoids contaminating the fingers, the dermatitis may also be located there. Patients allergic to formaldehyde usually have no problems when using nail lacquers based on TSFR, because the amount of free formaldehyde is minimal. Sculptured nails based on methyl methacrylate can cause a nail varnish dermatitis and nail dystrophy in sensitized individuals.[47]

LANOLIN (DERIVATIVES)

Lanolin and lanolin derivatives are used extensively in cosmetic products as emollients and emulsifiers. The allergens are the wool alcohols. In the United States, the NACDG found a prevalence rate of 1.5 percent positive reactions in eczema patients.[30] Most cases are caused by topical pharmaceutical preparations containing it, especially those used for treating varicose ulcers and stasis dermatitis. The presence of lanolin (derivatives) in cosmetics rarely sensitizes patients, but patients who have been presensitized may experience cosmetic allergy from using cosmetics containing lanolin or its derivatives.[48] Chemical modification may enhance its safety.[49] Avoidance of contact with lanolin (derivatives) often leads to disappearance of sensitivity.[50]

SUNSCREENS

As drugs, sunscreens are used to prevent sunburn and photosensitive dermatoses such as herpes labialis and chronic polymorphic light eruption (CPLE). In cosmetics, they are added to protect the user's skin but also to prevent the product from photodegradation. The main classes of sunscreens are PABA (*p*-aminobenzoic acid) and its esters (amyl dimethyl, glyceryl, octyl dimethyl), the cinnamates, the salicylates, the anthranilates, the benzophenones, and the dibenzoylmethanes.[51] The last category is gaining popularity, as it absorbs mainly in the UVA region (315 to 400 nm). UV filters have been identified with increasing frequency as allergens and photoallergens, but reactions to them remain uncommon. Photoallergic reactions can easily be overlooked, as the resulting dermatitis may be interpreted by the patient/consumer as failure of the product to protect against sunburn or as worsening of the photodermatosis for which the sunscreen was used. PABA is a common cause of photoallergic reactions. Recently, most such reactions have been caused by benzophenones[51] and the dibenzoylmethanes, isopropyl dibenzoylmethane, and butyl methoxydibenzoylmethane.[22,23] The literature on adverse reactions to sunscreens has been reviewed by Freeman[51] and Dromgoole and Maibach.[52]

OTHER ALLERGENS

Methyldibromoglutaronitrile is one of the active ingredients of the preservative system Euxyl K 400. Several cases of cosmetic allergy have recently been reported.[20,21,53] The negative publicity on methyl(chloro)isothiazolinone[12–14] has made many manufacturers of cosmetics look out for other preservatives, and Euxyl K 400 appears to be one of the most suitable candidates.

Cocamidopropyl betaine is a pseudo-amphoteric surfactant derived from trimethylglycine. It is reported as a sensitizer with increasing frequency in shampoos and other cosmetics.[24] A comprehensive literature review of cosmetic allergy is provided in Refs. 2 and 54.

DIAGNOSTIC PROCEDURES

The diagnosis of cosmetic allergy should strongly be suspected in any patient presenting with dermatitis of the face, eyelids, lips, and neck. Allergic contact dermatitis to cosmetics may develop on previously healthy skin of the face or on already damaged skin (irritant contact dermatitis, atopic dermatitis, seborrheic dermatitis, allergic contact dermatitis from other sources). Also, dermatitis of the arms and hands may be caused or worsened by skin-care products to treat or prevent dry skin and irritant or atopic dermatitis. Patchy dermatitis in the neck and around the eyes is suggestive of cosmetic allergy from nail lacquers or hardeners.[46] A thorough history of cosmetic usage should always be obtained. It must be stressed that most women think of "cosmetics" in terms of decorative cosmetics such as eye shadow, rouge, lipsticks, hair colors, and nail lacquers. Therefore, it is necessary to specifically inquire about products such as day and night cream, cleansers, removing pads, perfume, eye cream, etc. The "classic" cosmetic dermatitis of periorbital dermatitis may be caused by any product used on the hair, scalp, face, hands, and nails. Often, women are surprised to be informed about the possibility of cosmetic allergy, for three reasons: (1) they have already stopped using their cosmetics but without improvement; (2) they have already used the same products for many years without ill-effects; and (3) they have used "hypoallergenic products" or cosmetics which have been "dermatologically tested."

1. When specifically asked, patients often admit to having stopped using their eye cosmetics only (which is fairly logical in the case of dermatitis around the eyes), but they continued using other cosmetics on the face, such as skin-care products, which far more often are responsible for the reaction.[5,7] Skin-care products used on the face and/or hands may well cause dermatitis around the eyes in the absence of a reaction on the face. This may be explained by the extremely thin and sensitive skin of the eyelids.

2. Contact allergy is an acquired phenomenon; that is, the patient must have been in contact with the allergenic product for some time (and in the case of the weakly allergenic cosmetics, usually a long time) before sensitization takes place and allergic cosmetic dermatitis can develop.

3. Terms such as *hypoallergenic* and *dermatologically tested* have very little if any meaning. All cosmetic manufacturers obviously try to make their products as safe as possible, and such terms, which should be regarded as sales-promotion arguments, do not imply enhanced safety over other cosmetics bearing no such labels.

When the diagnosis of cosmetic allergy is suspected, patch tests should be performed to confirm the diagnosis and identify the sensitizer. Only in this manner can the patient be counseled about future use of cosmetic (and other) products and the prevention of recurrences of dermatitis from cosmetic or noncosmetic sources.[6] Patch tests should be performed with the NACDG routine series, a "cosmetic series" containing known cosmetic allergens and, of course, with all products used by the patient.

The NACDG routine series[30] contains a number of allergens which may cause allergic cosmetic dermatitis: rosin (colophony, an indicator for perfume allergy and a possible allergen in eyeshadow); the preservatives diazolidinyl urea, imidazolidinyl urea, formaldehyde, and quaternium-15; the fragrances cinnamic aldehyde, cinnamic alcohol, and balsam of Peru (indicator for perfume sensitivity); the hair color *p*-phenylenediamine; and lanolin alcohol. A suggested "cosmetic series" is shown in Table 32-4. Most of these allergens are available from Chemotechnique Diagnostics (Edvard Olsv. 2, P.O. Box 80, 230 42 Tygelsjö, Malmö, Sweden) or from Hermal Kurt Herrmann (D 21462 Reinbeck/Hamburg, Scholtzstrasse 3A, Federal Republic of Germany). Although the patient's products should always be tested (for test concentrations, see Table 32-5), patch testing with cosmetics has some important drawbacks. Patients often use many cosmetic products, which makes the investigation very laborious. More importantly, both false-negative and false-positive reactions occur frequently. A false-negative reaction means that the patient is allergic to a certain cosmetic but the patch-test reaction to the product itself remains negative. This is due to the low concentration of some allergens and the usually weak sensitivity of the patient. The product does cause allergic cosmetic dermatitis when applied repeatedly (e.g., daily), when applied to damaged (dry or eczematous) skin, or when applied to very sensitive skin (e.g., the eyelids). However, one application on the thick and intact skin of the back, even under occlusion (as is the case with patch testing) is insufficient to cause a positive patch-test reaction. Classic examples of false-negative reactions are with methyl(chloro)isothiazol-

(*text continues on page 349*)

ALLERGIC COSMETIC DERMATITIS—PATIENT HANDOUT

WHAT IS ALLERGIC COSMETIC DERMATITIS?

Allergic cosmetic dermatitis is an allergic reaction to a cosmetic product. Cosmetics include hair gel, permanent-wave solutions, hair color, skin-care products (creams, lotions, milks, tonics, both for moisturizing and cleansing purposes: face, eyelids, hands, body), eye makeup preparations (eye shadow, mascara, eyeliner), lipsticks, toothpastes, perfumes, personal cleanliness products (soap, shower and bath foam/gel), deodorants, and powder.

HOW LONG DOES IT TAKE TO BECOME ALLERGIC?

On first exposure, we are not allergic. We have to be in contact with a product for a considerable time (with cosmetics, usually months to years), before an allergic reaction can develop.

WHAT DOES ALLERGIC COSMETIC DERMATITIS LOOK LIKE?

Allergic contact dermatitis (eczema) can have many faces: in the acute form, it is characterized by redness and swelling of the skin, papules (pimples), vesicles (blisters), and weeping of the skin. Later, the dermatitis dries out, scaling develops, and painful chapping may be observed. In the case of allergic eczema caused by cosmetics, the dermatitis is usually localized around the eyes, with mild redness, swelling of the eyelids, and scaling. Itching is always present. The face and neck are also frequently involved. Dermatitis on the arms, hands, and armpits should also alert you to the possibility of a cosmetic reaction.

WHICH PRODUCTS CAUSE ALLERGIC REACTIONS?

"Wash-off" or "rinse-off" products such as soap, shampoo, and bath and shower foam rarely cause allergic reactions (however, they do frequently cause *irritant* reactions by irritating or drying out the skin, especially in the cold season and mainly in atopic persons, who have a familial tendency to eczema, asthma, or hay fever). Most allergic reactions are caused by skin-care products, hair cosmetics (colors, permanent waves), facial makeup, and perfumed products. Reactions around the eyes may be caused by any product used on the eyes, face, scalp/hair, or hands even if the rash is localized around the eyes only.

WHICH INGREDIENTS CAUSE THE ALLERGY?

The main ingredients in cosmetics which cause the allergic reaction (the "allergens") are fragrances (both in products used for their scent such as perfume, eau de cologne, and deodorant and in other scented cosmetics), preservatives, hair colors, glyceryl thioglycolate (in permanent waves), nail lacquer resins, and sunscreening agents (both in sunscreens to prevent sunburn and in other cosmetic products, notably skin-care products).

DO I HAVE TO CONSULT A DOCTOR WHEN I THINK I AM ALLERGIC TO COSMETICS?

Yes. First, a doctor can treat your condition, usually with a cortisone cream or ointment. This should clear the dermatitis in a few days, provided, of course, that you are no longer using the suspected cosmetics. Furthermore, your doctor will determine whether you are indeed allergic with the help of an allergologic examination. All cosmetic products used by you and many other possible allergens, both in cosmetics and other products, are applied to the skin of your back, fixed with tape and are left in place for 2 days. After 2 days, the materials are removed, and 20 minutes and 1 or 2 days later, the reactions are scored. Often, the dermatologist can tell you at that time to which products you are allergic, what the allergens are, which products you have to avoid in future to prevent new rashes. Sometimes, additional tests are necessary. Both the allergy investigations and the treatment are safe procedures.

HOW DO I PREVENT NEW RASHES?

This can only be done when you know to which substances (allergens) you are allergic. Your doctor will give you their names and lists of products to avoid. When you want to buy other cosmetic products, check their labels to make sure they do not contain the substances your dermatologist has instructed you to avoid.

TABLE 32–4. Suggested Allergens for a Cosmetic Screening Series

Allergen	Function	Test Concentration and Vehicle
Amerchol L 101	Emulsifier	50% pet
Benzophenone-3 (oxybenzone)	Sunscreen	2% pet
Benzophenone-10 (mexenone)	Sunscreen	2% pet
2-Bromo-2-nitropropane-1,3-diol (bronopol)	Preservative	0.5% pet
Cetearyl alcohol	Emulsifier	30% pet
Cocamidopropyl betaine	Surfactant	1% aqua
Fragrance-mix (ICDRG)	Fragrance	8 × 1% pet
Glyceryl thioglycolate	Permanent-waving agent	1% pet
4-Isopropyldibenzoylmethane	Sunscreen	2% pet
Methyl(chloro)isothiazolinone (Kathon CG)	Preservative	100 ppm in water
Methyldibromoglutaronitrile	Preservative	0.1% pet
Musk ambrette	Fragrance	5% pet
Octyl dimethyl PABA	Sunscreen	2% pet
PABA	Sunscreen	2% pet
Parabens	Preservatives	5 × 3% pet
Propylene glycol	Humectant	10% water
Toluenesulfonamide/formaldehyde resin	Nail lacquer resin	10% pet

TABLE 32–5. Recommended Test Concentrations for Cosmetic Products[a]

Cosmetic product	Test Concentration and Vehicle
Bleach	Ammonium persulfate 1% pet
Depilatory	Thioglycolate 1% pet
Foaming bath product	1% water
Foaming cleanser	1% water
Hair dyes	2% water
Mascara	Pure (allow to dry)
Nail cuticle remover	Individual ingredients
Nail glue	Individual ingredients
Nail polish	Pure (allow to dry)
Nail polish remover	Individual ingredients
Permanent-wave solution	Glyceryl thioglycolate 1% pet
Shampoo	1% water
Shaving lather or cream	1% water
Skin lightener	Hydroquinone 1% pet
Soap or detergent	1% water
Hair straightener	Individual ingredients
Toothpaste	2% water

[a]Most cosmetics not mentioned in this table can be tested undiluted.
Source: Adapted from de Groot, Weyland, and Nater[54] and Engasser and Maibach.[61]

TABLE 32–6. Possible Cross- or Pseudo-Cross-Reactions from Cosmetic Allergens

Allergen	Cross-Reactions
Balsam of Peru	Balsam of Tolu, beeswax, benzoin tincture, benzyl salicylate, fragrances, propolis, rosin (colophony), styrax
Benzophenones	Other benzophenones
Bronopol	Formaldehyde (donors)[a]
Cocamidopropyl betaine	Cocobetaine
Diazolidinyl urea	Formaldehyde (donors)[a], imidazolidinyl urea
DMDM hydantoin	Formaldehyde (donors)[a], MDM hydantoin

Formaldehyde	Formaldehyde donors:
	   bronopol
	   diazolidinyl urea
	   DMDM hydantoin
	   imidazolidinyl urea
	   quaternium-15

Glyceryl thioglycolate	Ammonium thioglycolate
Imidazolidinyl urea	Diazolidinyl urea, formaldehyde (donors)[a]

PABA (p-aminobenzoic acid)	PABA esters (amyl dimethyl, glyceryl, octyl dimethyl), other para-compounds:
	   azo colors
	   benzocaine and related local anesthetics
	   oral antidiabetics
	   p-phenylenediamine
	   sulfonamides

Perfume ingredients (some)	Balsam of Peru, rosin, turpentine oil, wood tars

p-Phenylenediamine	Other para- hair colors:
	   p-aminodiphenylamine
	   p-aminophenol
	   2-nitro-p-phenylenediamine
	   N-phenyl-p-phenylenediamine
	   p-toluenediamine
	Other para- compounds:
	   azo colors
	   benzocaine and related local anesthetics
	   oral antidiabetics
	   sulfonamides

Propylene glycol[29]	Butylene glycol,[59] ethylene glycol, hexylene glycol, polyethylene glycol
Rosin	Balsam of Peru, dihydroabietyl alcohol, fragrances, wood tars
Sorbic acid	Potassium sorbate
Wool alcohols	Cetearyl alcohol, eucerit, Eucerit, lanolin, lanolin alcohol and other lanolin-derivatives.

[a] If allergic to formaldehyde (see under formaldehyde).

Source: Adapted from de Groot, Weyland, and Nater.[54]

inone[12–14] and paraben sensitivity. Therefore, such allergens have to be routinely tested in the appropriate concentration in a cosmetic screening series. False-positive reactions may occur with any cosmetic product but especially with products containing detergents/surfactants such as shampoo, soap, or bath and shower foam. As a consequence, these products are usually diluted to 1% in water before testing. Even then, mild irritant reactions are observed frequently and, of course, the necessary dilution of these products may result in false-negative results in patients actually allergic to them. Testing these products therefore is highly unreliable.

TABLE 32–7. Noncosmetic Sources of Some Cosmetic Allergens

Allergen	Noncosmetic Sources
Balsam of Peru	See Chap. 28
Colophony (rosin)	See Chap. 12
Formaldehyde	See Chap. 20
Fragrances	Household products, and in foods as flavoring agents
Methyl(chloro)isothiazo-linone (Kathon CG)	Water cooling systems, paper mills, metalworking fluids,[60] hydraulic fluids, household detergents, fabric softeners, paints, adhesives, commerical photoprocessing chemicals
Parabens	Pharmaceutical preparations (topical, oral, parenteral) and in foods
p-Phenylenediamine	See Chap. 13
Propylene glycol[45]	Pharmaceutical preparations (topical, oral, parenteral), foods, antifreeze in dairies and breweries, production of varnishes and synthetic resins, automotive brake fluids and antifreeze preparations, solvent for flavors in baking and candy production, household cleansers
Quaternium-15	See Chap. 23
Triethanolamine	Topical pharmaceutical preparations
Wool alcohols (lanolin)	See Chap. 16

In many cases, as a result of testing with the NACDG routine series, the suspected products and a cosmetic screening series will establish the diagnosis of cosmetic allergy and identify one or more contact allergens. Often one can find on the label of the incriminated product whether or not the product actually contains the allergen or allergens. If not, the possibility of a false-positive reaction to the product should be suspected. The test should be repeated and/or control tests on nonexposed individuals performed. If allergy is confirmed, an ingredient of the product which was not tested in the NACDG series and the cosmetic screening series may have been responsible. In such cases, the manufacturer should be asked for samples of the ingredients, and these can be tested on the patient after proper dilution.[55]

In certain cases, allergy to cosmetics is strongly suspected but patch testing remains negative. In such cases, repeated open application tests (ROATs[56]) and/or usage tests can be performed. In the ROAT, the product is applied twice daily for a maximum of 7 days to the antecubital fossa. A negative reaction after a week makes sensitivity highly unlikely. This procedure should be performed with all suspected products. In the usage test, all cosmetic products are stopped until the dermatitis has disappeared. Then, cosmetics are reintroduced as normally used, one at a time, with an interval of 3 days for each product, until a reaction develops.

Photopatch testing should be performed whenever photoallergic cosmetic dermatitis is suspected (Ref. 57 and Chaps. 8 and 9). When all tests have remained negative, the possibility of seborrheic dermatitis (scalp, eyelids, face, axillae, trunk), atopic dermatitis (all locations), irritant contact dermatitis (also from cosmetic products), and allergic contact dermatitis from other sources should next be considered.

THERAPY AND PREVENTION

The therapy of allergic cosmetic dermatitis consists of discontinuation of the suspected allergenic product or products and, if necessary, topical (and rarely systemic) steroids (see also Chap. 42). To prevent recurrences, the patient should receive the CTFA names of the allergen or allergens identified and be instructed to avoid products containing them and possible cross-reacting (chemically related) substances (Table 32-6). Cosmetic ingredient labeling enables the patient to choose products not containing these. In the case of contact allergy to fragrances, balsam of Peru, and possibly colophony, fragrance-free products should be used. In some patients, a fragrance may sometimes be applied to clothing or hair without eliciting an allergic response. "Connubial contact" (i.e., from the partner) with fragrances should be avoided.[58] Many allergens in cosmetics are relatively easy to avoid, as they are used only or mainly in cosmetics. Others have many applications [e.g., methyl(chloro)isothiazolinone], and some are impossible to avoid (e.g., formaldehyde). The most common noncosmetic sources of such allergens are listed in Table 32-7.

A patient instruction handout on allergic cosmetic dermatitis appears on pages 346 and 347.

ACKNOWLEDGMENT

Photographs supplied by Dr. Henk van der Walle, Arnhem, The Netherlands.

REFERENCES

1. *Cosmetic Handbook.* Washington DC, Food and Drug Administration, 1986.
2. Groot AC, de: *Adverse Reactions to Cosmetics* (dissertation). University of Groningen, the Netherlands, 1988, pp 17–27, 39–42, 72–100. (Published by the author.)
3. Groot AC, de, Nater JP, van der Lende R, Rijcken B: Adverse effects of cosmetics and toiletries: A retrospective study in the general population. *Int J Cosm Science* 9:255–259, 1987.
4. Groot AC, de, Beverdam ECA, Tjong Ayong C, et al: The role of contact allergy in the spectrum of adverse effects caused by cosmetics and toiletries. *Contact Dermatitis* 19:195–201, 1988.
5. Groot AC, de, Bruynzeel DP, Bos JD, et al: The allergens in cosmetics. *Arch Dermatol* 124:1525–1529, 1988.
6. Groot AC, de: Labelling cosmetics with their ingredients. *Br Med J* 300:1636–1638, 1990.
7. Adams RM, Maibach HI: A five-year study of cosmetic reactions. *J Am Acad Dermatol* 13:1062–1069, 1985.
8. Schorr WF: Cosmetic allergy: Diagnosis, incidence, and management. *Cutis* 14:844–850, 1974.
9. Skog E: Incidence of cosmetic dermatitis. *Contact Dermatitis* 6:449–451, 1980.
10. Romaguera C, Camarasa JMG, Alomar A, Grimalt F: Patch tests with allergens related to cosmetics. *Contact Dermatitis* 9:167–168, 1983.
11. Ngangu Z, Samsoen M, Foussereau J: Einige Aspekte zur Kosmetika-Allergie in Strassburg. *Dermatosen* 31:126–129, 1983.
12. Groot AC, de, Herxheimer A: Isothiazolinone preservative: Cause of a continuing epidemic of cosmetic dermatitis. *Lancet* 1:314–316, 1989.
13. Groot AC, de, Weyland JW: Kathon CG: A review. *J Am Acad Dermatol* 18:350–358, 1988.
14. Groot AC, de: Methylisothiazolinone/methylchloroisothiazolinone (Kathon CG) allergy: An updated review. *Am J Contact Dermatitis* 1:151–156, 1990.
15. Marks JG, Moss JN, Parno JR, et al: Methylchloroisothiazolinone/methylisothiazolinone (Kathon CG) biocide—United States multicenter study of human skin sensitization. *Am J Contact Dermatitis* 1:157–161, 1990.
16. Fransway AF: Sensitivity to Kathon CG: Findings in 365 consecutive patients. *Contact Dermatitis* 19:342–347, 1988.

17. Rietschel RL, Nethercott JR, Emmett EA, et al: Methylchloroisothiazolinone-methylisothiazolinone reactions in patients screened for vehicle and preservative hypersensitivity. *J Am Acad Dermatol* 22:734–738, 1990.

18. Groot AC, de, Bruynzeel DP, Jagtman BA, Weyland JW: Contact allergy to diazolidinyl urea (Germall II). *Contact Dermatitis* 18:202–205, 1988.

19. Perret CM, Happle R: Contact sensitivity to diazolidinyl urea (Germall II), in Frosch PJ, Dooms-Goossens A, Lachapelle J-M, et al (eds): *Current Topics in Contact Dermatitis*. Berlin, Springer Verlag, 1989, pp 92–94.

20. Groot AC, de, Weyland JW: Contact allergy to methyldibromoglutaronitrile in the cosmetics preservative Euxyl K 400. *Am J Contact Dermatitis* 2:31–32, 1991.

21. Groot AC, de, Bruynzeel DP, Coenraads PJ, et al: Frequency of allergic reactions to methyldibromoglutar-onitrile (1,2-dibromo-2,4-dicyanobutane) in the Netherlands. *Contact Dermatitis* 25:260–261, 1991.

22. Groot AC, de, van der Walle HB, Jagtman BA, Weyland JW: Contact allergy to 4-isopropyldibenzoyl-methane and 3-(4'-methylbenzylidene)-camphor in the sunscreen Eusolex 8021. *Contact Dermatitis* 16:249–254, 1987.

23. Schauder S, Ippen H: Photoallergisches und allergisches Kontaktekzem durch Dibenzoylmethan-Verbin-dungen und andere Lichtschutzfilter. *Hautarzt* 39:435–440, 1988.

24. Taniguchi S, Katok J, Hisa T, et al: Shampoo dermatitis due to cocamidopropyl betaine. *Contact Dermatitis* 26:139, 1992.

25. Larsen WG: Perfume dermatitis. *J Am Acad Dermatol* 12:1–9, 1985.

26. Wojnarowska F, Calnan CD: Contact and photocontact allergy to musk ambrette. *Br J Dermatol* 114:667–675, 1986.

27. Fransway AF: The problem of preservation in the 1990s: I. Statement of the problem, solution(s) of the industry and the current use of formaldehyde and formaldehyde releasing biocides. *Am J Contact Dermatitis* 2:6–23, 1991.

28. Fransway AF, Schmitz NA: The problem of preservation in the 1990s: II. Formaldehyde and formalde-hyde-releasing biocides: Incidences of cross-reactivity and the significance of the positive response to formaldehyde. *Am J Contact Dermatitis* 2:78–88, 1991.

29. Fransway AF: The problem of preservation in the 1990s: III. Agents with preservative function indepen-dent of formaldehyde release. *Am J Contact Dermatitis* 2:145–174, 1991.

30. Nethercott JR, Holness DL, Adams RM, et al: Patch testing with a routine screening tray in North America, 1985 through 1989: I. Frequency of response. *Am J Contact Dermatitis* 2:122–129, 1991.

31. Rosen M, McFarland AG: Free formaldehyde in anionic shampoos. *J Soc Cosm Chem* 35:157–169, 1984.

32. Council on Scientific Affairs: Formaldehyde. *JAMA* 261:1183–1187, 1989.

33. Parker LU, Taylor JS: A 5-year study of contact allergy to quaternium-15. *Am J Contact Dermatitis* 2:231–234, 1991.

34. Jordan WP: Human studies that determine the sensitizing potential of haptens: Experimental allergic contact dermatitis. *Dermatol Clin* 2:533–538, 1984.

35. Storrs F, Bell DE: Allergic contact dermatitis to 2-bromo-2-nitropropane-1,3-diol in a hydrophilic ointment. *J Am Acad Dermatol* 8:157–164, 1983.

36. Peters MS, Connolly SM, Schroeter AL: Bronopol allergic contact dermatitis. *Contact Dermatitis* 9:397–401, 1983.

37. Frosch PJ, White IR, Rycroft RJG, et al: Contact allergy to bronopol. *Contact Dermatitis* 22:24–26, 1990.

38. Groot AC, de, Joost Th van, Bos JD, et al: Patch test reactivity to DMDM hydantoin: Relationship to formaldehyde. *Contact Dermatitis* 18:197–201, 1988.

39. Groot AC, de: Choosing preservatives: Dermatoallergenic considerations. *Cosmetics and Toiletries* 106:37–38, 1991.

40. Menné T, Hjorth N: Routine testing with paraben esters. *Contact Dermatitis* 19:189–191, 1988.

41. Holness DL, Nethercott JR: Epicutaneous testing results in hairdressers. *Am J Contact Dermatitis* 1:224–234, 1990.

42. Zviak C: *The Science of Hair Care*. New York, Dekker, 1986, pp 263–308, 409–424.

43. Guerra L, Bardazzi F, Tosti A: Contact dermatitis in hairdressers' clients. *Contact Dermatitis* 26:108–111, 1992.

44. Storrs F: Permanent wave contact dermatitis: Contact allergy to glyceryl monothioglycolate. *J Am Acad Dermatol* 11:74–85, 1984.

45. Catanzaro JM, Smith JG: Propylene glycol dermatitis. *J Am Acad Dermatol* 24:90–95, 1991.

46. de Wit FS, de Groot AC, Weyland JW, Bos JD: An outbreak of contact dermatitis from toluenesulfonamide formaldehyde resin in a nail hardener. *Contact Dermatitis* 18:280–283, 1988.
47. Fisher AA: Cross reactions between methyl methacrylate monomer and acrylic monomers presently used in acrylic nail preparations. *Contact Dermatitis* 7:345, 1980.
48. Kligman AM: Lanolin allergy: Crisis or comedy. *Contact Dermatitis* 9:99–107, 1983.
49. Edman B, Möller H: Testing a purified lanolin preparation by a randomized procedure. *Contact Dermatitis* 20:287–290, 1989.
50. Carmichael AJ, Foulds IS, Bradbury DS: Loss of lanolin patch-test reactivity. *Br J Dermatol* 125:573–576, 1991.
51. Freeman S, Frederiksen P: Sunscreen allergy. *Am J Contact Dermatitis* 1:240–243, 1990.
52. Dromgoole SH, Maibach HI: Sunscreen intolerance: Contact and photocontact sensitization and contact urticaria. *J Am Acad Dermatol* 22:1068–1078, 1990.
53. Tosti A, Guerra L, Bardazzi F, Gasparri F: Euxyl K 400: A new sensitizer in cosmetics. *Contact Dermatitis* 25:89–93, 1991.
54. De Groot AC, Weyland JW, Nater JP: *Unwanted Effects of Cosmetics and Drugs Used in Dermatology*, 3d ed. Amsterdam, Elsevier, 1994.
55. Groot AC, de: *Patch Testing: Test Concentrations and Vehicles for 3700 Allergens*, 2d ed. Amsterdam, Elsevier, 1994.
56. Hannuksela M, Salo H: The repeated open application test (ROAT). *Contact Dermatitis* 14:221–225, 1986.
57. Holzle E, Neumann N, Hausen B, et al: Photopatch testing: The 5-year experience of the German, Austrian and Swiss Photopatch Test Group. *J Am Acad Dermatol* 25:59–68, 1991.
58. Larsen WG: How to instruct patients sensitive to fragrances. *J Am Acad Dermatol* 21:880–885, 1989.
59. Fan W, Kinnunen T, Niinimaki H, Hannuksela M: Skin reactions to glycols used in dermatological and cosmetic vehicles. *Am J Contact Dermatitis* 2:181–183, 1991.
60. Nethercott JR, Rothman N, Holness DL, O'Toole T: Health problems in metal workers exposed to a coolant oil containing Kathon 886 MW. *Am J Contact Dermatitis* 1:94–99, 1990.
61. Engasser PG, Maibach HI: Dermatitis due to cosmetics, in Fisher AA (ed): *Contact Dermatitis*, 3d ed. Philadelphia, Lea & Febiger, 1986, pp 368–393.

33

PERFUMED PRODUCTS

Torkel Fischer

Often one thinks of a perfume as the concentrated alcoholic solution applied behind the ear and on the wrist, but a perfume can be any compound which induces a characteristic stimulation of the olfactory sense. These fragrance materials are used in almost every kind of product sold to create in the noses and minds of potential buyers a favorable impression, as there is a strong olfactory impression associated with a variety of products, ranging from cars to soaps. The materials used to create the desired illusion are volatile organic compounds of relatively low molecular weight. Most produce an odor so distinctive that it is recognized immediately. Other fragrance materials, such as the masking fragrances, are used to produce odor fatigue (masking other odors in a product) without producing a recognizable scent.

Until the nineteenth century, fragrances were manufactured from essential oils and alcohol extracts of plant products. A few—such as musk, ambergris curet, and castoreum—were of animal origin. Fragrances were luxury products which found use in perfumes, eaux de toilette, and soaps.

This situation has changed completely. Since the introduction of chemical compounds of characteristic scent produced from natural raw materials or in a synthetic process, it is almost impossible to avoid fragrances. They are used with increased sophistication to fit the needs of a large number of specific commercial products found in our household environment to produce a characteristic scent or to cover an unpleasant odor. The artistry, often as sophisticated as painting or music, creates an olfactory image that the seller wishes the user to associate with the product.

PRODUCTS WHERE FRAGRANCES ARE FOUND

Perfumes and eaux de cologne typically cause reactions in allergic persons wherever they have been applied (Fig. 33-1). They are commonly found in cosmetics and skin care products such as creams, lotions, soaps, cleansers, shampoos, cold permanents and other hair care products, antiperspirants, facial and eye makeup products, lip cosmetics, shaving preparations, sunscreen and suntan products, bath preparations, medical creams, ointments, and baby care products.

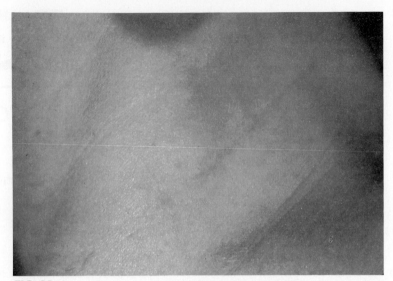

FIG. 33–1. A "perfume" or cologne is relatively easy to suspect when it occurs where the product is usually applied, as here, on the neck. (See color Plate 15.)

Flavors used in oral hygiene products[1]—toothpaste, mouthwash, dental floss, and fluoride treatments—are fragrance chemicals. Even eugenol, widely used by dentists, is a fragrance chemical. Scented household products include detergents, cleansers, softeners, deodorizing sprays, polishes, solvents, waxes. The list is very long.

Cutting fluids, electroplating fluids, paints, rubber, plastics, insecticides, herbicides, and additives used in air conditioning water may all be scented.

Paper and paper products—including diapers, facial tissue,[2] moist toilet paper,[3] and sanitary napkins[4]—may cause a reaction.

Fabrics and clothes may contain fragrance materials, especially after they are laundered or treated with a fabric softener. Perfume-sensitive individuals may also apply so much cologne to clothing that it soaks through (Fig. 33-2).

The distinction between fragrances and spices is often indistinct. Many synthetic fragrances are used as spices. Natural fragrances like cinnamon, clove, vanilla, and cardamon are added to foods, soft drinks, lozenges, chewing gums, candies, ice cream, tobacco, and snuff. Fragrance sensitivity in a patient with hand eczema should suggest the possibility of allergy to kitchen spices, such as sensitivity to alpha-amylcinnamic aldehyde and alpha-amylcinnamic alcohol.[5]

THE ART OF PERFUMERY

Perfumery is the art of making individuals and products attractive to the olfactory sense. Specific fragrances must be designed for individual products, as compatibility is essential and the product ingredients may affect the odor. To do this, the perfumer uses a blend of perfume, chemicals, and specialties. Among thousands of chemical substances which have an odor, about 5000 are used by a perfumer. He also uses specialties, which are more simple mixtures with a characteristic odor (e.g., tabac, for

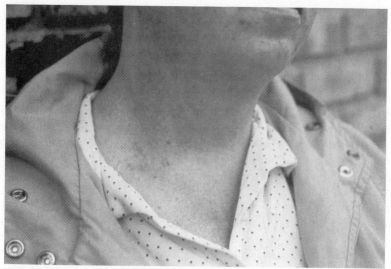

FIG. 33–2. Mild eczema of the neck from a perfume applied to the collar.

tobacco, used to add a masculine quality). These products may also be designed for a particular price range, which often determines the ingredients available to a perfumer.

Fragrances in cosmetics consist of natural or synthetic compounds or both. The number of ingredients may range from a few to more than 300. Synthetic chemicals may account for as much as 90 percent of the perfume composition. For technical products, synthetic ingredients dominate for reasons of cost, purity, compatibility, and quality control.

The amount of fragrance found in different products is 20 to 30 percent in fine fragrance, 4 to 5 percent in cologne and toilet water, 1 to 2 percent in soap, 0.5 percent in creams and lotions, and 0.1 to 0.01 percent to mask unpleasant odor.

FRAGRANCE MATERIALS

Natural fragrances are, with few exceptions, of botanical origin. A natural fragrance contains several hundred different chemicals, a few major and many minor ones, which are responsible for the complexity of the odor.

Synthetic fragrances are well defined chemical compounds with a simple odor.

Balsams are viscous, colored, and aromatic plant products soluble in alcohol but not in water. They are obtained from the exudate often artificially produced by incising the bark. Balsams with a characteristic odor can be obtained from trees rich in resins (e.g., balsam of Peru, balsam of Tolu, styrax, galbanum, myrrh, and benzoin).

Essential oils are obtained by stem distillation of various plant raw materials such as the blossoms, leaves, and fruits of roses, laurel, and lavender and of the wood and roots of cedar or sandalwood.

Concretes or absolutes are obtained by solvent extraction of plant materials (which for absolutes is alcohol), with evaporation of the solvent. Materials manufactured this way are subject to less change during their preparation than those distilled.

SENSITIZING FRAGRANCES AND REGULATIONS OF FRAGRANCE USE

Considering the extensive use of balsams, fragrances, spices, and flavor additives to food, the frequency of contact allergy to these groups of materials is relatively small. In absolute numbers, however, fragrance allergy is common.

It may seem impossible to find out which chemicals in fragrances cause disease. This problem is approached in different ways by dermatologists and fragrance manufacturers. Our knowledge of allergy to fragrance materials is based on testing to relatively few perfume ingredients. It received a boost when the ingredients of one product were used to test a sensitive patient, and this has been expanded in recent years.[6,12,17]

The dermatologists patch test with natural and synthetic fragrance materials either in patients chosen at random or in those with a history of cosmetic or perfume sensitivity or with hand eczema. If reactions are positive, one may elect to test to a larger fragrance test series. Walter Larsen, one of the pioneers in this area, developed a mix of eight common sensitizing fragrances which were included in Mycolog Cream. This mix detects 70 to 80 percent of fragrance sensitivity and has been used for standard tests of contact allergy for more than 15 years (see Tables 33-1 and 33-2).[6]

The industrial approach is somewhat different. Fragrance materials apparently have medical risks. The perfume industry therefore decided to organize to prevent undesired regulations. In 1966, the Research Institute for Fragrance Materials (RIFM) was founded, and some years later the International Fragrance Association (IFRA), both aiming to assure the quality and safety of fragrance materials.

TABLE 33–1. Natural Constituent Included in the Fragrance Mix and Test Concentrations Natural Fragrance Patch-Test Materials From Chemotechnique and Hermal Companies

Material	In fragrance mix	Chemotechnique, percent	Hermal, percent
Balsam of Peru		25.0	25.0
Cananga oil		2.0	
Cedarwood oil			10.0
Clove oil			2.0
Eucalyptus oil			2.0
Geranium oil of Bourbon		2.0	
Jasmine absolute of Egypt		2.0	
Laurel oil			2.0
Lavender absolute		2.0	
Lemon grass oil			2.0
Lemon oil		2.0	2.0
Neroli oil			2.0
Oak moss absolute	x[a]	2.0	1.0
Orange oil			2.0
Peppermint oil			2.0
Rose oil, Bulgarian		2.0	
Sandalwood oil		2.0	
Ylang ylang oil		2.0	

[a] "x" denotes presence of constituent in fragrance mix.

TABLE 33–2. Synthetic Constituents of the Fragrance Mix and Test Concentrations Fragrance Patch-Test Materials from Chemotechnique and Hermal Companies

Material	In fragrance mix	Chemotechnique, percent	Hermal, percent
Amyl cinnamicaldehyde	x[a]	1.0	1.0
Benzaldehyde			5.0
Benzyl alcohol		1.0	
Benzyl cinnamate			5.0
Benzyl salicylate		2.0	1.0
Cinnamic alcohol	x	2.0	1.0
Cinnamic aldehyde	x	1.0	1.0
Eugenol	x	2.0	1.0
Geraniol	x	2.0	1.0
Hydroxycitronellal	x	2.0	1.0
Isoeugenol	x	2.0	1.0
Jasmine synthetic		2.0	
Musk ambrette		1.0	
Musk ketone		1.0	
Musk moskene		1.0	
Musk tibetine		1.0	
Musk xylene		1.0	
Salicylaldehyde			2.0
Vanillin		10.0	10.0

[a]"x" denotes presence of constituent in fragrance mix.

The RIFM publishes recommendations for use of fragrance materials based on data from its own investigations as well as the evaluations of an international expert panel of toxicologists, pharmacologists, and dermatologists.

The IFRA is an international scientific organization working for safety in the perfume industry. They have formulated a Code of Practice about the use of fragrance materials. A committee with scientific advisers from member countries publishes regularly revised monographs of fragrance materials and recommendations for use.[7]

SKIN DISEASES CAUSED BY FRAGRANCES

Fragrances in perfumes and scented products are leading cosmetic allergens in both America and Europe.[8]

Contact allergic reactions to cosmetics and skin care products occur in about 5 percent of all patients with contact dermatitis. Positive patch-test reactions to fragrances and fragrance ingredients are responsible for the greatest number of these reactions. The majority of patients with cosmetic reactions are female (80 percent) and are equally distributed over the age groups between 20 and 60.

Fragrance ingredients may cause a wide spectrum of skin diseases. Allergic and irritant contact dermatitis is common, but pure pruritus is rare. Immunologic and nonimmunologic contact urticaria is probably also common but infrequently proved by tests. Photoreactions and pigmentary diseases are rare.

Cutaneous reactions associated with perfumed skin care products are often identified by the site of application. The body sites most frequently affected are the head and neck, including the eyelids and lips, followed by the hands.[8–10]

IRRITANT CONTACT DERMATITIS

Most fragrances have low levels of irritancy. An example of a fragrance with irritant properties is cinnamic aldehyde. The symptoms of irritant dermatitis from fragrances are persistent erythema, itching, and dryness of the facial skin.

ALLERGIC CONTACT DERMATITIS

The most common reaction to fragrance materials seen by practicing dermatologists is allergic contact dermatitis. The clinical picture varies from pruritus to various forms of eczema.

Perfume dermatitis typically is erythematous, although papular and even vesicular reactions occur. The dermatitis of a perfume or cosmetic product most commonly

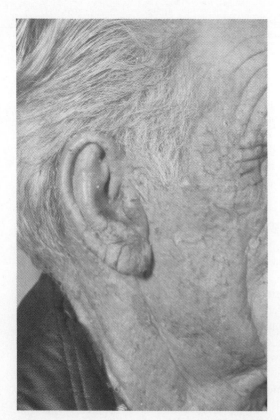

FIG. 33–3. Widespread eczema, probably from a product containing fragrance. This patient had multiple allergies, but only the fragrance reaction would explain a reaction in this location.

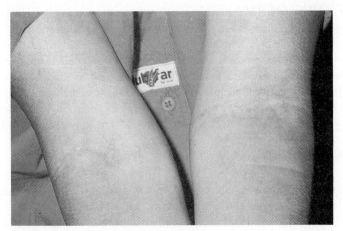

FIG. 33–4. Fragrance allergy simulating atopic eczema.

develops at the site of application. Examples are the retroauricular eczema which may appear after the application of perfume, and facial dermatitis from contact with aftershave.

Reactions to eau de cologne are often streaky, as is berloque dermatitis. A fragrance dermatitis may be generalized, may have multiple localizations, or may be situated at the upper chest, elbow flexures, or wrists. Dermatitis from perfumed products such as creams, lotions, and powders tends to spread outside the area of contact and to produce a diffuse dermatitis (Fig. 33-3).

Hand eczema occurs in about a quarter of patients with perfume sensitivity and is often of the dyshidrotic type.

Perfume eczema of the antecubital area may resemble atopic dermatitis (Fig. 33-4). Fragrance sensitivity may not be suspected until patch testing is done in atopic dermatitis and rarely changes the basic qualities of the atopic eczema. Fragrance sensitivity is overrepresented in patients with leg ulcers, and it may be the background of a seborrheic or psoriasisform dermatitis of the hair and face. Allergy may cause Koebnerization.

Rare clinical forms of fragrance sensitivity are pustular reactions similar to sycosis barbae, a lupus erythematosus-like eruption, and conjunctivitis.[9–17]

PIGMENTED COSMETIC DERMATITIS

Pigmented cosmetic dermatitis or melanosis faciei feminea has been reported in a large number of Japanese women since 1960. The background is contact sensitization to several different cosmetic ingredients: fragrances, colors, and preservatives.

The skin manifestations are diffuse or patchy brown hyperpigmentation on the cheeks and/or forehead, sometimes the entire face. In severe cases, the pigmentation may be black, blue-black, or purple; in mild cases, pale brown. It may attain lichenoid character.[18] The disease is controlled and heals within 1 or 2 years when known sensitizers from cosmetics are excluded using the "allergen control system" developed by Nakayama et al.[19]

PHOTOTOXIC DERMATITIS

The best-known phototoxic reaction to perfume is the berloque dermatitis caused by bergamot oil. The normal reaction is erythema and prickling pain at the site of perfume or eau de cologne application a few hours after exposure to sunlight. The dermatitis is often vesicular and is followed by a long-standing irregular hyperpigmentation.[20] The cause, 5-methoxypsoralen or bergapten, is today in greatly reduced use, at least in products manufactured in the United States, so that phototoxic reactions are rarely seen.

PHOTOALLERGIC DERMATITIS

Photoallergic reactions to musk ambrette and from different methyl coumarins are reported; these products are now prohibited by IFRA (Fig. 33-5).

Musk ambrette had been extensively used for 60 years as a fragrance ingredient and spice additive when suddenly, around 1980, numerous reports were published on photoallergic reactions in men using aftershave or men's colognes. A pruritic eruption was present on sun-exposed areas of the face, neck, and hands, followed by erythema, edema, and scaling.[21,22]

6-Methylcoumarin caused several cases of severe photoallergic reactions after being introduced as fragrance in a suntan product. 6-Methylcoumarin and related derivatives have been withdrawn from the market.[23,24]

PIGMENTATION AND DEPIGMENTATION

The background of pigmentation to perfumed cosmetics is as follows:

1. Berloque dermatitis, from a phototoxic perfume containing photosensitizers of the psoralen type, is characterized by sharply demarcated pigmentation at the site of application of the perfume and exposure to sunlight.

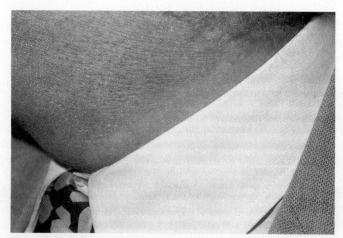

FIG. 33–5. Photosensitivity to musk ambrette in a man's cologne. This type of reaction is less common since levels of that ingredient have been reduced. (See color Plate 16.)

2. Photoallergic reactions from musk ambrette with long-standing diffuse brownish pigmentation of areas of the face and neck is mostly due to perfumed aftershave lotions.
3. Pigmented cosmetic dermatitis with diffuse or mottled pigmentation. Airborne contact dermatitis to musk ambrette in incense may be the cause of the pigmentation.

Depigmentation is a rare sequela of allergic contact dermatitis to flavor and fragrance ingredients.[25,26]

IMMEDIATE CONTACT REACTIONS

Contact urticaria has recently been included in a broader concept of immediate reactions which disappear within 24 h, including itching, tingling, and burning erythematous reactions, wheal and flare reactions, and eczematous reactions. Such reactions may be produced through an immunologic or nonimmunologic mechanism.[27]

Under optimal conditions, cinnamic aldehyde may cause erythema and edema reactions in more than half of the individuals exposed.

Balsam of Peru can provoke both nonimmunologic contact urticaria and urticarial immunologic reactions of the immediate type—even anaphylactic symptoms.[28,29] Other fragrances responsible for immediate contact reactions are cassia oil, clove oil, menthol, and vanillin.[13,30]

PREVENTION AND PROPHYLAXIS

Since it is seldom possible to obtain a detailed declaration of fragrance ingredients in a product, the problem of avoiding a fragrance allergen must be approached in one of three ways. One may use any or all of them in combination depending on the degree of sensitivity.

The first method is a total avoidance of perfumed products and reduction of the environmental burden of fragrance. However, a woman's perfume may still exacerbate her partner's dermatitis.[31] Patients with strong positive reactions to alpha amyl-cinnamic aldehyde responded to a careful program of avoidance[5] and substitution of laundry products free of that allergen (Fig. 33-6).

The second method is safe use of perfumed products. The patient may be permitted to use a favorite sensitizing perfume while taking certain precautions, such as applying it on the hair or clothing in such a way that there is no direct contact with the skin.[14]

The third method is to evaluate a set of personal cosmetic products by use tests and then to faithfully use these products only. The patient should obtain a sample of a desired perfume or cosmetic and apply the product twice daily on a circumscribed area of the lower arm for 7 days, checking for itch and erythema, before proceeding to use it routinely.

PATCH TESTING WITH FRAGRANCES

The fragrance mix composed by Walter Larsen includes eight common sensitizing fragrance materials—seven synthetic and one natural (oak moss absolute). (See Tables

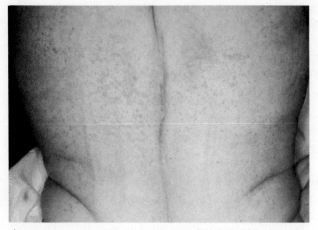

A

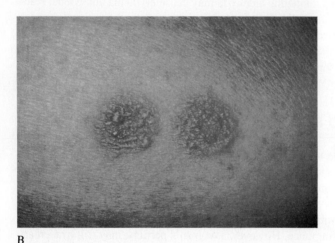

B

FIG. 33–6. *A.* Allergy to alpha-amylcinnamic aldehyde in a laundry detergent. (See color Plate 17.) *B.* Positive patch tests to alpha-amylcinnamic aldehyde and alpha-amylcinnamic alcohol.

33-1 and 33-2.) The fragrance mix is a valuable screening tool and detects 70 to 80 percent of fragrance sensitivity.[12]

Since the fragrance mix is a borderline irritant, weak positive tests reactions have to be controlled with a retest with the separate components of the mix at higher concentrations.[32]

The True Test (Glaxo Dermatology, Five Moore Drive, Research Triangle Park, NC 27709) includes the allergens of the Larsen mix in a slow-release vehicle and is therefore less irritant.[33,34]

Tables 33-1 and 33-2 present data on fragrance test materials not included in the fragrance mix, which may be used on strong suspicion of fragrance allergy when the mix test is negative.

Fragrance allergy is rarely detected by patch testing with cosmetic products because too small an amount of the causative fragrance is present in the ready product. Photopatch testing and tests for immediate contact reactions with fragrances do not differ from tests with other allergens.

The evaluation of the relevance of a positive fragrance reaction is important but difficult. There may be no actual relation between the reaction and fragrance exposure, but more often the exposure is neglected because perfumes are so widespread in our environment that we do not even notice them. Perfume dermatitis can be elicited by extremely low concentrations of fragrance. A positive test should, if possible, be confirmed with a use test.

COMPONENTS OF THE FRAGRANCE MIX

Oak moss absolute, extracted from *Evernia prunastri* (oak moss) and *Pseudevernia furfuracea* (tree moss), is found in perfumes, colognes, and aftershaves. It is in many scented products marketed to men. Oak moss is a moderately strong allergen and is also a photosensitizer[35,36] (see Fig. 33-7).

Alpha-amyl cinnamic aldehyde is a greenish-yellow liquid with an intense jasmine odor not found in nature. It may be a constituent of several synthetic essential oils (e.g., jasmine oil synthetic). Found in perfumes, cosmetics, soaps, and a wide range of industrial products, it is a weak sensitizer. It may cross react or coreact with alpha-amyl cinnamic alcohol.[5]

Cinnamic alcohol in pure form may produce crystalline needles with the odor of hyacinth. It occurs as an ester in natural fragrance materials such as balsam of Peru, storax, cinnamon leaves, hyacinth oil, and propolis. It is found in perfumed cosmetic products, deodorants, paper, and laundry products and is often used in flavors. It cross-reacts with cinnamic aldehyde and may cause pigmented cosmetic dermatitis.[18,37]

Cinnamic aldehyde is a yellowish oily liquid with a powerful, aromatic, warm, spicy odor and with the taste of cinnamon. It is a constituent of cinnamon oil, cinnamon

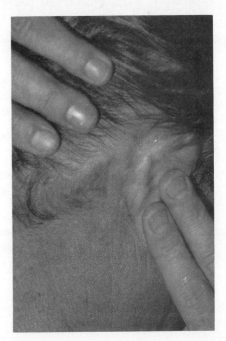

FIG. 33–7. Photoallergy to oak moss absolute in a man's aftershave. This patient was also compositae-allergic but improved dramatically after he stopped using the aftershave. (See color Plate 18.)

powder, and patchouli oil and is found in bath oils and salts, tonics, hair cosmetics, lipsticks, mouthwashes and breath fresheners, soaps, detergents, and as flavoring agent in toothpastes, sweets, soft drinks, and pastries. It is irritating in a concentration of 2%, is a moderately strong sensitizer, and is a common cause of contact dermatitis. It may also cause nonimmunologic contact urticaria. It is reported to be phototoxic to *Candida* and to cause photoallergic reactions in persistent light reactors.[38–40]

Eugenol is a colorless or light yellow viscous liquid which darkens and thickens on exposure to air. It has a powerful, spicy odor of clove, pungent taste—characteristic of the odor one associates with a dentist's office, where it is often used. It is found in oils of clove, bay, pimento, cinnamon leaf, sassafras, and patchouli. It is used in colognes, toilet waters, tonics, dressings, hair cosmetics, dentifrices, impression materials, and periodontal packings. It is a moderately strong sensitizer and it may cause pigmented cosmetic dermatitis or contact urticaria. It cross-reacts with balsam of Peru, isoeugenol, and benzoin.[18,41,42]

Geraniol is an oily, colorless liquid with a sweet, floral odor of rose. It constitutes the chief part of rose and palmarose oil, geranium oil, citronella oil, lavender oil, jasmine oil, and is present in most other essential oils. It is isomeric with linalool. It is used in perfumery, is an insect attractant, and is a moderately strong contact allergen. Patch-test sensitization has been described.

Hydroxycitronellal is a colorless viscous oil, a synthetic floral fragrance not found in nature. It has a sweet, fresh, green odor of lily of the valley. It is used in perfumes and many cosmetic products and is a moderately strong sensitizer that commonly causes allergic contact dermatitis and pigmented cosmetic dermatitis. It cross-reacts with citronellal and geranial.[16]

Isoeugenol is a colorless oily liquid which turns yellow, with an odor of clove weaker than that of eugenol. It is a constituent of ylang ylang oil and nutmeg oil. It is used in perfumery and is a moderately potent sensitizer. It cross-reacts with eugenol.[43]

DEFINITIONS OF FRAGRANCE TERMINOLOGY*

ABSOLUTE—A concentrated alcohol-soluble perfume material usually obtained by alcohol extraction of a concrete, pomade, or other hydrocarbon extract, followed by cold filtration and recovery of the solvent under a vacuum.

AROMA CHEMICAL—A synthetic product of organic chemistry (or a "pure" isolate) that is used as a fragrance ingredient.

ATTAR—A fragrance product from distillation of flower petals. The most prominent such product is attar of roses. Attar is derived from a Persian word meaning essence or, in its verb form, to smell sweet.

BALSAMS—Viscous, colored, and aromatic plant products, soluble in alcohol but not in water, and obtained by either spontaneous exudation or an artificially induced flow from an incision made through the bark of the plant. Examples are storax and balsams of Peru and Tolu.

*From Guin,[44] used by permission.

CONCRETE—The residue left following extraction and evaporation of the solvent (mostly the hydrocarbon type) used for that process.

ENFLEURAGE—Cold fat extraction of fragrance products from floral material.

ESSENTIAL OIL—Strictly speaking, a volatile fragrance material produced by distillation of a single botanical species, the name of which it will bear. Unfortunately, confusion has arisen because the term is often used to include expressed oils and other products.

EXPRESSED OIL—An "essential" oil obtained by pressure from plant material, usually citrus.

FRAGRANCE OIL—A finished fragrance product that is usually a composition of fragrance materials created to produce a desired aroma with qualities satisfactory for a particular use.

FRAGRANCE SPECIALTY—A combination of multiple raw materials made by the perfumer to be used as a basic working tool. It is often described as a rose, mossy, floral, or tabac creation. A perfumer may have specialties for different price ranges or applications.

GUM—A natural exudate of a plant that is water soluble and a good emulsifier (e.g., gum arabic). A gum resin (or more properly an oleo-gum resin) comprises gums, resins, and sometimes an essential oil and has different solubility properties. Examples are myrrh and olibanum (frankincense).

INFUSION—A solution of a botanical material following subjection to an organic solvent and heat.

ISOLATE—A fraction or chemical compound separated from an essential oil.

MACERATION—Removal of fragrance products from flowers by warm fat extraction.

PERFUME—A finished fragrance product ready for sale to the consumer.

PERFUME AND FLAVOR CHEMICALS—Chemical substances derived from natural sources, from chemical reaction with these substances, or from synthesis by organic chemistry.

POMADE—The fatty material containing the fragrance obtained by enfleurage or maceration.

QUENCHING—Interference with the sensitizing potential of certain aldehydes by other ingredients. The phenomenon, found in predictive testing, is much discussed but poorly understood.

TINCTURE—A product derived from subjecting natural raw material to a cold solvent, chiefly alcohol.

INFORMATION ON FRAGRANCE DERMATITIS—
PATIENT HANDOUT

WHAT CAUSES FRAGRANCE DERMATITIS?

The rash is caused by one or more chemicals contained in essential oils, other natural fragrance products, or synthetic fragrance chemicals which come into contact with your skin.

HOW DO I KNOW THAT IT IS A FRAGRANCE DERMATITIS?

The rash from fragrances is characteristically located on the face and on hands and arms. It may appear as an intense swelling and erythema within a few hours or a day after use of a fragrance or a scented cosmetic product. Often, the only symptoms are redness, dryness, and itching sometimes associated with pigmentation of the skin. Proof that the fragrance caused the problem may require patch testing or reexposure in a limited area on your neck or where your arm bends.

WHERE DO I FIND FRAGRANCES?

We are surrounded by fragrances. The main sources are fine perfumes and colognes and perfumed cosmetic products such as creams; ointments; hair, eye, and lip cosmetics; shampoos; sunscreens; and bath preparations. You will find fragrances in oral hygiene products, medicated skin products, and baby care products.

Household products such as detergents, cleaners, polishes, waxes, and air fresheners contain fragrances. Fabrics, clothes, paper, diapers, moist toilet paper, and sanitary pads may contain perfumes. We may find fragrances in paints and cutting fluids—even in the humidity produced by an air conditioner. The same or similar chemicals are found as flavoring in cough syrups, lozenges, chewing gum, candy, colas, ice cream, bakery products, and many other flavored foods.

WHICH FRAGRANCES PRODUCE ALLERGY?

Fragrance allergy is proved by patch testing. Your test indicates that you are sensitive to a fragrance chemical. Only a minor number of the fragrances are

This information is provided to help persons with contact dermatitis in the understanding of their problem. The contents are subject to change as more information becomes available and are not intended as a substitute for medical treatment.

common sensitizers. The most common are those behind cinnamic, clove, and citronella odors.

WHAT IS THE BEST WAY TO PREVENT THE RASH?

A complete fragrance is a complex mixture of several different components— often a secret formula. It is therefore necessary to avoid all kinds of fragrances even when you are sensitive to just one of them. Fragrance-free products are freely available; therefore, use only fragrance-free cosmetics and medical care products. Fragrance-free products should be free of fragrance, while nonscented and hypoallergenic products may contain a low concentration of fragrance to cover an undesired odor.

Flavors are often the same chemicals as fragrances, so ingesting these can cause oral discomfort or even a flare on the skin. If you are severely allergic, you should consider avoiding foods that contain citrus peel and spices such as cinnamon, clove, vanilla, and curry. Fragrance-free laundry products are available, and these should be used exclusively until you are in control of your problem. Basis soap is free of perfume. The most difficult product to substitute is shampoo. All of these have fragrance. You can often use Basis soap with soft water until your problem is under control. Then you may try products with a distinctly different scent. Daily use for a week will usually tell, but be prepared to treat the rash. Hundreds of fragrance materials are blended to make the "perfume" used for each product, so the same ingredient may be in many or even *most* products.

HOW IS THE RASH BEST TREATED?

Avoidance of all perfumed products is the best approach. Mild topical cortisone preparations are adequate for most patients, but for some a prescription for an oral cortisone is necessary.

HOW DO I TEST A PRODUCT FOR SAFETY?

Apply a small amount of the product you want to test on a 3- by 3-cm area on the inner aspect of the lower arm or elbow twice daily for 7 days. If no reaction of erythema or itching develops, you will probably tolerate the product.

REFERENCES

1. Andersen KE: Contact allergy to toothpaste flavours. *Contact Dermatitis* 4:195–198, 1978.
2. Guin JD: Contact sensitivity to perfume in paper products. *J Am Assoc Dermatol* 4:733–734, 1981.
3. de Groot AC, Baar TJ, Terpstra H, Weyland JW: Contact allergy to moist toilet paper. *Contact Dermatitis* 24:135–136, 1991.
4. Larsen WG: Sanitary napkin dermatitis due to the perfume. *Arch Dermatol* 115:363, 1979.
5. Guin JD, Haffley P: Sensitivity to alpha amyl cinnamic aldehyde and alpha amyl cinnamic alcohol. *J Am Assoc Dermatol* 8:76–80, 1983.
6. Larsen WG: Allergic contact dermatitis to the perfume in Mycolog cream. *J Am Assoc Dermatol* 2:131–133, 1979.
7. IFRA, 8 Rue Charles-Humbert, Ch-1205, Geneva, Switzerland.
8. Eiermann HJ, Larsen W, Maibach HI, Taylor JS: Prospective study of cosmetic reactions; 1977–1980. *J Am Assoc Dermatol* 6:909–917, 1982.
9. Adams RM, Maibach HI, and the North American Contact Dermatitis Group: A five year study of cosmetic reactions. *J Am Assoc Dermatol* 13:1062–1069, 1985.
10. de Groot AC, Liem DH, Nater JP, van Ketel WG: Patch tests with fragrance materials and preservatives. *Contact Dermatitis* 12:87–92, 1985.
11. Meynadier J-M, Meynadier J-L, Peyron J-L, Peyron L: Formes cliniques des manifestations cutanées d'allergie aux parfums. *Ann Dermatol Venereol* 113:31–39, 1986.
12. Larsen WG: Perfume dermatitis. *J Am Assoc Dermatol* 12:1–12, 1985.
13. Abifadel R, Mortureux P, Perromat M, et al: Contact sensitivity to flavourings and perfumes in atopic dermatitis. *Contact Dermatitis* 127:43–46, 1992.
14. Fisher AA: Perfume dermatitis: Part I. General considerations and patch testing. *Cutis* 26:438–463, 477, 1980.
15. de Groot AC, Liem DH: Facial psoriasis caused by contact allergy to linalool and hydroxycitronellal in an after-shave. *Contact Dermatitis* 9:230–232, 1983.
16. Calnan CD: Unusual hydroxycitronellal perfume dermatitis. *Contact Dermatitis* 5:123, 1979.
17. Larsen WG: Cosmetic dermatitis due to a perfume. *Contact Dermatitis* 1:142–145, 1975.
18. Nakayama H, Matsuo S, Hayakawa K, et al: Pigmented cosmetic dermatitis. *Int J Derm* 23:299–305, 1984.
19. Nakayama H, Hanaoka H, Ohshiro A: *Allergen Controlled System (ACS)*. Tokyo: Kanehara Shuppan (Tokyo), 1974, p 42.
20. Harber LC, Harris H, Leider M, Baer RL: Berloque dermatitis: A technique for its deliberate reproduction. *Arch Dermatol* 90:572–576, 1964.
21. Raugi GH, Storrs FJ, Larsen WG: Photoallergic contact dermatitis to men's perfumes. *Contact Dermatitis* 5:251–260, 1979.
22. Giovinazzo VJ, Harber LC, Armstrong RB, Kochevar IE: Photoallergic contact dermatitis to musk ambrette. *J Am Assoc Dermatol* 3:384–393, 1980.
23. Jackson RT, Nesbitt LT, DeLeo VA: 6-methylcoumarin photocontact dermatitis. *J Am Assoc Dermatol* 2:124–127, 1980.
24. Eiermann HJ: Regulatory issues concerning AETT and 6-MC. *Contact Dermatitis* 6:120–122, 1980.
25. Hayakawa R, Matsunaga K, Arima Y: Depigmented contact dermatitis due to incense. *Contact Dermatitis* 16:272–274, 1987.
26. Mathias CGT, Maibach HI, Conant MA: Perioral leucoderma simulating vitiligo from use of a toothpaste containing cinnamic aldehyde. *Arch Dermatol* 116:1172–1173, 1983.
27. Lahti A, Maibach HI: Immediate contact reactions, in Menné T, Maibach HI (eds): *Exogenous Dermatoses: Environmental Dermatitis*. Boca Raton, Fla, CRC Press, 1991, pp 21–35.
28. Hjorth N: Eczematous allergy to balsams, allied perfumes and flavouring agents. *Acta Derm Venereol* 41(suppl 46):1–216, 1961.
29. Forsbeck M, Skog E: Immediate reactions to patch tests to balsam of Peru. *Contact Dermatitis* 3:201–205, 1977.
30. Rietschel RL: Contact urticaria form synthetic cassia oil and sorbic acid limited to the face. *Contact Dermatitis* 4:347–349, 1978.
31. Swinyer LJ: Connubial contact dermatitis from perfumes. *Contact Dermatitis* 6:226, 1980.

32. Lachapelle JM, Bruynzeel DP, Ducombs G, et al: European multicenter study of the TRUE test. *Contact Dermatitis* 19:91–97, 1988.
33. Svensson AM, Enström S, Thurell L, Swanberg H: Chemical and pharmaceutical standardization of fragrance mix for patch testing, in Frosch PJ, et al (eds): *Current Topics in Contact Dermatitis*. Berlin, Springer-Verlag, 1989, pp 530–534.
34. Fischer T, Maibach HI: Improved but not perfect: Patch testing. *Am J Contact Dermatitis* 1:73–90, 1990.
35. Dahlquist I, Fregert S: Contact allergy to antranorin and oak moss in lichen and perfumes. *Contact Dermatitis* 6:168–169, 1980.
36. Ford RA, Api AM: An investigation of the potential for allergenic contact sensitization of several oakmoss preparations. *Contact Dermatitis* 23:249, 1990.
37. Weibel H: Kontakteksem: Biofarmaceutiske aspekter (thesis). Danmarks Farmaceutiska Højskole, 1988.
38. Maibach HI: Cheilitis: Occult allergy to cinnamic aldehyde. *Contact Dermatitis* 15:106–107, 1986.
39. Scorr WF: Cinnamic aldehyde allergy. *Contact Dermatitis* 1:108–111, 1975.
40. Guin JD, Meyer BN, Drake RD, Haffley P: The effect of quenching agents on contact urticaria caused by cinnamic aldehyde. *J Am Assoc Dermatol* 10:45–51, 1984.
41. Vilaplana J, Grimault F, Romaguera C, Conellana F: Contact dermatitis from eugenol in mouth wash. *Contact Dermatitis* 24:223–224, 1991.
42. Rothenstein AS, Booman KA, Dorsky J, et al: Eugenol and clove leaf oil: A survey of consumer patch test sensitization. *Food Chem Toxicol* 21:727–733, 1983.
43. Basketter DA, Basketter DA: Possible origin of the skin sensitization potential of isoeugenol and related compounds. *Contact Dermatitis* 27:98–104, 1992.
44. Guin JD: History, manufacture, and cutaneous reactions to perfumes, in Frost P, Horwitz SN (eds): *Principles of Cosmetics for the Dermatologist*. St. Louis, Mosby, 1982.

34

RUBBER

Donald V. Belsito

The term *rubber* refers to both natural rubber latex as well as a number of varying synthetic rubber materials. While natural rubber is based in the polymer 1,4-polyiso-prene, a variety of synthetic rubbers exist, each based on different polymers. Table 34-1 lists some of the more common synthetic rubbers. Readers interested in a more complete delineation are referred to standard texts.[1,2]

Rubber products may be natural, synthetic, or mixtures of the two. Since the vast majority of rubberized products are unlabeled, it is difficult to determine whether a product contains natural or synthetic rubber. The overlap between "rubber" and "plastic" further complicates the matter, especially since plastics contain many of the same catalysts, stabilizers, antioxidants and pigments/dyes present in rubber products.[3] Although completely cured, plastics are rare sensitizers; rubber products, even fully cured, do produce allergic reactions, given the ability of the sensitizers to leach out or "bloom" over time.

THE ALLERGENS

During the manufacturing process, the polymers of both natural and synthetic rubber must be mixed with additional chemicals to confer useful properties. For natural rubber, the principal additive is usually a sulfur mixture which, when heated with latex (by "vulcanization"), produces a product which does not soften when warm or stiffen when cold. Vulcanization also enhances the elasticity, resistance to abrasion, and strength of the final product. Since vulcanization with sulfur is a slow process, organic accelera-tors are added to speed the reaction. These accelerators, some of which are listed in Table 34-2, are the most significant causes of delayed-type hypersensitivity reactions to rubber products. Certain synthetic rubbers (i.e., butyl and nitrile rubber) can be vulcanized with organic peroxides; hence the addition of accelerators, which act as sulfur donors, is not necessary.

Another major group of allergens are the antioxidants, which are added to the manufacturing process to retard deterioration due to oxygen and ozone. Table 34-3 lists the antioxidants with the greatest potential for cutaneous sensitization. Additional

TABLE 34-1. Synthetic Rubbers Encountered in Nonoccupational Settings

Common Name	Polymer	Usage
Styrene-butadiene	Styrene + butadiene	Most widely used in industrial rubber products, especially tires
Butyl	Isobutylene + isoprene or butadiene	Inner tubes
Neoprene	Chloroprene	Clothing/gloves, latex foams, industrial products
Nitrile	Acrylonitrile + butadiene	Shoes/gloves, waterproof clothing, adhesives, artificial leathers, industrial products
Polyurethane (i.e., Spandex)	Isocyanates + polyesters	Elasticized clothing, shoes, sealants/caulkings, adhesives, industrial products

TABLE 34–2. Accelerators in Natural and Synthetic Rubbers Likely to Cause Allergic Contact Hypersensitivity[a]

Chemical Class	Allergen Present in Standard Patch-Test Kits[b]
Benzothiazoles	2-MBT and mercapto mix[c]
Thiurams	Thiuram mix[d]
Dithiocarbamates	Carba mix[e]
Guanidines	Carba mix[e]
Thioureas	No

[a]For a more complete listing of the many available accelerators, see Ref. 1.

[b]Based on the contents of the only presently available standard kit manufactured by Hermal Kurt Hermann, Reinbek, Germany, for sale in the United States.

[c]2-MBT: 2-mercaptobenzothiazole; mercapto mix contains N-cyclohexyl-2-benzothiazole-sulfenamide, 2, 2′-benzothiazyl disulfide and morpholinyl-2-benzothiazyl disulfide.

[d]Thiuram mix contains tetramethylthiuram disulfide, tetramethylthiuram monosulfide, tetraethylthiuram disulfide, and dipentamethylenethiuram disulfide.

[e]Carba mix contains zinc diethyldithiocarmate, zinc dibutyldithiocarbamate, and 1,3-diphenylguanidine.

chemicals which may be added to rubber during manufacture include fillers, reinforcing agents, ultraviolet inhibitors, pigments/dyes, softeners/extenders, plasticizers, stabilizers, retarders, and blowing agents. These chemicals, except for the phenol formaldehyde resins which can be used as plasticizers[2] and epoxy resins which can be used as stabilizers,[4] are rare causes of allergic contact dermatitis. Readers interested in a more

TABLE 34–3. Antioxidants in Natural and Synthetic Rubber Likely to Cause Allergic Contact Hypersensitivity[a]

Chemical Class	Allergen Present in Standard Patch-Test Kits[b]
Amines	
Phenylenediamines	Black rubber mix[c]
Quinolines	No
Phenols	
Hydroquinones	No

[a]For a more complete listing of the many available antioxidants, see Ref. 1.

[b]Based on the contents of the only presently available standard kit manufactured by Hermal Kurt Hermann, Reinbek, Germany, for sale in the United States.

[c]Black rubber mix contains N-phenyl-N′-cyclohexyl-p-phenylenediamine, N-isopropyl-N′-phenyl-p-phenylenediamine, and N, N′-diphenyl-p-phenylenediamine.

complete listing of the hundreds of chemicals that can be added to rubber during its manufacture are referred to Taylor.[1]

With the exception of two case reports of possible allergic contact dermatitis (ACD) to isocyanates present in a synthetic polyurethane wound dressing[5] and one report of a reaction to polyisoprene in natural rubber,[6] the polymers on which both natural and synthetic rubbers are based have not been reported to cause allergic reactions. However, contaminants present in the saps containing the polyisoprene from which natural rubber latex is manufactured can cause problems. A 3000- to 10,000-Da substance, the exact chemical nature of which remains unknown, has been said to cause the increasingly reported episodes of allergic contact urticaria (ACU) to natural rubber latex obtained from the *Hevea braziliensis* tree.[7] Since *H. braziliensis* accounts for over 99 percent of natural rubber used worldwide,[8–11] ACU to latex is potentially a significant problem.

Other commercial sources of natural rubber include *Parthenium argentatum* (guayule rubber) and plants of the Sapotaceae family (gutta-percha). Although it is unknown whether the polyisoprene-containing sap from these plants contains the chemical responsible for inducing ACU, it has been reported that the sap from *P. argentatum,* a member of the Compositae family, contains a cinnamic acid ester of sesquiterpene which proved to be a potent sensitizer for delayed-type hypersensitivity in the guinea pig maximization test.[12] Perhaps for this reason, guayule rubber has not become a significant source of rubber worldwide. Although the sap of the Sapotaceae plant is apparently free of sensitizers, it is highly irritating[13] and gutta-percha is little used except for covering athletic balls and dental fillings.[2]

INCIDENCE OF DELAYED-TYPE HYPERSENSITIVITY TO RUBBER

Rubber additives are among the more frequent causes of ACD. Of 274 nondermatologic patients undergoing hip arthroplasty at a Swedish general hospital from 1968 to 1977, 1.1 percent (3/274) had allergic reactions to thiuram mix and carba mix and 0.4 percent (1/274) had reactions to black rubber mix and mercapto mix upon routine patch testing.[14] Since these patients were more "randomly" selected than those usually referred for patch testing, the incidence rates of allergic reactions to rubber additives in this study are more representative of those in the Swedish population. Unfortunately, whether due to genetic variations in differing populations, exposure patterns within a population, or other factors, the incidence of a given allergic reaction can vary among countries. In the United States, no comparable study has been done. The only available data come from publications of the North American Contact Dermatitis Group,[15–17] where incidence rates are probably overstated, since the reported data are generated from patients referred for evaluation of suspected contact dermatitis.

As shown in Table 34-4, a significant percentage of North American patients referred for patch testing had positive reactions to one or more of the rubber additives tested. The percentage of patients reacting to the thiazoles and carbamates has been relatively constant over time. In contrast, the percentage reacting to black rubber and thiuram mixes seems to be increasing. Reactivity rates for black rubber mix ostensibly are indicative of the rate of sensitivity from industrial occupational exposure, while those for thiuram are indicative of the rate of sensitization from nonindustrial exposure, especially from gloves.[18] Thus, the data from Table 34-4 suggest that both industrial

TABLE 34–4. Incidence of Positive (Presumably Allergic) Reactions to Rubber-Related Chemicals in a Population of Patients Undergoing Patch Testing in North America: 1972–1989[a]

Test Substance	1972–1974[b] (n)	1984–1985[c] (n)	1985–1989[d] (n)
Thiuram mix	4.2%[e] (1200)	3.9% (1137)	5.5% (3986)
Carba mix	NT[f]	3.3% (1135)	3.1% (3988)
Mercapto mix	NT	2.6% (1132)	2.5% (3979)
Mercaptobenzothiazole	4.8% (1200)	2.9% (1141)	2.1% (3968)
Black rubber mix	NT	1.4% (1140)	2.1% (3985)

[a]Percentages given are for patients referred for patch testing with eczematous dermatitides and presumed allergic contact dermatitis.
[b]Data from Ref. 15.
[c]Data from Ref. 16.
[d]Data from Ref. 17.
[e]2% thiuram and not thiuram mix tested.
[f]NT = not tested.

production of rubber-related materials and usage of latex gloves has increased significantly in North America during the past decade. A similar increase in the rate of ACD to rubber chemicals, especially thiurams, has been reported worldwide.[8–11]

Allergic contact dermatitis to rubber additives is a significant cause of occupationally acquired dermatitis. From 1974 to 1983, allergic reactions to rubber-related chemicals accounted for 19.9 percent of all occupational ACD seen in Finland; only metals (28.4 percent) and plastic materials (27.7 percent) were more frequent offenders.[19] Similar results have been reported from other countries throughout Europe.[20–22] In studies performed outside the rubber and tire industry, the principal source of exposure to rubber-related chemicals among workers is gloves: in the Finnish study, gloves accounted for 58.3 percent of rubber-related eczema.[11] Similar results were seen in a general dermatology clinic in Germany where, out of 3851 patients evaluated between 1985 and 1990, allergic reactions to rubber were seen in 145 individuals (3.8 percent); in 80 of 145 (55 percent), the source of exposure was occupational.[23] Of the occupational cases, 67/80 (84 percent) acquired the dermatitis from use of rubber gloves.[23] Workers at greatest risk for developing ACD to rubber additives were those engaged in health/laboratory services (30 percent) or homemaking activities (18.8 percent). In these two groups of "wet workers" (hospital personnel, domestic personnel, food handlers, beauticians, etc.), gloves accounted for all but one of the cases of occupational exposure.[23]

Because of the association of rubber-related allergy with wet work, it is instructive to evaluate the incidence of dermatitis among wet workers. In a Finnish study of 536 randomly recruited hospital workers, 46.2 percent were found to have had a past or present hand dermatitis which they related to work.[24] Although many of these were considered irritant, ACD to rubber additives accounted for 2.4 percent (13/536) of all occupational hand dermatitis.[24] In a similar Danish study of 541 hospital cleaning personnel, 39.1 percent were found to have a present or past dermatitis.[25] Among 52 patients with active occupationally related dermatitis at the time of the study, 75.0 percent were thought to have primarily irritant and 21.2 percent primarily allergic contact dermatitis. Of the 11 cases of ACD, 4 (36.4 percent) were due to rubber accelerators.[25] In a prospective study over 20 months of 2452 newly employed Swedish hospital workers, 142 individuals (5.8 percent) developed occupationally related hand dermatitis.[26] Of the 142, 120 were evaluated by patch testing and 10 (8.3 percent) were found to be allergic to rubber additives, although the allergy was felt to be significant in only 2 patients.[26] Thus, although irritant contact dermatitis is the most likely cause of hand dermatitis in wet workers, a significant percentage of these individuals will have ACD, of which many are rubber-related.

In addition to wet workers, workers in basic rubber industries form another high-risk group. The annual risk of allergic plus irritant dermatitis in these workers ranges from 0.31 percent in Britain[27] to 0.56 percent in Finland.[28] The only available data from the United States state a risk of 0.7 percent for Californian workers, but this number includes workers in the plastics industry as well.[29] The apparently lower risk of developing ACD among workers in the rubber industry relates in part to the reporting of an annual risk rate rather than the total percentage of workers with occupationally related dermatitis as well as to the increasing automation within the rubber industry, which minimizes direct physical contact with the allergens. An important difference between the ACD seen in rubber workers and that seen in wet workers is the high percentage of ACD due to black rubber in the former. In a 5-year Finnish study of rubber workers, 15/21 (71.4 percent) of all occupationally related ACD was due to a component of black rubber mix.[28] In contrast, when allergic to a rubber material, wet workers are more likely to be allergic to thiuram present in gloves.[11,19,23–26,30]

In workers with occupational exposure to rubber, many other allergens are encountered. Among hospital wet workers, metals and fragrances were historically more common allergens than rubber-related chemicals.[24,25] Even among workers in rubber industries, reactions to contaminants such as dinitrochlorobenzene[31] or to other allergens such as cobalt[32] do occur. Individuals evaluating occupationally related dermatitides should consult standard texts delineating the likely allergens and irritants encountered.[2]

CLINICAL PATTERNS OF ALLERGIC CONTACT DERMATITIS TO RUBBER

ECZEMATOUS DERMATITIS

A vast majority of allergic reactions to rubber additives are subacute to chronic eczematous dermatitides presenting as a lichenified, scaling, occasionally fissured dermatitis with or without accompanying vesiculation (Fig. 34-1). In acute contact dermatitis, the presentation over most areas of the body is one of macular erythema with papules, vesicles, or bullae, depending on the intensity of the allergic response. However, in acute ACD on certain areas of the body, such as the eyelids and genital areas, erythema and edema predominate with or without papulovesiculation. The shape and location(s) of the rash provide the most important clues, especially as to the causal allergen(s). Since rubber-containing materials are ubiquitous, patients presenting with rubber-related ACD can have various combinations of the clinical patterns described below.

Hand Dermatitis

In one published report, 33 percent of patients referred for patch testing had a primary hand dermatitis.[12] Among these patients, 28.9 percent were found to have ACD, while

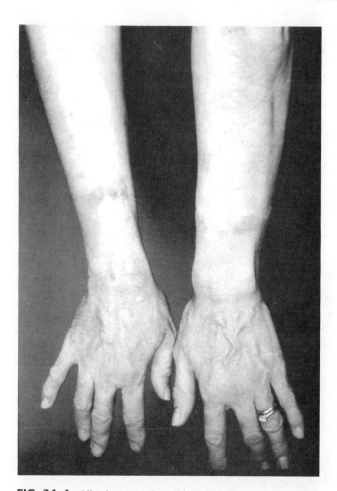

FIG. 34–1. Allergic contact dermatitis to thiurams and carbamates in a rubber glove. A middle-aged woman initially presented with a presumed dyshidrotic eczema of the fingers and was instructed to wear rubber gloves for household wet work. She returned several months later with this erythematous scaling dermatitis of the dorsal hands. Note the demarcation at the wrists, with patches of dermatitis about the mid-forearm, which is typical of allergic reactions to household gloves. Patch tests showed positive reactions to both the thiuram and carba mixes. Her dermatitis cleared with use of cotton liners and vinyl gloves. *(Reproduced with permission of the Ronald O. Perelman Department of Dermatology, New York University School of Medicine.)* (See color Plate 19.)

the bulk of the remainder had either irritant contact dermatitis (21.6 percent) or atopic dermatitis (10.3 percent). Not unusually, a secondary ACD of the hands will develop in a patient with an underlying, nonallergic hand dermatitis who begins utilizing rubber gloves and/or topical creams and becomes sensitized to a chemical in these products (Fig. 34-1).

Significantly greater involvement of the finger webs and dorsa of the hands rather than the palms suggests ACD, assuming that the allergen contacts all areas of the hand equally, as is the case for gloves (Fig. 34-1). Obviously, the truck driver who contacts

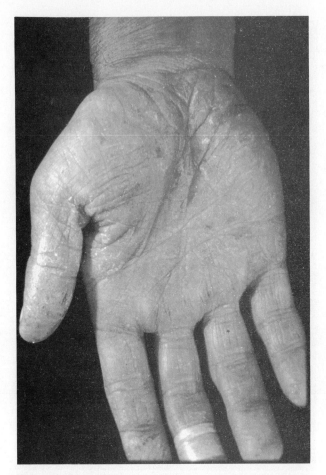

FIG. 34–2. Allergic contact dermatitis to *para*-phenylenediamine derivatives in a rubber shift handle. A middle-aged truck driver complained of this dermatitis over the volar aspect of the right hand which developed several months after purchasing a new truck. Patch test showed positive reactions to pieces of rubber taken from the shift handle as well as to black rubber mix. The dermatitis resolved when the rubber-coated knob was replaced with plastic. *(Reproduced with permission of the Ronald O. Perelman Department of Dermatology, New York University School of Medicine.)* (See color Plate 20.)

a rubber-coated shift handle with the palmar aspect of the right hand and fingers may present with dermatitis restricted primarily to these areas (Fig. 34-2). In seeking a rubber-related cause of ACD of the hands, one must pay particular attention to those materials which are encountered in the occupation(s) and hobbies of the patient. Office workers might have frequent contact with rubber bands, erasers, finger cots, and so on, while the hobbyist's exposure relates to use of rubber-based glues and adhesives. Thus, while most cases of rubber-related ACD of the hands result from thiuram in gloves,[11,19,23–26,30] carbamates, thiazoles, phenylenediamine derivatives, thioureas, and other rare but potential sensitizers that might be present in the many rubber products handled during the activities of modern life also produce a significant number of reactions.

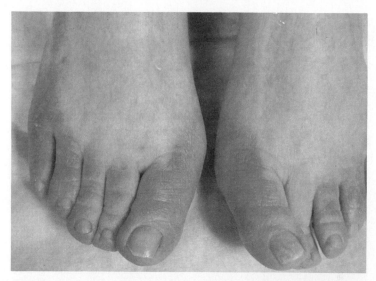

FIG. 34–3. Allergic contact dermatitis to *p-tert*-butylphenol formaldehyde resin in neoprene glues. A middle-aged woman presented with a many months' history of this erythematous scaling dermatitis limited only to the dorsal aspect of the toes bilaterally. Treatment with a variety of potent glucocorticoids ameliorated the pruritus but not the dermatitis. Patch tests showed positive reactions to the linings of several shoes as well as to *p-tert*-butylphenol formaldehyde resin. The dermatitis resolved upon purchase of shoes free of the neoprene adhesives which contain the allergen. (See color Plate 21.)

Foot Dermatitis

Like the palms of the hands, the soles of the feet are relatively resistant to the manifestations of ACD. Thus, the typical picture of pedal ACD is dermatitis over the dorsal parts of the feet, accentuated over the joints of the toes (Fig. 34-3). In a 12-year Portuguese study of 539 patients with shoe dermatitis, 75.7 percent of the patients presented with only dorsal dermatitis, the principal allergens being chromates in tanned leather and *para-tertiary*-butylphenol formaldehyde resin (PTBFR) in neoprene adhesives.[33] However, not all patients with ACD of the feet due to rubber will present with such a classic picture. As detailed by Storrs,[34] the manufacturing of shoes is in a state of constant flux, and rubber-based materials are continually being added and subtracted from the components (e.g., box toes are now made of celastic rather than rubber).

When ACD involves the soles, it tends to spare the flexural creases of the toes and the arch (Fig. 34-4). The dermatitis is usually bilateral, although not always, and it may be patchy.[35,36] Among 539 Portuguese patients, 22.3 percent were found to have dermatitis involving the soles, and the predominant allergens were mercaptobenzothiazoles, which accounted for 54.2 percent of these cases.[33] Chromates and PTBFR accounted, respectively, for 24.2 and 19.2 percent of volar dermatitis.[33]

Although 2-mercaptobenzothiazole and PTBFR are the usual rubber-related allergens in shoes, reactions to thiurams and carbamates can also be seen.[37] Rarely, the antioxidants in black rubber mix have been responsible for dermatitis related to rubber work

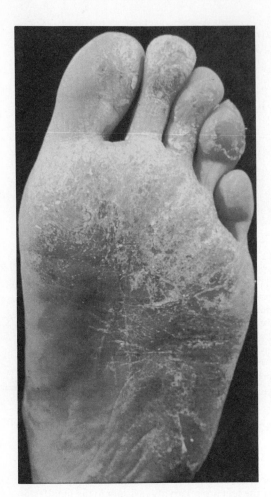

FIG. 34–4. Allergic contact dermatitis to mercaptobenzothiazole in shoe inserts. A young man presented with a several-year history of this hyperkeratotic dermatitis limited to the volar aspects of the feet. The condition had been treated with a variety of antipsoriatic regimens without success. Patch tests showed positive reactions to mercaptobenzothiazole, mercapto mix, and rubber inserts in several pairs of athletic shoes. Note the sparing of the arches and flexural creases of the toes typical of ACD to shoe inserts. The dermatitis eventually resolved when rubber-free shoes were purchased. *(Reproduced with permission of the Ronald O. Perelman Department of Dermatology, New York University School of Medicine.)* (See color Plate 22.)

boots.[38] In addition, sporadic reports of ACD to thioureas,[39] mercaptans,[40] and the many other rubber-related chemicals found in shoes pepper the literature. Individuals interested in detailed lists of these potential allergens are referred elsewhere.[37,41]

Facial Dermatitis

Allergic contact dermatitis of the face, ears, and neck can be difficult to diagnose, since many substances could potentially be responsible. One must consider not only the components of facial cosmetics (vehicles, preservatives, emulsifiers, fragrances, etc.), airborne allergens, or photocontact allergens but also rubber-related allergens, among others. Eyelash curlers lined with rubber have been among the more frequently reported, with the responsible allergens being thiurams, carbamates and *para*-phenylenediamine (PPD) derivatives.[42,43] Rubber makeup sponges can also cause facial dermatitis, which can be very patchy and may simulate seborrheic dermatitis (Fig. 34-5). Other causes of rubber-related facial dermatitis are swimming caps,[18] goggles,[44] respira-

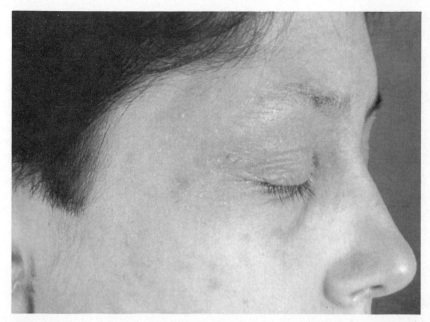

FIG. 34–5. Allergic contact dermatitis to thioureas in a makeup applicator. A middle-aged woman presented with this lichenified dermatitis of the eyelids of 1 year's duration. Initial evaluation with standard patch tests was negative, but she returned for further diagnostic workup when her dermatitis cleared upon discontinuation of all makeup. Patch tests were positive only to her makeup sponges and to a mix of di-alkyl thioureas (1% in petrolatum). The patient resumed use of cosmetics but without rubber sponges and remained free of her dermatitis. *(Reproduced with permission of the Ronald O. Perelman Department of Dermatology, New York University School of Medicine.)* (See color Plate 23.)

tors,[45] and balloons.[18] Readers interested in a more complete listing of additional sources of rubber exposure are referred to Taylor.[1]

In evaluating any patient with facial dermatitis, note that the hands can be an unwitting source of transmission of allergens to the face (especially the eyes) and yet may manifest no evidence of dermatitis themselves. This is typically seen with allergies to nail polish but can also be seen with rubber-related allergens. Jordan[46] reported several cases of eyelid dermatitis in hospital personnel with frequent use of rubber gloves. The patients were reactive to thiuram, which had leaked into the glove powder and was then transmitted to the eyelids, where it caused dermatitis.

Undergarment Dermatitis

Dermatitis about the brassiere area, waistband, girdle area, and garter strap area can be due to allergic reactions to rubber additives (Fig. 34-6). In evaluating such patients, it is important to be aware of the "bleached rubber syndrome."[47] This should be suspected when patch testing with standard rubber allergens is negative, since the allergen (*N,N'* dibenzylcarbamyl chloride) results from the effect of bleach on the rubber accelerator zinc dibenzyldithiocarbamate. Fortunately, patch testing with the bleached elastic of the garment usually produces a positive result.

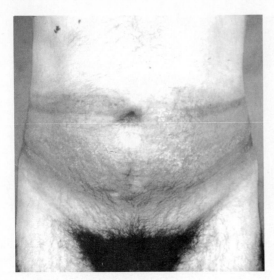

FIG. 34–6. Allergic contact dermatitis to bleached rubber. A middle-aged man presented with this waistband dermatitis of several months duration. Patch testing to a standard tray as well as to an expanded rubber series was negative. The only positive reaction was to the elasticized waistband of his underwear. This case of "bleached rubber" syndrome resolved when he purchased new underwear which remained unbleached. *(Reproduced with permission of the Ronald O. Perelman Department of Dermatology, New York University School of Medicine.)* (See color Plate 24.)

Mucosal Dermatitis

Despite widespread exposure of mucosal surfaces to allergens, it is obvious from the dearth of reports in the literature that patients only rarely react to delayed-type allergens presented mucosally. When allergic reactions do occur, the symptoms are usually seen in association with a related dermatitis elsewhere on the body, most frequently on the adjoining periorificial integument. Rubber-related allergens are not infrequently responsible for mucosal ACD. Among the many rubber-based items likely to contact mucosal surfaces are dental dams, balloons, endotracheal tubes, condoms, diaphragms, pessaries, catheters, and latex exam gloves. Readers seeking more detailed discussions of these and related materials are referred to Taylor[1] and Fisher.[48]

Systemic Contact Dermatitis

Systemic exposure to a delayed-type allergen to which an individual has been cutaneously sensitized can result in bizarre clinical patterns ranging from diffuse dermatitis with or without accentuation at sites of previous exposure[49] to the "baboon syndrome."[50] Systemic contact dermatitis to rubber accelerators has been reported in patients undergoing hemodialysis.[49] Since it has been shown that rubber accelerators can emigrate into foodstuffs stored in rubber containers[51] and into medications contained in vials topped with rubber seals,[52] rubber-related allergies must be suspected in patients with bizarre eczematous dermatitides whose history suggests such potential systemic exposures.

Other Rubber-Related Eczemas

Because rubber is ubiquitous, other locations on the body ranging from wrists (watch-strap dermatitis[53]) to amputation stumps (prosthesis dermatitis[54]) may be involved. Interested readers can find a more detailed listing of the many rubber-based consumer articles in Taylor.[1]

NONECZEMATOUS DERMATOSES

Hyperkeratosis Palmaris et Plantaris

Long-standing, chronic ACD of the palms and soles can present as a hyperkeratotic, fissured dermatitis. According to some,[55] hyperkeratosis palmaris et plantaris is particularly seen in association with ACD to the amine antioxidants.

Purpuric Contact Dermatitis

Pigmented purpuric ACD has been observed usually due to *para*-phenylenediamine (PPD) derivatives present in black rubber mix.[56–58]

Pustulosis Palmaris et Plantaris

Although pustular ACD of the palms and soles has been seen most frequently as a reaction pattern to metals, cases due to the benzothiazole accelerators present in mercapto mix[59] and PPD derivatives present in PPD mix[60] have been reported.

Erythema Multiforme

One case of erythema multiforme localized to the right forearm was reportedly caused by ACD to PPD derivatives present in a black rubber band wrapped about the wrist.[61]

Leukoderma/Vitiligo

Hydroquinone and its derivatives are known causes of leukoderma, and exposure to the monobenzyl ether in work boots represented the first reported cases of this disease in association with rubber products.[62] Subsequently, leukoderma has been reported following exposure to rubber goggles, although whether the condition was allergic or not was not proved.[44]

ALLERGIC CONTACT URTICARIA

Since 1979, when Nutter[63] first called attention to allergic contact urticaria (ACU) induced by rubber, more than several hundred additional cases have been reported. When investigated by scratch or RAST testing, a majority of cases have been ascribed to a component of the sap from *H. braziliensis*.[64–67] In other instances, natural latex from *H. braziliensis* has been implicated by a positive reaction to the rubber article and negative reactions to rubber additives.[11,68] Using a histamine-release assay and indirect enzyme-linked immunosorbent testing, researchers were able to document the allergen as a $\leq$ 30,000-Da trypsin-sensitive protein component of *H. braziliensis*.[69] In a subsequent study, the molecule has been further characterized as a 3000- to 10,000-Da water-soluble protein.[7]

Not all cases of ACU to rubber are due to reactions to the natural rubber itself. In their evaluation of 15 patients with symptoms related to rubber gloves, Wrangsjö and associates[70] found 6 of 15 to have contact urticaria, but only 3 of 6 were scratch-test positive to natural dried latex and only 2 of these 3 had a positive RAST test to *H. braziliensis*. Another patient who did not react to natural latex had a positive RAST test to latex. Of interest, one of the only two natural latex-RAST and latex scratch-test–positive patients had an urticarial response to zinc pentamethylene dithiocarbamate and to zinc dibutyl dithiocarbamate.[70] In their evaluation of one patient with contact urticaria secondary to rubber, Helander and Makela[71] found him to be sensitized to zinc diethyl dithiocarbamate. In another study of 7 patients with contact urticaria to rubber products, 3 reactions were attributable to *H. braziliensis* and 1 each to mercaptobenzothiazole, carba mix, black rubber mix, and cornstarch powder.[72] Thus, allergens other than natural latex that are found in rubber materials can precipitate contact urticaria.

Individuals at greatest risk for developing ACU are those who have repeated exposure to latex products, especially medical/dental personnel. In a study of 512 hospital workers, 2.9 percent were found to have ACU to rubber gloves. Indeed, 6 percent of operating room personnel had ACU.[67] In this same study, evaluation of 44 medical students and 130 controls with suspected atopy revealed that one student (2.3 percent) and one control (0.8 percent) also had ACU to rubber gloves. In other series, the rate of ACU among hospital wet workers has been reported to be 5.6 percent[26] while that among a general patch-test clinic population was 0.09 percent.[10]

Atopic dermatitis[63,67,70] and/or other preexisting dermatitis[72,73] predisposes to the development of ACU. In addition, mucosal exposure to latex appears to be a risk factor. In one study, 3 of 7 patients developed ACU following mucosal exposure[72]: 2 were paraplegics and the other was a young woman exposed to latex in a condom. In 2 of these 3 individuals, anaphylactic reactions developed within minutes of exposure. Similar results have been seen by other investigators.[66] Thus, in addition to hospital personnel, paraplegics, sexually active individuals exposed to latex condoms,[72] and others with repeated mucosal exposure to latex must be considered high-risk groups for development of ACU. The failure to detect ACU to latex can have grave consequences in the allergic patient during intraoperative contact with surgeons' latex gloves.[74]

The presentation of ACU from latex is varied. For many patients, the symptoms are immediate burning, stinging, or itching with or without localized urticaria upon contact with latex. In some, symptoms progress to disseminated urticaria, allergic rhinitis, asthma, and/or anaphylaxis (Fig. 34-7). Other patients may present with an eczematous-appearing dermatitis. This clinical pattern is usually due to concomitant ACD to a rubber additive which, in many cases, precedes the development of ACU.[72,73] However, some patients presenting with an eczematous pattern may have protein contact dermatitis.[75] In many patients with ACU from latex gloves, the palmar aspects of the hands are as involved or more involved than the dorsal surfaces. This may relate to the lipid composition of the palmar epidermis,[76] which allows it to be more easily penetrated by the water-soluble allergen of latex.

DIAGNOSIS

IN VIVO TESTS FOR ALLERGIC CONTACT DERMATITIS

The only useful and reliable method for the diagnosis of ACD remains the patch test. At the present time, only 20 commercially prepared allergens are readily available in

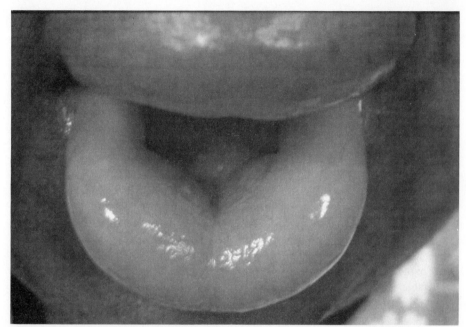

FIG. 34–7. Allergic contact urticaria to latex in a balloon. This young dental technician had a known history of atopic dermatitis and allergic contact dermatitis to thiurams in gloves. She presented with acute swelling of the lips, scattered hives of the face, hands, and arms, and respiratory distress. Her symptoms developed within minutes of blowing up several balloons. Subsequent prick testing to eluates from the balloons and several pairs of latex gloves were positive, although the RAST test for latex was equivocal. Prick testing to the rubber accelerators including thiurams was negative. (See color Plate 25.)

the United States. However, in recognition of the significant number of individuals allergic to rubber-related chemicals, 5 of these allergens are rubber-related. In fact, 4 of 5 are mixes; hence, on the standard tray, 14 rubber additives are tested. In addition, PTBFR and epoxy resin, plasticizers which can be added to specialty rubber items, are also included.

Given the vast number of additives in a given rubber product, dermatologists interested in fully evaluating at least some of their patients with ACD to rubber must be prepared to perform tests with the patient's own materials. In so doing, pieces of the suspected materials should be cut out to conform to the size of the patch; it is frequently helpful to soak the material in water for 15 min prior to testing. Furthermore, when testing for a rubber material as is, it may be necessary to leave the patch in place for longer than 48 h, perhaps up to 1 week. Patients unreactive to the rubber allergens on the standard tray who react to their own product will often require testing to an expanded rubber series either obtained abroad or privately compounded. Typical components of a commercially available rubber tray have been published elsewhere.[23,30] For physicians compounding their own allergens, texts detailing appropriate concentrations and vehicles are available.[77]

Like any in vivo assay, patch testing is subject to pitfalls, and practitioners are well advised to read the excellent review by Sulzberger.[78] Of primary concern is that even once a chemical is found to be allergenic for a given patient, one cannot de facto assume that it is the cause of ACD. This is particularly true for individuals with a suspected rubber-related dermatitis, since the ingredients of the offending product are almost never labeled. Thus, in an effort to determine whether an allergen is likely to be the culprit, the results of a positive patch test must always be correlated with the materials encountered by the involved areas of skin. In the case of thiurams and carbamates, simple office-based tests are available for detecting these chemicals in patient-provided material.[34] However, even in some instances where patients are allergic to chemicals present in products which they are using, the allergen may be present in only minimal amounts and may not be responsible for the dermatitis.[79] In this regard, "use testing" can also be helpful.[80]

Individuals performing patch tests must also be concerned with the possibility of false-positive reactions due either to the use of allergens at irritant concentrations or to the "excited skin syndrome."[81] The "false" nature of these reactions can usually be resolved by repeating the patch tests individually and/or in lower concentrations. Among the rubber additives present in the standard tray, carba mix seems to be the most frequent cause of false-positive irritant reactions.[17]

False-negative reactions are more problematic than false-positive reactions and require high levels of suspicion and diligence to uncover. One common and easily correctable cause of false-negative reactions is the failure to perform a second reading of the test sites after the initial 48-h inspection. This second reading, sometime between 3 and 7 days after application of the patches, is particularly important for elderly patients, in whom it takes longer to mount an allergic reaction.[82] Another cause of false-negative tests is the possibility that the reaction is a photoallergic contact dermatitis requiring light to elicit the positive response, as has been reported for at least one case of thiourea-induced dermatitis.[83] Finally, with so many potential rubber-related allergens, negative reactions may simply indicate that the responsible chemical has not been tested. This seems particularly true for shoe-related dermatitis, where estimates of the rate of false-negative reactions upon patch testing range around 20 percent.[35,37]

IN VITRO TESTS FOR ALLERGIC CONTACT DERMATITIS

Laboratory studies such as lymphocyte transformation or macrophage migration inhibition have been used as in vitro measurements of ACD in both humans and animals.[84] However, these in vitro assays have not been reliably standardized and are therefore not clinically useful for diagnosis. One of the major problems in developing in vitro systems is the lack of knowledge as to what is the antigenic moiety of a particular chemical. Thus, in vivo patch testing in which the skin can process the allergen for presentation remains the gold standard.

IN VIVO TESTS FOR ALLERGIC CONTACT URTICARIA

As with testing for ACD, in vivo tests for ACU are more reliable.[7,67,72] Various tests are available, including prick testing, closed-chamber testing with or without abrasion of the underlying skin, and use testing. In performing such tests, one ideally would want the purified allergen extracted from natural latex; however, since this has not been identified, others have found that the responsible allergen can be leached out of rubber by soaking the material in water at room temperature for 30 min.[7,85] In most but not all cases, use of such an eluate for prick or scratch testing will be sufficient for detecting ACU. Individuals interested in more detailed descriptions of the methods for in vivo testing are referred elsewhere.[67,72] They must be aware of the potential for life-threatening anaphylactic reactions during the course of such testing, especially in patients whose symptoms suggest prior systemic reactions to latex products. The author has seen such reactions even following prick testing.

As with patch testing, testing for ACU is subject to both false-negative and false-positive reactions. Appropriate positive (histamine, 1 to 10 mg/mL) and negative (physiologic saline) controls must always be tested concomitantly. False-negative reactions are usually due to limited exposure to the allergen and can be unmasked by abrading the skin and/or by allowing more of the allergen to leach out by properly moistening the sample with water prior to use. Additional causes of false-negative reactions include testing of patients depleted of IgE due to recent systemic reactions. False-positive reactions can occur for a variety of reasons, but among the most common is dermatographism.

IN VITRO TESTS FOR ALLERGIC CONTACT URTICARIA

RAST testing for latex allergy is available commercially, but these tests are notoriously unreliable. In one study, only 2 of 5 patients with ACU to latex were RAST-positive,[67] while, in another, only 1 of 3 patients reacting to natural dried latex resin had a positive RAST test.[72]

TREATMENT AND PREVENTION

ALLERGEN AVOIDANCE

The treatment of ACD and ACU lies in correctly identifying its cause and in properly instructing the patient in avoidance of the responsible allergen(s). Patients must be warned that the term *hypoallergenic* when applied to a latex article is meaningless unless they know the actual ingredients. Most "hypoallergenic" latex products contain carbamates, which have been regarded as less sensitizing than thiuram or benzothiazole derivatives[86]; these materials would be very allergenic for the individual with ACD to carbamates or ACU to latex. For many of the patient's needs, a variety of substitute plastic materials exist in the marketplace. When in doubt, the patient can always contact the manufacturer. Guidance is generally needed in selecting the following:

Gloves

A wide array of alternative gloves are available for individuals reacting to a component of latex gloves. Table 34-5 is a partial list of gloves which should be sufficient for most patients. A more detailed listing can be found in Heese et al.[30]

TABLE 34-5. A Partial Listing of Glove Ingredients Useful in Guiding the Allergic Patient[a]

Brand Name	Polymer	MBT	TH	CAR	TU	Powder
				Components[b]		
Sterile surgical	Latex					
Eudermic[c]	Latex	—	—	+	—	+ CS
Dermaguard Plus[d]	Latex	—	—	+	—	+ CS
Pristine[e]	Latex	—	+	—	+	—
Safeskin[f]	Neoprene	—	—	—	—	±[n]
Dermaprene[g]	Neoprene	—	—	—	+	+
Neolon[c]	Thermoplastic	—	—	+	—	+ LAS
Tactyl-1[h]	elastomer	—	—	—	—	+ CS
Nonsterile exam						
Safeskin[f]	Latex	—	—	—	—	±
Tru-Touch[i]	PVC	—	—	—	—	+ CS
Tactyl-1[h]	Thermoplastic elastomer	—	—	—	—	+ CS
SensiCare	PVC-plastic hybrid	—	—	—	—	+ CS
Household						
Bluette[j]	Neoprene	—	—	+	—	—
Task Handler[j]	Neoprene	—	—	—	+	—
Nimblefinger[j]	PVC	—	—	—	—	—
Allerderm vinyl[h]	PVC	—	—	—	—	—
Industrial						
N-Dex[k]	Nitrile	—	—	—	—	+ CS
Nitrile Decontam. Glove[l]	Nitrile	—	—	—	+	—
4-H Gloves[m]	Polyethylene	—	—	—	—	—

[a]The accuracy of components was verified in July 1992. The components of individual brands may have changed since then.
[b]MBT: 2-mercaptobenzothiazole; TH: tetramethylthiurams; CAR: carbamates; TU: thioureas; CS: cornstarch; LAC: lactose.
[c]Becton Dickinson AcuteCare; Tel.; #800-333-4813.
[d]Smith & Nephew Perry; Tel.; #800-321-9752; Dermaguard Plus has a polyurethane inner lining.
[e]World Medical Supply; Tel. #800-545-5475.
[f]Safeskin Corp.; Tel. #800-456-8379.
[g]Ansell, Inc.; Tel. #800-633-0909 or 800-327-8659.
[h]Allerderm Labs; Tel. #800-365-6868.
[i]Becton Dickinson Division; Tel. #201-460-2211.
[j]Pioneer Industrial Products; Tel. #800-537-2897 or 419-933-2211.
[k]Niche Research, Inc.; Tel. #800-788-8850.
[l]SmartPractice; Tel. #800-822-8956.
[m]Aca Derm; Tel. #415-854-6002.
[n]±: available in both powdered (cornstarch) and nonpowdered forms.

Shoes

Tracking the individual ingredients of commercially available shoes is a frustrating and time-consuming task which is rarely successful. Fortunately, specialty shoe manufacturers are available to custom-manufacture shoes (Table 34-6). Although expensive, custom-made shoes are the easiest way to assure that the shoes are devoid of the relevant allergen. Occasionally, commercially manufactured shoes can be identified:

TABLE 34–6. Manufacturers of Specialty Shoes

Company	Shoe Types
Eneslow Comfort Shoes 924 Broadway New York, NY 10010 Tel. #212-477-2300	Men's, women's, and children's shoes in all styles
The Cordwainer Shop P.O. Box 110 Deerfield, NH 03037 Tel. #603-463-7742	Men's and women's dress shoes and sandals
P.W. Minor Co. P.O. Box 678 Batavia, NY 14020 Tel. #716-343-1500	Limited men's and women's dress shoes; men's work boots; limited men's and women's athletic shoes
Loveless Custom Boots and Shoes 2434 SW 29th Street Oklahoma City, OK 73119 Tel. #800-637-9731	Men's dress shoes and women's dress flats (no heels); men's and women's western-style and hunting boots
Happy Feet, Inc. P.O. Box 1417 Corona, CA 91718 Tel. #714-734-6400	Women's sandal-style shoes in plastic
Servus Footwear Co. P.O. Box 3610 Rock Island, IL 61204 Tel. #800-451-1806	PVC work boot (catalog #18822); PVC work boot w/steel-reinforced toe (catalog #18821)

according to Storrs,[87] Air Mariah running shoes from Nike (model #10600017000) are free of rubber additives. Alternatively, one can patch test all components of the patient's existing shoes (including outer soles) and, if negative, have the patient use test only this pair of shoes for a period of several weeks. If this use test is negative, then the shoe is presumptively free of relevant allergens. Although this is not guaranteed, the patient will, by purchasing the same make and model shoe in the future, be able to avoid the allergen. Unfortunately, due to constant reformulation of shoe components, this can not always be depended upon, and patients should be advised to purchase only one new pair of shoes at a time. Patients with persistent dermatitis despite avoidance of the allergen in shoes should be advised to purchase new socks, since at least one investigator has found that, even when thoroughly washed, socks can be a reservoir for allergens.[88]

Medical Devices

Patients allergic to rubber need specific guidance in choosing contraceptive devices. Table 34-7 lists some alternatives for these patients. They must also warn their physicians against performing exams with rubber gloves to which they might react (Table 34-5). Finally, there are a vast number of other medical devices containing rubber

TABLE 34–7. Contraceptive Devices for Rubber-Sensitive Individuals[a]

Device	Comments
Condoms Fourex Natural Lamb Skins or Trojan Naturalamb	Made from processed sheep intestines; no rubber-related allergens; not completely effective in blocking transmission of HIV.
Tactylon Condom	Thermoplastic elastomer free of latex and rubber additives. Adequately prevents transmission of HIV. Presently unavailable and brand name not yet designated; estimated market date 1994.
Trojan Latex Condom	Natural latex and must be avoided by patients with ACU; contains carbamates but no mercaptobenzothiazole, thiurams, or antioxidants. Adequately prevents transmission of HIV.
Reality Vaginal Pouch	Vaginal condom made of polyurethane. No latex, MBT, thiurams, carbamates, or thioureas. Adequately prevents transmission of HIV. Presently unavailable.
Diaphragms[b] Koromex or Koro-Flex	Latex diaphragm supposedly containing dithiocarbamate accelerators and phenolic antioxidants but no mercaptobenzothiazole or thiurams.[c]
Sponges Today Vaginal Sponge	Polyurethane foam without mercaptobenzothiazole, thiurams, carbamates, or thioureas.

[a]The accuracy of components was verified in July 1992. The components of individual brands may have changed since then.

[b]Nonlatex diaphragms are not presently available.

[c]Information obtained from Ref. 1. The manufacturer refused to confirm the components for proprietary reasons, and therefore the reliability of this information cannot be assured.

which patients, especially those with ACU to latex, need to avoid. More complete listings of these devices can be found elsewhere.[1,48]

Nonrubber Materials Containing Rubber-Related Allergens

Rubber chemicals have varied uses outside of the rubber industry. 2-Mercaptobenzothiazole (2-MBT) and related thiazoles can be found in fungicides and algicides,[3] cutting oils,[89] antifreeze,[3] photographic film emulsions,[90] and veterinary products,[91] among others. Thiurams are extensively used as animal repellants and fungicides[92] and are the active ingredients in disulfiram (Antabuse). The carbamates are widely used as lawn and garden fungicides[93] as well as in the plastics industry.[3] *Para*-phenylenediamine derivatives may cross react with PPD-containing hair dyes and can be used in acrylic products.[1] The thioureas are found in detergents,[94] plastic-based adhesives,[95] photocopy paper,[83] and paint/glue removers.[96] Finally, the allergen responsible for ACU to natural latex may be present in or may cross react with a chemical present in bananas,[97,98] avocados,[98] chestnuts,[98] and possibly other fruits.

SYMPTOMATIC THERAPY

Allergic Contact Dermatitis

In addition to avoidance of further contact with the allergen and its cross-reactants, treatment of ACD should be directed to amelioration of symptoms. Acute, vesicular, weeping eruptions benefit from drying agents such as topical aluminum sulfate/calcium acetate; chronic, lichenified eruptions are best treated with emollients. Pruritus can be controlled with topical antipruritics or oral antihistamines; topical antihistamines or anesthetics are best avoided, given the risk of inducing a secondary allergy in existing dermatitic skin. Patients with glove and/or shoe dermatitis frequently suffer from hyperhidrosis; management of this condition is essential to complete resolution of the dermatitis.

Allergic Contact Urticaria

Patients with ACU to rubber can usually be managed with oral or parenteral antihistamines. Patients with symptoms of anaphylaxis should be managed in an appropriate setting, as indicated by their symptoms. All patients must purchase Medic-Alert tags indicating their allergy to rubber. It may be necessary to dispense epinephrine for self-administration to patients with histories of generalized urticarial reactions. Regardless of the prior pattern of urticarial response to rubber, patients with ACU should seek immediate medical attention when symptoms involving mucosal surfaces, especially respiratory ones, develop.

REFERENCES

1. Taylor JS: Rubber, in Fisher AA (ed): *Contact Dermatitis,* 3d ed. Philadelphia, Lea & Febiger, 1983, pp 603–643.
2. Adams RM: Natural and synthetic rubber, in Adams RM (ed): *Occupational Skin Disease.* New York, Grune & Stratton, 1983, pp 298–312.
3. Fregert S: *Manual of Contact Dermatitis,* 2d ed. Chicago, Yearbook, 1981, p 46.
4. Kilpikari I, Halme H: Contact allergy to Hypalon rubber. *Contact Dermatitis* 9:529, 1983.
5. Helland S, Nyfors A, Utne L: Contact dermatitis to Synthaderm. *Contact Dermatitis* 9:504, 1983.
6. Malten KE: Gummichemikalien und Akryl-Kunstharze als Kontaktallergene. *Allergologie* 2:285, 1979.
7. Turjanmaa K, Reunala T: Condoms as a source of latex allergen and cause of contact urticaria. *Contact Dermatitis* 20:360, 1989.
8. Nurse DS: Rubber sensitivity. *Austr J Dermatol* 20:31, 1979.
9. Themido R, Brandão FM: Contact allergy to thiurams. *Contact Dermatitis* 10:251, 1984.
10. Lammintausta K, Kalimo K: Sensitivity to rubber: Study with rubber mixes and individual rubber chemicals. *Dermatosen* 33:204, 1985.
11. Estlander T, Jolanki R, Kanerva L: Dermatitis and urticaria from rubber and plastic gloves. *Contact Dermatitis* 14:20, 1986.
12. Rodriguez E, Reynolds GW, Thompson JA: Potent contact allergen in the rubber plant guayule *(Parthenium argentatum). Science* 211:1444, 1981.
13. Mitchell JM, Rook A: *Botanical Dermatology.* Vancouver, Greengrass, 1979, p 286.
14. Magnusson B, Möller H: Contact allergy without skin disease. *Acta Derm Venereol* 59(suppl 85):113, 1979.
15. Rudner E, Clendenning WE, Epstein E, et al: Epidemiology of contact dermatitis in North America 1972–1974. *Contact Dermatitis* 6:309, 1980.
16. Storrs FJ, Rosenthal LE, Adams RM, et al: Prevalence and relevance of allergic reactions in patients patch tested in North America 1984 to 1985. *J Am Acad Dermatol* 20:1038, 1989.
17. Nethercott JR, Holness DL, Adams RM, et al: Patch testing with a routine screening tray in North America, 1985 through 1989: I. Frequency of response. *Am J Contact Dermatitis* 2:122, 1991.
18. Cronin E: *Contact Dermatitis.* Edinburgh, Churchill Livingstone, 1980, pp 714–770.
19. Estlander T: Occupational skin disease in Finland. Observations made during 1974–1988 at the Institute of Occupational Health, Helsinki. *Acta Derm Venereol* 70(suppl 155):1, 1990.

20. Budden MG, Kirton V, Wilkinson DS: An industrial dermatitis clinic: Results of a 5-year pilot study. *Trans St. John's Hosp Derm Soc* 59:261, 1973.
21. Lachapelle JM, Tennstedt D: Epidemiological survey of occupational contact dermatitis of the hands in Belgium. *Contact Dermatitis* 5:244, 1979.
22. Fregert S: Occupational dermatitis in a 10-year material. *Contact Dermatitis* 1:96, 1975.
23. von Hintzenstern J, Heese A, Koch HU, et al: Frequency, spectrum and occupational relevance of type IV allergies to rubber chemicals. *Contact Dermatitis* 24:244, 1991.
24. Lammintausta K, Kalimo K, Havu VK: Occurrence of contact allergy and hand eczemas in hospital wet work. *Contact Dermatitis* 8:84, 1982.
25. Hansen KS: Occupational dermatoses in hospital cleaning women. *Contact Dermatitis* 9:343, 1983.
26. Nilsson E: Contact sensitivity and urticaria in "wet" work. *Contact Dermatitis* 13:321, 1985.
27. Calnan CD: Dermatology and industry: Prosser White oration 1977. *Clin Exp Dermatol* 3:1, 1978.
28. Kilpikari I: Occupational contact dermatitis among rubber workers. *Contact Dermatitis* 8:359, 1982.
29. Baginsky E: Surveillance and reporting. A paper presented at Occupational, Industrial and Plant Dermatology Conference, U.S.A. March 26–29, 1979.
30. Heese A, von Hintzenstern J, Peters K-P, et al: Allergic and irritant reactions to rubber gloves in medical health services. *J Am Acad Dermatol* 25:831, 1991.
31. Zina AM, Bedello PG, Cane D, et al: Dermatitis in a rubber tyre factory. *Contact Dermatitis* 17:17, 1987.
32. Foussereau J, Cavelier C: Allergic contact dermatitis from cobalt in the rubber industry. *Contact Dermatitis* 19:217, 1988.
33. Correia S, Brandão FM: Contact dermatitis of the feet. *Dermatosen* 34:102, 1986.
34. Storrs FJ: Dermatitis from clothing and shoes, in Fisher AA (ed): *Contact Dermatitis,* 3d ed, Philadelphia, Lea & Febiger, 1986, pp 283–337.
35. Epstein E: Shoe contact dermatitis. *JAMA* 209:1487, 1969.
36. Angelini G, Vena GA, Meneghini CL: Shoe contact dermatitis. *Contact Dermatitis* 6:279, 1980.
37. deVries HR: Allergic dermatitis due to shoes. *Dermatologica* 128:68, 1964.
38. Ho VC, Mitchell J: Allergic contact dermatitis from rubber boots. *Contact Dermatitis* 12:110, 1985.
39. Roberts JL, Hanifin JM: Athletic shoe dermatitis, contact allergy to ethyl butyl thiourea. *JAMA* 241:275, 1976.
40. Grimalt F, Romaguera C: New resin allergens in shoe contact dermatitis. *Contact Dermatitis* 1:169, 1975.
41. Gaul LE: Results of patch testing with rubber antioxidants and accelerators. *J Invest Dermatol* 29:105, 1957.
42. Vestey JP, Buxton PK, Savin JA: Eyelash curler dermatitis. *Contact Dermatitis* 13:274, 1985.
43. Cabrita JC, Conçalo M, Azenha A, Gonçalo S: Allergic contact dermatitis of the eyelids from rubber chemicals. *Contact Dermatitis* 24:145, 1991.
44. Goette DK: Raccoon-like periorbital leukoderma from contact with swim goggles. *Contact Dermatitis* 10:129, 1984.
45. Fowler JF Jr, Callen JP: Facial dermatitis from a neoprene rubber mask. *Contact Dermatitis* 18:310, 1988.
46. Jordan WP Jr: Richmond VA, personal communication.
47. Jordan WP Jr, Bourlas MC: Allergic contact dermatitis to underwear elastic. *Arch Dermatol* 111:593, 1975.
48. Fisher AA: Iatrogenic allergic rubber reactions in medical and dental patients. *Cutis* 49:81, 1992.
49. Buxton PK, Going SM, Hunter JAA, Winney RJ: Allergic reactions to rubber chemicals in haemodialysis equipment. *Br Med J* 287:1513, 1983.
50. Anderson KE, Hjorth N, Menné T: The baboon syndrome: Systemically induced allergic contact dermatitis. *Contact Dermatitis* 10:97, 1984.
51. Stankevich VV, Vlasyuk MG, Prokof'eva LG: Hygienic assessment of organosulfur accelerators for vulcanization of rubbers for the food industry. *Gig Sanit* 10:88, 1980.
52. Hamilton G: Contamination of contrast agent by MBT in rubber vials. *Can Med Assoc J* 136:1020, 1987.
53. Romaguera C, Aguirre A, Diaz Perez JL, Grimalt F: Watch strap dermatitis. *Contact Dermatitis* 14:260, 1986.
54. Condé-Salazar L, Llinas Volpe MG, Guimaraens D, Romero L: Allergic contact dermatitis from a suction socket prosthesis. *Contact Dermatitis* 19:305, 1988.
55. Condé-Salazar L: Rubber dermatitis: Clinical forms. *Dermatol Clin* 8:49, 1990.
56. Batschvarov B, Minkov DM: Dermatitis and purpura from rubber in clothing. *Trans St. John's Hosp Derm Soc* 54:178, 1968.

57. Carlsen L, Anderson KEA, Egsgaard H: IPPD contact allergy from orthopedic bandage. *Contact Dermatitis* 17:119, 1987.
58. Roed-Petersen J, Clemmensen OJ, Menné T, Larsen E: Purpuric contact dermatitis from black rubber chemicals. *Contact Dermatitis* 18:166, 1988.
59. Pecegueiro M, Brandão M: Contact plantar pustulosis. *Contact Dermatitis* 11:126, 1984.
60. Schoel VJ, Frosch PJ: Allergisches Kontaktekzem durch Gummiinhaltsstoffe unter dem Bild einer Pustulosis palmaris. *Dermatosen* 38:178, 1990.
61. Foussereau J, Cavelier C, Protois JC, et al: A case of erythema multiforme with allergy to isopropyl-*p*-phenylenediamine of rubber. *Contact Dermatitis* 18:183, 1988.
62. Oliver EA, Schwartz L, Warren LH: Occupational leucoderma: Preliminary report. *JAMA* 113:927, 1939.
63. Nutter AF: Contact urticaria to rubber. *Br J Dermatol* 101:597, 1979.
64. Meding B, Fregert S: Contact urticaria from natural latex gloves. *Contact Dermatitis* 10:52, 1984.
65. Frosch PJ, Wahl R, Bahmer FA, et al: Contact urticaria to rubber gloves is IgE-mediated. *Contact Dermatitis* 14:241, 1986.
66. Axelsson JGK, Johansson SGO, Wrangsjö K: IgE-mediated anaphylactic reactions to rubber. *Allergy* 42:46, 1987.
67. Turjanmaa K, Reunala T: Contact urticaria from rubber gloves. *Dermatol Clin* 6:47, 1988.
68. Forstrom L: Contact urticaria from latex surgical gloves. *Contact Dermatitis* 6:33, 1980.
69. Carrillo T, Cuevas M, Muñoz T, et al: Contact urticaria and rhinitis from latex surgical gloves. *Contact Dermatitis* 15:69, 1986.
70. Wrangsjö K, Mellstrom G, Axelsson G: Discomfort from rubber gloves indicating contact urticaria. *Contact Dermatitis* 15:79, 1986.
71. Helander I, Makela A: Contact urticaria to zinc diethyldithiocarbamate (ZDC). *Contact Dermatitis* 9:327, 1983.
72. Belsito DV: Contact urticaria caused by rubber: An analysis of seven cases. *Dermatologic Clinics* 8:61, 1990.
73. van Ketel WG: Contact urticaria from rubber gloves after dermatitis from thiurams. *Contact Dermatitis* 11:323, 1984.
74. Goh CL: Contact dermatitis to surgeons' gloves in their patients. *Contact Dermatitis* 20:223, 1989.
75. Hjorth N, Roed-Petersen J: Occupational protein contact dermatitis in food handlers. *Contact Dermatitis* 2:28, 1976.
76. Lampe MA, Burlingame AL, Whitney J, et al: Human stratum corneum lipids: Characterization and regional variations. *J Lipid Res* 24:120, 1983.
77. deGroot AC: *Patch Testing: Test Concentrations and Vehicles for 2800 Allergens.* Amsterdam, Elsevier, 1986.
78. Sulzberger MB: The patch test: Who should and should not use it and why. *Contact Dermatitis* 1:117, 1975.
79. Marks JG Jr, Moss JN, Parno JR, et al: Methylchloroisothiazolinone/methylisothiazolinone (Kathon CG) Biocide-United States multicenter study of human skin sensitization. *Am J Contact Dermatitis* 1:157, 1990.
80. Epstein WL: The use test for contact hypersensitivity. *Arch Dermatol Res* 272:279, 1982.
81. Mitchell JC: Multiple concomitant positive patch test reactions. *Contact Dermatitis* 3:315, 1975.
82. Przybilla B, et al: Evaluation of the immune status in vivo by the 2,4-dinitro-1-chlorobenzene contact allergy time (DNCB-CAT). *Dermatologica* 167:1, 1983.
83. Van der Leun JC, et al: Photosensitivity owing to thiourea. *Arch Dermatol* 113:1611, 1977.
84. Dupuis G, Benezra C: *Allergic Contact Dermatitis to Simple Chemicals: A Molecular Approach.* New York, Dekker, 1982.
85. Turjanmaa K, Reunala T, Räsänen L: Comparison of diagnostic methods in latex surgical glove contact urticaria. *Contact Dermatitis* 19:241, 1988.
86. Fisher AA: "Hypoallergenic" surgical gloves and gloves for special situations. *Cutis* 15:797, 1975.
87. Personal communication, Frances J. Storrs, Portland OR.
88. Rietschel RL: Role of socks in shoe dermatitis. *Arch Dermatol* 120:398, 1984.
89. Fregert S, Skog E: Allergic contact dermatitis from mercaptobenzothiazole in cutting oil. *Acta Derm Venereol (Stockh)* 42:235, 1962.
90. Rudzki E, et al: Dermatitis from 2-mercaptobenzothiazole in photographic films. *Contact Dermatitis* 7:43, 1981.

91. Adams RM: Mercaptobenzothiazole in veterinary medications. *Contact Dermatitis Newsletter* 16:514, 1974.

92. Shelly WB: Golf-course dermatitis due to thiuram fungicide. *JAMA* 188:415, 1964.

93. Nater JP, Terpstra H, Bleumink E: Allergic contact sensitization to the fungicide Maneb. *Contact Dermatitis* 5:24, 1979.

94. Anderson KE: Diethylthiourea contact dermatitis from an acidic detergent. *Contact Dermatitis* 9:146, 1983.

95. Fregert S, Trulson L, Zimerson E: Contact allergic reactions to diphenylthiourea and phenylisothiocyanate in PVC adhesive tape. *Contact Dermatitis* 8:38, 1982.

96. Kanerva L, et al: Contact dermatitis from dibutylthiourea. *Contact Dermatitis* 10:158, 1984.

97. M'Raihi L, Charpin D, Pons A, et al: Cross-reactivity between latex and banana. *J Allergy Clin Immunol* 87:129, 1991.

98. Ceuppens JL, Durme PV, Dooms-Goossens A: Letter to the editor. *Lancet* 339:493, 1992.

35

DENTAL PROBLEMS

Lasse Kanerva
Tuula Estlander
Riitta Jolanki

Both dental health care workers and their patients are at risk to develop contact sensitivity to dental products, but the risk factor and clinical presentation are different. Dental workers especially develop fingertip dermatitis from handling noncured acrylic resin[1] (Fig. 35-1). This is perhaps more common than suspected, since as many as 40 percent of orthodontists and 43 percent of dental assistants reported work-related skin problems.[2] Patients can become sensitized from dental devices, dental products, or various dental "cosmetics," for instance toothpaste, and may develop mucosal allergy, such as allergic stomatitis, gingivitis, or cheilitis, e.g., from dental amalgams or dentures (Fig. 35-2). Jacobsen and Hensten-Pettersen[2] calculated that about 1 percent of orthodontists' patients exhibit adverse reactions from dental materials. Generalized systemic allergic contact dermatitis caused by dental devices has also been described.[1,3] Contact allergy also may be the cause of burning mouth syndrome.[4–4e]

FINDING THE CAUSE BY PATCH TESTING

From an allergological point of view, both dental workers and patients can be investigated using the same commercial dental screening series for diagnostic patch tests. For most, a practical test series can be assembled to look for the underlying causes. Several test series are listed in Tables 35-1 to 35-3, and a more complete listing is presented in Table 35-4 of dental antigens from multiple sources—we also present our own test series in Table 35-9.

In the majority of cases patch testing can be performed in the standard way, i.e., on the skin of the back, even though sensitization and symptoms have developed only on the mucosa.[1,5,6] In some cases, there may be sensitization of the mucous membrane but not the skin, and patch testing should be performed on the target organ, i.e., the oral mucous membrane.[6] We have no experience of performing patch testing on mucous membranes, and we feel that at least the less experienced patch tester should not perform patch testing on mucous membranes, because of the technical difficulties in reading the reactions. Clearly, more research and knowledge in this field is needed.[7]

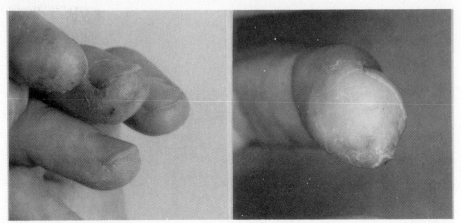

FIG. 35–1. Fingertip dermatitis from handling noncured acrylics. *Left,* allergic contact dermatitis caused by methyl methacrylate in an orthodontist who was remodeling children's dental devices with a two-component, cold-cured methyl methacrylate liquid and powder *Right,* a dentist allergic to 2-hydroxyethyl methacrylate from dentin primer.

If contact allergy from dental products is suspected, we patch test with the standard tray and the dental screening tray, and with additional haptens that we consider to be important, depending on the patient's history. Chemotechnique Diagnostics (P.O. Box 80, 230 42 Tygelsjö, Malmö, Sweden) has a rather extensive dental screening series of 30 haptens (Table 35-1),[8] and Hermal Kurt Herrmann (Trolab, D 21462 Reinbek/ Hamburg, Scholtzstrasse 3A, Federal Republic of Germany) has a smaller tray of 13 haptens (Table 35-2).[9] We usually use a modified Chemotechnique series. In the following, the haptens of both series are presented. Sometimes patch testing can be

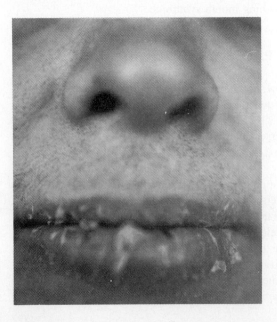

FIG. 35–2. Severe cheilitis from acrylic dental device. The patient had become sensitized to hydroquinone present in the acrylic dental device (courtesy of Dr. Torres).

TABLE 35–1. Dental Screening Series of Chemotechnique

Compound	Concentration, Percent
Methyl methacrylate	2.0 pet
Triethyleneglycol dimethacrylate	2.0 pet
Urethane dimethacrylate	2.0 pet
Ethyleneglycol dimethacrylate	2.0 pet
BIS-GMA	2.0 pet
N,N-Dimethyl-4-toluidine	5.0 pet
2-Hydroxy-4-methoxy-benzophenone	2.0 pet
1,4-Butanediol dimethacrylate	2.0 pet
BIS-MA	2.0 pet
Potassium dichromate[a]	0.5 pet
Mercury	0.5 pet
Cobalt chloride[a]	1.0 pet
2-Hydroxyethyl methacrylate	2.0 pet
Gold sodium thiosulfate	0.5 pet
Nickel sulfate[a]	5.0 pet
Eugenol	2.0 pet
Colophony[a]	20.0 pet
N-Ethyl-4-toluene sulfonamide	0.1 pet
Formaldehyde[a]	1.0 aq
4-Tolyldiethanolamine	2.0 pet
Copper sulfate	2.0 pet
Methylhydroquinone	1.0 pet
Palladium chloride	2.0 pet
Aluminum chloride hexahydrate	2.0 pet
Camphoroquinone	1.0 pet
N,N-Dimethylaminoethyl methacrylate	0.2 pet
1,6-Hexanediol diacrylate	0.1 pet
2 (2-Hydroxy-5-methylphenyl) benzotriazol	1.0 pet
Tetrahydrofurfuryl methacrylate	2.0 pet
Tin	50.0 pet

[a] Also present in standard series.

TABLE 35–2. Dental Materials Series of Trolab

	Concentration, Percent	
Benzoyl peroxide	1.0	pet
Tetracaine (amethocaine) hydrochloride	1.0	pet
Mercury	1.0	pet
Copper sulfate	1.0	pet
Potassium dicyanoaurate	0.002	aq
Methyl methacrylate	2.0	pet
Hydroquinone	1.0	pet
Bisphenol A	1.0	pet
N,N-Dimethyl-p-toluidine	2.0	pet
Eugenol	1.0	pet
Ethyleneglycol dimethacrylate (EGDMA)	2.0	pet
Triethyleneglycol dimethacrylate (TEGDMA)	2.0	pet
BIS-GMA	2.0	pet

TABLE 35–3. Dental Screening Series Suggested by Foussereau[11]

Compound	Concentration, Percent
Methyl methacrylate	2.0 pet
Triethyleneglycol dimethacrylate	2.0 pet
Ethyleneglycol dimethacrylate	2.0 pet
Potassium dichromate	0.5 pet
Cobalt chloride	1.0 pet
Nickel sulfate	5.0 pet
Eugenol	2.0 pet
Colophony	20.0 pet
Formaldehyde	1.0 aq
Benzoyl peroxide	1.0 pet
Mercury	1.0 pet
Bisphenol A	2.0 pet
Butyl acrylate	0.1 pet
Epoxy resin	1.0 pet
Epoxy acrylate (bis-GA)	0.5 pet
Ethyl acrylate (EA)	0.1 pet
Glutaraldehyde	1.0 pet
Glyoxal	1.0 aq
Methyl dichlorobenzene sulfonate (Impregum)	0.1 alc
Procaine hydrochloride	1.0 pet
Methyl-*p*-toluene sulfonate (Scutan)	0.1 pet

directed by the location of the patient, but screening with a battery of dental antigens is a good idea, as contact reactions are often multiple.

DESCRIPTION OF SELECTED HAPTENS

The haptens to be described have been selected from the suggestions made by Swedish investigators[10] and Chemotechnique (Table 35-1),[8] Hermal (Table 35-2),[9] Foussereau (Table 35-3),[11] Adams,[12] and Adams and Fischer.[13] The haptens and patch-test concentrations are given in Table 35-4. The more important haptens as regards dental problems are described in more detail in alphabetical order below. Most of the haptens are commercially available from Chemotechnique or Trolab. If material safety data sheets are available, it may be possible to look for the specific chemical to which the patient has been exposed.

ACRYLICS

Acrylates are esters of acrylic acid and methacrylates are esters of methacrylic acid. In the following, acrylates and methacrylates will be called *acrylics*. Three groups of acrylics are important in dentistry (1) monofunctional acrylics such as methyl methacrylate (MMA) and 2-hydroxyethyl methacrylate (2-HEMA), (2) polyfunctional acrylics such as triethylene glycol dimethacrylate (TREGDMA) and triethylene glycol diacrylate (TREGDA), and (3) acrylated and methacrylated prepolymers such as

TABLE 35–4. Compiled List of Dental Haptens Containing Haptens from the U.S. Standard Series, the European Standard Series, Chemotechnique Dental Screening Series, Trolab Dental Material Series, and Suggestions by Foussereau,[11] Adams,[12] and Adams and Fischer[13]

Aluminum, as is; aluminum chloride hexahydrate 2% aq.
Ammoniated mercury (see "Mercury Ammonium Chloride") (amalgam)
Ammonium tetrachloroplatinate, 0.25% pet
a-Amyl cinnamaldehyde, 1% pet
Balsam of Peru, 25% pet (medications)
Beeswax, 30% pet (impression materials)
Benzalkonium chloride, 0.01% aq (disinfectants)
Benzocaine, 5% pet
Benzophenone, 1% pet (light absorber in plastic materials)
Benzoyl peroxide, 1% pet
Benzyl-4-hydroxybenzoate (benzyl paraben), 3% pet
BIS-EMA (2,2-bis (4-(2-methacryloxyethoxy)phenyl)propane, 1% pet
BIS-GMA (2,2-bis(4-(2-hydroxy-3-methacryloxypropoxy)phenyl) propane, 2% pet
BIS-MA (2,2-bis(4-methacryloxy)phenyl) propane, 2% pet
Bisphenol A, 1% pet
Black rubber mix (standard series) (rubber gloves, rubber bands and dams)
Bronopol (2-bromo-2-nitropropane-1,3-diol), 0.25 to 0.5% pet (medications)
1,4-Butanediol diacrylate (BUDA), 0.1% pet
1,4-Butanediol dimethacrylate (BUDMA), 2% pet
n-Butyl acrylate, 0.1% pet
Butyl-4-hydroxybenzoate (butyl paraben), 3% pet
Butylmethacrylate, 2% pet
4-tert-Butylphenol formaldehyde (PTBF) resin, 1% pet
Caine mix, 8% pet (anesthetic agents)
Camphor, 10% pet
Carbamix, 3% pet (rubber gloves, rubber bands and dams)
Chlorhexidine digluconate, 0.05 to 0.5% aq (antiseptics)
4-Chloro-3-xylenol, 1% pet (antiseptic)
Chlorothymol, 2% pet (medications)
Chlorquinaldol (5,7-dichloro-2-methyl-8-quinolinol) (Sterosan), 5% pet (in "Quinoline Mix")
Cinnamic alcohol, 1 to 5% pet
Cinnamic aldehyde, 1% pet
Cinnamic oil, 0.5% pet (medications, toothpaste)
Cobalt (II) chloride hexahydrate, 0.5 to 1% pet
Colophony (rosin), 20% pet
Copper sulfate, 1% aq
N-Cyclohexylbenzothiazyl sulphenamide (CBS), 1% pet (see "Mercapto Mix")
N-Cyclohexyl-N'-phenyl paraphenylenediamine, 0.25% pet (see "Black Rubber Mix")
Diazolidinyl urea (Germall II), 1% aq
Dibenzothiazyl disulfide (MBTS) in mercapto mix, 1% pet
5,7-Dichloro-2-methyl-8-quinolinol (see "Chlorquinaldol"; in "Quinoline Mix")
N,N-Diethyl-2-methyl-1,4-phenylenediamine hydrochloride (CD-2, Color Developer 2)
4-N,N-Diethyl-1,4-phenylenediamine sulfate (monohydrate (CD-1, Color Developer 1)
N,N-dimethylaminoethyl methacrylate, 0.2% pet
N,N'-Dimethyl-4-toluidine, 2% pet
Dipentamethylene thiuram disulfide (PTD), 0.25% pet
1,3-Diphenylguanidine, 1% pet
N,N'-Diphenyl-4-phenylenediamine (DPPD), 0.25% pet
Epoxy acrylate, 0.5% pet
Epoxy resin (Bisphenol A-epichlorhydrin), 1% pet

(Continued)

TABLE 35–4 (Continued). Compiled List of Dental Haptens Containing Haptens from the U.S. Standard Series, the European Standard Series, Chemotechnique Dental Screening Series, Trolab Dental Material Series, and Suggestions by Foussereau,[11] Adams,[12] and Adams and Fischer[13]

Ethyl acrylate, 0.1% pet
Ethylene glycol dimethacrylate, 2% pet
Ethyl-4-hydroxy benzoate (ethyl paraben), 3% pet
4-(n-Ethyl-*n*-2-hydroxyethyl)-2-methyl-1,4-phenylenediamine sulfate monohydrate (CD-4, Color Developer 4)
4-*N*-Ethyl-*N*-(2-methane-sulfonamidoethyl)2-methyl-1,4-phenylene-diamine sesquisulfate hydrate (CD-3, Color Developer 3)
4-(*N*-ethyl-*N*-methoxyethyl)-2-methyl-phenylenediamine ditoluene sulfonate (CD-6, Color Developer 6)
N-Ethyl-4-toluenesulfonamide, 0.1% alc
Eucalyptus oil, 2% pet
Eugenol, 1% pet
Formaldehyde, 1% aq
Fragrance mix, 8% pet
Geraniol, 1% pet
Glutaraldehyde, 0.25 to 1.0% aq
Glycol dimethacrylate, 2% pet
Gold chloride, 0.1% aq
Gold sodium thiosulfate, 0.5% pet
Hexachlorophene, 1% pet (disinfectants)
1,6-Hexanedioldiacrylate (HDDA), 0.1% pet
Hexylresorcinol, 1% pet (medications)
Hydroquinone, 1% pet, or methylhydroquinone, 1% pet
Hydroquinone monobenzylether (monobenzone), 1% pet
Hydroxycitronellal, 1% pet
2-Hydroxyethyl methacrylate (HEMA), 2 to 5% pet
2-Hydroxy-4-methoxybenzophenone (Benzophenone 3)
2,2-bis(4-[2-Hydroxy-3-methacryloxypropoxy)phenyl] propane (see "BIS-GMA")
2(2'-Hydroxy-5'-methyl-phenyl) benzotriazole (Tinuvin P), 5% pet
8-Hydroxyquinoline, 5% pet
Imidazolidinyl urea (Germall 115), 2% pet
Isoeugenol, 1% pet
N-Isopropyl-*N*-phenyl-4-phenylene diamine (IPPD), 0.1% pet (rubber)
cl + me-Isothiazolinone (Kathon CG), 0.01 to 0.02% aq
Lanolin alcohols (wool alcohols), 30% pet
Lanolin (anhydrous), as is (medications)
Lidocaine hydrochloride (Xylocaine), 2 to 15% pet
MEK peroxide (see "Methyl Ethyl Ketone Peroxide")
Menthol, 1% pet (medications)
2-Mercaptobenzothiazole, 1% pet (rubber gloves, rubber bands, and rubber dams)
Mercapto mix, 1% pet (rubber gloves, rubber bands, and rubber dams)
Mercury, 1% pet
6-Methoxy-2-*N*-pentyl-4-benzoquinone (Primin), 0.01% pet
Methyl dichlorbenzene sulfonate (catalyst in Impregum), 0.1% pet (alc)
Methyl ethyl ketone peroxine (MEK peroxide), 1% pet (catalyst for acrylic resin systems)
Methyl-4-hydroxybenzoate (methyl paraben, in paraben mix), 3% pet
Methyl methacrylate (MMA), 2% pet
Methyl salicylate (oil of wintergreen), 2% pet (toothpastes)
Metol (4-methylaminophenol sulfate)
2-(4-Morpholinyl-mercapto)benzothiazole (MOR), 0.5 to 0.1% pet

(Continued)

TABLE 35-4 (Continued). Compiled List of Dental Haptens Containing Haptens from the U.S. Standard Series, the European Standard Series, Chemotechnique Dental Screening Series, Trolab Dental Material Series, and Suggestions by Foussereau,[11] Adams,[12] and Adams and Fischer[13]

Neomycin sulfate, 20% pet (medications, especially for root canal work)
Nickel sulfate hexahydrate, 2.5% pet
Oak moss absolute, 1% pet
Palladium chloride, 1% pet
Paraben mix, 15% pet (medications, toothpaste)
PCNB (Pentachloronitrobenzene)
N-Phenyl-N'-cyclohexyl-4-phenylenediamine, 1% pet
4-Phenylenediamine dihydrochloride, 0.5% pet (clients' recently dyed hair)
4-Phenylenediamine, 1% pet (clients' recently dyed hair)
Phenylmercuric acetate, 0.01% aq
Platinum chloride, 1% aq
Potassium dichromate, 0.5% pet (fillings)
Potassium dicyanoaurate, 0.002% aq
Procaine hydrochloride (Allocaine, Neocaine, Novocaine, Syncaine, Topocaine), 1% pet
Propyl-4-hydroxybenzoate (propyl paraben), 3% pet
Quarternium 15 (Dowicil 200; 1-(3-chloroallyl)-3,5,7-triaza-1-azoniaadamantane chloride), 1% pet
Quinoline mix, 6% pet
Rosin (colophony), 20% pet
Silver nitrate (lapis), 1% aq
Spearmint oil, 2% pet
Tetracaine hydrochloride (2-dimethylaminoethyl parabutylaminobenzoate), 5% pet
Tetrahydrofurfuryl methacrylate, 2% pet
Tetramethylthiuram disulfide (Thiram, TMTD), 1% pet
Tetramethylthiuram monosulfide, 1% pet
Thimerosal (merthiolate, sodium ethyl mercury thiosalicylate), 0.1% pet (disinfectants)
Thiuram mix, 1% pet
Tin, 2, 5% pet, as is
4-Tolyldiethanolamine, 2% alc
Triethylene glycol diacrylate (TREGDA), 0.1% pet
Triethylene glycol dimethacrylate (TREGDMA), 2% pet
Urethane dimethacrylate (UEDMA), 2% pet
Wool alcohols (lanolin alcohols, medications), 30% pet
Zinc dibutyldithiocarbamate (ZBC), 1% pet
Zinc diethyldithiocarbamate (ZDC), 1% pet

2, 2-bis [4-(2-hydroxy-3-methacryloxypropoxy)phenyl]propane (BIS-GMA) or ure-thane acrylate. The extensive (meth)acrylate series of Chemotechnique comprising 30 acrylics is seen in Table 35-5. The abbreviations in Table 35-5 are used in the text.

Stevenson[14] and Moody[15] in 1941 were the first to report hypersensitivity from MMA, and in 1948 Bradford[16] had a patient with stomatitis from a dental methacrylate prosthesis. The patient showed an allergic patch-test reaction with the prosthesis. In 1954, Fisher[17] encountered two dentists with dermatitis of the right hand, mainly of the first fingers, and two dental mechanics with dermatitis of both hands. The patients had occupationally been sensitized to methacrylates and had positive patch-test reactions to 100% MMA. The number of cases of occupational allergic contact dermatitis (ACD) caused by acrylates was, however, relatively small in the 1970s, partly because of the awareness of the sensitizing capacity of acrylates,[18] but possibly MMA was not very sensitizing.[19–21]

TABLE 35–5. Patch Test Results of (Meth)acrylate Series and Epoxy Resin of Six Patients Sentitized to Dental Composite Resins

ND[a]		Concentration, % (w/w)	Pat. 3	Pat. 4	Pat. 5	Pat. 6	Pat. 7	Pat. 8
Ethyl acrylate	(EA)	0.5–0.1	—	1+	—	—	3+	—
Butyl acrylate	(BA)	0.5–0.1	—	2+	—	—	3+	?+
2-Ethylhexyl acrylate	(2-EHA)	0.5–0.1	—	—	—	—	—	—
2-Hydroxyethyl acrylate	(2-HEA)	0.5–0.1	—	2+	—	—	3+	?+
2-Hydroxypropyl acrylate	(2-HPA)	0.5–0.1	—	2+	—	—	3+	—
Methyl methacrylate	(MMA)	2–10	3+	—	—	—	2+	—
Ethyl metacrylate	(EMA)	2.0	—	—	—	—	3+	—
n-Butyl methacrylate	(BMA)	2.0	—	—	—	—	2+	—
2-Hydroxethyl methacrylate	(2-HEMA)	2.0	—	1+	—	2+	3+	—
2-Hydoxypropyl methacrylate	(2-HPMA)	2.0	—	2+	—	2+	3+	—
Ethylene glycol dimethacrylate	(EGDMA)	2.0	—	—	—	3+	2+	—
Triethylene glycol dimethacrylate	(TREGDMA)	2.0	—	3+	—	4+	2+	3+
1,4-Butanediol dimethacrylate	(BUDMA)	2.0	—	—	—	—	1+	—
Urethane dimethacrylate	(UEDMA)	2.0	—	—	—	—	—	—
2,2-bis[4-(2-methacryloxyethoxy) phenyl] propane	(BIS-EMA)	1.0	—	3+	—	—	—	—
2,2-bis[4-(methacryloxy)phenyl] propane	(BIS-MA)	2.0	—	—	—	—	—	—
2,2-bis[4-(2-hydroxy-3-methacry-loxyproxy)phenyl] propane	(BIS-GMA)	2.0	4+	3+	2+	2+	—	—
1,4-Butanediol diacrylate	(BUDA)	0.1	—	2+	—	—	2+	2+
1,6-Hexanediol diacrylate	(HDDA)	0.1	—	2+	—	—	—	—
Diethylene glycol diacrylate	(DEGDA)	0.1	—	3+	—	—	2+	2+
Tripropylene glycol diacrylate	(TPGDA)	0.1	—	—	—	—	—	—
Trimethylolpropane triacrylate	(TMPTA)	0.1	—	—	—	—	—	—
Pentaerythritol triacrylate	(PETA)	0.1	—	—	—	—	—	?+
Oligotriacrylate 480	(OTA 480)	0.1	—	—	—	—	—	—
Epoxy diacrylate	(BIS-GA)	0.5	4+	2+	2+	2+	—	—
Urethane diacrylate (aliphatic)		0.1	—	—	—	—	—	—
Urethane diacrylate (aromatic)		0.1	—	—	—	—	—	—
Triethylene glycol diacrylate	(TREGDA)	0.1	—	3+	—	2+	3+	3+
N,N'-Methylenebisacrylamid		1.0	ND	ND	ND	ND	ND	—
Tetrahydrofurfuryl methacrylate		2.0	ND	ND	ND	ND	ND	—
Epoxy resin		1.0	3+	3+	3+	3+	—	—

[a]ND = not determined.

Methyl methacrylate was previously in widespread use as a standard allergen for patch-test screening for acrylate allergy.[18] However, both our and other studies[18,20–23] indicate that MMA is a poor screening substance for allergy to acrylates. The newer acrylates are much stronger sensitizers than MMA,[20–27] and the dental personnel seem to be at high risk to develop occupational allergy to acrylics. Extensive acrylics series have therefore been developed (Table 35-5). The main dental acrylic products that have caused allergy are described below.

Dental acrylic products can be divided into prostheses, dental composite resins (DCRs), and dentin primers.

TABLE 35–6. Components of the Powder and Liquid of an Acrylic Denture Base Material

Powder	Liquid
Polymethyl methacrylate or polymer[a]	Methyl methacrylate or monomer[b]
Organic peroxide initiator	Hydroquinone inhibitor
Titanium dioxide to control translucency	Dimethacrylate or cross-linking agent[c]
Inorganic pigments for color	Organic amine accelerator[d]
Dyed synthetic fibers for esthetics	

[a]Copolymers of other acrylates may be used.

[b]Other methacrylate monomers may be used.

[c]A cross-linking agent is present if the manufacturer indicates that the material is a cross-linked acrylic.

[d]The amine is present only if the material is labeled as a product to be processed at room temperature. These may be listed as cold-curing or self-curing materials.

Prostheses

In the manufacture of dental prostheses, polymethyl methacrylate powder is mixed with liquid MMA and the mass is molded manually or with technical devices. The components of the powder and liquid of an acrylic denture base material are given in Table 35-6. In addition, the powder may contain copolymers of polymethyl methacrylate, polyisobutyl acrylate, or polystyrene.[28] Instead of liquid methyl methacrylate, n-butyl methacrylate, isobutyl methacrylate, or lauryl methacrylate can also be used.[28] After molding, the acrylate mass polymerizes. The polymerization reaction is based on the use of heat, chemicals, or light (UV or visible).

The monomer solution used in the heat-networking (heat-polymerization) reaction contains polyfunctional acrylates, such as 1,4-butanediol dimethacrylate or ethylene glycol dimethacrylate. The chemically polymerizing monomer solutions usually contain N,N-dimethyl toluidine as an accelerator. Recently, dental technicians have started to use more modern and more complex light-cured acrylics similar in composition to dental composite resin.[29]

Dental Composite Resins

Dental composite resins (DCR) based on bisphenol A and (meth)acrylates (e.g., BIS-GMA) have been used since 1962.[30] Although BIS-GMA monomer is synthetized from glycidyl ethers containing epoxy groups, it does not contain epoxy groups. DCR contain several contact allergens: first, chemically reactive prepolymers, usually acrylated epoxies or acrylated urethanes[31]; second, mono- and especially multifunctional aliphatic acrylates (i.e., acrylates, methacrylates, diacrylates, and dimethacrylates)[30–32]; and third, additives that trigger the polymerization at an appropriate time such as initiators (e.g., benzoyl peroxide), activators (e.g., tertiary aromatic amines; see "Acrylic Resin Polymerization Activators", below) and inhibitors (e.g., hydroquinone).[31–32]

When sensitized patients were patch tested with the large methacrylate series of Chemotechnique,[8] variable results were obtained (Table 35-5). The interpatient cross-reactions to acrylics vary. Furthermore, concomitant sensitization to the various acrylics of the DCR also occurs. As dental personnel are often exposed to various DCRs and as differences in the composition of batches may occur,[22–24] it is sometimes difficult to detect the origin of the sensitization.

Several of our dental personnel patients developed epoxy acrylate allergy.[22,24] Epoxy acrylates are also used in many other compounds, but only a few reports on contact allergy have been published. The sensitized workers have mainly been in the ultraviolet-light printing industry.[33–35] Acrylated urethanes are used in dental composite and sealant applications, playing the same role as BIS-GMA,[30] and they are allergens.[36,37] The aliphatic urethane acrylates are the most common, but none of the urethane acrylates tested (i.e., aliphatic or aromatic urethane diacrylates or urethane dimethacrylates) gave positive patch tests in any of our patients.[22,29] Urethane acrylate allergy may be less common than epoxy acrylate allergy.

Dentin Primers

The increased use of composite resins as dental restorative materials[38] has made it necessary to develop substances that induce firm adhesion of the DCRs to the tooth. In 1988, Aasen and Oxman[39] patented a system based on maleic acid and 2-HEMA, called the Scotchbond 2 Dental Adhesive System (SB-2-DAS). We have had 10 patients who have become sensitized by components of SB-2-DAS.[23,29] These findings indicate that SB-2-DAS is an important sensitizer. It is important to use no-touch techniques when handling this adhesion promoter, since SB-2-DAS contains two known allergens, 2-HEMA and BIS-GMA. Our patients' allergy to SB-2-DAS was caused by 2-HEMA, and none of the patients had allergic reactions from BIS-GMA.[23,29]

Many acrylates quickly penetrate practically all surgical rubber and PVC gloves.[23,29] A commercial laminated disposable glove (4H-glove, Safety 4 A/S, Denmark) has recently been introduced, but it is expensive and does not fit well. We have recommended[29] the use of a fingertip-piece of 4H-glove under a disposable latex or PVC glove (Fig. 35-3).

Dental patients treated with SB-2-DAS are probably at a much less risk of contracting allergy than are dental personnel because they are exposed to uncured monomers for only a short time. Very few dental patients have been reported to have become sensitized to DCR.[40–43] However, uncured acrylics (e.g., those in the SB-2-DAS) are theoretically capable of sensitizing the patient even after a single exposure,[25–27] for which reason mucosal exposure should be avoided. Even though some of the acrylics from SB-2-DAS may remain uncured, they probably do not sensitize via the oral mucosa once the restoration has been finalized, because they are covered with DCR.

Other Aspects

In occupational dermatology, we consider it important to use the patients' own substances for patch testing, since this is the only way to detect new allergens. However, the possibility of sensitization when testing with own substances, especially acrylates, has to be taken into consideration. Recently we have seen one patient who was sensitized from patch testing (elsewhere) with 100% SB-2-DAS.[44]

The commercial patch-test substances may sensitize.[25–27] Chemotechnique lowered the patch-test concentration of the five acrylates (i.e., EA, BA, 2-EHA, 2-HEA, and

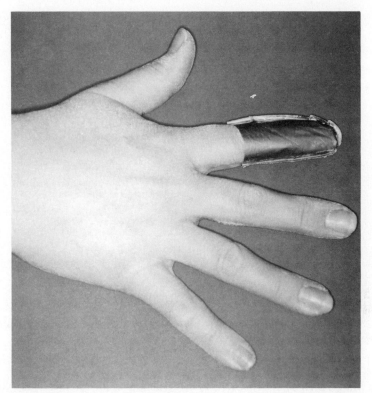

FIG. 35–3. Suggested use of a fingertip piece of laminated 4H-glove under a disposable latex or PVC glove to inhibit penetration of acrylics.

2-HPA) from 0.5% to 0.1% when three of our patients became sensitized.[25] EA, 2-HEA, and 2-HPA (0.1% pet.) sensitized one of our patients,[26] and we have deleted these three substances from our methacrylate series. We have added cyanoacrylate (2% pet., available from Epikon OY, Helsinki, Finland), which is also a sensitizing acrylate.[45-49] Chemotechnique recently added *N,N*-dimethylaminoethyl methacrylate (Table 35-1) to their dental series on the recommendation of the Scandinavian Institute of Dental Materials because it is frequently used in the light-cured dental composite materials. This compound sensitized one of our patients when patch tested at 2% pet.,[27] and Chemotechnique[8] has now lowered the concentration to 0.2% pet. (Table 35-1).

Immediate hypersensitivity, such as contact urticaria (see below), pharyngitis,[50] and/ or bronchial asthma[49] from cyanoacrylates, methyl methacrylate,[51] acrylic acid,[52] and nonspecified acrylics[53] has been reported.

Most DCRs contain the same (partly cross-reacting) acrylics,[22,29,31] and currently there are probably no alternatives which can be used by the affected dental personnel. In our experience, dermatitis from acrylics is often long-lasting (Fig. 35-4). Therefore the prevention of sensitization is very important. We think the 3M Corporation (Minnesota) did a good job when they gave new instructions regarding the precautions for dental personnel using primers (Table 35-7). Also, other manufacturers of dental acrylic resins should prepare similar instructions.

We suggest that the dental screening series should contain at least the following

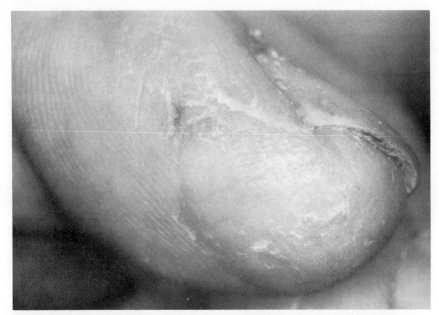

FIG. 35–4. Fingertip dermatitis from acrylics is long-lasting. This patient had been on sick leave for 4 weeks.

acrylics: MMA, 2-HEMA, TREGDA, EGDMA, and possibly urethane diacrylate, because it is used in DCR and very little is known about its cross-reactions (i.e., the allergy may not be revealed if it is not on the tray). The patients' own DCR (and primers) should probably not be tested at a higher concentration than 1% pet. because of the risk of active sensitization.[44]

Other groups have recently reported occupational allergy to acrylics in dental personnel.[54–57]

Detailed descriptions of dentin bonding system(s) can be found in a recent review.[29]

ACRYLIC RESIN POLYMERIZATION ACTIVATORS

Acrylic resins are produced by inducing polymerization of a mixture of MMA monomer and polymethyl methacrylate powder with benzoyl peroxide. The dough is hardened into shape by heating. At room temperature, the reaction needs an accelerator (activator). The one most widely used is the tertiary amine *N,N*-dimethyl-*p*-toluidine (DMT). Another amine accelerator is 4-tolyldiethanolamine.

N,N-Dimethyl-4-toluidine

Only a few case reports have been presented. Kaaber and coworkers[58] reported one positive skin reaction to DMT among 53 denture wearers. Tosti et al.[59] had a 62-year-old DMT patch-test-positive housewife with burning and soreness of mouth which had lasted 1 month. Clinically, she showed redness of the hard palate and aphthae.

TABLE 35–7. Precautions for Dental Personnel and Patients Using the Scotchbond 2 Dental Adhesive System

SB-2 and Scotchprep Precautions for Dental Personnel and Patients

1. *Etching precaution:* Avoid etching gel contact with oral soft tissue, eyes and skin. If accidental contact occurs, flush immediately with large amounts of water. Contains 35% phosphoric acid.

2. *Dentin primer and adhesive contain HEMA. HEMA is a known contact allergen. Use of protective gloves and a no-touch technique is recommended.* If adhesive contacts skin, wash immediately with soap and water. Acrylates may penetrate commonly used gloves. If adhesive contacts glove, remove and discard glove, wash hands immediately with soap and water, and then reglove.

3. *Dentin Primer Precautions:* Scotchprep dentin primer is a severe eye irritant. Avoid contact with eyes. If contact occurs, flush immediately with large amounts of water and consult a physician. Scotchprep dentin primer should be refrigerated. Failure to refrigerate can increase the possibility of mucosal tissue irritation if the primer contacts the tissue. May cause irritation to mucosal membranes with whitening and/or swelling followed by tissue sloughing in some individuals. Avoid mucosal tissue contact. Isolation with rubber dam is the best menas to avoid mucosal tissue contact and is highly recommended. If contact occurs, flush with large amounts of water. A small percentage of the population is known to have an allergic response to acrylate resins. To reduce the risk of allergic response, minimize exposure to these materials. If skin contact occurs, wash immediately with soap and water. Contains maleic acid, methacrylic acid and 2-hydroxyethylmethacrylate (HEMA).

4. *Adhesive precaution:* A small percentage of the population is known to have an allergic response to acrylate resins. To reduce the risk of allergic response, minimize exposure to these materials. In particular, exposure to uncured resins should be avoided. If accidental contact with eyes or prolonged contact with oral soft tissue occurs, flush with large amounts of water. If skin contact occurs, wash immediately with soap and water. Contains bisGMA and 2-hydroxyethylmethacrylate (HEMA).

Source: 3M Company, St. Paul, Minnesota.

Verschueren and Bruynzeel[60] also had a female patient with denture-related sore-mouth syndrome. After the diagnosis was made, she stopped using the dentures and became free of symptoms.

4-Tolyldiethanolamine

This amine is a less active accelerator than DMT. Farli and coworkers[56] had a dental technician with positive patch test reactions to *p*-tolyldiethanolamine.

ACRYLIC RESIN INHIBITORS

Hydroquinone

Hydroquinone is used in acrylic systems to prevent unintended spontaneous polymerization.[1] Hydroquinone has several other applications. It is used, for example, in bleaching creams, and has caused occupational depigmentation (vitiligo) in photographic development.[61–63] Monobenzyl ether of hydroquinone is both a stronger inducer of depigmentation[1] and a sensitizer.[64] Hydroquinone released from acrylic dentures has on rare occasions caused gingivostomatitis[65,66] (Fig. 35-2). Liden[67] had four patients at a film laboratory who were allergic to hydroquinone.

ALUMINUM

Aluminum is used as a pure metal or as an alloy for dental materials, utensils, aircraft, electrical conductors, etc. Aluminum salts are widely used in deodorants and antiperspirant preparations. Aluminum salts are also used in dental ceramics.

Allergic sensitivity is very rare, especially considering the amount of exposure (e.g., from antiperspirants).[68] The first allergic case was reported in 1980,[69] and now more than 50 cases have been reported.[70] When all patches in a Finn chamber test show red, infiltrated papular rings, contact sensitivity to aluminum should be suspected.[70-72]

AMPHOLYT (see "Tego")

AZULENE

Azulene (cyclopentacycloheptene) in toothpaste has caused allergic cheilitis.[98,99] In addition to its use in toothpaste, azulene is found in other cosmetic products such as mouthwashes, soaps, shampoos, creams, and lotions; 1% pet. has been considered the appropriate patch-test concentration.[98,99]

BENZOCAINE AND TETRACAINE

The local anesthetic benzocaine is included in the standard series because it is a common and potent sensitizer. Benzocaine is a derivative of *para*-aminobenzoic acid (PABA). It cross-reacts with local anesthetic agents such as procaine, tetracaine, piperocaine (Metycaine), and cocaine. Benzocaine also cross-reacts with hair dyes, aniline dyes, and drugs such as PABA, *p*-aminosalicylic acid, antidiabetic medications, and sulfonamides.[1] Tetracaine, as a PABA derivative, cross-reacts with benzocaine. Both benzocaine and tetracaine are used in a great number of products such as analgesics, antitussives, astringents, remedies for athlete's foot, burn remedies, corn, callus, and wart remedies, hemorrhoidal products, oral antibacterial preparations, oral topical medications, poison ivy medications, sunscreens, and preparations for toothache, teething, canker sores, cold sores, and denture irritation.[1]

Dentists are frequently sensitized to local anesthetics. Fisher[1] has described the two ways by which dentists are exposed to local anesthetics: First, they may rub with the finger a solution, spray, or ointment containing a "caine" onto the surface of the gums, prior to injecting local anesthetic or for various conditions in the mouth, such as relief from pain due to ulcers or traumatic injury, or they may handle medicated gauze packs or ointment for postextraction sockets. Second, by injecting a "caine" compound into the buccal areas, in which case skin contact arises when the solution spills over onto the fingers used in retraction or holding the syringe.

Different local anesthetics are used in different countries. Accordingly, the incidence of reactions to different anesthetics varies geographically. At St. John's Hospital in London, 52 patients were found during a 6-year period to be sensitive to local anesthetics. In 48 cases the source was a medicament, and for 4 dentists the source was occupational.[18]

The clinical picture of the four dentists sensitized by tetracaine (synonyms: Amethocaine, Pontocaine) was considered characteristic. Each had cracking and scaling of the finger pulps especially the thumb and the index and middle fingers. Each dentist reacted to tetracaine but not to procaine or to paraphenylenediamine.[18]

Occupational allergic contact dermatitis from tetracaine used by oculists has been reported.[73] A handout for ester-type anesthetics can be found in Chap. 10.

BENZOYL PEROXIDE

In addition to its use in the treatment of acne and stasis ulcers, benzoyl peroxide is a catalyst for acrylic and polyester resins. Hardening of the acrylic resin takes place by heating or self-curing at room temperature. For self-curing acrylic resins, polymerization of the mixture of liquid monomer and polymethyl powder (Table 35-6) is induced with an organic peroxide such as benzoyl peroxide and an accelerator such as DMT. Benzoyl peroxide is also used as a bleaching agent for flour, fats, oils, and waxes.

Benzoyl peroxide has been reported to cause stomatitis.[74] We had a dentist with occupational allergic contact dermatitis caused by benzoyl peroxide.[75] Benzoyl peroxide in acne preparations[75a,76] and as handled by bakers[77,78] is a rare sensitizer. Sensitization is more common when it is used on leg ulcers.[79,80]

Jager and Balda[81] reported loosening of a hip prosthesis due to an allergic reaction to benzoyl peroxide in the acrylic bone cement.

o-BENZYL-p-CHLOROPHENOL

We had an instrument attendant in a dental care unit who developed allergic contact dermatitis to this disinfectant.[82] This substance had earlier been reported to cause allergic contact dermatitis[82,83] and depigmentation.[84]

BISPHENOL A

Bisphenol A is the raw material used in the production of most epoxy and epoxy acrylate resins. Only few cases of allergic contact dermatitis have been reported. Krajewska and Rudzki[85] described positive patch tests to bisphenol A in 13 out of 17 Polish workers sensitized to epoxy resin by testing bisphenol A at a concentration of 2% in water. No data were given on how the positive reactions were scored. Additional data on the high incidence of bisphenol A allergy is lacking. The group of van Joost[86–88] did not find cases of bisphenol A allergy among workers at epoxy resin plants despite the fact that several patients had become sensitized to epichlorohydrin[86–88]— the other starting substance in the production of epoxy resin. Cases of allergy to bisphenol A have been reported from fiberglass made of epoxy resin,[89] semisynthetic waxes,[90] and plastic footwear containing bisphenol A.[91] Occupational allergic contact dermatitis caused by bisphenol A has been reported in a dental technician.[92] Van Joost et al.[4] reported a case with the burning mouth syndrome who had a denture of unknown composition and who had a positive reaction to bisphenol A (test concentration and vehicle not given) and epoxy resin. It was hypothesized that epoxy resin used for denture repair could have caused the sensitization. Bisphenol A has been reported to cross-react with stilbestrol-like chemicals.[92a]

CAMPHOROQUINONE

Camphoroquinone is an initiator for visible light–cured dental acrylic composite materials and primers, e.g., the Scotchbond 2 Dental Adhesive system.[23] It has been included in the dental screening series because it is widely used in dentistry. Patch testing has caused active sensitization.[92b]

CHROMIUM (see "Cobalt and Chromium")

CINNAMIC ALDEHYDE AND CINNAMIC ALCOHOL

Cinnamic aldehyde and alcohol are used as flavoring agents and fragrances in toothpastes, beverages (cola), vermouths, bitters, chewing gums, mouthwashes, toilet soaps, and sanitary napkins.[93] Cinnamic aldehyde is a common sensitizer in perfumes (see Eugenol). Cinnamic aldehyde in toothpaste has caused allergic stomatitis.[94–96] Fisher[1] had three patients who developed an allergic cheilitis and stomatitis from the use of toothpaste containing cinnamic aldehyde. Patch tests with 1% cinnamic aldehyde gave strongly positive reactions. Contact dermatitis from cinnamic aldehyde has resulted in depigmentation about the vermilion border.[96] Cinnamic aldehyde in lipstick may cause cheilitis.[97] A handout for persons allergic to cinnamic aldehyde can be found in Chap. 15.

COBALT AND CHROMIUM

Chromium and cobalt are common sensitizers, although the sensitization seldom arises from the dental products. A woman with severe dermatitis recovered only after removal of a cast chrome-cobalt denture.[100] Fisher[1] had a patient whose chrome-cobalt pins used to fasten porcelain teeth to acrylic dentures produced extensive stomatitis and cheilitis. The mucosa was exposed to the pins because the acrylic part had worn away. Hubler and Hubler[3] had a patient with generalized eczematoid dermatitis caused by allergy to chromium liberated from a metal dental plate. A handout for persons allergic to chromates can be found in Chap. 27.

COLOPHONY (ROSIN)

Colophony is a common sensitizer and an ingredient of many mixtures used for sealing pulp canals. Colophony has been added to zinc oxide or eugenol (see below) as an ingredient of pulp-capping preparations, surgical packs, impression pastes, and other preparations. Colophony in chloroform solution has been used as a varnish for pulp protection in deep cavities. Dawson[101] reported a dental mechanic who developed colophony allergy from a dental impression compound. Colophony used in dental preparations may cross-react with perfume, balsams, and fragrances. The North American contact Dermatitis Group has a listing of over 300 products that contain rosin.[1]

COPPER

Dental amalgams may contain copper, but allergic reactions to copper have been considered rare.[102] Dermatitis from copper intrauterine devices has been reported.[103-107] The copper patch-test substance may, however, contain nickel as an impurity, and some of the reactions reported to have been caused by copper may have represented nickel allergy.[108] Barkoff[104] had a patient with an acute urticarial reaction from a copper intrauterine device. Another woman developed a widespread urticarial rash within 2 h of having a tooth temporarily filled with black copper cement.[109] Frykholm et al.[110] reported lichen planus of the buccal mucosa and tongue in a patient allergic to metallic copper. Replacement of the copper-containing amalgam fillings cleared the lichenoid eruption.

N,N-DIMETHYL-4-TOLUIDINE (see "Acrylic Resin Polymerization Inhibitors")

DODECYL-DI-(AMINOETHYL)GLYCINE (see "Tego")

EPOXY RESIN

Epoxy resins based on diglycidylether of bisphenol A (DGEBA) are strong contact sensitizers.[92,111] DGEBA-based epoxy resins (DGEBA-ER) are used in adhesives, surface coatings, electrical insulations, plasticizers, and polymer stabilizers as well as in the building industry, electron microscopy, sculpture, etc. DGEBA-ER epoxy resin is a common occupational allergen[92,111] and it belongs to the standard tray.

DGEBA-ER is probably not widely used in dentistry but it can be used in the production of DCR. Most DCR are based on the type of aromatic dimethacrylate monomer introduced by Bowen.[30,31] This monomer can be produced by a reaction between DGEBA-ER and (meth)acrylic acids. BIS-GMA is the most commonly used monomer in DCR.

Some of the patients sensitized to DCR also show a positive patch-test reaction to DGEBA-ER (Fig. 35-5). The explanation for this is not known.[21,22] One reason may be that DCR contain DGEBA-ER as an impurity. Traces of DGEBA-ER have been revealed in Concise[22] but not in Miradapt/R, Delton, or Bonding Agent Universal Resin[24]; about 0.001 percent of oligomer DGEBA-ER, molecular weight 340, was present in one Concise batch analyzed.[22] In other words, some batches may contain sensitizing amounts of DGEBA-ER as an impurity. Another possibility is that DGEBA-ER and epoxy acrylates cross-react in some individuals, although there is also evidence that they do not cross-react.[35] Van Joost and coworkers[4] had a patient with allergic patch-test reactions to DGEBA-ER. The allergy had probably developed from the epoxy glue which had been used to repair the patient's dental plate. A handout for epoxy-allergic patients can be found in Chap. 22.

N-ETHYL-4-TOLUENE SULFONAMIDE

N-Ethyl-4-toluene sulfonamide is a resin carrier in dental materials used for isolating cavities underneath restorations. Chemotechnique has included it in its dental screening

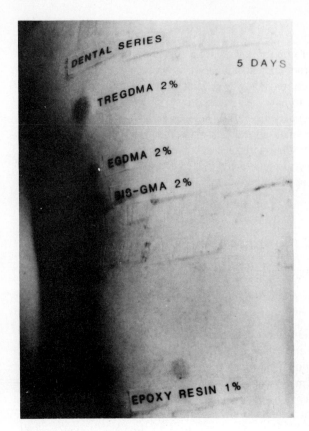

FIG. 35–5. A patient allergic to several acrylics also shows an allergic patch-test reaction to epoxy resin.

series. In a Swedish multicenter study, 9 of 1657 patients with oral symptoms had an allergic patch test reaction to *N*-ethyl-4-toluene sulfonamide (unpublished). In a literature search, we did not find published cases of allergic contact dermatitis but recently we reported a dentist with an allergic patch-test reaction caused by *N*-ethyl-4-toluene sulfonamide.[111a].

EUGENOL AND ISOEUGENOL

Eugenol is the essential chemical constituent of clove oil and is also present in cinnamon oil, perfumes, soaps, bay rum, oil of carnation (hyacinth), pimento oil (allspice), flower oils, food spices, and flavors. In dentistry, eugenol is used in the zinc oxide–eugenol cement, toothache drops, and antiseptics. It may also be combined with colophony.[1]

Eugenol is one of the eight components in the fragrance mixture which belongs to the standard patch-test tray. The fragrance mixture is irritant and may give false-positive (allergic-appearing irritant) reactions. Therefore, before making a final diagnosis of allergy to a perfume (including eugenol), a perfume screening series containing individual perfume components should be used for patch testing. Eugenol is both a primary irritant and a sensitizer; for patch testing, a 10% solution in olive oil or a 5% solution in petrolatum has been suggested.[1] Recently, lower concentrations have been preferred, and Chemotechnique uses a 2% concentration.

When eugenol is used in dental preparations, such as impression pastes, surgical packing, and cements, it may produce stomatitis venenata and allergic eczema in dental personnel.[112] Göransson et al.[112] observed three cases of eugenol hypersensitivity. In one patient, a eugenol impression paste produced allergic cheilitis and stomatitis. In the other two, an allergic eczematous reaction was produced from handling eugenol. Koch et al.[113] demonstrated that eugenol is a potent sensitizer. Eugenol may cross-react with iso-eugenol, balsam of Peru, cinnamon, diethylstilbestrol, and benzoin.[1]

Eugenol seems to be a less common sensitizer than, for example, cinnamic aldehyde, cinnamic alcohol, and isoeugenol. Calnan and coworkers[114] patch tested 2461 patients; the fragrance mixture induced a positive reaction in 7 percent. The individual components gave positive patch-test reactions as follows: cinnamic aldehyde, 4 percent; cinnamic alcohol, 2 percent; isoeugenol, 2 percent; hydroxycitronellal, 1.4 percent; oak moss, 1.2 percent; eugenol, 1 percent; geraniol, 0.2 percent; and *alpha*-amyl cinnamic alcohol, 0.2 percent.

FORMALDEHYDE

Formaldehyde is used in dentistry for sterilizing, as a disinfectant, or as a tissue-fixing solution. In addition to being a significant sensitizer, formaldehyde is also an irritant, and formaldehyde solution (formalin) may cause paronychia and nail changes. After sensitization, formaldehyde may cause widespread airborne dermatitis. Because formaldehyde is an irritant even at the patch-test concentrations used, an irritant reaction is often misinterpreted as being allergic. We usually confirm our formaldehyde allergy by performing patch testing with a small formaldehyde dilution series (2%, 1%, 0.32%, 0.1% in water). In this way the patch-test reactions are easier to read.[115]

Formaldehyde in Formo-Cresol may cause allergic stomatitis in patients undergoing root canal therapy.[1] Formaldehyde in toothpaste may cause allergic cheilitis.[116] According to Fisher,[1] formaldehyde is also present in Thermodent dentrifice. The formaldehyde releasers (see Ref. 117) may be responsible for the allergic symptoms.

Formaldehyde has also been suspected of causing anaphylaxis after dental treatment with paraformaldehyde-containing filling materials.[118] Finally, denture base polymers may release formaldehyde.[119]

GLUTARALDEHYDE

Glutaraldehyde is used as a germicidal agent in the cold sterilization of dental and dialysis equipment. Glutaraldehyde is also a hardener for photographic gelatin, a tanning agent for leather, and a fixative for electron microscopy. Glutaraldehyde is moderately irritant, and Cronin[18] considered it a weak sensitizer. More recent reports, however, indicate that it may be a stronger sensitizer.[120,121]

Sensitization to glutaraldehyde has occurred mainly through its use as a cold sterilizing solution in hospitals and dental clinics. Contact dermatitis has been reported in operating theater staff,[122-124] in an assistant at a renal dialysis unit,[125] in an inhalation therapy aide,[126] and in dental assistants.[11,22,121,127,128]

Glutaraldehyde and formaldehyde usually do not cross-react. If a subject is allergic to both, it indicates concomitant sensitization.[1,18]

GLYOXAL

Glyoxal is used in dentistry to disinfect instruments. Foussereau[11] has suggested that glyoxal be incorporated in the dental tray, although allergy to glyoxal has been reported to be induced only by a polyvinyl resin emulsion.[129]

GOLD

Gold salts can be strong sensitizers,[130] but allergy to metallic gold is rare. Metallic gold in dental applications has caused allergic stomatitis and gingivitis.[131-137] Gold is not entirely safe for piercing the ears.[138] Patch tests for gold allergy should include gold salts, because gold leaf, metallic gold, or gold scrapings may yield false-negative results.[1] Fowler[139] has suggested the use of gold sodium thiosulfate (0.5% aq.; also present in the Chemotechnique dental screening series) for patch testing, but even this salt may give long-lasting allergic patch-test reactions,[137] in contradiction to what Fowler[139] believed. Metals other than gold may be the cause of gold jewelry dermatitis or stomatitis, since gold jewelry is not made of pure 24-carat gold but contains nickel, copper, zinc, silver, or palladium (14- or 18-carat gold).

HYDROQUINONE (see "Acrylic Resin Inhibitors")

2-HYDROXY-4-METHOXY-BENZOPHENONE (see "UV Absorbers")

2-(2-HYDROXY-5-METHYLPHENYL)BENZOTRIAZOLE (see "UV Absorbers")

IODOFORM AND IODINE

Bismuth subnitrate and iodoform (BIPP) gauze is a dressing commonly used for the packing of tooth sockets after dental extraction. The iodoform component is antiseptic and bismuth subnitrate astringent. Severe cheilitis, stomatitis, and perioral dermatitis was reported from iodoform by Maurice and coworkers.[140] Potassium iodide (5% pet.) gave an allergic patch-test reaction. A patient described by Goh and Ng[141] was allergic to both bismuth and iodoform. The commonly used povidone (polyvinylpyrrolidone) iodide (Betadine) is also a sensitizer.[142,143]

LIDOCAINE (XYLOCAINE)

Lidocaine is used as a local anesthetic and as an antiarrhythmic agent. It does not cross-react with benzocaine or tetracaine. Lidocaine is usually safe to use because allergic reactions are rare, but they have been reported.[144-147]

MERCURY

Metallic mercury is used in dental amalgam, thermometers, pharmaceuticals, antifouling paints, agricultural chemicals, etc. Mercury unites with many metals to form amalgams. Amalgams composed of zinc, tin, and mercury are used as dental cements, and amalgams of mercury with tin, zinc, silver, or copper are used as fillings for teeth.[1] Dermatitis from amalgams may be caused by metallic mercury or the mercury compound.

Mercury amalgam allergy has created much public controversy but has been reported relatively seldom. According to Vernon et al.[148] only 39 cases had been reported by 1986, but other investigators think it is more common.[149–151] It is possible that amalgam fillings cause lichen planus or lichenoid reactions on the buccal mucosa without an allergic mechanism.

Many of the mercury compounds are irritant on patch testing and easily give false-positive (i.e., irritant) patch-test reactions.[1]

Occupational amalgam allergy is rare. Ancona et al.[152] reported a dentist, and Goh and Ng[153] and we[154] encountered a dental nurse who developed allergic occupational dermatitis caused by uncured amalgam handled with bare hands. Recently, we reported on a dentist with occupational allergic contact dermatitis caused by mercury in dental amalgam.[75] Totally different frequencies of mercury allergy have also been reported. A dental student and two biochemists patch tested dental students to an aqueous solution of mercuric chloride and obtained positive reactions in one-third of the subjects.[155] They stated that these reactions indicated allergy to mercury,[155] but the reactions may have been irritant in part, and mercury amalgam allergy cannot be evaluated from a patch test with mercuric chloride. Rudzki et al.[156] reported that 5.4 percent of the dentists, 7.2 percent of the surgeons, and 2.4 percent of other physicians had positive patch tests from mercury compounds. In the material of Berova et al,[157] 1 dental nurse out of 84 had a positive patch-test reaction with 5% amalgam. It was recently shown that possibly the best way to diagnose an allergic patch-test reaction to amalgam would be to use 5 or 10% pulverized amalgam in petrolatum.[158] The commercially available 1% amalgam seems to give false-negative results.[158]

Currently, the mercury compound thimerosal is among the most common causes of allergic contact dermatitis in some countries.[159] One would expect occupational mercury allergy to develop in a group of patients sensitized from thimerosal, because up to 60 percent of the patients with thimerosal allergy cross-react with at least one mercury-containing patch test substance.[160]

Spilled mercury droplets from a broken thermometer can cause severe allergic reactions.[161–163] Exanthem or erythema mulitforme has been reported in patients who, at work, have been exposed to mercury from broken thermometers.[164,165] This clinical picture is believed to represent systemic allergic contact dermatitis and has also been called the baboon syndrome.[166] Immediate mercury allergy[167–171] is also known.

METALS

A wide variety of metals for fillings and prostheses has been used by dentists, but many of these are currently replaced by plastics. The metals used include aluminum, antimony, chromium, cobalt, copper, gold, iridium, mercury, nickel, osmium, palladium, platinum, rhodium, ruthenium, silicon, silver, tin, tungsten, and zinc.[1,172]

METHYL-*p*-TOLUENE SULFONATE AND METHYL DICHLOROBENZENE SULFONATE (SCUTAN AND IMPREGUM)

Contact allergy from the catalysts in two dental impression compounds has been reported in both patients and dental personnel.

Scutan is an epimin plastic that polymerizes in the cold and hardens quickly. It is used for temporary crowns and bridges together with a separate liquid cross-linking agent (the so-called catalyst). It contains no monomers and is not an acrylic derivative. The catalyst is methyl-*p*-toluene sulfonate and the solvent is dibenzyl toluene. The catalyst has caused contact dermatitis in dentists' fingers.[173] For testing, 1% in acetone[1] or 0.1% in petrolatum has been suggested.

Impregum is an impression rubber material used for the construction of inlays, crowns, and bridges. It usually comes in contact with the oral mucosa for only a short period but nevertheless has caused allergic contact dermatitis both in dental patients and personnel.[174-178]

Impregum is supplied in two tubes of a base and a catalyst. The base consists of a low-molecular-weight polymer where the backbone is polyether, usually ethylene oxide and tetrahydrofuran with a three-membered aziridine terminal group. The catalyst is methyl dichlorobenzene sulfonate and the solvent is dibenzyl toluol. Allergic reactions have been caused by the catalyst, but aziridine is also a sensitizer.[179] Foussereau[11] suggests a patch test concentration of 0.1% in acetone. According to Chemotechnique[8] methyl dichlorobenzene sulfonate is no longer an ingredient in Impregum; consequently new cases of allergy may not develop.

The intraoral tissue hypersensitivity reactions to Scutan and Impregum (see Ref. 180) have occurred surprisingly quickly, appearing in some hours. This may reflect the rapid penetration of the hapten through the oral mucosa. However, many of the reactions have been associated with fever (see Ref. 180) and may thus represent other mechanisms than pure type IV allergy.

NICKEL

This most common contact allergen may cause dental problems from dentures.[181-184] Nickel is usually the sensitizing metal in chromium-nickel dentures, because metallic chromium is not a sensitizer.[1] Allergic contact dermatitis and cheilitis may also develop from nickel-plated instruments that are used in dental procedures.[181] On the other hand, there is recent evidence that nickel dentures, in patients who are not nickel-allergic may induce immunologic tolerance to nickel. It was shown in a European multicenter study that if orthodontic treatment had preceded the event of ear-piercing (which often induces nickel allergy), the frequency of nickel hypersensitivity was significantly reduced.[185]

ORAL HYGIENE PRODUCTS

Dentrifices and mouthwashes are often incriminated as causing allergic contact dermatitis. Fisher[1,186] has reviewed the concentrations for patch-testing ingredients found in toothpastes and mouthwashes. Reports on allergic sensitization to toothpastes have mostly involved flavoring agents.[187] Cinnamic aldehyde has been the most frequent cause.[187-190] Tartar-control toothpaste may cause an irritant reaction.

PALLADIUM

Palladium is found most commonly in ore combined with platinum, gold, and copper. It is used in alloys for dental plates, relays, and switching systems in telecommunications equipment and as a catalyst in white gold, as well as in aircraft and ornamental work.[68]

Previously palladium dermatitis was considered rare.[68] Van Ketel and Nieboer[191] reported a patient with mouth irritation and systemic symptoms. The symptoms cleared when the patient stopped wearing a dental bridge that contained palladium. The patient had an allergic patch-test reaction to both palladium and nickel. Recently, quite a number of patients allergic to nickel also have shown positive patch-test reactions to palladium.[192-196] Currently it is not known whether the patients have a concomitant sensitization to nickel and palladium analogous to concomitant sensitization to, for example, nickel and cobalt, or whether nickel and palladium cross-react.

PLATINUM

Metallic platinum is used in dentistry, jewelry, photography, and the chemical and electrical industries. It rarely causes allergic contact dermatitis.[197,198] Soluble platinum salts have caused dermatitis but more often occupational contact urticaria, allergic rhinoconjunctivitis, and asthma.[197-203]

Already in 1955,[197] Sheard claimed that reactions to dentists' platinum wiring may be allergic in nature.

PROCAINE

Procaine (Allocaine, Ethocaine, Neocaine, Novocaine, Syncaine, Topocaine) is a local anesthetic which cross-reacts with benzocaine and tetracaine. Allergy to procaine used to be common among dentists.[204,205] More recently, occupational allergic contact dermatitis has been reported among veterinary surgeons.[206] A handout for benzocaine and other *para*-aminobenzoic acid esters (including procaine) can be found in Chap. 10.

PROFLAVINE

Proflavine dihydrochloride, an acridine dye, was used in the past as a preoperative surgical application and caused many cases of pigmented allergic dermatitis.[207] Currently, it is commonly used as an antiseptic in the tropics and developing countries and is one of the most common contact sensitizers (e.g., in Singapore).[208,209] Lim and coworkers[210] reported a case of cheilitis. Following a dental extraction, proflavine had been used in a mouthwash. Proflavine may cause an erythema multiforme–like eruption.[211] Proflavine 0.5% pet was suggested for patch testing.[210]

RUBBER

Rubber products, from rubber bands used with orthodontic braces to rubber dams or gloves, cause reactions from periodontitis and stomatitis to contact urticaria and anaphylaxis (see below).[211a-d]

SILVER

Dental amalgam contains silver, but metallic silver should not cause allergic contact dermatitis. Silver nitrate (lapis) is used as an antiseptic agent and also in photography, silver plating, coloring porcelain, mirror manufacture, ivory etching, and as an analytical agent. Gaul[212] reported a patient with allergic reactions to silver coins, pure silver, and silver nitrate (lapis). In another old report, silver nitrate also sensitized.[213] Silver nitrate becomes an irritant when aged or exposed to light.[214] Topical silver nitrate and other silver salts may cause localized or generalized argyria.[198,215-217]

TARTAR-CONTROL TOOTHPASTES

Tartar-control toothpastes cause common forms of irritation from dental products. These include cheilitis and circumoral dermatitis around the angles of the mouth.[236a] Intraorally, these preparations may cause burning mouth, erythema, desquamation, erosions, or an increased frequency of migratory glossitis.[236b]

TEGO

Tego is the commercial name of certain disinfectants. The active ingredient of Tego is dodecyl-di-(aminoethyl)glycine (DDAG). Not all Tego products contain DDAG.[11] Tego is widely used in Finland as an antiseptic for instruments in hospitals and especially in dental practice.[22,82] Based on material from a 10-year period at our clinic, it was found to be the most common antimicrobial which caused allergic occupational eczema.[218] Allergic contact dermatitis has been reported from several products containing DDAG and sold under the trade names Tego,[219-221] Tego 103G,[222] Tego 51,[223] Desimex i,[22,82,224] Ampholyt G, and Ampholyte 103G.[225] We have included DDAG in our dental screening series (0.5% aq.).

TETRACAINE (see "Benzocaine")

TIN

Tin is used in dental metal preparations including amalgam, in tin-plating, materials, soldering alloys, and collapsible tubes. Before the study of Menne and coworkers[226] in 1987, tin allergy had not been reported, but patch tests with metallic tin in 73 nickel-sensitive patients revealed 6 positive reactions. Menne et al.[226] believe that tin is a common sensitizer.

4-TOLYL DIETHANOLAMINE (see "Acrylic Resin Polymerization Activators")

UV ABSORBER

2-(2'-Hydroxy-5'-methylphenyl)benzotriazole (Trade Name Tinuvin P)

Tinuvin P is a UV light absorber for dental materials, acrylics, plastics, cosmetics, dyes, etc. Allergic contact dermatitis has been reported from Tinuvin P in cosmetics,[227–230] plastic watch straps,[231] an ostomy bag,[232] and Spandex tape sewn onto underwear.[230] Tinuvin P and other benzotriazoles did not cross-react.[230]

2-Hydroxy-4-methoxy-benzophenone (Oxybenzone; Trade Name Eusolex 4360)

Benzophenones are incorporated as UV absorbers in dental composite materials, other plastics, textiles, and sunscreens. Allergic[233–235] and photoallergic[236] contact dermatitis has been reported from sunscreens. All Eusolex products do not contain benzophenones.[8]

XYLOCAINE (see "Lidocaine")

IRRITANTS

Dental personnel wash their hands up to 100 times per day; this causes drying of the skin.[19,29] Other irritant factors[12] are listed in Table 35-8.

CONTACT URTICARIA

Contact urticaria is a local immediate urticarial and/or erythemal or pruritic reaction at the site of epidermal or mucosal contact with the causative agent. Generalized cutaneous reactions, rhinitis, asthma, or anaphylaxis may be associated. As even death has been reported, the symptoms range from mild erythema and/or itching[237] to death. Contact urticaria may be allergic or nonallergic. The best-known allergic reactions are the IgE-mediated immediate (type I allergic) reactions.

CONTACT URTICARIA CAUSED BY PROTEINS

Probably most proteins that have caused type I respiratory allergy may also cause contact urticaria, especially if the exposed skin is injured from, for example, irritation, and thus is more permeable than intact skin. This also applies to the oral mucosa, (e.g., after eating vegetables and fruits). Extensive lists of causative agents can be found in recent review articles.[1,238,239]

TABLE 35–8. Irritants in Dental Work

Abrasives in polishing materials (pumice, silica, calcium carbonate)
Acrylics
Adhesives (epoxy and cyanoacrylates)
Amalgam mixtures
Coumarone-indene resins
Essential oils
Etching compounds (e.g., phosphoric acid)
Germicidal solutions
Orthodontic plasters
o-Phosphoric acid
Soaps and detergents
Sodium hypochlorite
Solvents (alcohol, chloroform, methyl cellusolve)
Resins and catalysts
X-rays
Thymol-iodide (root canal sealer)

NATURAL RUBBER (LATEX) CONTACT URTICARIA

This entity was not appreciated before 1979,[240] but currently latex is probably the most important cause of contact urticaria. More than 10 deaths have recently been reported. As mucosal contact usually gives a stronger reaction than skin contact, dental patients are a special risk group. If latex allergy is present, no rubber equipment (such as rubber gloves or a dental rubber dam[241]) can be used. Dental personnel may themselves develop contact urticaria from work. On the other hand, they should remember that contact urticaria from rubber latex may be life-threatening during dental examinations. Dental patients should always be asked about a possible latex allergy.

Latex contains at least 10 allergenic protein fractions,[242] and the allergy is IgE-mediated. Unfortunately, the current commercial prick-test substances are not optimal, and a negative prick test or a radioallergosorbent test (RAST) does not exclude latex allergy.[243]

Latex is an important occupational allergen, and health personnel,[243] including dental personnel, constitute a special high-risk group.

CONTACT URTICARIA CAUSED BY LOW-MOLECULAR-WEIGHT CHEMICALS (LMWC)

Dermatologists are familiar with haptens, since they are the main cause of type IV allergic reactions, such as allergic contact dermatitis. Dermatologists, however, usually have limited experience of skin-prick testing to detect type I allergic reactions. There is increasing evidence that haptens may also cause IgE-mediated type I allergic reactions.[244-246] In most cases it is believed that the hapten binds to a protein or another macromolecule and that the resulting hapten-carrier conjugate acts as the allergen.

SKIN TESTING WITH LMWC

As the allergen is believed to be a hapten-carrier conjugate, the skin testing should ideally be performed with a hapten-carrier conjugate, not the hapten. In some cases positive skin-test reactions may be obtained with the hapten without conjugation (e.g., by using patch-test substances in petrolatum). Belsito[247] reported rubber chemical contact urticaria in four patients from mercaptobenzothiazole, carba mix, mercapto mix, and black rubber mix, respectively, and obtained positive open scratch reactions with patch-test substances (in petrolatum) to the above chemicals.

However, haptens in petrolatum (e.g., the patch-test substances) often do not give an allergic prick-test reaction.[246] Preformed hapten-carrier systems have therefore been developed. Human serum albumin (HSA) has generally been used as the carrier.[244,245] Preparing the hapten-protein conjugate is unfortunately currently much on the "trial and error" level.[244] For example, concentration, pH, and temperature affect the forming of the hapten-protein conjugate. The diagnostics in this field should be improved. For instance, although acrylics have caused immediate skin reactions and asthma,[49-53] skin prick tests have not been positive, possibly because an appropriate hapten-protein conjugate has not been available.

SUGGESTED DENTAL SCREENING SERIES

We recommend the use of the "medium-sized" dental screening series for relatively advanced patch testing (Table 35-9). The standard tray should also be used for testing,

TABLE 35–9. Recommended Dental Screening Series—Together with the U.S. Standard Tray

Compound	Concentration, Percent	
Methyl methacrylate	2.0	pet
Triethyleneglycol dimethacrylate	2.0	pet
Urethane dimethacrylate	2.0	pet
Ethyleneglycol dimethacrylate	2.0	pet
BIS-GMA	2.0	pet
N,N-dimethyl-4-toluidine	5.0	pet
Mercury	0.5	pet
Cobalt chloride	1.0	pet
2-Hydroxyethyl methacrylate	2.0	pet
Gold sodium thiosulfate	0.5	aq
Eugenol	2.0	pet
Copper sulfate	2.0	aq
Methylhydroquinone	1.0	pet
Palladium chloride	1.0	pet
Tin	50.0	pet
Benzoyl peroxide	1.0	pet
Tetracaine (Amethocaine) hydrochloride	1.0	pet
Glutaraldehyde	1.0	aq
Lidocaine hydrochloride	15.0	pet
Fragrance mix	8.0	pet
Kathon CG	0.02	aq

if this has not been done earlier. For example, rubber chemicals are a common cause of occupational skin disease in health personnel, and rubber chemicals in the standard series plus possibly a series of rubber chemicals and patch testing with own glove may be needed.[248,249] For the more experienced, the "own" substances (brought in by the patient) should also be tested, because this is the only way to detect new allergens. Different disinfectants, anesthetics, etc., are used in different countries or areas and may necessitate the use of other dental screening trays to optimize the diagnostics.

ACKNOWLEDGMENT

This research is part of the Allergy and Work program under way at the Finnish Institute of Occupational Health. The Allergy and Work program is headed by one of the authors (LK).

REFERENCES

1. Fisher AA: *Contact Dermatitis*, 3d ed. Philadelphia, Lea & Febiger, 1986.
2. Jacobsen N, Hensten-Pettersen AO: Occupational health problems and adverse patient reactions in orthodontics. *Eur J Orthod* 11:254, 1989.
3. Hubler WR Jr, Hubler WR Sr: Dermatitis from a chromium dental plate. *Contact Dermatitis* 9:377, 1983.
4. Van Joost TH, van Ulsen J, van Loon LAJ: Contact allergy to denture materials in the burning mouth syndrome. *Contact Dermatitis* 18:97, 1988.
4a. Ali A, Bates JF, Reynolds AJ, et al: The burning mouth sensation related to wearing of acrylic dentures: An investigation. *Br Dent J* 161:444, 1987.
4b. Kaaber S: Allergy to dental materials with special reference to the use of amalgam and polymethylmethacrylate. *Int Dent J* 40:359, 1990.
4c. Dutree-Meulenberg ROGM, Kozel MMA, van Joost Th: Burning mouth syndrome: A possible etiologic role for local contact hypersensitivity. *J Am Acad Derm* 26:935, 1992.
4d. Fowler JF Jr: Burning mouth caused by dentures. *Am J Contact Dermatitis* 3:3, 1992.
4e. Guerra L, Vincenzi C, Peluso AM, et al: Role of contact sensitizers in the burning mouth syndrome. *Am J Contact Dermatitis* 4: 154, 1993.
5. McCarthy PL, Shklar G: *Diseases of the Oral Mucosa: Diagnosis, Management, Therapy*, New York, McGraw-Hill, 1964, p 157.
6. Zegarelli EV, Kutcher AH, Hyman GA: *Diagnosis of Diseases of the Mouth and Jaws*. Philadelphia, Lea & Febiger, 1969, p 306.
7. Larsson Å, Kinnby B, Könsberg R, et al: Irritant and sensitizing potential of copper, mercury and tin salts in experimental contact stomatitis of rat oral mucosa. *Contact Dermatitis* 23:146, 1990.
8. Chemotechnique Diagnostics: *Patch Test Allergens: Product Catalogue*. Chemotechnique Diagnostics AB, Malmö, Sweden, 1992.
9. *The Trolab Guide to Patch Testing*: Reinbek/Hamburg, Federal Republic of Germany, Hermal Kurt Herrmann, 1987, chap. 6.
10. Axell T, Björkner B, Fregert S, Niklasson B: Standard patch test series for screening of contact allergy to dental materials. *Contact Dermatitis* 9:82, 1983.
11. Foussereau J: *Guide de Dermato-Allergologie Professionnelle*. Paris, 1991.
12. Adams RM: *Occupational Skin Disease*, 2d ed. Philadelphia, Saunders, 1990.
13. Adams RM, Fischer T: Diagnostic patch testing, in Adams RM (ed): *Occupational Skin Disease*, 2nd ed. Philadelphia, Saunders, 1990, p 223.
14. Stevenson WJ: Methyl-methacrylate dermatitis. *Contact Point* 18:171, 1941.
15. Moody WL: Severe reaction from acrylic liquid, *Dent Digest* 47:305, 1941.
16. Bradford EW: Case of allergy to methyl-methacrylate, *Br Dent J* 84: 195, 1948.

17. Fisher AA: Allergic sensitization of the skin and oral mucosa to acrylic denture materials. *JAMA* 156:238, 1954.
18. Cronin E: *Contact Dermatitis*. Edinburgh, Churchill Livingstone, 1980.
19. Estlander T, Rajaniemi R, Jolanki R: Hand dermatitis in dental technicians. *Contact Dermatitis* 10:201, 1984.
20. Van der Walle HB: Sensitizing potential of acrylic monomers in guinea pig. Thesis, Katholieke Universiteit te Nijmegen, Krips Repro Meppel, 1982, pp 1–112.
21. Björkner B: Sensitizing capacity of ultraviolet curable acrylic compounds, MD Thesis, Lund, Sweden, 1984, pp 1–78.
22. Kanerva L, Estlander T, Jolanki R: Allergic contact dermatitis from dental composite resins due to aromatic epoxy acrylates and aliphatic acrylates. *Contact Dermatitis* 20:201, 1989.
23. Kanerva L, Turjanmaa K, Estlander T, Jolanki R: Occupational allergic contact dermatitis from 2-hydroxyethyl methacrylate (2-HEMA) in a new dentin adhesive. *Am J Contact Dermatitis* 2:24, 1991.
24. Kanerva L, Jolanki R, Estlander T: Occupational dermatitis due to an epoxy acrylate. *Contact Dermatitis* 14:80, 10986.
25. Kanerva L, Estlander T, Jolanki R: Sensitization to patch test acrylates. *Contact Dermatitis* 18:10, 1988.
26. Kanerva L, Estlander T, Jolanki R: Double active sensitization caused by acrylics, *Am J Contact Dermatitis* 3:23, 1992.
27. Kanerva L, Estlander T, Jolanki R: Active sensitization caused by 2-hydroxyethyl methacrylate, 2-hydroxypropyl methacrylate, ethyleneglycol dimethacrylate and *N,N*-dimethylaminoethyl methacrylate, *J Eur Acad Derm Venerol* 1:165, 1992.
28. Finnish Advisory Board of Chemicals. *Acrylate Compounds: Uses and Evaluation of Health Effects*. Helsinki, Government Printing Centre, 1992.
29. Kanerva L, Estlander T, Jolanki R, Tarvainen K: Dermatitis from acrylates in dental personnel, in Menne T, Maibach HI (eds): *Hand Eczema*. Boca Raton, FL, CRC Press, 1994, 231–254.
30. Bowen RL: Dental filling material comprising vinyl silane treated fused silica and a binder consisting of the reaction product of bis phenol and glycidyl acrylate, *US Pat*, 3,066,112, 1962.
31. Ruyter IE, Sjövik IJ: Composition of dental resin and composite materials. *Acta Odontol Scand* 39:133, 1981.
32. Rietschel RL: Contact allergens in ultraviolet-cured acrylic resin systems, in Adams RM (ed): *Occupational Medicine: State of the Art Reviews*. Hanley & Belfus, Inc, Philadelphia, 1986, pp 1–301.
33. Emmett EA, Kominsky JR: Allergic contact dermatitis from ultraviolet cured inks, *J Occup Med* 19:2, 113, 1977.
34. Björkner B: Allergic contact dermatitis from acrylates in ultraviolet curing inks. *Contact Dermatitis* 6:405, 1980.
35. Nethercott JR: Allergic contact dermatitis due to an epoxy acrylate, *Br J Dermatol* 104:697, 1981.
36. Nethercott JR, Jakubovic HR, Pilger C, Smith JW: Allergic contact dermatitis due to urethane acrylate in ultraviolet cured inks. *Br J Industr Med* 40:241, 1983.
37. Maurice PDL, Rycroft RJG: Allergic contact dermatitis from UV-curing acrylate in the manufacture of optical fibers. *Contact Dermatitis* 15:92, 1986.
38. Vanherle G, Smith DC: *Posterior Composite Resin Dental Restorative Materials*. Holland, Peter Szule, 1985.
39. Aasen SM, Oxman JD: Method for priming hand tissue. *US Patent*, 4719,149, Jan 12, 1988.
40. Nathanson P, Lochart P: Delayed extraoral hypersensitivity to dental composite material. *Oral Surg Oral Med Oral Pathol* 47:329, 1979.
41. Tinkelman DG, Tinkelman CL: An unusual etiology of urticaria. *Pediatrics* 63:339, 1979.
42. Niinimäki A, Rosberg J, Saari S: Allergic stomatitis from acrylic compounds: Report of a case, *Contact Dermatitis* 9:148, 1983.
43. Malten KE: Dermatological problems with synthetic resins and plastics in glues: Part II. *Derm Beruf Umwelt* 32:118, 1984.
44. Kanerva L, Turjanmaa K, Jolanki R, Estlander T: Occupational allergic contact dermatitis from iatrogenic sensitization by a new acrylate dentin adhesive. *Eur J Dermatol* 1:25, 1991.
45. Shelley ED, Shelley WB: Chronic dermatitis simulating small-plaque parapsoriasis due to cyanoacrylate adhesive used on fingernails. *JAMA* 252:2456, 1984.
46. Pigatto PD, Ghacchetti A, Altomare CF: Unusual sensitization to cyanoacrylate ester. *Contact Dermatitis* 14:193, 1986.

47. Belsito D: Contact dermatitis to ethyl cyanoacrylate containing glue. *Contact Dermatitis* 17:234, 1987.

48. Fisher AA: Adverse reactions to acrylate sculptured nails with particular reference to prolonged paresthesia. *Am J Contact Dermatitis* 2:38, 1991.

49. Savonius B, Keskinen H, Tuppurainen M, Kanerva L: Occupational respiratory disease caused by acrylics. *Clin Exp Allergy* 23:416, 1993.

50. Kanerva L, Estlander T, Jolanki R, Pekkarinen E: Occupational pharyngitis associated with allergic patch test reactions from acrylics. *Allergy* 47:571, 1992.

51. Lozewicz S, Davison AG, Hopkirk A, et al: Occupational asthma due to methyl methacrylate and cyanoacrylates. *Thorax* 40:836, 1985.

52. Fowler JF Jr: Immediate contact hypersensitivity to acrylic acid. *Dermatol Clin* 8:193, 1990.

53. Taylor JS: Acrylic reactions—ten years' experience, in Frosch PJ, Dooms-Goossens A, Lachapelle J-M, et al (eds): *Current Topics in Contact Dermatitis*. Berlin, Springer Verlag, 1989, pp 346–351.

54. Riva F, Pigatto PD, Altomare GF, Riboldi A: Sensitization to dental acrylic compounds, *Contact Dermatitis* 10:245, 1984.

55. Blichmann CW, Roed-Petersen J: Occupational skin problems in dental technicians. *Ugeskrife Laeger* 148:1370, 1986.

56. Farli M, Gasperini M, Francalanci S, et al: Occupational contact dermatitis in 2 dental technicians. *Contact Dermatitis* 22:282, 1990.

57. Tosti A, Rapacchiale S, Piraccini BM, Peluso AM: Occupational airborne contact dermatitis due to ethylene glycol dimethacrylate. *Contact Dermatitis* 24:152, 1991.

58. Kaaber S, Thulin H, Nielsen E: Skin sensitivity to denture base materials in the burning mouth syndrome. *Contact Dermatitis* 5:90, 1979.

59. Tosti A, Bardazzi F, Piancastelli E, Brasile GP: Contact stomatitis due to *N,N*-dimethyl-paratoluidine. *Contact Dermatitis* 22:113, 1990.

60. Verschueren GLA, Bruynzeel DP: Allergy to *N,N*-dimethyl-*p*-toluidine in dental materials. *Contact Dermatitis* 24:149, 1991.

61. Arndt KA, Fitzpatrick TB: Topical use of hydroquinone as a depigmenting agent. *JAMA* 194:965, 1965.

62. Frenk E, Loi-Zedda P: Occupational depigmentation due to a hydroquinone-containing photographic developer. *Contact Dermatitis* 6:238, 1980.

63. Duffield JA: Depigmentation of the skin by quinol and its monobenzyl ether. *Lancet* 1:1164, 1952.

64. Van Ketel WG: Sensitization to hydroquinone and the monobenzyl ether of hydroquinone. *Contact Dermatitis* 10:253, 1984.

65. Langer H: Das Schleimhautbrennen beim Tragen von Akrylatplatten. *Dtsch Zahnärzt Z* 5:1321, 1956.

66. Torres V, Mano-Azul A, Correia T, Soares AP: Allergic contact cheilitis and stomatitis from hydroquinone in an acrylic dental prosthesis. *Contact Dermatitis* 29:102, 1993.

67. Lidén C: Occupational dermatoses at a film laboratory: Follow-up after modernization. *Contact Dermatitis* 20:191, 1989.

68. Burrows D, Adams RM: Metals, in Adams RM (ed): *Occupational Skin Disease*, 2d ed. Philadelphia, Saunders, 1990, p 349.

69. Clemmensen OJ, Knudsen HE: Contact sensitivity to aluminium in a patient hyposensitized with aluminium precipitated grass pollen. *Contact Dermatitis* 6:305, 1980.

70. Böhler-Sommeregger K, Lindemayr H: Contact sensitivity to aluminium. *Contact Dermatitis* 15:278, 1986.

71. Fischer T, Rystedt I: A case of contact sensitivity to aluminium. *Contact Dermatitis* 8:343, 1982.

72. Kotovirta ML, Salo OP, Visa-Tolvanen K: Contact sensitivity to aluminium. *Contact Dermatitis* 11:135, 1984.

73. Rebandel P, Rudzki E: Occupational contact sensitivity in oculists. *Contact Dermatitis* 15:92, 1986.

74. Danilewich-Stysiak Z: Allergy as a cause of denture sore mouth. *J Prosthet Dent* 25:16, 1971.

75. Kanerva L, Tarvainen K, Eslander T, Jolanki R. Occupational allergic contact dermatitis caused by mercury and benzoyl peroxide. *Eur J Dermatol* 4:359–361, 1994.

75a. Cunliffe WJ, Burke B: Benzoyl peroxide: Lack of sensitization. *Acta Derm Venereol (Stockh)* 62:458, 1982.

76. Rietschel RL, Duncan SH: Benzoyl peroxide reactions in an acne study group. *Contact Dermatitis* 8:323, 1982.

77. Fisher AA: Dermatitis of the hands from food additives, *Cutis* 30:304, 1982.

78. Lindemayr H, Drobil M: Contact sensitization to benzoyl peroxide. *Contact Dermatitis* 7: 137, 1981.

79. Angelini G, Rantuccio F, Meneghini CL: Contact dermatitis in patients with leg ulcers. *Contact Dermatitis* 1:81, 1975.
80. Jensen O, Petersen SH, Vesteroger L: Contact sensitization to benzoyl peroxide following topical treatment of chronic leg ulcers. *Contact Dermatitis* 6:179, 1980.
81. Jager M, Balda BR: Loosening of a total hip prosthesis at contact allergy due to benzoyl peroxide. *Arch Orthop Traumat Surg* 94:175, 1979.
82. Estlander T, Kanerva L, Jolanki R: Occupational skin sensitization to the antimicrobials orthobenzyl parachlorophenol (oBpCP) and Ampholyte 103 G, in Frosch PJ, Dooms-Goossens A, Lachapelle JM, et al (eds): *Current Topics in Contact Dermatitis*. Berlin, Springer-Verlag, 1989, pp 88–91.
83. Sonnex TS, Rycroft RJG: Allergic contact dermatitis from orthobenzyl parachlorophenol in a drinking glass cleaner. *Contact Dermatitis* 14:247, 1986.
84. Kahn G: Depigmentation caused by phenolic detergent germicides. *Arch Dermatol* 102:177, 1970.
85. Krajewska D, Rudzki E: Sensitivity to epoxy resin and triethylenetetramine. *Contact Dermatitis* 2:135, 1976.
86. Prens EP, De Jong G, Van Joost T: Sensitization to epichlorohydrin and epoxy resin system components. *Contact Dermatitis* 15:85, 1986.
87. Van Joost T: Occupational sensitization to epichlorohydrin and epoxy resin. *Contact Dermatitis* 19:178, 1988.
88. Van Joost T, Roesyanto ID, Satawan I: Occupational sensitization to epichlorohydrin (ECH) and bisphenol-A during the manufacture of epoxy resin. *Contact Dermatitis* 22:125, 1990.
89. Gaul LE: Sensitivity to bisphenol A. *Arch Dermatol* 82:1003, 1960.
90. Freeman K, Warin AP: Contact dermatitis due to bisphenol A in semisynthetic waxes. *Contact Dermatitis* 11:259, 1984.
91. Srinivas CR, Devadiga R, Aroor AR: Footwear dermatitis due to bisphenol A. *Contact Dermatitis* 2:150, 1989.
92. Jolanki R: Occupational skin diseases from epoxy compounds. Epoxy resin, epoxy acrylates and 2,3-epoxypropyl trimethyl ammonium chloride. *Acta Derm Venereol (Stockh) Suppl* 169:1, 1991.
92a. Fregert S, Rorsman H: Hypersensitivity to epoxy resins with reference to the role played by bisphenol A. *J Invest Dermatol* 39:471, 1962.
92b. Malanin K: Active sensitization to camphoroquinone and double active sensitization to acrylics with long-lasting patch test reactions. *Contact Dermatitis* 29:284, 1993.
93. Larsen W: Perfume dermatitis, in Fisher AA (ed): *Contact Dermatitis*, 3d ed. Philadelphia, Lea & Febiger, 1996, p 394.
94. Drake TE, Maibach HI: Allergic contact dermatitis and stomatitis caused by a cinnamic-aldehyde flavored toothpaste. *Arch Dermatol* 112:202, 1976.
95. Magnusson B, Wilkinson DS: Cinnamic aldehyde in toothpaste: I. Clinical aspects and patch tests. *Contact Dermatitis* 1:70, 1975.
96. Mathias CGT, Maibach HI, Conant MA: Perioral leukoderma simulating vitiligo from use of a toothpaste containing cinnamic aldehyde. *Arch Dermatol* 116:1172, 1980.
97. Maibach HI: Cheilitis: Occult allergy to cinnamic aldehyde. *Contact Dermatitis* 15:106, 1986.
98. Angelini G, Vena GA: Allergic contact cheilitis to guaiazulene. *Contact Dermatitis* 10:311, 1984.
99. Balato N, Lembo G, Nappa P, Ayala F: Allergic cheilitis to azulene. *Contact Dermatitis* 13:39, 1985.
100. Brendlinger DL, Tarsitano JJ: Generalized dermatitis due to sensitivity to a chrome-cobalt removable partial denture. *J Am Dent Assoc* 81:392, 1970.
101. Dawson TAJ: Colophony sensitivity in dentistry. *Contact Dermatitis* 3:343, 1977.
102. Saltzer EI: Allergic contact dermatitis due to copper. *Arch Dermatol* 98:37, 1968.
103. Barranco VP: Eczematous dermatitis caused by internal exposure to copper. *Arch Dermatol* 106:386, 1972.
104. Barkoff JR: Urticaria secondary to a copper intrauterine device. *Int J Dermatol* 15:594, 1976.
105. Jouppila P, Niinimäki A, Mikkonen M: Cooper allergy and copper IUD. *Contraception* 6:631, 1979.
106. Frenz G, Teilum D: Cutaneous eruptions and intrauterine contraceptive copper devices. *Acta Derm Venereol (Stockh)* 60:69, 1980.
107. Romaguera C, Grimalt F: Contact dermatitis from a copper-containing intrauterine contraceptive device. *Contact Dermatitis* 7:163, 1981.
108. Karlberg A, Boman A, Wahlberg JE: Copper-A rare sensitizer. *Contact Dermatitis* 9:134, 1983.
109. Reid DJ: Allergic reaction to copper cement. *Br Dent J* 124:92, 1968.

110. Frykholm KO, Frithiof L, Fernstorm AI, et al: Allergy to copper derived from dental alloys as a possible cause of oral lesions of lichen planus. *Arch Derm Venereol (Stockh)* 49:268, 1969.
111. Jolanki R, Kanerva L, Estlander T, Tarvainen K: Epoxy dermatitis, in Nethercott J (ed): *Occupational Medicine: State of the Art Reviews.* Hanley & Belfus, Inc, Philadelphia, 1994, pp 97–112.
111a. Kanerva L, Jolanki R, Estlander T: Dentist's occupational allergic contact dermatitis caused by coconut diethanolamide, N-ethyl-4-toluenesulfonamide and 4-tolyldiethanolamine. *Acta Derm Venereol (Stockh)* 73:126–129, 1993.
112. Göransson K, Karltorp N, Ask H, Smedberg O: Några fall av eugenolöverkänslighet (Some cases of eugenol hypersensitivity). *Svensk Tandläkaretidskrift* 60:545, 1967 (in Swedish with English summary).
113. Koch G, Magnusson B, Nyquist G: Contact allergy to medicaments and materials used in dentistry: II. Sensitivity to eugenol and colophony. *Odont Rev* 22:275, 1971.
114. Calnan CD, Cronin E, Rycroft RJG: Allergy to perfume ingredients. *Contact Dermatitis* 6:500, 1980.
115. Jahkola A, Estlander T, Jolanki R, Kanerva L: Formaldehydi ammatti-ihotautien aiheuttajana (Formaldehyde as cause of occupational dermatoses; in Finnish with English and Swedish summaries.) Työ ja Ihminen. Työympäristötutkimuksen aikakauskirja 1:189, 1987.
116. Ormerod AD, Main RA: Sensitization to "sensitive teeth" toothpaste. *Contact Dermatitis* 13:192, 1985.
117. Flyvholm M-A, Menne T: Allergic contact dermatitis from formaldehyde: A case study focussing on sources of formaldehyde exposure. *Contact Dermatitis* 27:27, 1992.
118. Ebner H, Kraft D: Formaldehyde-induced anaphylaxis after dental treatment: *Contact Dermatitis* 24:307, 1991.
119. Ruyter IE: Release of formaldehyde from denture base polymers. *Acta Odont Scand* 38:17, 1980.
120. Bardazzi F, Melino M, Alagna G, Verienesi S: Glutaraldehyde dermatitis in nurses. *Contact Dermatitis* 15:319, 1986.
121. Nethercott JR, Holness DL, Page E: Occupational contact dermatitis due to glutaraldehyde in health care workers. *Contact Dermatitis* 18:193, 1988.
122. Sanderson KV, Cronin E: Glutaraldehyde and contact dermatitis. *Br Med J* 3:802, 1968.
123. Skog E: Sensitivity to glutaraldehyde. *Contact Dermatitis Newsletter* 4: 79, 1968.
124. Harman RRM, O'Grady KJ: Contact dermatitis due to sensitivity to Cidex (activated glutaraldehyde). *Contact Dermatitis Newsletter* 11:279, 1972.
125. Neering H, Ketel Van WG: Glutaraldehyde and formaldehyde allergy. *Contact Dermatitis Newsletter*, 16:518, 1974.
126. Gordon HH: Glutaraldehyde contact dermatitis. *Contact Dermatitis Newsletter* 15:442, 1974.
127. Lyon TC: Allergic contact dermatitis due to Cidex. *Oral Surgery* 32:895, 1971.
128. Jordan WP, Dahl MV, Albert HL: Contact dermatitis from glutaraldehyde. *Arch Dermatol* 105:94, 1972.
129. Hindson C, Lawlor F: Allergy to glyoxal in a polyvinyl resin emulsion. *Contact Dermatitis* 8:213, 1989.
130. Kligman A: The identification of contact allergies by human assay. *J Invest Dermatol* 47:393, 1966.
131. Schöpf E, Wex O, Schulz KH: Allergische Kontaktdermatitis mit spezifischer Lymphozytenstimulation durch Gold. *Hautarzt* 21:422, 1970.
132. Elgart ML, Higdon RS: Allergic contact dermatitis to gold. *Arch Dermatol* 103:649, 1971.
133. Klaschka F: Contact allergy to gold. *Contact Dermatitis* 1:264, 1975.
134. Young E: Contact hypersensitivity to metallic gold. *Dermatologica* 149:29, 1974.
135. Fregert S, Kollander M, Poulsen J: Allergic contact stomatitis from gold dentures. *Contact Dermatitis* 5:63, 1979.
136. Wiesenfeld D, Ferguson MM, Forsyth A, et al: Allergy to dental gold. *Oral Surg* 57:158, 1984.
137. Aro T, Kanerva L, Häyrinen-Immonen R, et al: Long-lasting allergic patch test reaction caused by gold. *Contact Dermatitis* 28:276, 1993.
138. Fisher AA: Ear piercing hazard of nickel-gold sensitization (letter). *JAMA* 228:1226, 1974.
139. Fowler JF: Selection of patch test materials for gold allergy. *Contact Dermatitis* 17:23, 1987.
140. Maurice PDL, Hopper C, Punnia-Moorthy A, Rycroft RJG: Allergic contact stomatitis and cheilitis from iodoform used in a dental dressing. *Contact Dermatitis* 18:114, 1988.
141. Goh CL, Ng SK: Contact allergy to iodoform and bismuth subnitrate. *Contact Dermatitis* 16:109, 1987.
142. Marks JG: Allergic contact dermatitis to povidone-iodine. *J Am Acad Derm* 6:473, 1982.
143. Ancona A, Suarez de la Torre R, Macotela E: Allergic contact dermatitis fom povidone-iodine. *Contact Dermatitis* 13:66, 1985.
144. Fregert S, Tegner E, Thelin I: Contact allergy to lidocaine. *Contact Dermatitis* 5:185, 1979.

145. Chin TM, Fellner MJ: Allergic hypersensitivity to lidocaine hydrochloride. *Int Soc Trop Derm* 19:147, 1980.
146. Soesman-van Waadenoden Kernekamp A, van Ketel WG: Contact allergy to licocaine (Xylocaine, Lignocaine). *Contact Dermatitis* 5:403, 1979.
147. Klein CE, Gall H: Type IV allergy to amide-type local anesthetics. *Contact Dermatitis* 25:45, 1991.
148. Vernon C, Hildebrand HF, Martin P: Amalgames dentaires et allergie. *J Biol Buccale* 14:83, 1986.
149. Finne K, Göransson K, Winckler L: Oral lichen planus and contact allergy to mercury. *Int J Oral Surg* 11:236, 1982.
150. Lind PO, Hurlen B, Lyberg T, Aas E: Amalgam-related oral lichenoid reaction. *Scand J Dent Res* 94:448, 1986.
151. James J, Ferguson MM, Forsyth A, et al: Oral lichenoid reaction releated to mercury sensitivity. *Br J Oral Maxillofac Surg* 25:474, 1987.
152. Ancona A, Ramos M, Suarez R et al: Mercury sensitivity in a dentist. *Contact Dermatitis* 8:218, 1982.
153. Goh CL, NG SK: Occupational allergic contact dermatitis from metallic mercury. *Contact Dermatitis* 19:232, 1988.
154. Kanerva L, Komulainen M, Estlander T, Jolanki R: Occupational allergic contact dermatitis caused by mercury. *Contact Dermatitis* 28:26, 1993.
155. Miller EG, Perry WL, Wagner MJ: Prevalence of mercury hypersensitivity among dental students. *J Prosthet Dent* 58:235, 1987.
156. Rudzki E, Rebandel P, Grzywa Z: Patch tests with occupational contactants in nurses, doctors and dentists. *Contact Dermatitis* 20:247, 1989.
157. Berova N, Stransky L, Krasteva M: Studies on contact dermatitis in stomatological staff. *Dermatol Monatschr* 176:15, 1990.
158. Von Mayenburg J, Rakoski J, Szliska C: Patch testing with amalgam at various concentrations. *Contact Dermatitis* 24:266, 1991.
159. Aberer W: Topical mercury should be banned—Dangerous, outmoded, but still popular. *J Am Acad Derm* 24:150, 1991.
160. Cox NH, Forsyth A: Thiomersal allergy and vaccination reactions. *Contact Dermatitis* 18:229, 1988.
161. Frykholm KO, Wahlberg F: A fatal a case of mercurial dermatitis with complication. *Acta Derm Syph* 44:362, 1964.
162. Miedler LH, Forbes JD: Allergic contact dermatitis due to metallic mercury. *Arch Environ Health* 17:960, 1964.
163. Swinyer LJ: Allergic contact dermatitis from metallic mercury. *Contact Dermatitis* 6:226, 1980.
164. Vermeiden I, Oranje AP, Vuzekski VD, et al: Mercury exanthem as occupational dermatitis. *Contact Dermatitis* 6:88, 1980.
165. Nakayama H, Niki F, Shono M, et al: Mercury exanthem. *Contact Dermatitis* 9:411, 1983.
166. Andersen K, Hjorth N, Menné T: The baboon syndrome: Systematically induced allergic contact dermatitis. *Contact Dermatitis* 10:97, 1984.
167. Mathews KP, Pan PM: Immediate type hypersensitivity to phenylmercuric compounds. *Am J Med* 44:310, 1968.
168. Corrales JL, Fernandez De Corres L: Anaphylactic hypersensitivity to mercurochrome (merbromium). *Ann Allergy* 54:230, 1985.
169. Temesvári E, Daroczy J: Histological examination of immediate and delayed contact allergy provoked by mercuric chloride. *Contact Dermatitis* 21:271, 1989.
170. Sanz PB, Munoz FM, Serrano CL, et al: Hypersensitivity to mercuric fluorescein compounds. *Allergol Immunopathol* 17:219, 1989.
171. Spector LS: Allergic manifestations to mercury. *JAMA* 42:320, 1951.
172. Oshima H, Kawahara D, Kosugi H, et al: Epidemiologic study on occupational allergy in the dental clinic. *Contact Dermatitis* 24:138, 1991.
173. Malten KE: Recently reported causes of contact dermatitis due to synthetic resins and hardeners. *Contact Dermatitis* 5:11, 1979.
174. Van Ketel WG: Reactions to dental impression materials. *Contact Dermatitis* 3:55, 1977.
175. Cronin E: Impregum (dental impression material). *Contact Dermatitis Newsletter* 13:362, 1973.
176. Groeningen van G, Nater JP: Reaction to dental impression materials. *Contact Dermatitis* 1:373, 1975.
177. Nally FS, Storrs J: Hypersensitivity to a dental impression material. *Br Dent J* 134:244, 1973.
178. Kulenkamp D, Hausen BM, Schulz K-H: Kontaktallergie durch neuartige, zahnärztlich verwendete Abdruckmaterialien. *Hautartz* 28:353, 1977.

179. Kanerva L, Autio P, Estlander T, et al: Immediate and delayed polyfunctional aziridine allergy in *First Congress of the European Society of Contact Dermatitis*, Brussels, October 8–10, 1992, p 52.

180. Duxbury AJ, Turner EP, Watts DC: Hypersensitivity to epimine containing dental materials. *Brit Dent J* 147:331, 1979.

181. Fisher AA, Shapiro A: Allergic eczematous contact dermatitis due to metallic nickel. *JAMA* 161:717, 1956.

182. Fernandez JP, Veron C, Hildebrand HF, Martin P: Nickel allergy to dental prostheses. *Contact Dermatitis* 14:312, 1986.

183. Temesvari E, Racz I: Nickel sensitivity from a dental prosthesis. *Contact Dermatitis* 18:50, 1988.

184. Wilson AG McT, Gould DJ: Nickel dermatitis from a dental prosthesis without buccal involvement. *Contact Dermatitis* 21:53, 1989.

185. Van Hoogstraten IMW, Andersen KE, von Blomberg BME, et al: Preliminary results of a multicenter study on the incidence of nickel allergy in relationship to previous oral and cutaneous contacts, in Frosch PJ, Dooms-Goossens A, Lachapelle J-M, et al (eds): *Current Topics in Contact Dermatitis*. Berlin, Springer-Verlag, Heidelberg New York 1989; 178–183.

186. Fisher AA: Patch tests for allergic reactions to dentifrices and mouthwashes. *Cutis* 6:554, 1970.

187. Anderson KE: Contact allergy to toothpaste flavors. *Contact Dermatitis* 4:195, 1978.

188. Drake TE, Maibach HI: Allergic contact dermatitis and stomatitis caused by a cinnamic aldehyde-flavored toothpaste. *Arch Dermatol* 112:202, 1976.

189. Magnusson B, Wilkinson DS: Cinnamic aldehyde in toothpaste: I. Clinical aspects and patch tests. *Contact Dermatitis* 1:70, 1975.

190. Kirton V, Wilkinson DS: Sensitivity to cinnamic aldehyde toothpaste: II. Further studies. *Contact Dermatitis* 1:77, 1975.

191. Van Ketel WG, Nieboer C: Allergy to palladium in dental alloys. *Contact Dermatitis* 7:331, 1981.

192. van Loon LAJ, van Elsas PW, van Joost T, et al: Contact stomatitis and dermatitis to nickel and palladium. *Contact Dermatitis* 11:294, 1984.

193. van Loon LAJ, van Elsas PW, van Joost T, Davidson CL: Test battery for metal allergy in dentistry. *Contact Dermatitis* 14:158, 1986.

194. Downey D: Contact mucositis due to palladium. *Contact Dermatitis* 21:54, 1989.

195. Camarasa JG, Serra-Baldrich E: Palladium contact dermatitis. *Am J Contact Dermatitis* 1:114, 1990.

196. Wahlberg JE, Boman A: Palladium chloride—A potent sensitizer in the guinea pig. *Am J Contact Dermatitis* 1:112, 1990.

197. Sheard S Jr: Contact dermatitis from platinum and related metals: Report of case. *Arch Dermatol* 71:357, 1955.

198. Conde-Salazar L, Cannavo A, Meza B, et al: Occupational argyrosis and platinosis. *Am J Contact Dermatitis* 3:44, 1992.

199. Marshalla J: Toxicity of platinum. *S Afr Med J* 26:8, 1952.

200. Roberts AE: Platinosis. *Arch Industr Hyg* 4:549, 1951.

201. Levene GM: Platinum sensitivity. *Br J Dermatol* 85:590, 1971.

202. Key MM: Some unusual allergic reactions in industry. *Arch Dermatol* 83:3, 1961.

203. Levene GM: Platinum sensitivity. *Br J Dermatol* 85:590, 1971.

204. Lane CG: Occupational dermatitis in dentists: Susceptibility to procaine. *Arch Dermatol* 3:235, 1921.

205. Laden EL, Wallace DA: Contact dermatitis due to procaine: A common occupational disease in dentists. *J Invest Dermatol* 12:299, 1949.

206. Falk E, Hektorn H, Thune PO: Skin and respiratory tract systems in veterinary surgeons. *Contact Dermatitis* 12:274, 1985.

207. Mitchell JC: Contact dermatitis from proflavine dihydrochloride. *Arch Dermatol* 106:924, 1972.

208. Goh CL: Contact sensitivity to proflavine. *Int J Dermatol* 23:449, 1986.

209. Goh CL: Contact sensitivity to topical antimicrobials: I. Epidemiology in Singapore. *Contact Dermatitis* 21:46, 1989.

210. Lim J, Goh CL, Lee CT: Perioral and mucosal oedema due to contact allergy to proflavine. *Contact Dermatitis* 25:195, 1991.

211. Goh CL: Erythema multiforme-like and purpuric eruption due to contact allergy to proflavine. *Contact Dermatitis* 17:53, 1987.

211a. Blinkhorn AS, Leggate EM: An allergic reaction to a rubber dam. *Br Dent J* 156:402, 1984.

211b. Davenport JC: An adverse reaction to a silicone-rubber soft lining material. *Br Dent J* 128:545, 1970.

THE COLOR PLATES

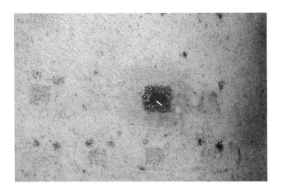

Plate 1. Angry back (spillover phenomenon). A strong positive allergic reaction is surrounded by several (weaker) false-positive reactions. (The plate is cited in Chap. 7.)

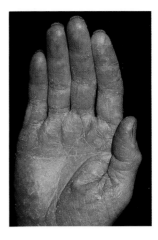

Plate 2. Hand dermatitis in MBT-positive carpet maker. (The plate is cited in Chap. 11.)

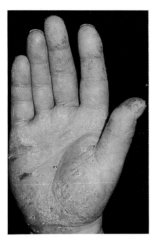

Plate 3. Rubber dermatitis of the hands in MBT-sensitive person with shoe dermatitis. (The plate is cited in Chap. 11.)

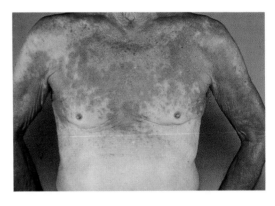

Plate 4. Severe generalized dermatitis of over 10 years' duration in a patient with brisk patch-test responses to formaldehyde, quaternium-15, and imidazolidinyl urea. (The plate is cited in Chap. 14.)

A   B

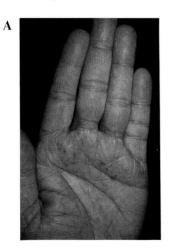

Plate 5. *A.* Hand eczema in doughnut maker exposed to cinnamon. *B.* Closeup of the finger web area in the previous patient. (The plate is cited in Chap. 15.)

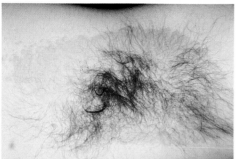

← **Plate 6.** Contact dermatitis to spice-scented deodorant in cinnamic aldehyde-allergic patient. (The plate is cited in Chap. 15.)

A

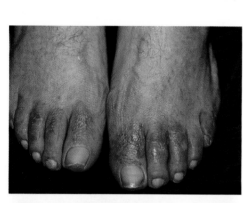

B

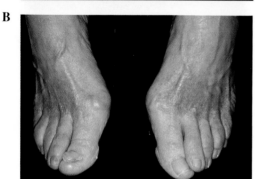

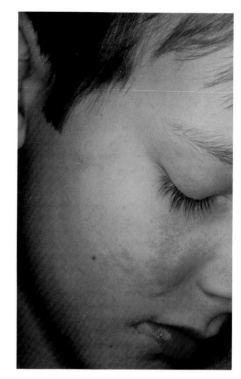

Plate 7. Reaction to perfumed facial tissue and toothpaste in a 10-year-old boy allergic to both cinnamic aldehyde and cinnamic alcohol. The toothpaste contained cinnamic aldehyde. (The plate is cited in Chap. 15.)

C

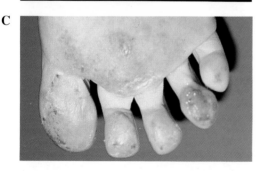

Plate 8. *A.* Eczema of the dorsum of the toes but sparing the plantar surfaces is typical of rubber-box-toe dermatitis. This was formerly a common form of shoe allergy. *B.* Allergic contact dermatitis to elastic in stretch loafers. *C.* Insole dermatitis in a rubber-allergic patient. (The plate is cited in Chap. 31.)

Plate 9. Allergic cosmetic dermatitis of the face with strong periorbital edema due to hair-dye allergy. (The plate is cited in Chap. 32.)

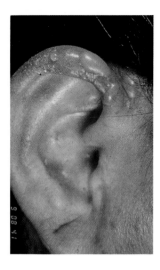

Plate 10. Bullous cosmetic dermatitis of the ears due to hair dye allergy. (The plate is cited in Chap. 32.)

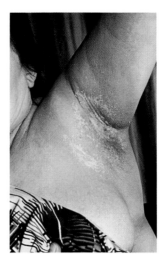

Plate 11. Allergic contact dermatitis from a deodorant. (The plate is cited in Chap. 32.)

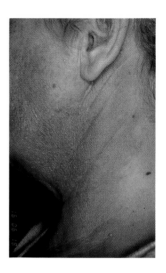

Plate 12. Allergic contact dermatitis from perfume. (The plate is cited in Chap. 32.)

← **Plate 13.** Allergic cosmetic dermatitis: typical example of mild involvement of the eyelids. (The plate is cited in Chap. 32.)

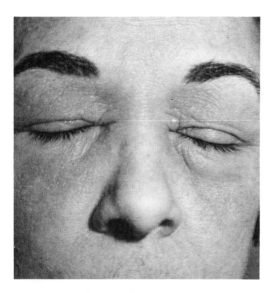

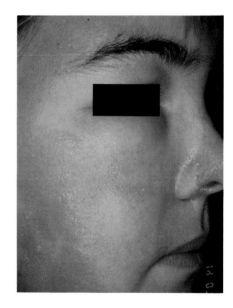

Plate 14. Allergic cosmetic dermatitis involving the face. (The plate is cited in Chap. 32.)

← **Plate 15.** A "perfume" or cologne is relatively easy to suspect when it occurs where the product is usually applied, as here, on the neck. (The plate is cited in Chap. 33.)

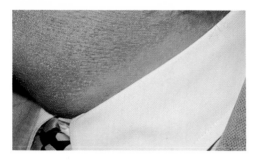

Plate 16. Photosensitivity to musk ambrette in a man's cologne. This type of reaction is less common since levels of that ingredient have been reduced. (The plate is cited in Chap. 33.)

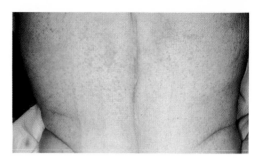

Plate 17. Allergy to alpha-amylcinnamic aldehyde in a laundry detergent. (The plate is cited in Chap. 33.)

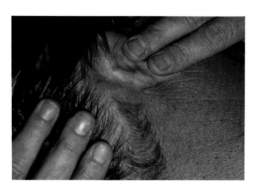

Plate 18. Photoallergy to oak moss absolute in a man's aftershave. This patient was also compositae-allergic but improved dramatically after he stopped using the aftershave. (The plate is cited in Chap. 33.)

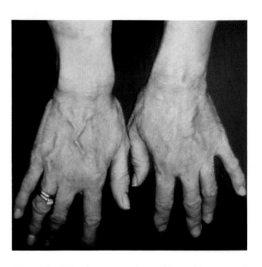

Plate 19. Allergic contact dermatitis to thiurams and carbamates in a rubber glove. A middle-aged woman initially presented with a presumed dyshidrotic eczema of the fingers and was instructed to wear rubber gloves for household wet work. She returned several months later with this erythematous scaling dermatitis of the dorsal hands. Note the demarcation at the wrists, with patches of dermatitis about the midforearm, which is typical of allergic reactions to household gloves. Patch tests showed positive reactions to both the thiuram and carba mixes. Her dermatitis cleared with the use of cotton liners and vinyl gloves. *(Reproduced with permission of the Ronald O. Perelman Department of Dermatology, New York University School of Medicine.)* (The plate is cited in Chap. 34.)

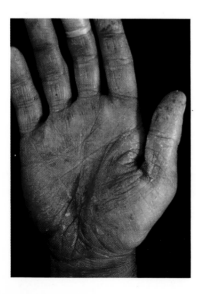

Plate 20. Allergic contact dermatitis to *para*-phenylenediamine derivatives in a rubber shift handle. A middle-aged truck driver complained of this dermatitis over the volar aspect of the right hand which developed several months after purchasing a new truck. Patch test showed positive reactions to pieces of rubber taken from the shift handle as well as to black rubber mix. The dermatitis resolved when the rubber-coated knob was replaced with plastic. *(Reproduced with permission of the Ronald O. Perelman Department of Dermatology, New York University School of Medicine.)* (The plate is cited in Chap. 34.)

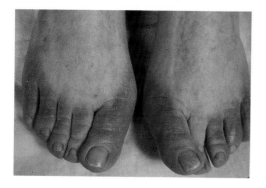

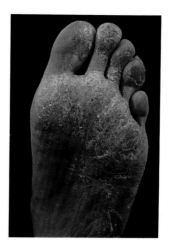

Plate 21. Allergic contact dermatitis to *p-tert*-butylphenol formaldehyde resin in neoprene glues. A middle-aged woman presented with a many months' history of this erythematous scaling dermatitis limited only to the dorsal aspect of the toes bilaterally. Treatment with a variety of potent glucocorticoids ameliorated the pruritus but not the dermatitis. Patch tests showed positive reactions to the linings of several shoes as well as *p-tert*-butylphenol formaldehyde resin. The dermatitis resolved upon purchase of shoes free of the neoprene adhesives which contain the allergen. *(Reproduced with permission of Donald V. Belsito, M.D., New York, New York.)* (The plate is cited in Chap. 34.)

Plate 22. Allergic contact dermatitis to mercaptobenzothiazole in shoe inserts. A young man presented with a several-year history of this hyperkeratotic dermatitis limited to the volar aspects of the feet. The condition had been treated with a variety of antipsoriatic regimens without success. Patch tests showed positive reactions to mercaptobenzothiazole, mercapto mix, and rubber inserts in several pairs of athletic shoes. Note the sparing of the arches and flexural creases of the toes typical of ACD to shoe inserts. The dermatitis eventually resolved when rubber-free shoes were purchased. *(Reproduced with permission of the Ronald O. Perelman Department of Dermatology, New York University School of Medicine.)* (The plate is cited in Chap. 34.)

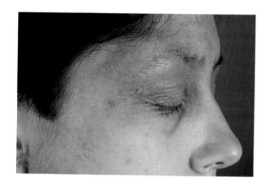

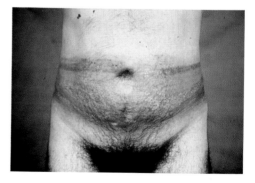

Plate 23. Allergic contact dermatitis to thioureas in a make-up applicator. A middle-aged woman presented with this lichenified dermatitis of the eyelids of 1 year's duration. Initial evaluation with standard patch tests was negative, but she returned for further diagnostic workup when her dermatitis cleared upon discontinuation of all makeup. Patch tests were positive only to her makeup sponges and to a mix of dialkyl thioureas (1% in petrolatum). The patient resumed use of cosmetics but without rubber sponges and remained free of her dermatitis. *(Reproduced with permission of the Ronald O. Perelman Department of Dermatology, New York University School of Medicine.)* (The plate is cited in Chap. 34.)

Plate 24. Allergic contact dermatitis to bleached rubber. A middle-aged man presented with this waistband dermatitis of several months' duration. Patch testing to a standard tray as well as to an expanded rubber series was negative. The only positive reaction was to the elasticized waistband of his underwear. This case of "bleached rubber" syndrome resolved when he purchased new underwear which remained unbleached. *(Reproduced with permission of the Ronald O. Perelman Department of Dermatology, New York University School of Medicine.)* (The plate is cited in Chap. 34.)

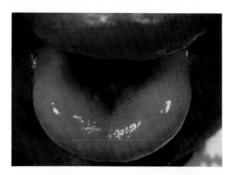

Plate 25. Allergic contact urticaria to latex in a balloon. This young dental technician had a known history of atopic dermatitis and allergic contact dermatitis to thiurams in gloves. She presented with acute swelling of the lips, scattered hives of the face, hands, and arms, and respiratory distress. Her symptoms developed within minutes of blowing up several balloons. Subsequent prick testing to eluates from the balloons and several pairs of latex gloves was positive, although the RAST test for latex was equivocal. Prick testing to the rubber accelerators including thiurams was negative. *(Reproduced with permission of Donald V. Belsito, M.D., New York, New York.)* (The plate is cited in Chap. 34.)

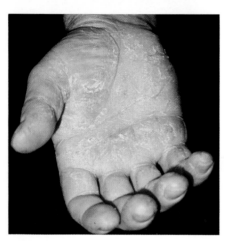

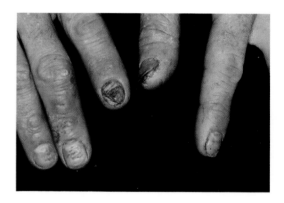

Plate 26. Body shop repairman with a history of reacting to paint. Patch testing showed him to be allergic to epoxy, and the source proved to be an adhesive used on bumpers. (The plate is cited in Chap. 36A.)

Plate 27. Rubber stamp worker who used an ultraviolet-cured lettering process. He was allergic to hydroxyethyl acrylate, hydroxypropyl acrylate, hydroxyethyl methacrylate, hydroxypropyl methacrylate, and ethylene glycol dimethacrylate. (The plate is cited in Chap. 36B.)

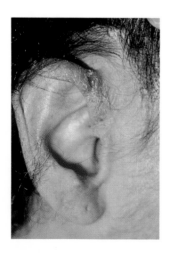

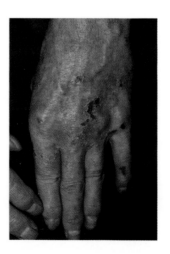

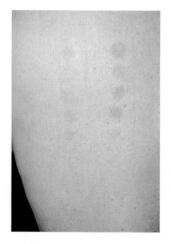

Plate 28. Contact dermatitis to a hearing aid wire covered with a polyethylene sleeve. (The plate is cited in Chap. 36B.)

Plate 29. Reaction to spicules of metal containing cobalt in a cobalt-allergic metal worker. (The plate is cited in Chap. 37.)

Plate 30. Aluminum reaction to Finn chambers. All chambers caused a ringed eruption where contact occurred. (The plate is cited in Chap. 37.)

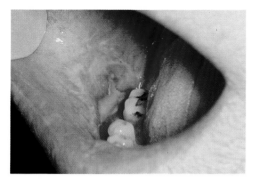

Plate 31. Erosive oral lichen planus in a patient allergic to copper in his dental amalgams. (The plate is cited in Chap. 37.)

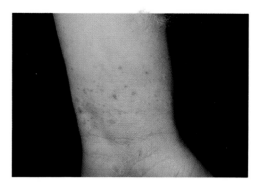

Plate 32. Papular gold dermatitis. (The plate is cited in Chap. 37.)

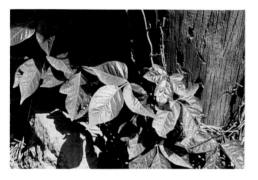

Plate 33. Poison Ivy, *Toxicodendron radicans* spp. *negundo.* (The plate is cited in Chap. 38.)

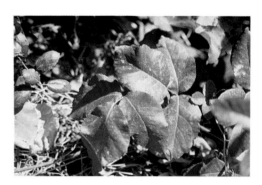

Plate 34. *Toxicodendron diversilobum,* or western poison oak. This is a much larger plant than the eastern species, which does not climb trees. Both have three leaflets per leaf. (The plate is cited in Chap. 38.)

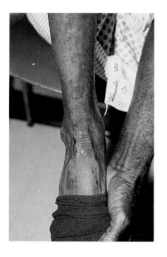

Plate 35. Compositae dermatitis resembling atopic eczema. (The plate is cited in Chap. 38.)

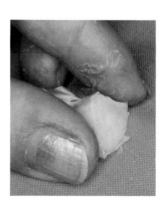

Plate 36. Garlic dermatitis in the area where garlic was held. *(Courtesy Dr. Luis Conde-Salazar and Dr. Robert Adams.)* (The plate is cited in Chap. 39.)

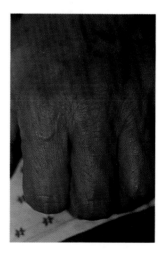

Plate 37. Immediate positive rub test to shrimp. This was seen in a waitress with hand eczema regularly precipitated by the handling of shrimp. (The plate is cited in Chap. 39.)

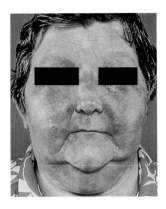
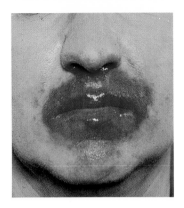
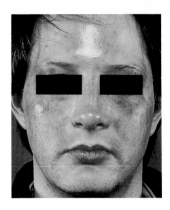

Plate 38. Allergic contact dermatitis of face sensitive to parabens in topical antibacterial silver sulfadiazine cream applied to foot abrasions and inadvertently spread to face. (The plate is cited in Chap. 40.)

Plate 39. Erosive perioral dermatitis due to paraben-containing lip balm; irritant and secondary monilial invasion factors complicate this situation. (The plate is cited in Chap. 40.)

Plate 40. Allergic contact dermatitis of face from MCI/MI in shampoo; positive patch test and resolution of dermatitis with change of shampoo confirm relevance. (The plate is cited in Chap. 40.)

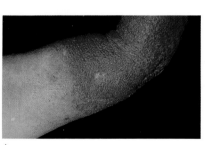
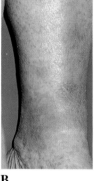
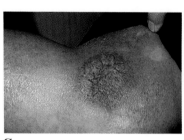

A
B
C

Plate 41. *A.* Typical spreading eczema from allergy to a topical agent. This can be a medication, a home remedy, or a cosmetic lotion used to treat an underlying eczema. *B.* Contact dermatitis to a moisturizer used to treat stasis eczema. The only positive patch test was to the moisturizer itself, and withdrawal cleared the eruption. *C.* Allergic contact dermatitis to mustargen applied to a plaque of cutaneous T-cell lymphoma. The eruption cleared locally in the plaques where the patient had experienced allergic contact dermatitis. (The plate is cited in Chap. 41.)

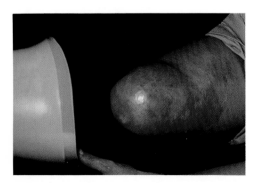
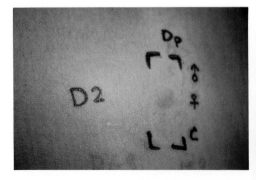

Plate 42. Allergic contact dermatitis of an amputation stump from an antibiotic ointment. (The plate is cited in Chap. 41.)

Plate 43. Strong positive reactions to three crushed *Dermatophagoides* in a patient with atopic dermatitis on day 2 of the patch test. (The plate is cited in Chap. 46.)

211c. Vandersall DC: Contact stomatitis resulting from the use of orthodontic rubber elastics. *J Am Dent Assoc* 88:1030, 1974.

211d. March PJ: An allergic reaction to latex rubber gloves. *J Am Dent Assoc* 117:590, 1988.

211e. Cohen DM, Hoffman M: *Oral Surg Oral Med Oral Pathol* 52:491, 1981.

212. Gaul LEO: Incidence of sensitivity to chromium, nickel, gold, silver and copper compared to reactions to their aqueous salts including cobalt sulphate. *Ann Allergy* 12:429, 1954.

213. Marcussen PV: Variations in the incidence of contact hypersensitivities. *Trans St John's Hosp Derm Soc* 48:40, 1962.

214. Gaul LE, Underwood GB: The effects of aging of solution of silver nitrate on its cutaneous reaction. *J Invest Dermatol* 11:7, 1948.

215. Marshall JP, Schneider RP: Systemic argyria secondary to topical silver nitrate. *Arch Dermatol* 113:1077, 1977.

216. Buckley WR: Localized argyria. *Arch Dermatol* 88:531, 1963.

217. Johansson EA, Kanerva L, Niemi KM, et al: Generalized argyria with low ceruloplasmin and copper levels in the serum: A case report with clinical and microscopical findings and a trial of penicillamine treatment. *Clin Exp Dermatol* 7:169, 1982.

218. Kanerva L, Estlander T, Jolanki R: Occupational skin disease in Finland: An analysis of 10 years of statistics from an occupational dermatology clinic. *Int Arch Occup Health* 60:89, 1988.

219. Bowers RE: Tego (dodecylic aminoethyl glycine hydrochloride). *Contact Dermatitis Newsletter* 4:76, 1968.

220. Fregert S, Dahlquist I: Allergic contact dermatitis from Tego (dodecylic aminoethyl glycine hydrochloride). *Contact Dermatitis Newsletter* 5:103, 1969.

221. Calnan CD: Tego dermatitis (telephone cleaner). *Contact Dermatitis Newsletter* 15:439, 1974.

222. Lachapelle JM, Reginster JP: Occupational contact dermatitis from an ampholytic soap (TEGO). *Contact Dermatitis* 3:211, 1977.

223. Valsecchi R, Leghissa P, Piazzolla S: Tego allergy in food industry. *Contact Dermatitis* 20:23, 188.

224. Suhonen R: Contact allergy to dodecyl-di-(aminoethyl)glycine (Desimex i). *Contact Dermatitis* 6:290, 1980.

225. Foussereau J, Samsoen M, Hecht MT: Occupational dermatitis to Ampholyt G in hospital personnel. *Contact Dermatitis* 9:233, 1983.

226. Menne T, Andersen KE, Kaaber K, et al: Tin: An overlooked contact sensitizer? *Contact Dermatitis* 16:9, 1987.

227. Hayakawa R, Matsunaga K, Kobayashi M: Leukomelanoderma from Tinuvin P. *Allergy Pract* 21:38, 1983.

228. Grout AC, Lien DH: Contact allergy to Tinuvin P. *Contact Dermatitis* 9:324, 1983.

229. Hecke EV, Vossaert K: Allergic contact dermatitis from an ostomy bag. *Contact Dermatitis* 21:330, 1988.

230. Arisu K, Hayakawa K, Ogino Y, et al: Tinuvin P in a spandex tape as a cause of clothing dermatitis. *Contact Dermatitis* 26:311, 1992.

231. Niklasson B, Björkner B: Contact allergy to the UV-absorber Tinuvin P in plastics. *Contact Dermatitis* 21:330, 1989.

232. Kaniwa M, Isama K, Kojima S, et al: Chemical approach to contact dermatitis caused by household products: VIII. UV absorber Tinuvin P in polyurethane elastomers for fabric products. *Jpn J Tox Envir Health* 37:218, 1991.

233. Thompson G, Maibach H, Epstein J: Allergic contact dermatitis from sunscreen preparations complicating photodermatitis. *Arch Dermatol* 113:1252, 1977.

234. Pariser RS: Contact dermatitis to dioxybenzone. *Contact Dermatitis* 3:172, 1977.

235. Ramsay DL, Cohen HS, Baer RL: Allergic reaction to benzophenone. *Arch Dermatol* 105:906, 1972.

236. Burry JN: Photo allergies from benzophenones and beta carotene in sunscreens. *Contact Dermatitis* 6:211, 1980.

236a. Beacham BE, Kurgansky D, Gould WM: Circumoral dermatitis and cheilitis caused by tartar-control dentifrices. *J Am Acad Dermatol* 22:1029, 1990.

236b. Kowitz G, Jacobson J, Meng Z, Lucatorto F: The effects of tartar-control toothpaste on the oral soft tissues. *Oral Surg Oral Med Oral Pathol* 70:529, 1990.

237. Kligman A: The spectrum of contact urticaria: Wheals, erythema, and pruritus. *Dermatol Clin* 8:57, 1990.

238. Lahti A, Maibach HI: Immediate contact reactions, in Menné T, Maibach HI (eds): *Exogenous Dermatoses; Environmental Dermatitis.* Boca Raton, FL, CRC Press, 1991, pp 21–35.

239. Kanerva L, Estlander T, Jolanki R: Skin testing for immediate hypersensitivity in occupational allergology, in Menné T, Maibach HI (eds): *Exogenous Dermatoses: Environmental Dermatitis.* Boca Raton, FL, CRC Press, 1991, pp 103–126.

240. Nutter A: Contact urtucaria to rubber. *Br J Dermatol* 101:597, 1979.

241. Taylor J, Evey P, Helm T, Wagner W: Contact urticaria and anaphylaxis from latex. *Contact Dermatitis* 23:277, 1990.

242. Alenius H, Turjanmaa K, Palosuo T, et al: Surgical latex glove allergy: Characterization of rubber protein allergens by immunoblotting. *Int Arch Allergy Appl Immunol* 96:376, 1991.

243. Turjanmaa K: Latex glove contact urticaria. Thesis. University of Tampere, Tampere, Finland, 1988.

244. Wass U: Studies on IgE antibodies induced by low-molecular-weight chemicals. Thesis, University of Göteborg, Göteborg, Sweden, 1989.

245. Welinger H: Occupational airways hypersensitivity to some small organic molecules: Exposure, response, and pathomechanism. Thesis, University of Lund, Lund, Sweden, 1989.

246. Kanerva L: Contact urticaria, in Burgdorf WHC, Katz SI, Hood AF, Malkinson FD, Peters MS, Robinson JK, Swerlick R (eds): *Dermatology. Progress and Perspectives. The Proceedings of the 18th World Congress of Dermatology, New York.* Lancaster, Parthenon Publishing, 1993, pp 745–749.

247. Belsito DV: Contact urticaria caused by rubber: Analysis of seven cases. *Dermatol Clin* 8:61, 1990.

248. Estlander T, Jolanki R, Kanerva L: Dermatitis and urticaria from rubber and plastic gloves. *Contact Dermatitis* 14:20, 1986.

249. Estlander T, Jolanki R, Kanerva L: Allergic contact dermatitis from rubber and plastic gloves, in Mellström G, Walhlberg JE, Maibach HI (eds). Boca Raton, FL, CRC Press, 1994, pp 221–239.

36A

PLASTICS: EPOXY RESINS

Jere D. Guin
William J. Work

CHEMISTRY

Epoxy resins are a broad class of (plastic) materials widely used in industry, including aerospace, electronics, and coatings manufacturing. Despite their name, the epoxy compound is only one of the chemicals used in epoxy resins. Epoxy resins always incorporate a hardener and often contain diluents, modifiers, fillers, and reinforcements. Epoxy resin systems derive their name from the cyclic three-membered ring structure containing oxygen, the epoxide group (Fig. 36A-1). Although many other ring sizes exist for epoxides, those containing three-membered rings usually undergo chemical reactions to form plastics most easily. Many chemical routes may be employed to prepare epoxides, but the most common involve oxidation of dienes with oxidizing agents such as peracetic acid and chemical substitution reactions between an alcohol or amine and 3-chloro-1,2-epoxypropane, also known as epichlorohydrin. Both types of chemistry are used commercially. Most epoxy resin monomers have two or more epoxy groups in the molecule, permitting chemical reactions to form the high-molecular-weight and cross-linked polymers which have proved to be so effective and useful.

The most commonly used epoxy resins are those derived from bisphenol A, a product of the reaction of an acetone molecule with two molecules of phenol. When reacted with epichlorohydrin, an epoxy ether is formed (Fig. 36A-2) by loss of a hydrogen ion from the bisphenol A and a chloride from the epichlorohydrin; the product is often referred to as the diglycidyl ether of bisphenol A or DGEBPA. By varying the ratio of epichlorohydrin to bisphenol A, the molecular weight of the formed diepoxide may be changed. The simplest epoxy resin monomer in that series is a bisphenol A molecule coupled to two glycidyl or epoxy propane groups bound by an ether linkage to each side,[1] with a molecular weight of about 340.

Higher-molecular-weight homologues of this resin, up to about 8000 g/mole, are used in the epoxy industry, and even higher-molecular-weight plastics that contain epoxy groups (phenoxy resins, with molecular weights to 45,000 g/mole) are used without reactive curing. Some other representative structures of commercially available epoxy resins are presented in Fig. 36A-3 and a list of chemical names of commercially available epoxy resins is provided in Table 36A-1. The resin or mixture of resins chosen for a particular application depends upon the desired balance of properties. The

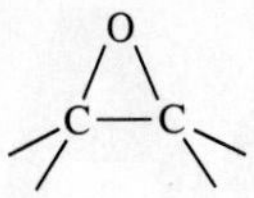

FIG. 36A–1. Epoxy functional group.

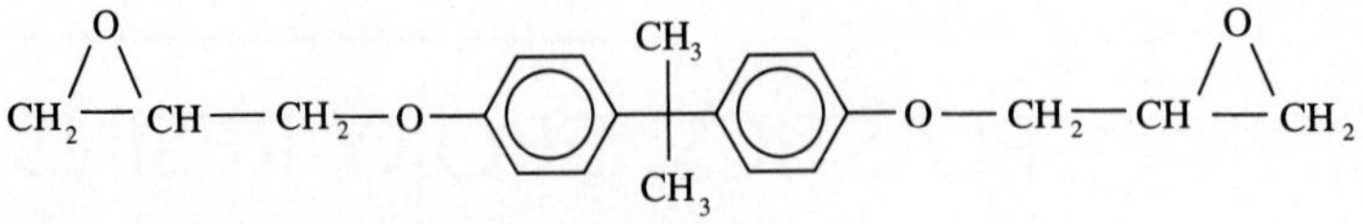

FIG. 36A–2. Diglycidyl ether of bisphenol A.

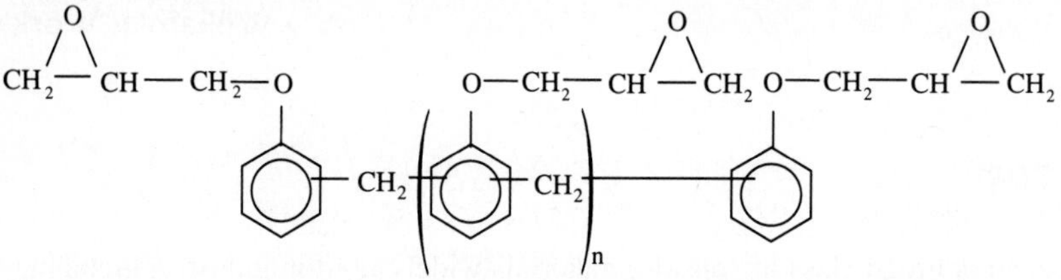

Epoxy phenol novolac resin

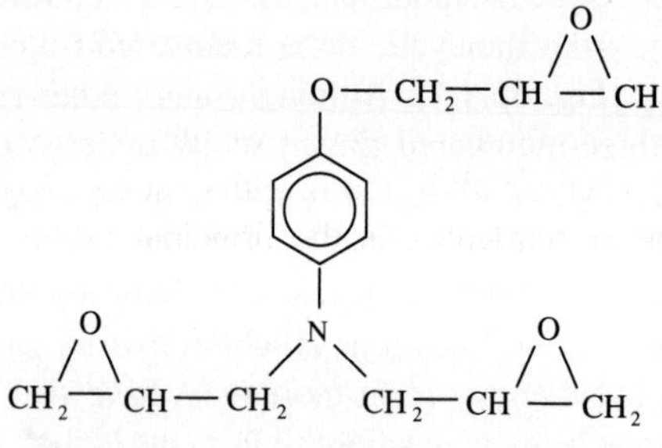

Gylcidyl ether or N, N-diglycidyl-p-aminophenol

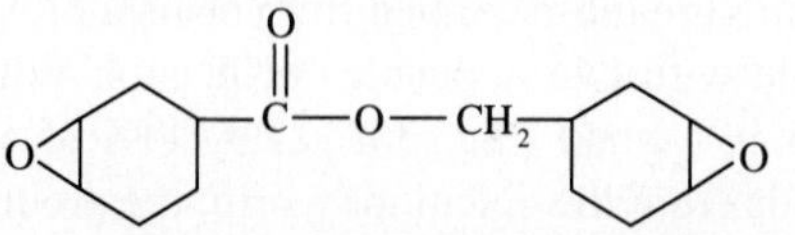

3', 4'-Epoxycyclohexyl-3,4-epoxycyclohexanecarboxylate

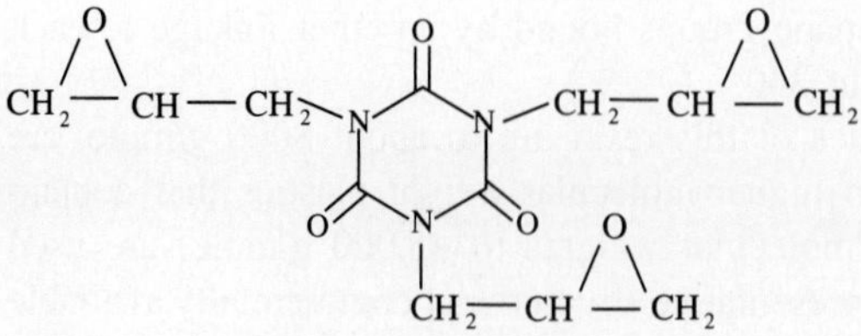

Triglycidyl isocyanurate

FIG. 36A–3. Representative epoxy resin chemical structures.

TABLE 36A–1. Chemical Names for Commercially Available Epoxy Resins

Diglycidyl ether of tetrabromobisphenol A
Diglycidyl ether of bisphenol A
Butanediol diglycidyl ether
Neopentylglycol diglycidyl ether
Bisphenol F epoxy monomer
Diglycidyl hexahydrophthalate
3',4'-Epoxycyclohexylmethyl-3,4-epoxycyclohexanecarboxylate
3,4-Epoxycyclohexyloxirane
2-(3',4'-Epoxycyclohexyl)-5,1"-spiro-3",4"-epoxycyclohexane-1,3-dioxane
Bis(3,4-epoxy-cyclohexylmethyl) adipate
Poly(propylene glycol) diglycidyl ether
Epoxidized phenol novolac resin
Epoxidized o-cresol novolac resin
Tetraglycidyl ether of p,p'-methylene dianiline
Triglycidyl isocyanurate
Glycidyl ether of N,N-diglycidyl-p-aminophenol
Multi-glycidyl ether of tetraphenylol ethane

trade names and major manufacturers of epoxy resins are provided in Table 36A-2. However, many small manufacturers and repackagers of epoxy resins may market their products under trade names different from those listed.

Some published series use monomers of various molecular weights, but in one series the 340-molecular-weight monomer picked up all of the reactors,[2] suggesting that the uncured 340-molecular-weight monomer remaining is the principal problem. Other epoxy monomers which are not based on bisphenol A, such as those shown in Fig. 36A-3, may be missed by routine patch testing[3] and qualitative tests for the more common chemical structure. Persons allergic to epoxy may also react to epichlorohydrin, the chemical used to synthesize the glycidyl (epoxy) component of the molecule. Some workers in epoxy resin manufacture may react to epichlorohydrin without being allergic to epoxy.[4] Occupational allergy to epichlorohydrin may or may not be picked up with a patch test to the diglycidylether of bisphenol A, a type of epoxy monomer.[5] Two other components are found in epoxy resins, a hardener and reactive diluents. Either may be a sensitizer alone or together with the monomer.

TABLE 36A–2. Trade Names and Major Manufacturers of Epoxy Resins

Trade Name	Manufacturer
Epi-Rez	Hoechst-Celanese Chemical
Epon Resin	Shell Chemical
Araldite	Ciba-Geigy Chemical
Dow D.E.R. & D.E.N.	Dow Chemical
Bakelite ERL & ERR	Union Carbide Chemical

HARDENERS

Hardeners are curing agents which polymerize and cross-link epoxy monomers. A wide variety of chemicals serve either as coreactive hardeners (such as polyamines and anhydrides), which become incorporated into the plastic after chemical reaction, or as catalysts for hardening chemical reactions (such as tertiary amines, dicyandiamide, imidazoles, and boron trihalide amine complexes), which may not become chemically bound to the plastic after curing the epoxide. Representative examples of chemically coreactive amine hardeners, anhydride hardeners, and catalysts are reported in Tables 36A-3, 36A-4, 36A-5, and 36A-6, respectively. Curing of epoxides by hardeners may occur at room temperature or with external heat applied. The chemical reactions responsible for transforming the epoxy resin into a hard plastic vary according to the type of hardener used; however, in all cases the three-membered epoxide ring is opened to form the product. (For example, Fig. 36A-4 shows anhydride cured epoxy chemistry.) Amine functional hardeners yield products with tertiary amino-alcohol products, anhydrides cure the resins to make polyesters, and catalyzed curing results in polyether formation. Polyethers are also likely to be found in cured plastics from amine and anhydride hardeners. In a two-pack epoxy glue, one package will contain the monomer and another the hardener. There are also one-component systems which contain one rather than two products and generally need to be heated to polymerize.

During the chemical hardening reaction, a series of physical changes take place sequentially, liquid to gel to vitrified solid to cured plastic, transforming the monomers into hard plastics. Accompanying these physical changes are chemical changes in which the number of epoxy groups and chemically coreactive groups from the hardener diminish with time. However, as the transformation proceeds, both epoxide and other chemically active groups will be present until the plastic is fully cured. The number of residual groups present at any stage in the transformation will depend upon the chemical reactivity of the formulation and the ratio of reacting species. Even after complete curing, there are usually some residual reactive groups, owing to the inability to measure the correct amount of each substance perfectly.

Testing is done to the monomer, generally, as allergy to the hardener occurs together with allergy to the resin. There are a few exceptions.

Sensitivity to the hardener is thought to occur more often on the face because of the relative volatility of the hardener compared with the monomer.[6] However, sensitivity to the hardener usually accompanies allergy to the resin.[2] If one is to patch test to these materials, the concentration and vehicle are important, as some hardeners, especially the aliphatic amines, are extremely irritating, and many are potent sensitizers as well. The potential for sensitization for hardeners depends upon the structure[7]:

HARDENER—PERCENT SENSITIZED

1. Aliphatic polyamines	55–93
2. Cycloaliphatic polyamines (e.g., isophorone damine)	0–100
3. Aromatic amine (e.g., diaminodiphenylmethane)	20
4. Polyaminoamides (based on TETA and TEPA)	20–67
5. Adduct of TETA	0
6. Adduct of phenol-accelerated TETA	47
7. Adduct of DETA and epoxy	0
8. Adduct of isophoronediamine and epoxy	73

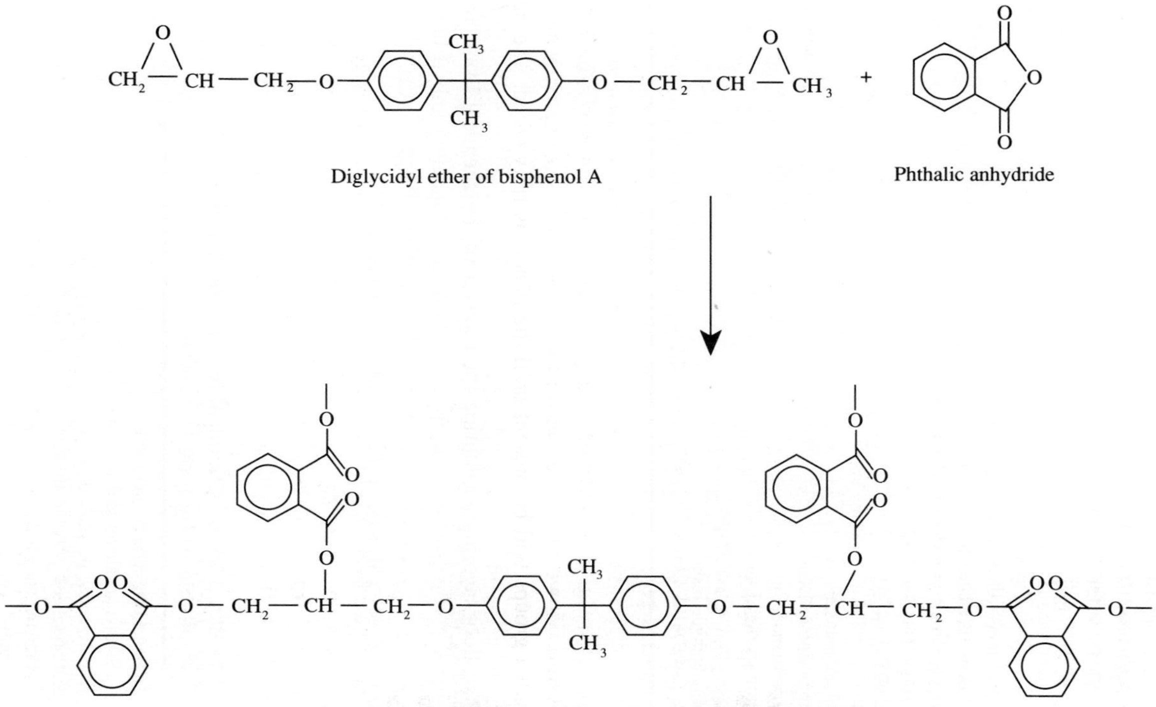

FIG. 36A–4. Epoxy curing reaction with phthalic anhydride.

Phthalic anhydride

Diglycidyl ether of bisphenol A

Segment of phthalic anhydride cross-linked polyepoxide

TABLE 36A–3. Chemical Names for Commercially Available Amine Hardeners

Polymeric amido-amine alkoxylated triethylene tetramine
4,4'-Diaminodiphenyl methane
4,4'-Diaminodiphenyl sulfone
Diethylenetriamine (DETA)
Triethylenetetramine (TETA)
Tetraethylenepentamine (TEPA)
N-aminoethylpiperazine
Diethyltoluenediamine
Cyanoethyl modified aliphatic amine
Diethylenetriamine-ethylene oxide adduct
Ethylene diamine adduct to solid epoxy
Triethylenetetramine-propylene oxide adduct
Poly(oxypropylene diamine)
Poly(oxypropylene triamine)
Diethylene glycol diaminopropyl ether
Ortho-tolylbiguanide
1,8-Diamino-p-menthane
Isophorone diamine
1,2-Diaminocyclohexane
Melamine-formaldehyde resin
Urea-formaldehyde resin
2,4-Diamino-6-(2'-alkylimidazolyl-(1'))ethyl-s-triazines (several alkyl groups available)

Isophorone diamine as a hardener has caused problems in the manufacture of plastic tennis racquets[8]; floor layering and during the transfer of the chemical from larger to smaller containers[9,10]; electron microscopy, due to dodecyl succinic anhydride.[11] The cycloaliphatic epoxy vinyl cyclohexene diepoxide caused an allergic contact dermatitis in an electron microscopist, said to be the first such instance.[12]

TABLE 36A–4. Chemical Names for Commercially Available Anhydride Hardeners

Hexahydrophthalic anhydride
Methyl hexahydrophthalic anhydride
Polyazelaic polyanhydride
Polysebacic polyanhydride
Phthalic anhydride
Methyl tetrahydrophthalic anhydride
Methyl endo-methylene-tetrahydrophthalic anhydride
Nadic methyl anhydride
Chloroendic anhydride
Succinic anhydride
Alkyl succinic anhydride (alkyl groups with 5 to 18
   carbon atoms available)

TABLE 36A–5. Chemical Names for Commercially Available Epoxy Curing Catalysts

2,4,6-Tri(dimethylaminomethyl)phenol
Dicyandiamide
Ketimine
Imidazoline
Alkyl imidazoles (alkyl groups of varying length available)
2-Phenylimidazole
1-Cyanoethyl-2-(alkyl or phenyl)imidazoles (alkyl groups of varying length available)
1-Cyanoethyl-2-(alkyl or phenyl)imidazole-trimellitates
1-Cyanoethyl-2-phenyl-4,5-di(cyanoethoxymethyl)imidazole
2-(Methyl or phenyl)imidazole-isocyanuric acid adduct
4,4'-Methylene-bis(2-ethyl-5-methylimidazole)
Morpholine salt of p-toluenesulfonic acid
Dimethylaminomethylphenol
Tris(dimethylaminomethyl)phenol-tri(2-ethylhexoate)
N,N-dimethyl benzyl amine
Thioether
Aliphatic thioester
Trifunctional mercaptan terminated polymer
Boron trichloride-amine complex
Boron trifluoride:benzylamine
Boron trifluoride:monomethylamine

Sometimes reactions occur in persons already allergic to chemically related products. Such cross-reactions may occur between ethylenediamine and diethylenetriamine and triethylenetetramine,[13] a potent sensitizer in some countries.[14] Cross-reactions have occurred between Mycolog and ethylenediamine epoxy hardener,[15] but m-phenylenediamine is not prone to react in those allergic to PPD.[16]

TABLE 36A–6. Trade Names of Commercially Available Hardeners

Amicure	Azamide
Araldite Accelerator	Versamid
Capcure	Genamid
YSE-CURE	Ciba Geigy Hardener
Lindax	Apco Hardeners
Epi-Cure	Tonox
CMD	Sumicure
Versamine	Dow Chemical D.E.H.
Millamine	Ethacure
Curezol	Apco
Resicure	Milldride
Actiron	Ancadride
Ancamine	AZcure
DMP-10	Lindride
DMP-30	Resicure
Armocure	Anchor

REACTIVE DILUENTS

These chemicals are added to epoxy resin compounds to reduce viscosity and to control how tightly the cured resin is cross-linked. The most common structures are the aromatic glycidyl ethers (e.g., cresyl glycidyl ether and butylglycidyl ether), usually present in a concentration of 0.1% to 20%.[17] Most reactive diluents are glycidyl ethers of fatty acids.[18] Even though these materials contain fewer epoxide groups per unit weight, they may still be more sensitizing than epoxies.[14] Because these materials can be quite sensitizing, care is indicated in patch testing.[19] The reactive diluent Epoxide 8, an aliphatic monoglycidyl ether with mostly C-12 and C-14, was more sensitizing than butylglycidyl ether and cresylglycidyl ether.[20] They may also be present in the finished product.[21]

Allergy to reactive diluents may occur without concomitant allergy to DEGBA or other common epoxy resins. These materials are more volatile than bisphenol A, and may cause an airborne dermatitis pattern.

SOURCES OF EXPOSURE

Many cases (some 7.7 percent[22] to 13 percent[23] to 20 percent[24]) of occupational dermatitis are caused by epoxy resins. The component causing sensitivity, while most often the resin, is probably determined more by opportunity for exposure. In one plant manufacturing epoxy resins, the sensitized employees were all allergic to epichlorohydrin and not bisphenol A.[25]

Dental laboratory workers developed sensitivity to tetraglycidylmethylene dianiline 9/11 and epoxy 4/11. The former is a condensation product between ECH and diaminodiphenylmethane.[26] Aircraft workers became allergic to composite material containing TGMDA and o-diglycidyl phthalate, and graphite coated with 4-glycidyloxy-N, N-diglycidylaniline.[27] Bisphenol A picked up only 3 of 12 cases.[28] There is a single case of a dental assistant who reacted to patch tests to both bis-GMA and epoxy, but there was no epoxy in the composite material with which she worked.[29] In another case, a hearing-aid worker became allergic to an adhesive applied from a syringe.[30] This proved to be epoxy on analysis, which was apparently not expected, since this was a change in product composition. Testing for bisphenol A is outlined in Table 36A-7.

Obviously occupations with high exposure pose a higher risk; but many industries employ epoxies in manufacturing because of the quality obtained in the final product. Almost any task with exposure is a possibility, but the following jobs or products have been reported to be associated with development of sensitivity: oil painting[31]; epoxy-coated glass fiber[32-35]; ski-stick sawdust[36]; taxidermy[37]; solvent cement[38]; application of a (contaminated) hand-applied lens[39]; a soil fumigant[40]; PVC tubes for shampoo[41]; stained-glass window manufacture[42]; electrical insulation[43]; capacitors; fishing rods; varnish[44]; electron microscopy[11]; drug industry (pouring into a vat)[45]; paints/lacquers; fillers; cleaning agents; binders; glues/adhesives (Fig. 36A-5); castings; coloring agents; corrosion inhibitors; construction materials; fillings; flooring materials; hardeners; metal coatings; printing inks[46,47]; tool (screwdriver) handles; cellulose acetate handles[48]; prefabrication work[49]; insulation material (coated)[50]; and gemstone polishing.[51]

Prognosis for those sensitized in industry is guarded. Of 80 persons who changed occupation because of allergy, 50 had relapses within a year, especially if they continued to work with the chemical after 3 months.[52]

TABLE 36A-7. Testing for Bisphenol A Type Epoxy—TLC Method

Chloroform/acetonitrile 90:10% is solvent system.
1 Molar sulfuric acid is first spray reagent.
Anisaldehyde in methanol 2.5% in acetone is second spray reagent.
A standard of 1% resin is used as the positive control.

Alcohol extraction is made of solid samples and evaporated to a few milliliters.
2 to 5 mL of standard solution is applied to the edge of the TLC silica plate.
2 to 5 mL is also applied next to the standard spot.
Dilutions of the unknown may be used for unknown concentrations.
Allow the solvent of the samples to evaporate (a few minutes).
Develop in chloroform/acetonitrile in a glass tank.
Air dry.
Examine by UV-light, looking for darker spots as evidence of lower-molecular-weight oligomers.
Spray with sulfuric acid until moist.
Spray lightly with acetaldehyde.
Dry 10 min at 110°C.
Violet spots appear with smaller epoxy oligomers at the top.
Weight corresponds to the standard(s).

Note: More details are given in Refs. 92 and 93.
Source: Ref. 93, with permission.

NONOCCUPATIONAL EXPOSURE

Nonoccupational exposure may take place almost anywhere. The home is mentioned, and this is accurate. However, there are an increasing number of case reports of medical and dental exposure as well. Some of the reactions were to finished products, which ostensibly occurred because the resin was not totally cured. At room temperature, curing is often not total immediately, with some reports of monomer being detectable for several months.

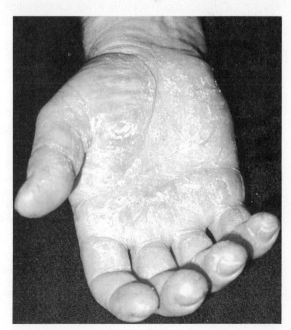

FIG. 36A-5. Body shop repairman with a history of reacting to paint. Patch testing showed him to be allergic to epoxy and the source proved to be an adhesive used on bumpers. (See color Plate 26.)

Reported products associated with nonoccupational epoxy contact dermatitis include hemodialysis needles[53]; ostomy pouch with plastic bag[54-57]; a pacemaker[58]; signboards[59]; brass door handles; twist-off bottle caps; a metal calendar on a watch strap[60]; nasal cannulae[61,62] (must test to the same batch in finished products); dentures (burning mouth syndrome)[63]; dental restorations,[64] both clinical and experimental[65]; varnish on a wooden amputation stump[66]; paint; printing ink; and PVC plastics.[67]

CLOTHING

Wearing apparel is not an expected cause of epoxy resin dermatitis, but reactions to it certainly occur. On clothing, epoxy is sometimes used as an adhesive and sometimes as an ink. Those allergic to epoxy acrylate products may react to epoxy resin. The filter-paper method for screening for presence of bisphenol A epoxies is possible even in finished products, as reported by Fregert. It is found in Table 36A-8.

Clothing products causing epoxy resin dermatitis include footwear[68]; a motorcycle helmet (facial dermatitis)[69]; printing on textile labels[70]; pockets of trousers[71]; and knee pads in jeans.[72] In the last two reports, the manufacturer denied that epoxy was in the product. In the last report, two inaccurate letters were sent to one of the dermatologists who had written the company giving details. The epoxy had been used as an adhesive, however, and it was finally admitted. In questionable cases the filter-paper test can be useful.

False-negative tests can be obtained when the epoxy is not based on bisphenol A, when sensitivity is caused by a reactive diluent, when epichlorohydrin is the sensitizer and bisphenol A is not, and in rare cases where hardener allergy is present without allergy to GEBA. The usual causes of false-negative patch tests (e.g., the test falling off) may also be a cause.

Another possibility is photosensitivity, which has been reported in a persistent light reactor.[73] Phototesting to epoxies is not a routine test antigen for most dermatologists, so it may not be suspected. Purpura from allergic contact to epoxy[74] would be rather easy to miss, as one might not think to test for it.

PROTECTIVE MEASURES

Use of less sensitizing products may reduce the opportunity to develop allergy to epoxy. Sensitization occurs in proportion to the number of epoxide groups. Epoxy

---

TABLE 36A–8. Filter Paper Method

Dissolve about 0.1 g of the sample in 2 mL of concentrated sulfuric acid by heating 40 to 50°C on a water bath. Dilute as necessary to produce a color (orange) equivalent to that of 0.1 M potassium dichromate solution.
Using a glass rod, streak a drop of epoxy solution across a filter paper.
A positive test will turn purple in 1 min, and ultimately it turns blue.
A bisphenol A monomer should be used as a positive control.
Both cured and uncured epoxy resins should show a positive test. Certain oils (fish, tung, and linseed treated with cyclopentadiene), rosin, and certain phenolic resins also give positive tests, so the test is used for screening purposes.

Source: Ref. 93, with permission.

resin monomers with a molecular weight over glycidyl ethers make up a greater percentage of the smaller molecules. Reactions are more influenced by the molecular weight than modifications, but reactions occur ostensibly to products of molecular weight as high as 3000,[75] as there are lower-molecular-weight contaminants in higher-molecular-weight products.[76,77] There is not supposed to be any sensitizer left in cured products,[78] but there are a number of case reports of that happening.[56,63,67] These are usually explained on the basis of uncured monomer being present.[56] Gloves used to protect the hands must be of the proper material or they can be counterproductive. This is especially true of rubber and cloth gloves.[79] Epoxies readily penetrate polyethylene, rubber, and to a lesser degree PVC,[80] as some individuals seem to tolerate exposure better with than without PVC gloves as protection. All epoxy resins penetrate rubber, but some are reduced by PVC and neoprene. Nitrile and nitrile butatoluene gloves are totally protective.[81]

Two barrier creams and a methacrylate spray reduced the severity of patch-test reactions to epoxy.[82]

Adams recommends antigen substitution where possible to avoid the sensitizing potential of epoxies,[83,84] including the use of higher-molecular-weight resins and a variety of other synthetic resins, which are less sensitizing[79] as well as less irritating, and less sensitizing hardeners.[12] While higher-molecular-weight epoxies do not sensitize as readily,[85,86] they nevertheless may elicit reactions because of their content of some lower-molecular-weight contaminants. Exposure is lessened with one-bag epoxies which mix in the package.[79] A patch-test series has to be used, as many epoxy resin products do not cross-react with the diglycidyl ether of bisphenol A.[87]

EPOXY ACRYLATES

The epoxy acrylate products are ultraviolet-cured materials commonly used for bonding. In dentistry these are commonly diglycidyl ethers (the epoxy component) linked to a vinyl acid (e.g., acrylic or methacrylic groups). Several years ago BIS-GMA [2,2-bis-(4-(2-hydroxy-3-methacryloxypropoxy)phenyl)propane], the addition reaction product of bisphenol A and glycidyl methacrylate or an epoxy resin and methacrylic acid, was the most commonly used bonding material, but that seems to have changed recently with the appearance of dimethacrylates based on bisphenol A, with various chain lengths.[88] Those sensitive to epoxy acrylates may[89] or may not[90] react to epoxy products but are not as likely to be allergic to acrylates.

These products are especially useful as fillers in dentistry because the epoxies do not polymerize when wet. They also are commonly found in ultraviolet printing processes.[90] Such workers may be allergic to epoxy or aliphatic acrylates (e.g., methyl methacrylate, triethylene glycol dimethacrylate, or triethylene diglycol diacrylate).[91] Sensitivity may also be seen to additives (e.g., hydroquinone).

REFERENCES

1. Cronin E: *Contact Dermatitis*. Churchill Livingstone, Edinburgh, 1980, pp 595–615.
2. Fregert S, Dahlquist I, Persson K: Sensitizing capacity of substances related to epoxy resin oligomer MW 340, (DGEBA). *Contact Dermatitis* 10:47–48, 1984.

3. Kanerva L, Jolanki R, Estlander T: Allergic contact dermatitis from non-diglycidyl-ether-of-bisphenol-A epoxy resins. *Contact Dermatitis* 24:293–300, 1991.
4. Calnan C: Epoxy resin dermatitis. *J Soc Occup Med* 25:123–126, 1975.
5. Thorgeirsson A, Fregert S: Allergenicity of epoxy resins in the guinea pig. *Acta Derm Venereol* 57:253–256, 1977.
6. Dahlquist I, Fregert S: Allergic contact dermatitis from volatile epoxy hardeners and reactive diluents. *Contact Dermatitis* 5:406–407, 1979.
7. Thorgeirsson A: Sensitization capacity of epoxy resin hardeners in the guinea pig. *Acta Derm Venereol* 58:322–336, 1978.
8. Lachapelle JM, Tennstedt D, Dumont-Fruytier M: Occupational allergic contact dermatitis to isophorone diamine (IPD) used as an epoxy resin hardener. *Contact Dermatitis* 4:109–112, 1978.
9. Dahlquist I, Fregert S: Contact allergy to the epoxy hardener isophoronediamine (IPD). *Contact Dermatitis* 5:120–121, 1979.
10. Camarasa JG, Serra-Baldrich E: Isophoronediamine (IPD) dermatitis in Spain. *Contact Dermatitis* 20:382, 1989.
11. Göransson K: Allergic contact dermatitis to an epoxy hardener: Dodecenyl-succinic anhydride. *Contact Dermatitis* 3:277–278, 1977.
12. Dannaker CJ: Allergic sensitization to a non-bisphenol A epoxy of the cycloaliphatic class. *J Occup Med* 30:641–643, 1988.
13. Rudzki E, Krajewska D: Cross-reactions between ethylenediamine, diethylenetriamine and triethylenetetramine. *Contact Dermatitis* 2:311–313, 1976.
14. Rudzki E, Krajewska D, Grzywa Z, Napiorkowska T: Contact allergy to epoxy resin hardeners. *Medycyna Pracy* 32:59–62, 1981.
15. Van Hecke E: Ethylenediamine sensitivity from exposure to epoxy resin hardeners and Mycolog cream. *Contact Dermatitis* 1:344–348, 1975.
16. Rudzki E, Krajewska D, Grzywa Z: Sensitivity to *m*-phenlenediamine. *Berufs Derm* 25:85–88, 1977.
17. Jolanki R, Estlander T, Kanerva L: Contact allergy to an epoxy reactive diluent: 1,4-butanediol diglycidyl ether. *Contact Dermatitis* 16:87–92, 1987.
18. Dahlquist I, Fregert S: Contact allergy to Cardura E, an epoxy reactive diluent of the ester type. *Contact Dermatitis* 5:121–122, 1979.
19. Björkner B, Dahlquist I, Fregert S, Magnusson B: Contact allergy to Epoxide 8, an epoxy reactive diluent. *Contact Dermatitis* 6:156, 1980.
20. Thorgeirsson A, Fregert S, Magnusson B: Allergenicity of epoxy-reactive diluents in the guinea pig. *Berufs Derm* 23:178–183, 1975.
21. Lovell CR, Rycroft RJ, Matood J: Isolated Cardura E10 sensitivity in an epoxy resin chemical process. *Contact Dermatitis* 11:190–191, 1984.
22. Jolanki R: Occupational skin diseases from epoxy compounds: epoxy resin compounds, epoxy acrylates and 2,3-epoxypropyl trimethyl ammonium chloride. *Acta Derm Venereol Suppl* 159:1–80, 1991.
23. Jolanki R, Estlander T, Kanerva L: Occupational contact dermatitis and contact urticaria caused by epoxy resins. *Acta Derm Venereol Suppl* 134:90–94, 1987.
24. Rudzki E: Occupational contact dermatitis in 100 consecutive patients. *Berufs Derm* 24:100–104, 1976.
25. Prens EP, de Jong G, van Joost T: Sensitization to epichlorohydrn and epoxy system components. *Contact Dermatitis* 15:85–90, 1986.
26. Ayala F, Lembo G, Balato N, et al: The use of laboratory methods in contact dermatitis induced by composite materials. (Published erratum appears in *Contact Dermatitis* 23:384, 1990.) *Contact Dermatitis* 22:262, 1990.
27. Mathias CG: Allergic contact dermatitis from a nonbisphenol A epoxy in a graphite fiber reinforced epoxy laminate. *J Occup Med* 29:754–755, 1987.
28. Burrows D, Fregert S, Campbell H, Trulsson L: Contact dermatitis from the epoxy resins tetraglycidyl-4,4'-methylene dianiline and *o*-diglycidyl phthalate in composite material. *Contact Dermatitis* 11:80–82, 1984.
29. Kanerva L, Jolanki R, Estlander T: Occupational dermatitis due to an epoxy acrylate. *Contact Dermatitis* 14:80–84, 1986.
30. Romaguera C, Grimalt F, Vilaplana J: Occupational dermatitis from epoxy resin. *Contact Dermatitis* 14:187, 1986.
31. Conde-Salazar L, Romero L, Guimaraens D, Harto A: Contact dermatitis in an oil painter. *Contact Dermatitis* 8:209–210, 1982.

32. Dahlquist I, Fregert S, Trulsson L: Allergic contact dermatitis from epoxy resin finished glass fiber. *Contact Dermatitis* 5:190, 1979.
33. Cuypers JM, Bleumink E, Nater JP: Dermatologic aspects of glass-fiber production. *Berufs Derm* 23:143–154, 1975.
34. Bruze M, Almgren G: Occupational dermatoses in workers exposed to epoxy-impregnated fiberglass fabric. *Derm Beruf Umwelt* 37:171–176, 1989.
35. Holness DL, Nethercott JR: Occupational contact dermatitis due to epoxy resin in a fiberglass binder. *J Occup Med* 31:87–89, 1989.
36. Suhonen R: Epoxy-dermatitis in a ski-stick factory. *Contact Dermatitis* 9:131, 1983.
37. Bjorkner B: Allergic contact dermatitis from (foxy) epoxy. *Contact Dermatitis* 6:499, 1980.
38. Beck MH, King CM: Allergic contact dermatitis to epichlorhydrin in a solvent cement. *Contact Dermatitis* 9:315, 1983.
39. Hambly EM, Wilkinson DS: Unusual presentation of epoxy resin sensitivity. *Contact Dermatitis* 4:114, 1978.
40. Nater JP, Gooskens VH: Occupational dermatosis due to a soil fumigant. *J Contact Dermatitis* 2:227–229, 1976.
41. Ancona-Alayon A, Jimenez-Castilla JL, Gomez-Alvarez EM: Dermatitis from epoxy resin and formaldehyde in shampoo packers. *Contact Dermatitis* 2:356, 1976.
42. Heskel NS: Epoxy resin dermatitis in a stained glass window maker. *Contact Dermatitis* 18:182–183, 1988.
43. Niinimäki A, Hassi J: An outbreak of epoxy dermatitis in insulation workers at an electric power station. *Derm Beruf Umwelt* 31:23–25, 1983.
44. Tosti A, Guerra L, Toni F: Occupational airborne contact dermatitis due to epoxy resin. *Contact Dermatitis* 19:220–222, 1988.
45. Rebandel P, Rudzki E: Dermatitis caused by epichlorohydrin, oxprenolol hydrochloride and propranolol hydrochloride. *Contact Dermatitis* 23:199, 1990.
46. Flyvholm MA: Contact allergens in registered chemical products. *Contact Dermatitis* 25:49–56, 1991.
47. Nethercott JR: Allergic contact dermatitis due to an epoxy acrylate. *Br J Dermatol* 104:697–703, 1981.
48. Fischer T, Fregert S, Thulin I, Trulsson L: Unhardened epoxy resin in tool handles. *Contact Dermatitis* 16:45, 1987.
49. Goh CL, Gan SL, Ngui SJ: Occupational dermatitis in a prefabrication construction factory. *Contact Dermatitis* 15:235–240, 1986.
50. Fisher AA: Fiberglass vs mineral wool (rockwool) dermatitis. *Cutis* 29:412–422, 1982.
51. O'Brien TJ: Epoxy resin and gemstone polishing (letter). *Australas J Dermatol* 28:43, 1987.
52. Krajewska D, Rudzki E: Sensitivity to epoxy resins and triethylenetetramine. *Contact Dermatitis* 2:135–138, 1976.
53. Brandao FM, Pinto J: Allergic contact dermatitis to epoxy resin in hemodialysis needles. *Contact Dermatitis* 6:218–219, 1980.
54. Fregert S, Meding B, Trulsson L: Demonstration of epoxy resin in stoma pouch plastic. *Contact Dermatitis* 10:106, 1984.
55. Mann RJ, Stewart E, Peachey RD: Sensitivity to urostomy pouch plastic. *Contact Dermatitis* 9:80–81, 1983.
56. O'Brien TJ: Contact dermatitis to epoxy resin in ileostomy bag. *Australas J Dermatol* 27:94–95, 1986.
57. Beck MH, Burrows D, Fregert S, Mendelsohn S: Allergic contact dermatitis to epoxy resin in ostomy bags. *Br J Surg* 72:202–203, 1985.
58. Romaguera C, Grimalt F: Pacemaker dermatitis. *Contact Dermatitis* 7:333, 1981.
59. Fregert S, Persson K, Trulsson L: Allergic contact dermatitis from unhardened epoxy resin in a finished product. *Contact Dermatitis* 5:277–278, 1979.
60. Fregert S, Persson K, Trulsson L: Hidden sources of unhardened epoxy resin of bisphenol A type. *Contact Dermatitis* 6:446–447, 1980.
61. Wright RC, Fregert S: Allergic contact dermatitis from epoxy resin in nasal cannulae. *Contact Dermatitis* 9:387–389, 1983.
62. Mørk NJ: Contact sensitivity from epoxy resin in a hemodialysis set. *Contact Dermatitis* 5:331–332, 1979.
63. van Joost T, van Ulsen J, van Loon LA: Contact allergy to denture materials in the burning mouth syndrome. *Contact Dermatitis* 18:97–99, 1988.
64. Nathanson D, Lockhart P: Delayed extraoral hypersensitivity to dental composite material. *Oral Surg Oral Med Oral Pathol* 47:329–333, 1979.

65. Kallus T, Hensten-Pettersen A, Mjör IA: Tissue response to allergenic leachables from dental materials. *J Biomed Mater Res* 17:741–755, 1983.

66. Kenkinson HA, Burrows D: Pitfalls in the demonstration of epoxy resins. *Contact Dermatitis* 16:226–227, 1987.

67. Malten KE: Tracing back a positive reaction to epoxy resin. *Contact Dermatitis* 3:217, 1977.

68. Srinivas CR, Devadiga R, Aroor AR: Footwear dermatitis due to bisphenol A. *Contact Dermatitis* 20:150–151, 1989.

69. Malanin G, Kalimo K: Facial dermatitis from epoxy resin in a helmet. *Contact Dermatitis* 12:221, 1985.

70. Fregert S, Orsmark K: Allergic contact dermatitis due to epoxy resin in textile labels. *Contact Dermatitis* 11:131–132, 1984.

71. Grimalt F, Romaguera C: Contact dermatitis caused by polyamide trouser pockets. *Derm Beruf Umwelt* 29:35–39, 1981.

72. Taylor JS, Bergfeld WF, Guin JD: Contact dermatitis to knee patch adhesive in boys' jeans: A nonoccupational cause of epoxy resin sensitivity. *Cleveland Clin Q* 50:123–127, 1983.

73. Allen H, Kaidbey K: Persistent photosensitivity following occupational exposure to epoxy resin. *Arch Dermatol* 115:1307–1310, 1979.

74. Laurberg G, Christiansen JV: Purpuric allergic contact dermatitis to epoxy resin. *Contact Dermatitis* 11:186–187, 1984.

75. Bokelund F, Fregert S, Trulsson L: Sensitization from epoxy resin powder of high molecular weight. *Contact Dermatitis* 6:144, 1980.

76. Fregert S, Trulsson L: Patch testing with brominated epoxy resins. *Contact Dermatitis* 10:112–113, 1984.

77. Fregert S, Thorgeirsson A: Patch testing with low molecular oligomers of epoxy resins in humans. *Contact Dermatitis* 3:301–303, 1977.

78. Broughton WE: Epoxy resins in industry—the hazards and their control. *Ann Occup Hyg* 8:131–142, 1965.

79. van Putten PB, Coenraads PJ, Nater JP: Hand dermatoses and contact allergic reactions in construction workers exposed to epoxy resins. *Contact Dermatitis* 10:146–150, 1984.

80. Pegum JS: Penetration of protective gloves by epoxy resin. *Contact Dermatitis* 5:281–283, 1979.

81. Blanken R, Nater JP, Veenhoff E: Protection against epoxy resins with glove materials. *Contact Dermatitis* 16:46–47, 1987.

82. Blanken R, Nater JP, Veenhoff E: Protective effect of barrier creams and spray coatings against epoxy resins. *Contact Dermatitis* 16:79–83, 1987.

83. Adams RM: Allergen replacement in industry. *Cutis* 20:511–516, 1977.

84. Thorgeirsson A: Sensitization capacity of epoxy reactive diluents in the guinea pig. *Acta Derm Venereol* 58:329–331, 1978.

85. Thorgeirsson A, Fregert S: Allergenicity of epoxy resins in the guinea pig. *Acta Derm Venereol* 57:253–256, 1977.

86. Thorgeirsson A, Fregert S, Ramnäs O: Sensitization capacity of epoxy resin oligomers in the guinea pig. *Acta Derm Venereol* 58:17–21, 1978.

87. Behrbohm P, Nehring A, Nehring P: False negative tests with epoxy resin. *Contact Dermatitis* 1:267, 1975.

88. Björkner B, Niklasson B, Persson K: The sensitizing potential of di-(meth)acrylates based on bisphenol A or epoxy resin in the guinea pig. *Contact Dermatitis* 10:286–304, 1984.

89. Björkner B: Sensitization capacity of acrylated prepolymers in ultraviolet curing inks tested in the guinea pig. *Acta Derm Venereol* 61:7–10, 1981.

90. Nethercott JR: Allergic contact dermatitis due to an epoxy acrylate. *Br J Dermatol* 104:697–703, 1981.

91. Kanerva L, Estlander T, Jolanki R: Allergic contact dermatitis from dental composite resins due to aromatic epoxy acrylates and aliphatic acrylates. *Contact Dermatitis* 20:201–211, 1989.

92. Fregert S, Trulsson L: Simple methods for demonstration of epoxy resins of bisphenol A type. *Contact Dermatitis* 4:69–72, 1978.

93. Fregert S: Physicochemical methods for detection of contact allergens. *Dermatol Clin* 6:97–104, 1988.

36B

OTHER PLASTICS

Jere D. Guin
William J. Work

ACRYLICS

CHEMISTRY

Acrylic plastics are familiar to most people from their uses in a wide variety of transparent applications where good outdoor durability is required. However, the characteristics of the chemistry of acrylics that make them attractive for hard, transparent plastics also make them attractive for many applications including adhesives, coatings, contact lenses, additives to other plastics, additives for construction materials such as concrete, additives for high-quality motor oil, resins for water purification, additives for detergents, and water-absorbent resins for diapers. Although many of these uses may not be considered plastics, the chemistry of the materials that serve these diverse markets is very similar, making clear demarcation of the limits difficult.

The term *acrylic* refers to chemicals that are derived from acrylic acid, a carboxylic acid with a carbon-carbon double bond connected to the acid functionality. The carbon-carbon double bond is the reactive group responsible for the formation of plastics by polymerization. Acrylic monomers differ in the types of groups attached to the double bond at the carbon atom closest to the acid group and in the types of group substituted on the carboxylic acid. The chemical structures of acrylic acid and a representative group of other monofunctional acrylates and related chemical structures grouped under the generic name of *acrylic* are shown in Figs. 36B-1 and 36B-2. By monofunctional acrylates (Fig. 36B-1), we mean those which possess only a single double bond capable of undergoing polymerization to form a plastic; from the standpoint of organic chemistry, most of these molecules have more than one functional group, but only those that participate in forming the polymer are considered. A number of multifunctional acrylates—that is, those possessing two or more polymerizable double bonds—are also available commercially. Some representative examples of these are shown in Fig. 36B-2.

Formation of the polymer that becomes the familiar plastic from the acrylic monomers proceeds by a simple repetition of a few basic chemical reactions shown in Fig. 36B-3, called *chain polymerization* by chemists. In this reaction, a small amount of initiator is added to the acrylic monomer, usually along with a small amount of a chain-length regulator to limit the molecular weight of the resulting polymer. Polymerization occurs when an initiator adds to the carbon-carbon double bond of the monomer, producing

Acrylic acid   Ethyl acrylate   Butyl acrylate

Methyl methacrylate   Ethyl-2-cyanoacrylate

2-Hydroxyethyl methacrylate   Acrylonitrile   Acrylamide

FIG. 36B–1. Monofunctional acrylic monomers.

a radical or anion. Following initiation, monomer units add to the reactive end of the chain, forming a sequence of carbon-carbon single bonds that ultimately becomes a very high-molecular-weight polymer. Initiators are usually used in amounts from 0.1 to 1% compared to the amount of monomer used and are most commonly either peroxides such as benzoyl peroxide, azo compounds such as azo-bisisobutyronitrile, or photoinitiators of which chemical derivatives of benzophenone, xanthone, and benzoin ethers are examples. In the case of the α-cyanoacrylates, even water can serve as an initiator. A wide variety of chemicals are effective in controlling the molecular weight of the resulting polymers; however, due to their efficiency, mercaptans are commonly

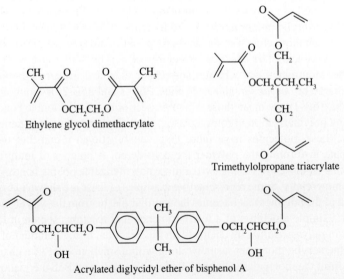

Ethylene glycol dimethacrylate

Trimethylolpropane triacrylate

Acrylated diglycidyl ether of bisphenol A

FIG. 36B–2. Representative monomers with multiple acrylic functional groups.

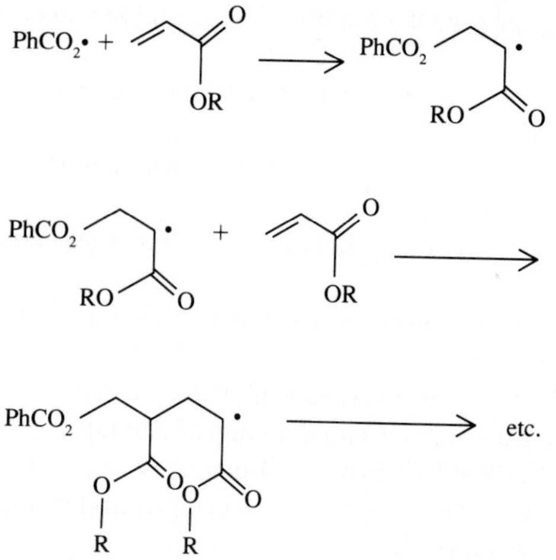

FIG. 36B–3. Peroxide-initiated acrylic polymerization.

used in amounts <1% based on monomer. During polymerization, monomer is present at all times until complete conversion to polymer, thus care must be taken during handling of partially polymerized product to avoid exposure to the monomer.

The acrylic plastics with which we are most familiar are usually manufactured by polymerization of methyl methacrylate and supplied either as a pellet or a sheet. These raw materials are sold to a fabricator to be formed into parts which are sold to consumers. Forming those parts usually involves heating the plastic to temperatures where it becomes soft enough to be reshaped. In processes that require the plastic to flow to form a complex shape, such as extrusion or injection molding at high processing temperatures, the amount of heat applied may result in a small amount of decomposition of the plastic back to its constituent monomer (methyl methacrylate).

In other uses, such as coatings and adhesives, the product that ultimately forms what we would call a plastic may be supplied as a polymer dispersed in water (acrylic latex), a polymer dissolved in an organic solvent, or as the undiluted monomer. In the first two cases, the amount of residual acrylic monomer is quite low, but other organic compounds may be present. Some examples of the uses for acrylic plastics either after polymerization or as undiluted monomer supplied to a customer (who then polymerizes it in place to form the plastic) are as follows:

1. Monofunctional acrylates and methacrylates (e.g., methyl methacrylate). Used after polymerization in plastic sheet and pellets, additives for polyvinyl chloride and other plastics, latex coatings, solution coatings. Monomeric products in this category may also be added to ultraviolet cured systems to reduce viscosity and enhance cross-linking (2-hydroxyethyl acrylate)[1] and in hydrophilic soft-contact lenses (2-hydroxyethyl methacrylate).

2. Acrylic and methacrylic acid. Polymerized and used in resins for water treatment, coatings, adhesives, and water absorption.

3. Diacrylates and methacrylates (e.g., polyethylene glycol dimethacrylate). These products are used as monomers in anaerobic adhesives and sealants—e.g., polyethylene glycol (PEG) dimethacrylate,[2] and dental composites, ethylene glycol dimethac-

rylate, and trimethylene glycol dimethacrylate,[3-5] and to reduce viscosity in ultraviolet cured systems.

4. Cyanoacrylates are used as monomers in adhesives for industrial, biomedical, and consumer applications.

5. Acrylo- and methacrylonitriles are a component polymerized to form ABS plastics; finger splints[6]; nitrile rubber; or textile fiber.[7]

6. Polyfunctional acrylates. Used as monomers in ultraviolet-cured coatings and printing inks.

7. Acrylamide. Used in polymers to provide cross-linking of coatings, adhesives, component in contact lenses.

8. Combinations with other system types (e.g., epoxyacrylates). Traditional composite materials in dentistry used resins based on dimethacrylates, BIS-GMA, an epoxy dimethacrylate,[8,9,10] [2,2-bis-(4-(2-hydroxy-3-methacryloxy-propoxy)phenyl)propane], the addition reaction product of bisphenol A and glycidyl methacrylate or an epoxy[8]; or dimethacrylated polyester.[11]

9. Urethane di(meth)acrylates, epoxy di(meth)acrylates, polyether diacrylates, and polyester diacrylates are used as prepolymers in ultraviolet-curable inks, varnishes, and coating formulations for industrial purposes[12] as well as dental composites and floor coverings.[1]

RECOGNIZING CONTACT DERMATITIS FOR ACRYLATES

One should suspect contact to acrylates when a worker in printing, rubber stamp making (Fig. 36B-4), painting, dentistry, or orthopedic surgery presents with a contact dermatitis in exposed areas, especially the hands, and, for many occupations, on the fingertips in a grip location (e.g., the first three digits). In the printing industry, one expects the hands and forearms to be involved, and usually this is the case. Some have experienced involvement of the face and/or eyelids.[13]

In a dental technician or orthopedic surgeon, the hands are commonly involved, often associated with glove allergy.[14] Reports of allergic stomatitis continue to appear[15] despite improvement in the curing process by employing heat, which is supposed to leave insufficient monomer to elicit a response.[16] The self-curing products which polymerize at room temperature,[17,18] are still reported to cause reactions, but heat-curing is said to polymerize the resin, preventing reactions even in sensitive subjects.[19-22] Reports of stomatitis and burning-mouth syndrome[23,24] have been attributed to use of self-curing resins used in repair,[16] to chronic wear (as with plastic spectacle frames), or to "seaming," which result from heat and/or pressure.[25] There are probably multiple reasons, but with the widespread usage, throughout the world, some mistakes in the production of the polymer are bound to occur.

Suspecting the cause should not be too difficult, as the eruption is often prominent and may be severe,[26] even when localized. Common sense will usually alert the clinician to the object(s) in contact with the affected area, and patch testing should help to confirm one's clinical impression.

Where there is contact to a nail product, one may see onycholysis as well as eczema around the nails and on the fingertips. Spread to other areas can occur, especially the eyelids due to hand transfer. Chronic exposure can result in permanent damage to the nail matrix, paresthesia, and Raynaud's syndrome.

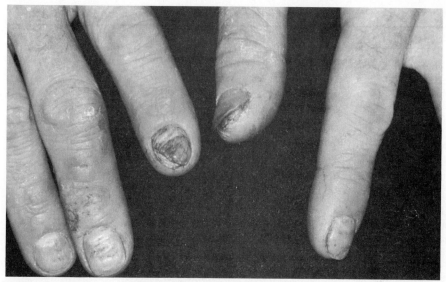

FIG. 36B–4. Rubber stamp worker who used an ultraviolet-cured lettering process. He was allergic to hydroxyethyl acrylate hydroxypropyl acrylate, hydroxyethyl methacrylate, hydroxypropyl methylacrylate, and ethylene glycol dimethacrylate. (See color Plate 27.)

CONFIRMATION

Patch testing is the best way to confirm that you are confronted with allergy to these products. Without a commercial kit, this can be more easily said than done, as the ideal concentration for each acrylic monomer can be greatly different,[27] and there seems to be no rational way to predict the concentration without looking it up. Petrolatum seems to be the best vehicle,[28,29] although some use olive oil. Preparing the antigen is a problem, as many acrylates are quite volatile and the odor can permeate the office for months. One needs to test to a broad group of these materials. It may be difficult to find the contents of the product in question. Methyl methacrylate is not adequate as a screening agent.[13,30–32] Another problem is that the commercial-grade chemical may contain impurities which are the sensitizers, rather than the chemical itself.[33] A good commercial patch test series is invaluable, but one may also have to test to the substances to which the patient is exposed.

Table 36-1 can be used in combination with positive reactions to components of the acrylate series. The uses are quite complex, but the patch-test data along with a good history can make even a dilettante look expert. Sometimes the pattern one sees on reading a patch test series does not seem logical, and this can be worrisome. Therefore the table and the section on cross-reactions are provided to help in interpreting the results.

Patch testing to cyanoacrylate is done by applying the glue to an adhesive plaster and allowing to dry (it takes 30 mins to be safe). This produces a bit milder erythema, which is spread over a larger area than a Finn chamber.

Obviously there are predictions which can be made based on the job, and perhaps the material safety data sheet, but many of these processes are secret and the active ingredient is frequently not available, even with a call to the company. There is also

TABLE 36–1. Associations of Acrylate Patch-Test Reagents[a]

1,4-Butanediol-diacrylate $C_{10}H_{14}O_4$	Cross-linking monomer for use in inks, adhesives, textile product modifiers, photoresists, etc. (BUDA)
1,4-Butanediol-dimethacrylate $C_{12}H_{18}O_4$	Cross-linking methacrylic monomer for use in dental composite materials, sealants, prostheses, etc. (BUDMA)
n-Butyl acrylate $C_7H_{12}O_2$	Cross-linking acrylic monomer for use in textile and leather finishes, paint formulations, etc. (BA)
n-Butyl methacrylate $C_8H_{14}O_2$	Cross-linking methacrylic monomer for use in dental composite materials, artificial nails, etc. (BMA)
Diethyleneglycol diacrylate $C_{10}H_{14}O_5$	Cross-linking acrylate monomer for use in coatings, adhesives, and printing plates of prepolymer type (DEGDA)
Epoxy acrylate	Acrylate oligomer for use in UV-reactive inks and varnishes
Ethyl acrylate $C_5H_8O_2$	Acrylic monomer in the production of textile and paper coatings, leather finish resins and adhesives (EA)
Ethyleneglycol dimethacrylate $C_{10}H_{14}O_4$	Cross-linking methacrylic monomer is dental composites, sealants, prostheses, etc. (EGDMA)
2-Ethylhexyl acrylate $C_{11}H_{20}O_2$	Acrylic monomer for use in UV-curable coatings and inks; ingredient in some acrylic based adhesive tapes (EHA)
1,6-Hexanediol diacrylate $C_{12}H_{18}O_4$	Common acrylic monomer in UV-cured adhesives, coatings, photoresists, castings, etc. (HDDA); monomer in dental composite materials
2-Hydroxyethyl acrylate $C_5H_8O_3$	Acrylic monomer for use in UV-inks, adhesives, lacquers, etc. (HEA)
2-Hydroxyethyl methacrylate $C_6H_{10}O_3$	Methacrylic monomer for use in UV-inks, adhesives, lacquers, etc. (HEMA)
2-2-Bis(4-(2-hydroxy- 3-methacryloxypropoxy) phenyl-propane $C_{29}H_{36}O_8$	Common methacrylic monomer in dental composite and sealant materials (BIS-GMA)
Hydroxypropyl acrylate $C_6H_{10}O_3$	Acrylic monomer for use in UV-inks, lacquers, adhesives, etc. (2-hydroxyl-1-propylacrylate, 67% + 1-hydroxy-2- propylacrylate, 33%)
2,2-Bis(4-(2-methacryl- oxyethoxy)phenyl)propane $C_{27}H_{32}O_6$	Methacrylic monomer based on bisphenol A; in dental restorative composite materials; as reactive monomer in adhesive products (BIS-EMA)
2,2-Bis(4- methacryloxy)phenyl)propane $C_{23}H_{24}O_4$	Methacrylic monomer based on bisphenol A; in dental restorative composite materials (BIS-MA)
N,N-Methylene-bis-acryalamide $C_7H_{10}N_2O_2$	Acrylamide compound cross-reacting with unidentified primary sensitizers in NAPP and Nyloprint UV-cured printing plates
Methyl methacrylate $C_5H_8O_2$	Methacrylic monomer in plastics for dentures, bone cement, artificial nails, hearing aids, etc. (MMA)
Oligotriacrylate	Multifunctional acrylic monomer for use in lithographic inks, overprinting varnishes, coatings on wood, paper etc.; cured by UV-light (OTA 480)
Pentaerythritol-triacrylate $C_{14}H_{18}O_7$	Trifunctional crosslinking acrylic monomer for use in adhesives, coatings, inks, photoresists, castings, etc. cured by UV-radiation
Tetrahydrofurfuryl-methacrylate $C_9H_{15}O_3$	Methacrylic component in dental materials such as crown and bridge products; also a component in artificial nails
Triethyleneglycol-diacrylate $C_{12}H_{18}O_6$	Cross-linking acrylate monomer for use in coatings, adhesives and in printing plates of photoprepolymer type (TEGDA)

(Continued)

TABLE 36–1 (Continued). **Associations of Acrylate Patch-Test Reagents**[a]

Triethyleneglycol-dimethacrylate $C_{10}H_{14}O_4$	Methacrylic monomer for use as cross-linking agent for, e.g., dental restorative materials (TREGDMA)
Trimethylol propane-triacrylate $C_{15}H_{20}O_6$	Triacrylate for use in UV-curable lithographic inks, varnishes, wood-finish, solder, and etch resists in the electronic industry
Tripropyleneglycol-diacrylate $C_{15}H_{24}O_6$	Diacrylate monomer for use in UV-curable flexographic and silk screen inks, wood finish varnishes, coatings on plastics, etc. (TPGDA)
Urethane diacrylate, aliphatic	UV-reactive prepolymer based on an acrylated aliphatic isocyanate; for use in curable coatings, inks, and varnishes (Ebecryl 270)
Urethane diacrylate, aromatic	UV-reactive prepolymer based on an acrylated aromatic isocyanate; for use in curable coatings, inks, and varnishes (Ebecryl 220)
Urethane dimethacrylate $C_{24}H_{40}N_2O_8$	Methacrylate based on a methacrylated aliphatic isocyanate; for use in dental bonding agents, resin veneering, and restorative materials (UEDMA)

[a]Information furnished by Chemotechnique Diagnostics regarding acrylate antigens was reproduced with permission.

good reason not to test to unknown acrylate products, as the proper concentration for some is extremely low,[27] and sensitization is not a remote possibility. Concentrations published in the literature are not entirely reliable either. One of us (JDG) sensitized himself (as a control subject for irritancy and safety) some 20 years ago when trying to standardize an acrylate series.

PATTERNS OF CROSS-REACTIVITY

Rules for patterns of cross-reactivity may not always prove to be true, but a number of patterns are suggested; especially in animal studies:

1. Closely related chemicals may cause a reaction equal to the sensitizing chemical.[30]
2. Animals sensitized to monoacrylates react to other monoacrylates but not monomethacrylates.[3] This means that acrylates cross-react with other acrylates which are close in structure, but they do not tend to cross-react with the corresponding methacrylates.[34] When methyl, ethyl, and butyl methacrylates are each used to sensitize individually and all animals are challenged with all four, each tends to elicit a cross-reactions equal in prominence to that of the original sensitizer, whichever one it was.[35]
3. Many animals sensitized to methacrylates react to other monomethacrylates and *also to* monoacrylates.
4. In an animal study epoxy acrylates cross-reacted with epoxy in 25 percent of cases, but not with acrylic acid.[36]
5. Animals sensitized to di(meth)acrylates do not tend to cross-react.[3]
6. The polyfunctional *acrylate,* trimethylol propane *triacrylate* (TMPTA), cross-reacts with pentaerythritol *triacrylate,* but not *trimethylol propane trimeth*acrylate.[37]
7. Reactions to tetraethylene glycol *acrylate* were solved in a printing plant by substituting tetraethylene glycol di*meth*acrylate.

8. Cross-reactivity among polyfunctional acrylates may depend more on the core structure than the substitutions.[38]
9. An epoxyacrylate-sensitive patient did not react to epoxy resin and cross-reacted incompletely to four epoxy acrylate resins.

WHERE DOES ONE COME IN CONTACT?

Contact problems have been reported from paint,[39] prostheses,[40–42] dental prostheses[43] and bonding materials[44]; hearing aids[45]; artificial nail "sculpturing,"[45] elongation,[47] and wrapping[48]; orthopedic devices[49]; ultraviolet-cured inks[13]; adhesives for machinery vibration[50]; surgical tape[30]; rubber stamp making; and many other areas. One should look for this category of synthetic materials in molded products, paints, and dental materials. Ultraviolet-cured inks and dental restorations also probably have this type chemical composition. In one series 4.5 percent of those tested for epoxy allergy, and 3 of 36 allergic to epoxy reacted to epoxy acrylates.[51] One should understand that epoxy acrylates, which are the product of the reaction of an epoxide with acrylic or methacrylic acid, do not contain "epoxy" groups but may cause a reaction in epoxy-allergic persons because of similarities in chemical structure.

Occupations where one must look for acrylate sensitivity include printing, rubber-stamp making, manufacturing (e.g., inks, anaerobic sealants), construction (windows, sealant, floor covering), electron microscopy, dentists and dental assistants, dental technicians,[52] orthopedic surgery, painting, and machine repair.

SURGICAL TAPE

Tape reactions in one brand were caused by ethylhexyl acrylate which may be associated with cross-reactivity to other acrylates[30,53] or *t*-butyl maleamic acid. Some acrylic adhesives are quite hypoallergenic and are widely used in patch testing.[30,54,55] Such adhesives are also used in the manufacturing of diaper adhesive for diapers.[56] It has been postulated that tape allergy could lead to more widely occurring sensitivity to acrylates, but there is no evidence for this happening. To the contrary, the incidence even in the patch-test population is quite low.[57]

PAINTS AND VARNISHES AND MEDICAL PRODUCTS

Acrylic paint containing cyclohexanone resin,[58] a primer for wood siding containing TMPTA and aziridine cross-linkers[39] and a floor covering (aziridine and TMPTA)[51] caused contact dermatitis. One may also see reactions from electron microscopy[60]; wound treatment (Neobecutan)[61]; or contact with spectacle frames.[62]

ANAEROBIC SEALANT[50,63–68]

These adhesives are used in high-performance industrial machinery where vibration can affect the retention of nuts and caps to shafts of gears, pulleys, collars, etc. The adhesive polymerizes under anaerobic conditions, permitting the nut or cap to be tightened before the adhesive effect takes place and reducing the tendency for one of these parts to become loose inadvertently.[50] Application is often automated in industry. For home, hobby, and some commercial uses, this type glue is supplied with an applicator nozzle, which helps. However, it is still rather easy to contaminate the fingers when applying the glue to small objects. The acrylates used are commonly diacrylates and dimethacrylates, but alkyl acrylates and methacrylates (hydroxyethyl, hydroxypropyl, etc.), and polyfunctional acrylates and methacrylates reportedly may be present. The known chemical may not be what you think. For example, "polyethylene glycol dimethacrylate" listed as an ingredient can range from ethylene glycol dimethacrylate to hexethylene glycol dimethacrylate, with most being tetraethylene glycol dimethacrylate.[50]

NAIL COMPLICATIONS

Nail involvement from use of acrylic resins to extend nail length or to create "sculptured" nails can cause a very severe allergic reaction[71,72] especially with periungual and fingertip eczema[48] and onycholysis[47]—sometimes with tragic consequences,[71] including paresthesia,[72] Raynaud's syndrome, or even permanent loss of the nails with resultant inability to pick up small objects, open clasps, and perform other tasks with the fingernails.[71] When methyl methacrylate was removed from such preparations, ethyl, butyl, isobutyl, and tetrahydrofurfuryl methacrylates, and ethylene glycol, and diethylene glycol dimethacrylates, and trimethylolpropane trimethacrylate, and methacrylic acid were substituted.[71] This may not solve the problem, as there is more cross-reactivity in some reports[48,69,73] than predicted.[30,74]

Nail sculpturing[46] or extending is used to make nails thicker or longer and can be used to produce essentially "artificial" nails. This is no longer done with methyl methacrylate, but today ethyl, butyl, and isobutyl methacrylates, methacrylic acid, ethylene glycol and diethylene glycol dimethacrylate, trimethylolpropane trimethacrylate, and tetrahydrofurfuryl methacrylate are used in various products.[71] Some processes use ultraviolet cured resins.[70]

Nail wrapping employs application of silk or linen to the nail with application of a cyanoacrylate glue, and the resultant "nail" is filed to a more natural shape and polished. Cyanoacrylates, used both with artificial nails and to repair nails, can also sensitize.[75]

ORTHOPEDIC SURGERY

Sensitization of orthopedic surgeons to methyl methacrylate has posed a problem since the advent of joint replacement, especially because surgical gloves are not adequate protection from exposure to methyl methacrylate. When methyl methacrylate is used in joint replacement, there is a much greater likelihood that the orthopedic surgeon rather than the patient will become allergic. However, allergic contact dermatitis can occur following surgery, and where the acrylate is located,[76,77] approximately 25 percent of patients tested some time later will have a positive patch test.[78]

LIGHT-SENSITIVE ACRYLATES

Because light activators can be used to polymerize acrylates following exposure to UV light, polymer chemistry can be used to print images. It is possible to polymerize only the monomer not protected by the darker parts of the negative, so that a positive image is left. This is especially useful in printing metallic and similar surfaces. It is also in commercial printing. In rubber stamp making the ultraviolet-cured polymer protects the rubber where it is treated so that the desired image is left raised. The usual ultraviolet-cured inks used in commercial printing contain some 50 to 70 percent of the acrylated "prepolymer," with photoinitiators and cross-linking agents, pigments, fillers, and inert polymers.[1]

The chemical structure is available for some ultraviolet-cured inks, but others are a trade secret. However, there are generally three basic components: a reactive base prepolymer, a photoinitiator (often a benzophenone), and a multifunctional (cross-linking) acrylic monomer.[36] The first, which may constitute as much as 80 percent of the total, may be an acrylated polyester, polyether, polyurethane, etc. However, when it is an epoxy acrylate, some of these can be extreme sensitizers.[36]

The chemicals are usually polyfunctional acrylics (i.e., they have multiple acrylic moieties). Sometimes more than one of these are used. There are also light-absorbing activators. The multifunctional acrylates in UV-curable resins are usually based on di(meth)acrylate esters of dialcohols or tri- and tetra-acrylate esters of polyalcohols. In UV-curable coatings, the most commonly used are pentaerythritol triacrylate (PETA), trimethylolpropane triacrylate (TMPTA), and 1,6-hexanediol diacrylate (HDDA).[5]

Nethercott[13] reported pentaerythritol triacrylate, trimethylolpropane triacrylate, and hexanedioldiacrylate all to be multifunctional monomers used in this process. Patch tests to two caused reactions but the third did not in those studied, which paralleled what had been found by Emmett.[31] In another plant, Emmett reported reactions to trimethylol propane triacrylate (7), 1,6-hexanediol diacrylate (6), pentaerythritol triacrylate (4), and epoxy acrylate oligomers (3). Whether this was due to a cross-reaction or was a concomitant allergy is not known.[79] Triacryl-(tris-2-hydroxyethyl) isocyanurate was the sensitizer in another printing plate.[80]

In Björkner's series the number-sensitive were ethyl (1); butyl (2); and 2-ethylhexyl acrylate (2); epoxy diacrylate (3); polyester diacrylate (3); TMPTA (4); TMPMA (none); stabilizer (3).[81] From data on cross-reactions, the sensitizing potential is known to be different for these compounds, so Björkner believes that it may be possible to substitute safer products for many of these applications.[82] Sometimes the equivalent methacrylate can be substituted with less sensitizing or irritant potential. This was effective in one printing plant where tetraethylene glycol diacrylate was replaced by tetrathylene glycol dimethacrylate, and the problem was eliminated.[83]

The active ingredients of some printing processes have been published, although some may well be out of date by now. The published contents are as follows:

1. NAPP printing uses 2-hydroxyethyl methacrylate and N,N'-methylene-bis-acrylamide.[84]
2. Nyloprint WD also uses 2-hydroxyethyl methacrylate.
3. Letterflex contained a polythiol sensitizer identified as pentaerythritol-tetrakis-3-mercaptoproprionate.[85]

Photodermatitis has been reported,[86] but is apparently not common.

IRRITATION

The irritant quality of these chemicals is at least partly predictable based upon structure. Methacrylates are less irritating than the corresponding acrylates,[34] and the diacrylates are much more irritating than the corresponding dimethacrylates. In one printing plant investigated by Nethercott, the irritant properties of tetraethylene glycol diacrylate used in ultraviolet curing inks[13] affected four workers, while only one became allergic. That chemical produced a delayed onset some 12 to 36 h after exposure.[87] Another multifunctional acrylate, trimethylpropane triacrylate, was the probable source of irritation in urethane acrylate ink.[88]

PROTECTION

The hands are perhaps the problem area, so protective gloves are an obvious solution. Unfortunately there is not an ideal protective material for many acrylates. However, contact with the American Industrial Hygiene Association, the National Institute of Occupational Safety and Health (NIOSH), the Occupational Safety and Health Association (OSHA), or glove manufacturers themselves can provide information on the best choices for gloves. The monomers readily penetrate rubber gloves, and tests show that not only latex but also neoprene is inadequate.[89,90] Nitrile gloves[91] and 4-H gloves[92] are rather helpful provided one does not try to leave them in contact with the monomer more than a few hours,[92] and the less time the better.

4-H gloves (polyethylene in two layers and ethylene vinyl alcohol copolymer) gave 20 min protection from methylmethacrylate monomer.[93] Viton butyl rubber 0.27 mm prevented absorption for 15 min.[93] Components penetrate gloves faster than the whole product. Nitrile rubber gloves are better for some types of monomer, but they are not perfect.

For persons allergic to an object such as a dental prosthesis, heat curing of methyl methacrylate resins tends to prevent or at least greatly reduce the chance of reactivity.[27] Antigen substitution has also been effective in some cases. Since methacrylates are less irritating[94] and less sensitizing than the corresponding acrylates and since methacrylates do not tend to cross-react in those allergic to the corresponding straight-chain acrylate, the methacrylate equivalent may substitute for the acrylate causing the problem.[95] Patch testing the sensitive worker to the proposed substitute in advance might help to prevent unpleasant surprises.

For protection in electron microscopy one needs a hood, protective clothing, goggles, and a respirator. The 2-hydroxyethyl acrylate penetrates rubber and vinyl and does not polymerize when not anaerobic. The pungent odor tells you there was an oxygen leak.[96]

For print shops, Malten[85] has ten rules:

1. Keep equipment together to minimize contaminated area.
2. Cover the floor of that area with paper to help in cleaning.
3. Use disposable, protective clothing.
4. Do not scrape the printing plates.
5. Use care in handling the protective sheet (which catches the ink).
6. Use care in collection of prepolymer in equipment.
7. Wash skin immediately when contaminated.
8. Use protective gloves for cleaning the machinery.
9. Educate personnel and control their activity.
10. Hire workers without skin problems.

POLYURETHANE

Reactions to isocyanates, the building blocks of the polyurethanes, are not common despite commercial availability of testing materials. There are reports of allergy to the coating of spectacle frames[97] and car badges,[98] to a covering for leg ulcers.[99] Reactions have been found in woodworkers,[100] a research chemist,[101] and a laboratory technician.[102]

AMINO FORMALDEHYDE POLYMERS

This category of resins includes urea and melamine formaldehyde resins. Exposure (and sometimes reactions) to urea formaldehyde resins have been seen from fiberboard[103] and foam insulation, but as Hjorth and Fregert[104] found in 1967, most reactions seen to these agents have been to textile finishes. Such patients often, but not always, are also allergic to formaldehyde.[104] Of course, most of those tested are suspected of having a clothing dermatitis.

Melamine formaldehyde resin has been associated with plaster casts used in orthopedics, where the plastic material forms a protective coating over the plaster cast.[105] In one series these reactions were assumed to be caused by formaldehyde, but testing to melamine formaldehyde resin was not done.[106] It has also been used in a glaze for clay pots.[107] This also is more often found in persons with clothing dermatitis.

NYLON

Nylon plastics are a class of materials based on polyamide polymers. Chemically, polyamides may be made by a variety of routes, but the most common methods involve either the reactions of diamines with dicarboxylic acids or ring opening of cyclic lactams to form polymers. Figure 36B-5 illustrates these two reaction routes. Although a number of different nylon plastics are commercially available, the most common are nylon 6, prepared by polymerization of ϵ-caprolactam, and nylon 6/6, prepared by the polymerization of hexamethylene diamine and adipic acid. Other commercially available nylons may use 1,4-butane diamine, azelaic acid, dodecanoic acid, 11-aminoundecanoic acid, or dodecanolactam as starting materials.

Nylons are usually supplied to customers as plastic pellets that are thermally transformed into shapes by either injection molding or extrusions. A wide variety of names are used for nylon plastics because they are easily compounded with glass fibers, mineral fillers, and other property modifiers to change their balance of properties. Some trade names used include Zytel, Bexloy (DuPont), Ultramid (BASF), Rilsan (Atochem), Trogamid (Huls), Amilon (Toray), Akulon (Akzo), Capron (Allied-Signal), and Grilon (Emser). In recent years there have also been efforts to commercialize a new process, reaction injection molding (RIM), for making shaped nylon by polymerization of the ϵ-caprolactam to polymer in the mold.

Most cases of "nylon dermatitis" are actually caused by dyes or fabric finishes.[108] True reactions to nylon occur, but they are not common. Both contact dermatitis and contact urticaria are reported. The eruption may be localized to the area of contact or widespread, involving areas where hand transfer may have occurred.[109] Patterns include nylon stocking dermatitis, attributed in almost all cases to dyes, usually disperse dyes.

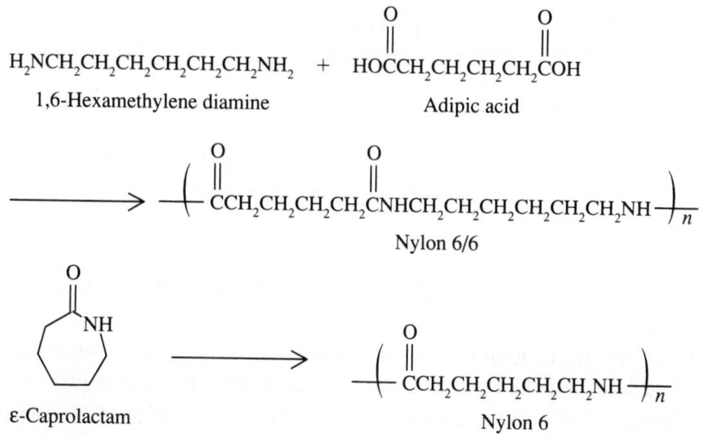

FIG. 36B–5. Chemical routes to nylon plastics.

There the patient develops a fine rash, worse in areas of pressure, especially above the knees. The pressure areas on the thigh also are prominent sometimes, and obviously the eruption can be anywhere that pantyhose come into contact.[110] A bullous dermatitis of the feet was shown to be caused by nylon by patch testing to undyed and untreated nylon and a spontaneous flare following exposure.[111] Six cases with positive patch tests to "raw" nylon had eczematous dermatoses, confined to the area of exposure. A seventh may have had stocking dermatitis (possibly due to an additive, as she was not tested).[112,113]

Another pattern involves the primary area, with lesions in exposed areas. This could be hand transfer. Several cases where there was no patch-test confirmation leave some doubt about allergy to fabric finishes and dyes.[114–116]

When this allergy is suspected, patch testing should be done with nylon which has no color and no fabric finishes. The subject has been reviewed recently by Hatch and Maibach.[108]

Contact urticaria also has been reported to raw (untreated) nylon, localized closely to the area of contact where a colorless nylon undergarment and white nurse's stockings were worn.[117] In another report an eruption developed both in and out of the area of exposure.[118]

CELLULOSE POLYMERS

Cellulose polymers comprise a wide range of products from rayon and acetate textiles to cellophane used in packaging and cellulosic hard plastics used in toothbrush handles, spectacle frames, and toys. Cellulose itself is a naturally occurring polysaccharide that is found in plants. In its natural state, it is a highly crystalline material that cannot be used as a plastic because it decomposes rather than melts upon exposure to heat. To make cellulose into a processable plastic, the chemistry of the polymer is modified by reactions with acetic, propanoic, and butyric acids, their mixtures, or their corresponding anhydrides—ethyl chloride or nitric acid. Figure 36B-6 summarizes the reaction that

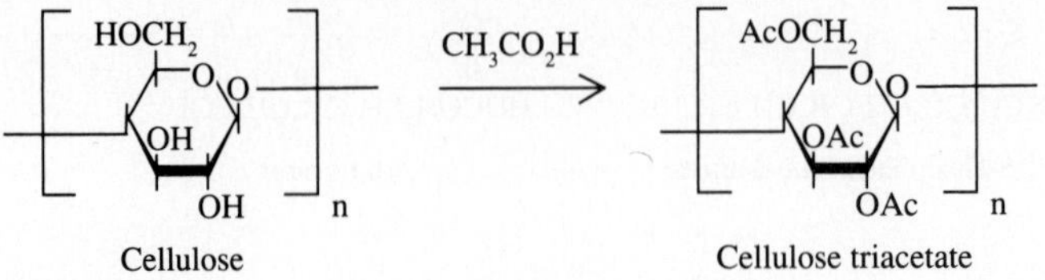

FIG. 36B-6. Cellulose triacetate formation from cellulose.

takes place between cellulose and acetic acid to form a triester. Analogous reactions take place with the other acids transforming the hydroxy groups in the cellulose, responsible for the high degree of crystallinity and resistance to melting, into ester groups as in cellulose acetate-butyrate and cellulose nitrate or ether groups as in ethyl cellulose. Commercially available under the name Tenite (Eastman Chemical) are cellulose acetate, cellulose triacetate, cellulose acetate propionate, cellulose acetate butyrate. Also available are ethyl cellulose and cellulose nitrate. Substitution on the glucoside ring can range from less than one ester or ether group per repeating unit up to three ester or ether groups per repeating unit.

Cellulosic plastics are usually mixed with plasticizers, such as esters of phthalic, adipic, sebacic, phosphoric, or citric acid, to improve their melt flow. Camphor may be used in cellulose nitrate as a plasticizer.

Reports of allergy are not common, and even then additives are suspect. In one case cellophane (along with propylene glycol) was positive.[119] In another report of six patients, an ultraviolet "stabilizer," resorcinol monobenzoate, caused the problem in three, *an antioxidant, p-tertiary*-butylphenol was positive in one, an azo dye was positive in that same one and another, and the sixth was allergic to an ingredient in an adhesive.[120] All but one allergen were found in eyeglass frames, and the site of the eruption was at least in part under the glasses, as determined by the object contacted. A hearing aid caused eczema behind the ear, a fountain pen caused dermatitis of the hand, and one patient broke out on the chest from carrying a pen in his pocket! Allergy to resorcinol monobenzoate might be suspected when reactions to balsam of Peru are seen in the standard series.[121] Patch testing is often positive to the object, such as the earpiece of the eyeglass frames, which is a convenient way to test. When a reaction is suspected, plasticizers, sunscreens, antioxidants, dyes, etc. should be suspected as possibilities, especially if all such products do not cause a problem.

VINYL

Strictly speaking, what is called *vinyl* can be any one of several polymers that are prepared from vinyl monomers such as acrylates, styrene, acrylonitrile, ethylene, or propylene. However, vinyl has become synonymous with *polyvinyl chloride* in the plastics industry. Vinyl is a very versatile plastic and may be found in automobile seat covers and hard plastic panels, in edible oil and water packaging, in TV and computer housings, in siding for houses, in water pipes and tubing, in medical devices, and in electric wire insulation, to name a few.

Vinyl is prepared by the reaction, shown in Fig. 36B-7, of vinyl chloride monomer

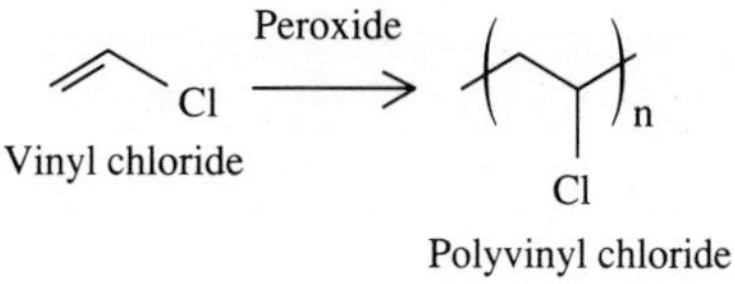

FIG. 36B–7. Vinyl chloride polymerization to polyvinyl chloride.

with a peroxide initiator to yield polyvinyl chloride. As formed, polyvinyl chloride has insufficient thermal stability to be processed by most commonly used plastics processing techniques. When vinyl decomposes thermally, hydrogen chloride is produced. To be processed without decomposition, polyvinyl chloride is normally mixed with either plasticizers, such as dibutyl phthalate or dioctyl phthalate, or acrylic polymer processing aids. Besides plasticizers and processing aids, a wide variety of thermal stabilizers are used in the formulations. It is beyond the scope of this chapter to present a list of all the different types of stabilizers used; however, they may include organic salts of zinc, calcium, tin, barium, lead and cadmium, organophosphites, and epoxies.

Some common trade names found for vinyl resins include Tenneco (Burlington-Frank), Geon (B. F. Goodrich), Oxy (Occidental Chemical), Polyvin (A. Shulman Inc.), and Vista PVC (Vista Chemical Co.).

Vinyl polymers are generally regarded as relatively nonsensitizing,[122] but allergies to additives in the finished product can occur. The concept that this is a rare sensitivity may be inaccurate due to underreporting of reactions. Two reports of reactions to gloves show that about 10 percent of reactions to medical/dental gloves are caused by PVC rather than latex gloves[123,124] (Fig. 36B-8). Additives usually have been assumed to be the ultimate cause, but this was not proved in most cases. One patient reacted to a dye rather than the vinyl monomer.[124] Jolanki et al.[125] found that a pigment additive was responsible in one case, but only one of five reactions in the same series was caused by this dye, while dimethyl glyoxal[126] and dibutyltin maleate and sebacate were incriminated in another report.[126] These are still cited as causes, although they were found some 50 years ago and may well be an anachronism.

Plasticizers, substances added to the monomer to control the temperature of the process and the flexibility of the final product,[127] include dibutyl and dioctylphthalates (but not diethyl phthalate, which is apparently relatively nonsensitizing), and tricresyl phosphate.[122,127] Some vinyl examination gloves contain low levels of formaldehyde in one of our laboratories (JDG). It is not known whether this can cause a reaction in formaldehyde-allergic patients. For other patients, the patch tests to reported additives are usually negative, but the number of such chemicals is long and few are usually included in even a good screening series. Both ethyl and isopropyl alcohols degrade vinyl gloves and tend to penetrate the material in 10 min or less.[128]

One of us evaluated an industrial problem in a plant worker exposed to PVC monomer (which had unnamed additives included in the formula according to the material safety data sheet). A patch test to the diluted monomer was a prominent 3 + reaction. He then remembered that he had to wear a plastic-coated disposable suit as a protective garment and had experienced a reaction in the areas this contacted, but he had never suspected it, as plastic materials were regarded as "safe." Tests to the suit material were also 3 + . A change in his work clothing solved a chronic problem.

Patch-test reactions to vinyl gloves are not that uncommon; they vary from the more common mild or doubtful readings to less common severe responses. Perhaps the most

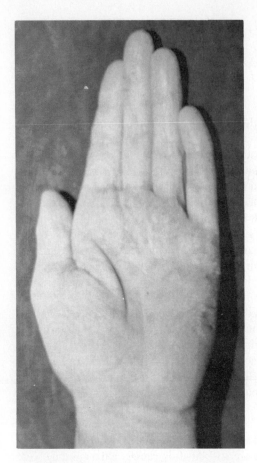

FIG. 36B–8. Hairdresser who had a chronic hand dermatitis. She was primarily allergic to glycerylmonothioglycolate but she also had a 2 + patch test to vinyl gloves.

reliable way to pick up this type reaction is to test to the specific product the patient has used. Lacking this, a vinyl examination glove will uncover many such allergies when applied for 48 h under the light pressure of an elastic bandage. Remember that every "vinyl" will not have the same additives, and testing with the objects to which the patient is exposed is more likely to accurately reflect that individual's ability to tolerate exposure to it.

One should suspect this type of sensitivity in patients with unresponsive hand eczema, perhaps with a long history of treatment with occlusion or working with a substance which is known to readily penetrate vinyl gloves (e.g., epoxy, acrylates, glyceryl monothioglycolate, etc.). Most have used vinyl (and often rubber) gloves and perhaps were sensitized concomitantly. For most nonindustrial applications, Tactylon gloves can be substituted or 4-H gloves (which have polyethylene on the inside layer) if exposure to penetrating allergens is a problem (e.g., acrylates).

POLYETHYLENE

Polyethylene is ubiquitous. It is used in garbage bags, milk cartons and other food packaging, plastic trash cans, electrical cable, toys, fuel tanks in automobiles and trucks to name a few. The chemistry of polyethylene is superficially very simple as one simply polymerizes a simple monomer, ethylene ($CH_2\!=\!CH_2$), to form a high-molecular-weight polymer. However, the simplicity is deceiving, as the variety of products found will testify. Polyethylene is produced to have a variety of structures dictated by the process used to prepare it and the comonomers used. By itself, polymerization of ethylene produces low-density polyethylene (LDPE) and high-density polyethylene (HDPE) that differ in the amount of branching of the polymer backbone. The more linear the backbone, the higher the density. Copolymerization of ethylene with 1-butene yields linear low density polyethylene (LLDPE) and recently products based on copolymerization of ethylene with 1-hexene have been introduced.

Some of the trade names used for polyethylene and its copolymers include Escorene (Exxon), Microthene and Petrothene (Quantum Chemical), Rexene (Rexene), Dowlex (Dow Chemical), and Marlex (Phillips 66 Co.).

Reports of allergy to polyethylene are rare. Recently a patient presented with an extreme (3 +) reaction to polyethylene products on patch testing to the whole products. This patient had an allergy to the protective tubing on her hearing aid, which was a polyethylene sleeve (Fig. 36B-9). She had reacted to nasal catheters when hospitalized, and testing to polyethylene tubing and flat products showed extreme reactivity (Fig. 36B-10). This patient also had a 2 + reaction to polyvinylidene (Saran) (Fig. 36B-11). So many patients with obvious contact allergy fail to conform to published "rules" that one must be wary of outliers in every case. Testing such patients to products to

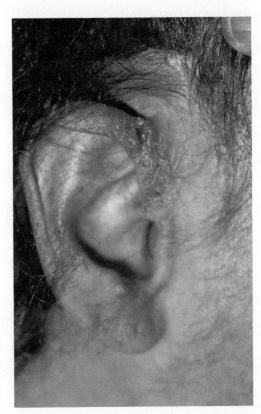

FIG. 36B–9. Contact dermatitis to a hearing aid wire covered with a polyethylene sleeve. (See color Plate 28.)

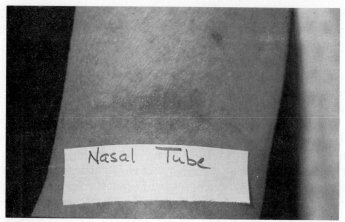

FIG. 36B–10. Positive patch test to polyethylene nasal tube in the patient in the preceding figure. She also reacted to IV tubing.

which they have been exposed and especially those to which they have a history of a reaction can be critical. In short, being thorough is often much more effective than being clever.

PHENOLIC RESINS

Some of us old enough to remember the early "plastics" think of Bakelite, the product of the original patent given for the productions of such plastic materials.[129–131] The electrical nonconductivity caused this material to be used with electrical insulation, and its heat resistance made the characteristic dark-colored "plastic" handle a familiar sight on small appliances. These materials are widely used in electronics (knobs, integrated circuits, etc.), adhesives (wood, especially plywood), binders, and coatings.[130]

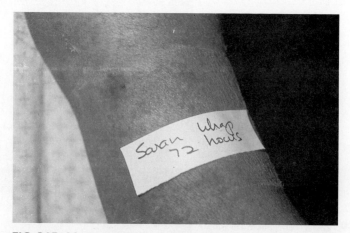

FIG. 36B–11. Positive patch test to Saran Wrap. The causative component is not known.

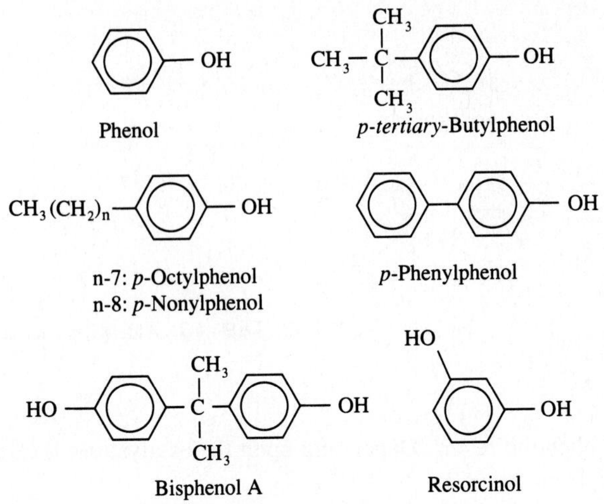

FIG. 36B–12. Phenol derivatives in phenolic resins.

Phenol-formaldehyde resins (PFR) also are sometimes combined with other materials such as rubber.[132]

CHEMISTRY

Phenolic resins derive their name from the use of phenol as a raw material in the manufacture of the most widely used resins. However, beyond phenol there are a number of other chemically similar raw materials that are used. Besides phenol, other phenols such as cresols, *p-tertiary*-butylphenol, *p*-octylphenol, *p*-nonylphenol, *p*-phenylphenol, bisphenol A, and resorcinol may all be used in plastics or adhesives. The chemical structures of these raw materials are shown in Fig. 36B-12. To become the familiar plastics we encounter, these raw materials must be polymerized by chemical reaction with aldehydes. Formaldehyde is most commonly used in its aqueous form as formalin, but acetaldehyde, glyoxal, or furfural may also be used. The chemical structure of these chemical reactants is shown in Fig. 36B-13.

Depending upon the type of chemistry used to polymerize these raw materials and their ratio, the products differ. The chemistry involves steps in synthesis of intermediates—i.e., resins (which often are the sensitizers)—but simplistically the end product is a polymer of (substituted) phenolics cross-linked by methylene or ether linkage.[131,132] Resins produced by strong acid catalysis, such as would be made if sulfuric, sulfonic, oxalic, or phosphoric acid were used, are called novolac resins and have chemical structures shown in Fig. 36B-14. These types of resins are also produced when divalent metal catalysts, such as zinc or calcium acetate are used. When strongly alkaline catalysts, such as sodium, calcium, or barium hydroxide, are used, the product is called a resole. A resole is chemically similar to the product shown in Fig. 36B-14, but a wider variety of chemical structures are found. In novolak resins there is a shortage of aldehyde groups while in resol resins there is a surplus. Besides hydroxide based alkaline catalysts, amines such as ammonia and hexamethylenetetramine may also be

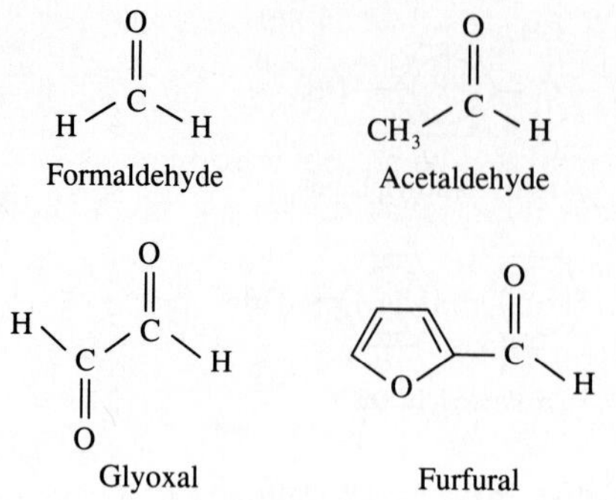

FIG. 36B–13. Aldehydes used in phenolic resins.

used to prepare phenolic resins. Depending upon the catalyst used, catalyst concentrations may range from about 1% to <10%.

Phenolic resins are highly cross-linked in their applications. The chemical reactions responsible for cross-linking are similar to those shown in Fig. 36B-14. In the novolak type resin, phenol is in excess in an acid medium and a cross-linker or hardener plus heat is used in curing. Formaldehyde added produces methylol groups which then bind to another substituted phenolic molecule to produce a low molecular weight product of two phenolics linked to methylene. In the presence of additional formaldehyde, further methylolation occurs, and these groups are, in turn, similarly linked to form a polymer.[131] With excess phenol, the novolaks lack methylol groups following heat

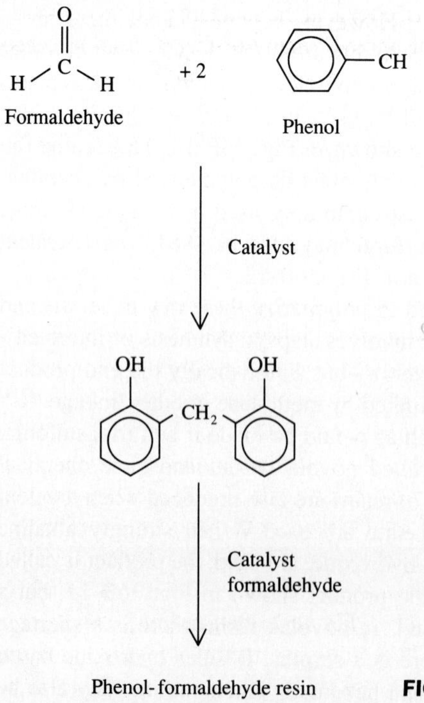

FIG. 36B–14. Phenolic resin polymerization.

curing. Completely cured resins are relatively free of reactive groups, but under extreme conditions they may break down to produce, among other things, the allergenic material.[133]

Other species, both reactive and nonreactive, may also be present in phenolic resins. These include reactive chemicals such abietic acid, dicyclopentadiene, and unsaturated oils or unreactive fillers such as wood flour.

Some of the trade names found for phenolic resins include Polychem (Budd Company), Fiberite (ICI/Fiberite), Durez (Occidental Chemical), Plenco (Plastics Engineering Co.), Pyrotex (Raymark Industrial Div.), and Tecolite (Toshiba Chemical Products).

These systems can produce contact dermatitis from either the resin or a component in its manufacture. They may or may not also react to p-tertiarybutyl phenol formaldehyde resin, but in those allergic to PFR (and not PTBPFR) the sensitizer was a methylol phenol[134] or dimethylol phenol[135] or a methoxy substituted methylene bisphenol.[136]

RECOGNITION

The usual patient with PFR dermatitis has hand dermatitis and perhaps facial involvement as well. Most develop it from occupational exposure. There are many places where exposure can occur other than the plastics manufacturing industry, including plywood manufacture, construction, paper materials of all kinds, textiles, and many other things.[131] The incidence of PFR dermatitis from sources other than p-tertiary-butylphenol (PTBP) is less than PTBP reactivity,[131] but this is at least partly caused by the antigens chosen to screen for allergy to this type chemical,[137–139] as the test for p-tertiary-butylphenol formaldehyde resin (PTBPFR) is in the standard patch-test series. That test is good for PTBPFR, but it does not uncover many of the reactors to other PFR resins.[140]

METHYLOL PHENOLS ARE ALLERGENS

The causative allergen in PFR dermatitis was a mystery until Rycroft[134] investigated a worker with an industrial sensitivity and isolated the potentially allergenic components from the final product. This patient reacted strongly to 2-monomethylol phenol, weakly to 2,4,6-trimethylol phenol, but not at all to 4-monomethylol phenol.

Bruze et al.[136] using MS and NMR, looked at the contact allergens in 11 patients with this type allergy and found that methoxy phenolics linked to methylene were the cause in 6 of the 11. The most potent allergen was 4,4'-dihydroxy-3,3'-di-(hydroxymethyl)-diphenyl methane, but two other methylene di(methoxy) phenolics were also allergens. Five of these patients reacted to the industrial resin P-F-R-2, but not to the three methylol substituted phenolics. Only 2 of 14 allergens, both methylene bisphenols, did not possess methylol groups on the aromatic ring(s). These PFR-allergic persons seem primarily to have been sensitized by industrial exposure.

The meaning of these data is that (nonPTBP) PFR will often be missed with the standard test series. To test for sensitivity, a PFR with free methylols present should be used, perhaps one present on the job. Monomethylol phenol is available as a commercial test material from Chemotechnique, which also sells P-F-R-2, the specific resin described by Bruze as uncovering all reactors of this type. Trolab markets a "resol-type" PFR patch-test antigen, which is probably equivalent.

p-TERTIARY-BUTYLPHENOL FORMALDEHYDE RESIN

RECOGNITION

This antigen is part of the standard test series, which is reviewed in that section. Persons allergic to PTBPFR often present with plantar dermatitis from the chloroprene (Neoprene) cement in the sponge rubber insoles of shoes,[141] especially athletic shoes. One may also see hand eczema.[142] Women[143] and children patch tested not infrequently react to PTBPFR,[144] perhaps from footwear.

The macromolecular end product of PTBPFR fills in gaps and crevices on opposing surfaces, and with its natural tackiness it becomes an excellent adhesive for chloroprene rubber. Allergy to PTBPFR has been responsible for a number of cases of shoe dermatitis where PTBPFR is a component of the insole adhesive.

HOW CAN A FINISHED RESIN BE ALLERGENIC?

According to Malten and Seutter,[145] the polymer is large for transdermal absorption and the chemistry suggests relatively little of the original ingredients remain in the finished product. How then does one explain allergy to the polymerized material? Although a trace of PTBP is still around in a fresh sample of the finished resin, fewer than 20 percent of those sensitive to PTBPFR are allergic to PTBP (the original chemical before formaldehyde and polymerization). Additional products appear after aging and environmental challenge, and they theorize that some deterioration of the resin may occur in the long-term presence of acid and water. This may explain why some patients seem to break out more to old shoes than new shoes.

PTBPFR can also produce a nail-bed reaction similar to that seen from acrylates and cyanoacrylate adhesive.[146] That eruption is reportedly almost identical to those seen with contact allergy to acrylic nail preparations and cyanoacrylate adhesives.

Contact reactions to PTBPFR can occur either as an occupational or a consumer-type problem. The traditional occupational association with cobblers[47] may now be an anachronism. Other occupational associations are seen in automobile workers working with weather stripping, from paper,[148] and, of course, where the chemical is manufactured.

Reactions in consumers may occur to a prosthesis,[149] an adhesive for watchbands[149] and other leather objects and to athletic tape,[150,151] and adhesive labels.[152] The chemical p-tertiary-butylphenol is widely used as an antioxidant, an antiseptic, a plasticizer for plastics, a pour-point depressant and emulsion breaker for petroleum, a plasticizer for cellulose acetate, in deodorants as a germicide, as a fumigant, in manufacture of varnish and lacquer resins, and as a soap antioxidant.

PATCH-TESTING RESULTS

Reactions to PTBPFR are somewhat more commonly reported than sensitivity to PTBP,[131] perhaps because the former is a standard patch-test antigen, while testing to the latter would have to be done either deliberately or as part of a "plastics and glues" series.

The PTBPFR patch-test antigen used is a polymer rather than the PTBP monomer used to produce the resin. PTBP is also used as an antioxidant, as a germicide, and for many other uses. According to most published reports, most reactors are not formaldehyde-allergic.[138,153,154] However, in Bruze's series, the prevalence of formaldehyde allergy was higher in those allergic to two different (nonPTBPFR) PFR,[155] and there is a significant quantity of free formaldehyde in many commercial resins.[137,156,157] There is also the possibility of variation from one batch to the next,[158] so one may wish to test to the one used on the job, as screening tests may miss allergy to that product.

Many years ago persons allergic to PTBPFR were assumed to be allergic to PTBP. However, some of those allergic did not fit, as they were allergic to PTBPFR *without* allergy to PTBP. Modern production of PTBPFR is done mostly without excess PTBP[132] in the final product, so today concomitant allergy is not as common.[145]

Because formaldehyde is such a prominent sensitizer, one might assume that it is the problem in these systems. However, the data does not bear this out, at least not in most centers.

DEPIGMENTATION FROM PTBP

Depigmentation may be a complication of exposure to PTBP even without contact dermatitis, with pigment loss similar to that seen with monobenzyl ether of hydroquinone. The problem with this chemical was first noticed in Russian workers,[159,160] and it was confirmed in a number of studies.

PTBP and *p-tertiary*-amylphenol (PTAP) in phenolic germicides is known to cause such problems in hospital workers exposed to adequate concentrations. This type depigmentation is also seen in *p-tertiary*-butylcatechol, monomethyl ether of hydroquinone, and hydroquinone.[161,162] Such reactions are mostly reported from industrial exposure but may also occur from exposure to shoes, bindi adhesive,[163] or a watchband.[164]

A few cases of vitiligo with hepatitis and euthyroid gland enlargement have been reported.[165-167] PTBP can cause depigmentation indistinguishable from idiopathic vitiligo, with or without systemic signs and symptoms of hepatitis and thyroiditis. Onset varies from 2 months to several years.[168] This may start without inflammation or obvious irritation, but the more irritating concentrations are probably necessary.[171] The onset may be where locally exposed or the location may suggest systemic origin.[166,167-169] Repigmentation occurs following PTBP depigmentation, but with continued use of PTAP (in Ves-Phene with 0.8% PTAP), no return of the pigment was evident (with continued exposure). PTAP at 1% was more irritating, but depigmentation was essentially equivalent to PTBP in a concentration of 6.0% (O-Syl had a 3.0% concentration of PTBP). Kahn's[172] patients mostly experienced only a local effect, but two had lesions at distant sites. The depigmentation in O-Syl (a phenolic germicide) was probably caused by the 3% PTBP component. This chemical can also experimentally produce depigmentation without local inflammation.

WHAT ARE THE IMPLICATIONS OF THE DATA?

1. Neither PTBP nor PTBPFR alone will suffice to uncover the great majority of reactors. Adding a resol-type PFR (e.g., P-F-R-2) and perhaps monomethylol phenol to the PTBPFR in the standard series is recommended for this type problem.
2. PTBPFR is in the standard test series, so that is not a problem. Bruze found a PFR (P-F-R-2) which picked up the other reactors.
3. Methylol derivatives are major sensitizers, especially the methylene bisphenolics.
4. Guinea pig studies show multiple antigens which have not been found clinically, at least not yet.
5. These chemicals also have irritant and toxic effects, including the widely reported depigmentation effect of PTBP.

REFERENCES

1. Rietschel RL: Contact allergens in ultraviolet-cured acrylic resin systems. *Occup Med* 1:301–306, 1986.
2. Mathias CG, Maibach HI: Allergic contact dermatitis from anaerobic acrylic sealants. *Arch Dermatol* 120:1202–1205, 1984.
3. van der Walle HB, Bensink T: Cross reaction pattern of 26 acrylic monomers on guinea pig skin. *Contact Dermatitis* 8:376–382, 1982.
4. Niinimäki A, Rosberg J, Saari S: Allergic stomatitis from acrylic compounds. *Contact Dermatitis* 9:148, 1983.
5. Björkner B: The sensitizing capacity of multifunctional acrylates in the guinea pig. *Contact Dermatitis* 11:236–246, 1984.
6. Balda BR: Acrylonitril as a contact allergen *Hautarzt* 26:599, 1975.
7. Uzunova S, Kruleva P, Kolusheva T, Ikonomova Z: Cleansing of the skin of metabolic products and microorganisms by the wearing of children's outer clothing made of polyacrylonitrile fibers. *Problemi Na Khigienata* 10:108–116, 1985.
8. Björkner B, Niklasson B, Persson K: The sensitizing potential of di-(meth)acrylates based on bisphenol A or epoxy resin in the guinea pig. *Contact Dermatitis* 10:286–304, 1984.
9. Kanerva L, Jolanki R, Estlander T: Occupational dermatitis due to an epoxy acrylate. *Contact Dermatitis* 14:80–84, 1986.
10. Jolanki R: Occupational skin diseases from epoxy compounds. Epoxy resin compounds, epoxy acrylates, and 2,3-epoxypropyl trimethyl ammonium chloride. *Acta Derm Venereol Suppl* 159:1–80, 1991.
11. Björkner B: Sensitization capacity of polyester methacrylate in ultraviolet curing inks tested in the guinea pig. *Acta Derm Venereol* 62:153–154, 1982.
12. Björkner B: Sensitizing potential of urethane (meth)acrylates in the guinea pig. *Contact Dermatitis* 11:115–119, 1984.
13. Nethercott JR: Skin problems associated with multifunctional acrylic monomers in ultraviolet curing inks. *Br J Dermatol* 98:541, 1978.
14. Kanerva L, Estlander T, Jolanki R: Allergic contact dermatitis from dental composite resins due to aromatic epoxy acrylates and aliphatic acrylates. *Contact Dermatitis* 20:201–211, 1989.
15. Olveti E: Contact dermatitis from an acrylic-metal dental prosthesis. *Contact Dermatitis* 24:57, 1991.
16. Rycroft RJ: Contact dermatitis from acrylic compounds. *Br J Dermatol* 96:685–687, 1977.
17. Giunta J, Zablotsky N: Allergic stomatitis caused by self-polymerizing resin. *Oral Surg Oral Med Oral Pathol* 41:631–637, 1976.
18. Maibach H: Allergic stomatitis caused by a self-polymerizing resin (letter). *Oral Surg Oral Med Oral Pathol* 43:106–107, 1977.

19. van Joost T, van Ulsen J, van Loon LA: Contact allergy to denture materials in the burning mouth syndrome. *Contact Dermatitis* 18:97–99, 1988.

20. Kanzaki T, Kabasawa Y, Jinno T, Isayama K: Contact stomatitis due to methyl methacrylate monomer. *Contact Dermatitis* 20:146–148, 1989.

21. Simm R, Anderseck E, Seyfarth M: Allergic reaction of the oral mucosa in a patient with a synthetic denture. *Contact Dermatitis* 24:313–315, 1991.

22. Kaaber S, Thulin H, Nielsen E: Skin sensitivity to denture base materials in the burning mouth syndrome. *Contact Dermatitis* 5:90–96, 1979.

23. Fernström AI, Oquist G: Location of the allergenic monomer in warm-polymerized acrylic dentures: Part I. Causes of denture sore mouth, incidence of allergy, different allergens and test methods on suspicion of allergy to denture material—a survey of the literature. Case report, allergenic analysis of denture and test casting. *Swedish Dental J* 4:241–252, 1980.

24. Pevny I, Binzenhöfer A: Contact allergies of the oral mucosa *Zeitsch Hautkrank* 59:245–251, 1984.

25. Malten KE: Recently reported causes of contact dermatitis due to synthetic resins and hardeners. *Contact Dermatitis* 5:11–23, 1979.

26. Jacobsen N, Hensten-Pettersen A: Occupational health problems and adverse patient reactions in orthodontics. *Eur J Orthodont* 11:254–264, 1989.

27. Calnan CD: Acrylates in industry. *Contact Dermatitis* 6:53–54, 1980.

28. Björkner B, Niklasson B: Influence of the vehicle on elicitation of contact allergic reactions to acrylic compounds in the guinea pig. *Contact Dermatitis* 11:268–278, 1984.

29. Clemmensen S: Sensitizing potential of 2-hydroxyethylmethacrylate. *Contact Dermatitis* 12:203–208, 1985.

30. Jordan WP Jr: Cross-sensitization patterns in acrylate allergies. *Contact Dermatitis* 1:13–15, 1975.

31. Emmett EA: Contact dermatitis from polyfunctional acrylic monomers. *Contact Dermatitis* 3:245–248, 1977.

32. Jordan WP Jr: Cross-sensitization patterns in acrylate allergies. *Contact Dermatitis* 1:13–15, 1975.

33. Waegemaekers TH, van der Walle HB: alpha, beta-Diacryloxypropionic acid, a sensitizing impurity in commercial acrylic acid. *Dermatosen Beruf Umwelt* 32:55–58, 1984.

34. Cavelier C, Jelen G, Hervë-Bazin B, Foussereau J: Irritation and allergy to acrylates and methacrylates: Part II: Polyfunctional acrylic monomers. *Ann Dermatol Venereol* 108:559–566, 1981.

35. Chung CW, Giles AL: Sensitization potentials of methyl, ethyl, and *n*-butyl methacrylates and mutual cross-sensitivity in guinea pigs. *J Invest Dermatol* 68:187–190, 1977.

36. Björkner B: Sensitization capacity of acrylated prepolymers in ultraviolet curing inks tested in the guinea pig. *Acta Derm Venereol* 61:7–10, 1981.

37. Björkner B: Allergenicity of trimethylol propane triacrylate in ultraviolet curing inks in the guinea pig. *Acta Derm Venereol* 60:528–531, 1980.

38. Clemmensen S: Cross-reaction patterns in guinea pigs sensitized to acrylic monomers. *Drug Chem Toxicol* 7:527–540, 1984.

39. Cofield BG, Storrs FJ, Strawn CB: Contact allergy to aziridine paint hardener. *Arch Dermatol* 121:373–376, 1985.

40. Fisher AA: Identifying prosthesis components. *Arch Dermatol* 107:774, 1973.

41. Pilliar RM, Cameron HU, Macnab I: Porous surface layered prosthetic devices. *Bio-Med Eng* 10:126–131, 1975.

42. Romaguera C, Vilaplana J, Grimalt F, Ferrando J: Contact sensitivity to meth(acrylates) in a limb prosthesis. *Contact Dermatitis* 21:125, 1989.

43. Olveti E: Contact dermatitis from an acrylic-metal dental prosthesis. *Contact Dermatitis* 24:57, 1991.

44. Jacobsen N, Hensten-Pettersen A: Occupational health problems and adverse patient reactions in orthodontics. *Eur J Orthodont* 11:254–264, 1989.

45. Dahl MV, Jordan WP Jr: Hearing aid dermatitis (letter). *Arch Dermatol* 115:676, 1979.

46. Marks JG Jr, Bishop ME, Willis WF: Allergic contact dermatitis to sculptured nails. *Arch Dermatol* 115:100, 1979.

47. Goodwin P: Onycholysis due to acrylic nail applications. *Clin Exp Dermatol* 1:191–194, 1976.

48. Belsito DV: Contact dermatitis to ethyl-cyanoacrylate-containing glue. *Contact Dermatitis* 17:234–236, 1987.

49. Massone L, Anonide A, Borghi S, et al: Allergic contact dermatitis from Codivilla's spring. *Contact Dermatitis* 24:231–232, 1991.

50. Ranchoff RE, Taylor JS: Contact dermatitis to anaerobic sealants. *J Am Acad Dermatol* 13:1015–1020, 1985.

51. Jolanki R, Kanerva L, Estlander T, et al: Occupational dermatoses from epoxy resin compounds. *Contact Dermatitis* 23:172–183, 1990.

52. Kanerva L, Estlander T, Jolanki R: Allergic contact dermatitis from dental composite resins due to aromatic epoxy acrylates and aliphatic acrylates. *Contact Dermatitis* 20:201–211, 1989.

53. Waegemaekers TH, van der Walle HB: The sensitizing potential of 2-ethylhexyl acrylate in the guinea pig. *Contact Dermatitis* 9:372–376, 1983.

54. Fischer T, Maibach HI: Easier patch testing with TRUE test. *J Am Acad Dermatol* 20:447–453, 1989.

55. Waegemaekers TH, van der Walle HB: The sensitizing potential of 2-ethylhexyl acrylate in the guinea pig. *Contact Dermatitis* 9:372–376, 1983.

56. Whittington CV: Dermatitis from UV acrylate in adhesive. *Contact Dermatitis* 7:203–204, 1981.

57. Maibach H, Hjorth N, Fregert S, et al: Butyl methacrylate monomer and ethyl methacrylate monomer—frequency of reaction. *Contact Dermatitis* 4:60, 1978.

58. Bruze M, Boman A, Bergqvist-Karlsson A, et al: Contact allergy to a cyclohexanone resin in humans and guinea pigs. *Contact Dermatitis* 18:46–49, 1988.

59. Dahlquist I, Fregert S, Trulson L: Contact allergy to trimethylolpropane triacrylate (TMPTA) in an aziridine plastic hardener. *Contact Dermatitis* 9:122–124, 1983.

60. Kanerva L, Verkkala E: Electron microscopy and immunohistochemistry of toxic and allergic effects of methylmethacrylate on the skin. *Arch Toxicol Suppl* 9:456–459, 1986.

61. Pock-Steen B: Contact allergy to Nobecutan. *Contact Dermatitis* 18:52–53, 1988.

62. Hambly EM, Wilkinson DS: Contact dermatitis to butyl acrylate in spectacle frames. *Contact Dermatitis* 4:115, 1978.

63. Guerra L, Vincenzi C, Peluso AM, Tosti A: Prevalence and sources of occupational contact sensitization to acrylates in Italy. *Contact Dermatitis* 28:101–3, 1993.

64. Conde-Salazar L, Guimaraens D, Romero LV: Occupational allergic contact dermatitis from anaerobic acrylic sealants. *Contact Dermatitis* 18:129–132, 1988.

65. Mathias CG, Maibach HI: Allergic contact dermatitis from anaerobic acrylic sealants. *Arch Dermatol* 120:1202–1205, 1984.

66. Allardice JT: Dermatitis due to an acrylic resin sealer. *Trans St Johns Hosp Dermatol Soc* 53:86–89, 1967.

67. Dempsey KJ: Hypersensitivity to Sta-Lok and Loc-Tite anaerobic sealant. *J Am Acad Dermatol* 7:779–782, 1982.

68. Magnusson B, Mobacken H: Contact allergy to a self-hardening acrylic sealer for assembling metal parts. *Berufs Dermatosen* 20:198–199, 1972.

69. Fisher AA: Cross reactions between methyl methacrylate monomer and acrylic monomers presently used in acrylic nail preparations. *Contact Dermatitis* 6:345–347, 1980.

70. Fisher AA: Adverse nail reactions and paresthesia from "photobonded acrylate 'sculptured' nails." *Cutis* 45:293–294, 1990.

71. Fisher AA: Permanent loss of fingernails due to allergic reaction to an acrylic nail preparation: A sixteen-year follow-up study. *Cutis* 43:404–406, 1989.

72. Baran RL, Schibli H: Permanent paresthesia to sculptured nails: A distressing problem. *Dermatol Clin* 8:139–141, 1990.

73. Mathias CGT, Caldwell TM, Maibach HI: Contact dermatitis and gastrointestinal symptoms from hydroxyethyl methacrylate. *Br J Dermatol* 100:447–449, 1979.

74. Maibach H, Hjorth N, Fregert S, et al: Butyl methacrylate monomer and ethyl methacrylate monomer—frequency of reaction. *Contact Dermatitis* 4:60, 1978.

75. Belsito DV: Contact dermatitis to ethyl-cyanoacrylate-containing glue. *Contact Dermatitis* 17:234–236, 1987.

76. Foussereau J, Cavelier C, Protois JP, Deviller J: Contact dermatitis from methyl methacrylate in an above-knee prosthesis. *Contact Dermatitis* 20:69–70, 1989.

77. Romaguera C, Grimalt F, Villaplana J, Mascaro JM: Contact dermatitis caused by Septopal. *Med Cutan Ibero-Latino-Americana* 14:43–47, 1986.

78. Clementi D, Surace A, Celestini M, Pietrogrande V: Clinical investigations of tolerance to materials and acrylic cement in patients with hip prostheses. *Ital J Orthop Traumatol* 6:97–104, 1980.

79. Emmett EA, Kominsky JR: Allergic contact dermatitis from ultraviolet cured inks: Allergic contact sensitization to acrylates. *J Occup Med* 19:113–115, 1977.

80. Widström L: Contact allergy to acrylate monomer in a printing plate. *Contact Dermatitis* 8:68–69, 1982.

81. Björkner B, Dahlquist I: Contact allergy caused by UV-cured acrylates. *Contact Dermatitis* 5:403–404, 1979.

82. Björkner B, Niklasson B, Persson K: The sensitizing potential of di-(meth)acrylates based on bisphenol A or epoxy resin in the guinea pig. *Contact Dermatitis* 10:286–304, 1984.

83. Beurey J, Mougeolle JM, Weber M: Cutaneous manifestations due to acrylic resins used in printing. *Ann Dermatol Syphil* 103:423–430, 1976.

84. Pedersen NB, Senning A, Nielsen AO: Different sensitizing acrylic monomers in Napp printing plate. *Contact Dermatitis* 9:459–464, 1983.

85. Calas E, Castelain PY, Lapointe HR, et al: Allergic contact dermatitis to a photopolymerizable resin used in printing. *Contact Dermatitis* 3:186–194, 1977.

86. Tilsley DA: Contact and photo-dermatitis from Nyloprint. *Contact Dermatitis* 1:334–335, 1975.

87. Nethercott JR, Gupta S, Rosen C, et al: Tetraethylene glycol diacrylate: A cause of delayed cutaneous irritant reaction and allergic contact dermatitis. *J Occup Med* 26:513–516, 1984.

88. Nethercott JR, Jakubovic HR, Pilger C, Smith JW: Allergic contact dermatitis due to urethane acrylate in ultraviolet cured inks. *Br J Indust Med* 40:241–250, 1983.

89. Rietschel RL, Huggins R, Levy N, Pruitt PM: In vivo and in vitro testing of gloves for protection against UV-curable acrylate resin systems. *Contact Dermatitis* 11:279–282, 1984.

90. Pegum JS, Medhurst FA: Contact dermatitis from penetration of rubber gloves by acrylic monomer. *Br Med J* 2:141–143, 1971.

91. Rietschel RL, Huggins R, Levy N, Pruitt PM: In vivo and in vitro testing of gloves for protection against UV-curable acrylate resin systems. *Contact Dermatitis* 11:279–282, 1984.

92. Fisher AA: Management of hairdressers sensitized to hair dyes or permanent wave solutions. *Cutis* 43:316–318, 1989.

93. Darre E, Vedel P, Jensen JS: Skin protection against methylmethacrylate. *Acta Orthop Scand* 58:236–238, 1987.

94. Björkner B: The sensitizing capacity of multifunctional acrylates in the guinea pig. *Contact Dermatitis* 11:236–264, 1984.

95. Björkner B: Contact allergy to 2-hydroxypropyl methacrylate (2-HPMA) in an ultraviolet curable ink. *Acta Derm Venereol* 64:264–267, 1984.

96. Tobler M, Wüthrich B, Freiburghaus AU: Contact dermatitis from acrylate and methacrylate compounds in Lowicryl embedding media for electron microscopy. *Contact Dermatitis* 23:96–102, 1990.

97. Vilaplana J, Romaguera C, Grimalt F: Allergic contact dermatitis from aliphatic isocyanate on spectacle frames. *Contact Dermatitis* 16:113, 1987.

98. White IR, Stewart JR, Rycroft RJ: Allergic contact dermatitis from an organic di-isocyanate. *Contact Dermatitis* 9:300–303, 1983.

99. Helland S, Nyfors A, Utne L: *Contact dermatitis* to Synthaderm. *Contact Dermatitis* 9:504–506, 1983.

100. Fasani F, Pisati A, La Manna A: Allergic risk factors in wood working. *G Ital Med Lavoro* 4:211–214, 1982.

101. Malten KE: Recently reported causes of contact dermatitis due to synthetic resins and hardeners. *Contact Dermatitis* 5:11–23, 1979.

102. Hjorth N: Dermatitis from trimethyl hexamethylene diisocyanate. *Contact Dermatitis* 1:59, 1975.

103. Vale PT, Rycroft RJ: Occupational irritant contact dermatitis from fiberboard containing urea-formaldehyde resin. *Contact Dermatitis* 19:62, 1988.

104. Hjorth N, Fregert S: Sensitivity to formaldehyde and formaldehyde resins. *Contact Dermatitis Newsletter* 2:18, 1967.

105. Ross JS, Rycroft RJ, Cronin E: Melamine-formaldehyde contact dermatitis in orthopaedic practice. *Contact Dermatitis* 26:203–204, 1992.

106. Logan WS, Perry HO: Cast dermatitis due to formaldehyde sensitivity. *Arch Dermatol* 106:717–721, 1972.

107. Fregert S: Formaldehyde dermatitis from a gypsum-melamine resin mixture. *Contact Dermatitis* 7:56, 1981.

108. Hatch KL, Maibach HI: Textile fiber dermatitis. *Contact Dermatitis* 12:1–11, 1985.

109. Grimalt F, Romaguera C, Piñol Aguade J: Contact dermatitis caused by plastic pockets on trouser. *Med Cutan Ibero-Latino-Americana* 4:7–14, 1976.

110. Grimalt F, Romaguera C: Contact dermatitis caused by polyamide trouser pockets. *Dermatosen Beruf Umwelt* 29:35–39, 1981.

111. Prassus MN: Bullous dermatitis of the feet caused by pure nylon (in French). *Bull Soc Franc Derm Syph* 62:508, 1955.

112. Morris GE: Nylon dermatitis. *N Engl J Med* 263:30–32, 1960.

113. Morris GE: Nylon dermatitis. *Berufs Dermatosen* 8:155–160, 1960.

114. Jansson H: On the question of the occurrence of sensitivity to perlon and nylon based substances. *Zertschr Haut Gschlkr* 26:37–39, 1959.

115. Braitman M: Dermatitis and fabrics. *J Med Soc NJ* 52:575–579, 1955.

116. Martin-Scott I: Contact textile dermatitis. *Br J Dermatol* 632–635, 1966.

117. Dooms-Goossens A, Duron C, Loncke J, Degreef H: Contact urticaria due to nylon. *Contact Dermatitis* 14:63, 1986.

118. Müller EM: Urticaria externa und urticarielle dermatitis durch perlon hufthalter. *Z Hautkr* 16:5, 1954.

119. Smith EL, Meara RH: Allergic dermatitis from sellotape. *Br Med J* 2:239, 1966.

120. Jordan WP, Dahl MV: Contact dermatitis from cellulose ester plastics. *Arch Dermatol* 105:880–885, 1972.

121. Jordan WP Jr: Resorcinol monobenzoate, steering wheels, Peruvian balsam. *Arch Dermatol* 108:278, 1973.

122. Cronin E: *Contact Dermatitis*. Churchill-Livingstone, Edinburgh 1982.

123. Estlander T, Jolanki R, Kanerva L: Dermatitis and urticaria from rubber and plastic gloves. *Contact Dermatitis* 14:20–25, 1986.

124. Frosch PJ, Born CM, Schütz R: Contact allergy to rubber, surgical and vinyl gloves. *Hautarzt* 38:210–217, 1987.

125. Jolanki R, Kanerva L, Estlander T: Organic pigments in plastics can cause allergic contact dermatitis. *Acta Derm Venereol Suppl* 134:95–97, 1987.

126. Schwartz L: Dermatitis from synthetic resins. *J Invest Dermatol* 6:239–255, 1945.

127. Malten KE: Occupational dermatoses in the processing of plastics. *Trans St Johns Hosp Dermatol Soc* 59:78–113, 1973.

128. Mellström G: Protective gloves of polymeric materials: Experimental permeation testing and clinical study of side effects. *Acta Derm Venereol Suppl* 163:1–54, 1991.

129. Bruze M: Contact dermatitis from phenol formaldehyde resins, in Maibach HI (ed): *Occupational and Industrial Dermatology*. Chicago, Year Book Medical Publishers, 1986, pp 430–435.

130. Cronin E. *Contact Dermatitis*. Edinburgh, Churchill-Livingstone, 1980.

131. Bruze M: Contact sensitizers in resins based on phenol and formaldehyde. *Acta Derm Venereol Suppl* 119:1–83, 1985.

132. Malten KE: Occupational dermatoses in the processing of plastics. *Trans St Johns Hosp Dermatol Soc* 59:78–113, 1973.

133. Malten KE: Old and new, mainly occupational dermatological problems in the production and processing of plastics, in Maibach HI (ed): *Occupational and Industrial Dermatology*. Chicago, Year Book Medical Publishers, 1986, pp 290–340.

134. Rycroft RJ: Contact sensitization to 2-monomethylol phenol in phenol formaldehyde resin as an example of the recognition and prevention of industrial dermatoses. *Clin Exp Dermatol* 7:285–290, 1982.

135. Bruze M, Zimerson E: Contact allergy to 3-methylol phenol, 2,4-dimethylol phenol and 2,6-dimethylol phenol. *Acta Derm Venereol* 65:548–551, 1985.

136. Bruze M, Fregert S, Persson L, Zimerson E: Contact allergy to 4,4'-dihydroxy-(hydroxymethyl)-diphenyl methanes: Sensitizers in a phenol-formaldehyde resin. *J Invest Dermatol* 87:617–623, 1986.

137. Bruze M, Fregert S, Zimerson E: Contact allergy to phenol-formaldehyde resins. *Contact Dermatitis* 12:81–86, 1985.

138. Bruze M: Detection of contact allergy to phenol formaldehyde resins. *Contact Dermatitis* 14:127, 1986.

139. Bruze M, Persson L, Trulsson L, Zimerson E: Demonstration of contact sensitizers in resins and products based on phenol-formaldehyde. *Contact Dermatitis* 14:146–154, 1986.

140. Bruze M: Patch testing with a mixture of 2 phenol-formaldehyde resins. *Contact Dermatitis* 19:116–119, 1988.

141. Angelini G, Vena GA, Meneghini CL: Shoe contact dermatitis. *Contact Dermatitis* 6:279–283, 1980.

142. Adams RM: "Spontaneous flare" to *p-tert*-butylphenol formaldehyde resin. *Contact Dermatitis* 1:321, 1975.

143. Geldof BA, Roesyanto ID, van Joost T: Clinical aspects of *para-tertiary*-butylphenolformaldehyde resin (PTBP-FR) allergy. *Contact Dermatitis* 21:312–315, 1989.

144. Barros MA, Baptista A, Correia TM, Azevedo F: Patch testing in children: A study of 562 schoolchildren. *Contact Dermatitis* 25:156–159, 1991.
145. Malten KE, Seutter E: Allergenic degradation products of *para-tertiary* butylphenolformaldehyde plastic. *Contact Dermatitis* 12:222–224, 1985.
146. Rycroft RJ, Wilkinson JD, Holmes R, Hay RJ: Contact sensitization to *p-tertiary* butylphenol (PTBP) resin in plastic nail adhesive. *Clin Exp Dermatol* 5:441–445, 1980.
147. Malten KE: Occupational eczema due to *p-tertiary* butylphenol in a shoe adhesive. *Dermatologica* 117:103, 1958.
148. Malten KE, Seutter E: Phenolformaldehyde resin in paper. *Contact Dermatitis* 11:127–128, 1984.
149. Romaguera C, Grimalt F, Vilaplana J: *Paratertiary* butylphenol formaldehyde resin in prosthesis. *Contact Dermatitis* 12:174, 1985.
150. Foussereau J, Petitjean J, Barre JG: Eczema due to wristwatch bands induced by allergy to formol-p.t. butylphenol resins of leather glue (resins of the C.K.R. 1634 type). *Bull Soc Francaise Dermatol Syphil* 75:630–635, 1968.
151. Foussereau J, Cavelier C, Selig D: Occupational eczema from *para-tertiary*-butylphenol formaldehyde resins: A review of the sensitizing resins. *Contact Dermatitis* 2:254–258, 1976.
152. Dahlquist I: Contact allergy to *para-tertiary* butylphenol formaldehyde resin in an adhesive label. *Contact Dermatitis* 10:54, 1984.
153. Hjorth N, Fregert S: Sensitivity to formaldehyde and formaldehyde resins. *Contact Dermatitis Newsletter* 2:18–19, 1967.
154. Gaul LE: Absence of formaldehyde sensitivity in phenol-formaldehyde resin dermatitis. *J Invest Dermatol* 48:485–486, 1967.
155. Bruze M: Simultaneous reactions to phenol-formaldehyde resins colophony/hydroabietyl alcohol and balsam of Peru/perfume mixture. *Contact Dermatitis* 14:119–120, 1986.
156. Bruze M: Sensitizers in PTBP-formaldehyde resins (letter). *Contact Dermatitis* 14:132–133, 1986.
157. Foussereau J, Cavelier C, Selig D: Occupational eczema from *para-tertiary*-butylphenol formaldehyde resins: A review of the sensitizing resins. *Contact Dermatitis* 2:254–258, 1976.
158. Fregert S: Batch-consciousness in dermatologic management. *Acta Derm Venereol* 59(suppl 85):63–65, 1979.
159. Chumakov NN, Babanov GP, Smirnov AG: Vitiliginous dermatoses in working with phenol-formaldehyde resins. *Bulletin of Dermatology.* Moscow, State publishing firm of Medical Literature, 1962.
160. Bobanov GP, Chumakov NN: Etiology and pathogenesis of occupational vitiligo. *Vestn Dermatol Vener* 11:44–48, 1966.
161. Stevenson CJ: Occupational vitiligo: Clinical and epidemiological aspects. *Br J Dermatol* 105(suppl 21):51–56, 1981.
162. Romaguera C, Grimalt F: Occupational leukoderma and contact dermatitis from *para-tertiary*-butylphenol. *Contact Dermatitis* 7:159–160, 1981.
163. Mathur AK, Srivastava AK, Singh A, Gupta BN: Contact depigmentation by adhesive material of bindi. *Contact Dermatitis* 24:310–311, 1991.
164. Malten KE: Paratertiary butylphenol depigmentation in a "consumer." *Contact Dermatitis* 1:181–182, 1975.
165. Budde J, Stary A: Skin and systemic disease caused by occupational contact with *p-tert*-butylphenol: Case reports. *Dermatosen Beruf Umwelt* 36:17–19, 1988.
166. Rodermund OE, Wieland H: Vitiligo, hepato-splenomegaly, and goitre after working with *para-tertiary* butylphenol. *Deutsche Med Wochensch* 100:2216–2222, 1975.
167. Goldmann PJ, Thiess AM: Occupational vitiligo caused by *paratertiary*-butylphenol, a triad of vitiligo, hepatosis and struma. *Hautarzt* 27:155–159, 1976.
168. Malten KE, Seutter E, Hara I, Nakajima T: Occupational vitiligo due to *paratertiary* butylphenol and homologues. *Trans St Johns Hosp Dermatol Soc* 57:115–134, 1971.
169. Kahn G: Depigmentation caused by phenolic detergent germicides. *Arch Dermatol* 102:177–187, 1970.

37

METAL ALLERGY

Jyoti B. Burruss
Joseph F. Fowler

The metals that most commonly cause allergic contact dermatitis (ACD) are nickel, chrome, and cobalt. In addition, many other metals have occasionally been shown to cause ACD, although with a much lower incidence than the first three. Gold and palladium have been responsible for ACD from jewelry and sometimes industrial exposure. Platinum may cause ACD in industrial settings as well as allergic and irritant respiratory problems. Many metals and metal salts are irritating to the skin, even in the absence of ACD, and may be irritating to the mucous membranes and respiratory tract as well.

Nickel is by far the most common metal allergen and is more often a problem in women than in men. This is possibly related to the wearing of jewelry, especially pierced earrings. In nature, cobalt is frequently found along with nickel and therefore is frequently present in metal objects that contain nickel, either intentionally or accidentally. In addition, cobalt is commonly used in many other metal alloys and in clay and pottery. It may be present in manufacturing processes for paint, polyester resins, glass, pigments. In contrast, chromate is not normally found in hard metal objects but is found in the form of chromium salts which are present in cement, concrete, and similar construction materials. It is also used to tan leather goods.

Patients with known metal allergies will find the information in Table 37-1 useful in preventing exacerbations of their dermatitis. They may also benefit from the sources (addresses and phone numbers) of companies/suppliers of products made specifically for metal-sensitive individuals. This information may be found in Table 37-2.

INCIDENCE AND PREVALENCE

NICKEL (see also Chap. 29)

The incidence of nickel allergy has increased over the years, especially among young females. The overall rate of positive patch tests to nickel was 6.7 percent in 1976 and

TABLE 37–1. Preventing/Avoiding Contact with Sensitizing Metals

Various measures can be employed to decrease contact with known sensitizers.

Nickel

Ears should be pierced only with hypoallergenic surgical steel parts.

Avoid wearing pierced earrrings if any inflammation develops.

Clear nail polish can be used to coat jewelry and clothing buttons, etc. This should be repeated weekly to maintain the barrier.

A jeweler can plate the jewelry with rhodium or platinum (not palladium).

All metal jewelry or objects with which prolonged contact occurs should be tested with the DMG spot test.

Keys can be made of aluminum instead of nickel.

Cobalt

Essentially the same principles used for nickel apply.

Chromates

Wear only vegetable-tanned leather or nonleather shoes (e.g., plastic or canvas).

Wear heavy socks if leather shoes are unavoidable.

Change the shoes and socks often to inhibit perspiration effects.

Wear cotton gloves under leather work gloves; change them often.

Use Aliplast, Dr. Scholl's, or other shoe liner between the skin and the leather parts.

Avoid direct contact with the skin of cement and other similar construction materials.

Add ferrous sulfate (which complexes with the chromates) to cement during use.

TABLE 37–2. Sources of Products Helpful to Metal-Sensitive Individuals

Skin and Allergy Shop
310 East Broadway
Louisville, KY 40202
800-366-6483
Suppliers of a wide range of products for skin and respiratory allergy sufferers including protective cotton gloves, DMG test, Aliplast shoe liners, hypoallergenic cosmetics, nickel free jewelry (Whispers earrings), Happy Feet shoes (plastic shoes), etc.

Allerderm Laboratories
P.O. Box 931
Mill Valley, CA 94942-0931
800-365-6868
Supply the DMG spot test (Allertest NI), cotton gloves, and 4H gloves.

Dermatologic Lab and Supply, Inc.
608 13th Avenue
Council Bluffs, IA 51507
800-831-6273
Supply the DMG spot test, gloves, etc.

Roman Research
33 Riverside Drive
Pembroke, MA 02359-1910
800-451-5700
Makers of Whispers earrings.

Happy Feet
P.O. Box 1417
Corona, CA 0666
714-674-0666
Supply plastic shoes without leather additives.

9.1 percent in 1986 in one study.[1] Women are affected much more commonly than men. Various studies have shown female-to-male ratio of ACD to nickel to be anywhere from 2:1 up to 10:1. In two different studies, the incidence of nickel hypersensitivity was 15 percent and 20 percent among teenage girls with pierced ears; only 2 percent of the patients without pierced ears were affected.[2,3] In girls with more than one hole per earlobe, the incidence was 35 percent, compared with 16 percent in those with only one hole.[3] In men, occupational exposure seems to be a greater risk factor. As more men pierce their ears, an increase in nickel allergy may be seen among males. Based on logistic regression statistical techniques to analyze for multiple variables, individual risk factors for positive patch tests to nickel sensitivity are sex (female), age (0 to 29 years), absence of atopy, and a history of eczema (usually hand eczema).[4]

COBALT

Data on the incidence of cobalt sensitization is somewhat lacking, at least in the United States, since it is not among the agents commonly tested. However European data show that simultaneous reactions to nickel and cobalt do occur, also with a greater female preponderance.[5] The incidence of cobalt sensitization roughly parallels that of nickel, although at a lower level. A prior history of nickel sensitivity may increase the risk of subsequent cobalt sensitization.[6] The risk is greater in the younger population (0 to 29 years old) among females; among males, slightly older persons (30 to 59 years old) are affected.[4] Although many cobalt-sensitive individuals are also allergic to nickel, up to 30 percent of those with a positive patch test to cobalt may be negative to nickel.

CHROMATE (see also Chap. 27)

Chromate allergy is seen somewhat more commonly in men, presumably because of occupational exposure from construction materials. In addition, chromate positivity is found more often in older individuals than in younger age groups. This either suggests that prevention strategies (such as adding iron sulfate to cement to reduce the level of free chromates) are worthwhile in protecting against chromate allergy or that long-term exposure is needed before chromate allergy is likely to develop.

SUSPECTING A METAL ALLERGY

The most classic clinical presentation of metal allergy is jewelry dermatitis; among the types of jewelry, earrings seem to be the greatest culprit. Presumably this is because the pierced earring actually penetrates the epidermal barrier, allowing potential exposure to tissue fluids at the time of piercing and again thereafter should trauma or infection occur. Some metal-sensitive individuals react only to earrings and are able to wear rings, necklaces, or other jewelry without difficulty. Wristwatch buckles and bands and eyeglass frames should not be forgotten as likely causes of metal jewelry dermatitis (Figs. 37-1 and 37-2).

There is a high correlation of positive history and patch testing in nickel hypersensitiv-

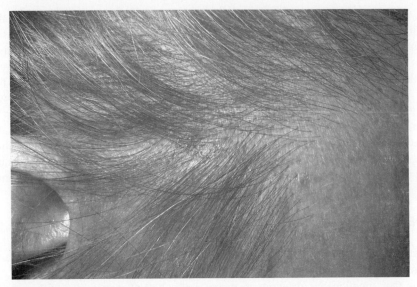

FIG. 37–1. Contact dermatitis to nickel in the scalp.

ity. There is a poor correlation however, of positive patch tests to nickel in atopics giving a history of metal allergy.[2] A negative test to nickel in a patient suspected of metal allergy may be accounted for in several ways: (1) cobalt, gold, or another metal may be the true culprit; (2) poor patch-testing technique, such as use of outdated allergens or failure to perform a delayed reading, may give a false-negative result; or (3) some other entity such as irritant or seborrheic dermatitis may be the actual diagnosis, rather than ACD.

The distribution of the dermatitis may give insight as to the type of metal allergy.

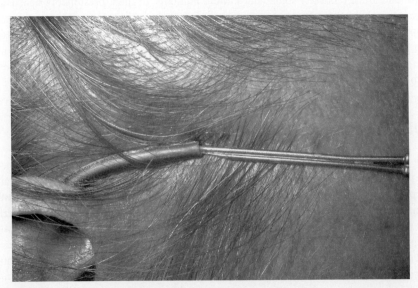

FIG. 37–2. The frames of the eyeglasses fit over the area in Fig. 37-1.

TABLE 37–3. Sites and Sources of Nickel Dermatitis

Location	Nickel Source
Scalp	Hairpins, curlers, and bobby pins
Eyelids	Eyelash curler
Earlobes	Earrings
Backs of ears	Eyeglass frames
Sides of face	Bobby pins, curlers, dental instruments, transfer from hands
Lips	Metal pins held in mouth and in metal lipstick holder
Neck	Clasp of necklace and zipper
Upper chest	Medallions and metal identification tags
Abdomen	Metal buttons on blue jeans
Breast	Wire brassiere support
Thighs	Garter clasps, metal chairs, and metal coins in pockets, etc.
Palms	Handles of doors, handbags, metal tools or parts in workplace
Fingers	Rings, thimbles, needles, scissors, coins and pens, paper clips, etc.
Wrist	Watchbands, bracelets, metal buttons
Arms	Bracelets
Ankles	Bracelets
Dorsum of foot	Metal eyelet of shoes
Leg	Zipper of boots

Table 37-3 relates the location of the dermatitis to the possible source of nickel resulting in the dermatitis.[6] Earlobe dermatitis is very suggestive of a contact hypersensitivity to nickel in jewelry. The hands tend to be involved more frequently in males. Occupational histories should be elicited in all cases of hand eczema, especially in males, as this is more often the source of exposure (Fig. 37-3).

The type of reaction may be helpful in suspecting an allergic contact dermatitis to metals. The lesions are most commonly eczematous but may occasionally be papular, urticarial, bullous, or of the pompholyx type. Granulomatous lesions may also occur, especially in gold allergy. The lesions may be confined to the specific site of contact or may spread from direct touch or as a secondary id reaction. Most patients complain of pruritus, which tends to be especially severe in the pompholyx variants.

A history of waxing and waning dermatitis at various times or seasons may be a helpful clue. Symptoms are often worse during times of increased perspiration. This occurs because sweat can cause the leaching or dissolving of chemicals out of the metal. The use of powders (talcum or other) under the jewelry or object in question can help for short periods of time by creating an absorbent barrier.[6] Black dermographism is a common discoloration that can occur under jewelry from the reaction of sulfides and chlorides in perspiration with the gold alloy. This may be more common at times of hormonal changes, such as pregnancy. This is a discoloration or smudging and should not be mistaken for an allergic reaction.[6]

Chromate allergy usually manifests itself as either foot dermatitis due to shoe leather or hand dermatitis due to chromates in cement or other building materials. Most leather is tanned in chromate solution. Therefore, any leather object such as a wallet, belt, pair of gloves, etc. may be implicated in chromate allergy. Chromates are present in cement, drywall, plaster, and similar building materials. Hand dermatitis from chromate exposure may become persistent even after all contact to the allergen is stopped, presenting a frustrating challenge to both the physician and patient. Some cosmetics

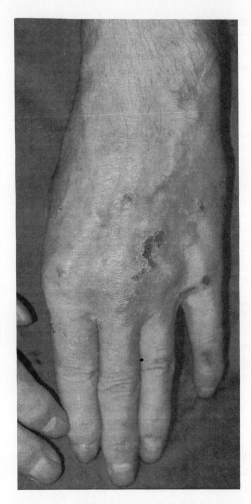

FIG. 37–3. Reaction to spicules of metal containing cobalt in a cobalt-allergic metal worker. (See color Plate 29.)

contain chromium as a coloring agent (e.g., chrome green) and may therefore cause a facial dermatitis in chrome-allergic patients.

PATCH TESTING/INTRADERMAL TESTING

Patch testing is very important in documenting the presence of a metal allergy. The common metals and the various concentrations used for patch testing are shown in Table 37-4.[1]

Patch tests with metals may be difficult to interpret because of irritant reactions. A strong nickel reaction has been suggested to cause an "angry back" reaction when tested near other metals, although this has not been conclusively proven. It is therefore recommended that patch tests be placed at least 6 in apart if a strong reaction is anticipated, so as to decrease false-positive reactions.

Intradermal testing is not often needed but has been used in some cases of negative patch tests. The indications for intradermal testing in doubtful cases of metal contact

TABLE 37–4. Suggested Patch-Test Concentrations

Concentrations	Comment
Nickel Nickel sulfate, 2.5% pet	Even at this concentration, occasional nonallergic pustular reactions may occur
Cobalt Cobalt chloride, 1% pet	A nonallergic "poral" reaction that resembles a sprinkling of cayenne pepper is not unusual

Chromate
  Potassium dichromate,
    0.25% pet
	A higher concentration will give more positives, but many will be irritant false-positives

Gold
  Gold sodium thiosulfate,
    0.5% pet
  Gold sodium thiomalate,
    1.0% pet
	Persistent (2–3 weeks) reactions may occur

hypersensitivity include (1) difficult-to-interpret patch test at 72 h or later, (2) negative patch tests to various metals with a positive history of a metal allergy, and (3) the need to confirm a doubtful patch test.[7]

Even in cases where metal allergy is highly probable on clinical grounds, patch testing should be performed for complete documentation. This will aid in reinforcing the exact nature of the dermatitis and may increase compliance in avoidance of contact with the specific metal. If occupational exposure is the source and a change of occupation may be necessary, documentation of the allergen(s) is critical for medical/legal purposes.

DIETARY ROLE

The dietary role of nickel in metal hypersensitivity has been highly researched.[8–10] It is apparent that flares of pompholyx can be induced with oral nickel challenge and can be prevented or attenuated with a diet low in nickel. Veien states that reduction of nickel intake by 50 percent has helped a number of his patients (personal communication). However, the practicality of diet modification is variable, depending on the patient's willingness to take the necessary measures. It is also difficult because the nickel content of various foods can vary greatly. Further complicating this issue is variable absorption of nickel from the gastrointestinal tract and individual variations in immunologic state. Patients may be referred to a dietician if a low-nickel diet is to be attempted or may use the lists in Table 37-5.[8] Also supporting the hypothesis that dietary nickel is relevant to flares of hand eczema are studies in which the use of disulfiram (a chelating agent) has resulted in improvement.

Dietary chromates as well as cobalt may aggravate the dermatitis in allergic individuals. See Table 37-6 for foods high in these metals.[6]

OCCUPATIONAL EXPOSURE

Men have a greater frequency of sensitization to nickel at work than women. Cobalt is also a cause of ACD in the workplace in some individuals. Wet work tends to

TABLE 37-5. Foods High in Nickel

Baking powder
Cocoa/chocolate
Gelatin
Kippered herring
Nuts (walnuts, almonds, hazelnuts)
Oats
Peas
Red kidney beans
Rye
Soya beans/legumes
Tea
Whole wheat
Canned foods are higher in nickel than fresh-
food equivalents

increase the likelihood of a sensitization. The sources of and occupations at risk for exposure are listed in Tables 37-7 and 37-8[11] for nickel and in Tables 37-9 and 37-10 for cobalt.[6] Rubber gloves are relatively protective against exposure to nickel, but vinyl gloves are not as protective.

TABLE 37-6. Foods High in Cobalt

Apricots	Coffee
Beans	Liver
Beer	Nuts
Beets	Scallops
Cabbage	Tea
Cloves	Whole-grain flour
Cocoa/chocolate	

TABLE 37-7. Some Sources of Occupational Exposure to Nickel

Alkaline batteries
Blackening zinc and brass
Ceramics
Coatings (electroplating)
Duplicating fluids and fluxes (brazing)
Dyes
Electrical wiring
Enamel (green: nickel oxides)
Fuel additives
Hardening of fats (acts as a catalyst)
Insecticides
Magnet cores
Mordant in dyeing and printing fabrics
Nickel alloys
Nickel plating
Paint for glass
Pigments for wallpaper and paint
Reagents and catalysts (plastics)

**TABLE 37–8. Jobs at Risk
for Nickel Exposure**

Metal workers
Electroplater
Hairdresser
Nurse, medical or dental assistant
Tailor
Cook, waitress
Cleaning person
Office worker
Electronics worker
Dairy worker
Librarian
Chemical cleaner
Engine fitter
Locksmith
Chemical worker
Electrician
Construction worker

**TABLE 37–9. Sources
of Cobalt Exposure**

Paint
Cement
Pottery
Ceramics
Pigments
Glass alloys
Lubricating alloys
Bricklayers
Hair dyes of light brown shades
Printing ink
Vitamin B_{12}

**TABLE 37–10. Jobs at Risk
for Cobalt Exposure**

Masons
Tile workers
Dentists
Printers
Mechanics
Machinists
Workers in galvanizing industry
Polyester resin workers
Workers with hard metal
Construction workers

DIMETHYLGLYOXIME TEST

Important to treatment success is patient recognition of objects containing the metals to which they have a specific ACD. Nickel-sensitive patients should be made aware of the dimethylglyoxime (DMG) spot test to detect the presence of nickel in jewelry, household utensils, etc. The spot-test kit can be obtained from multiple sources (Table 37-2). It contains 1% DMG in alcohol solution and 10% ammonium hydroxide. A positive reaction indicates the presence of available nickel in a concentration of at least 1:10,000. The test chemicals do not harm the item being tested.

OTHER METAL ALLERGIES

ALUMINUM

Contact sensitivity to aluminum is uncommon but rather easily suspected because reactions occur to all Finn chambers in a ringlike pattern (Fig. 37-4). It may be secondary to aluminum precipitated immunization materials[97] or deodorants,[98] and it may be an accidental finding on patch testing which has no clinical relevance.[99,100]

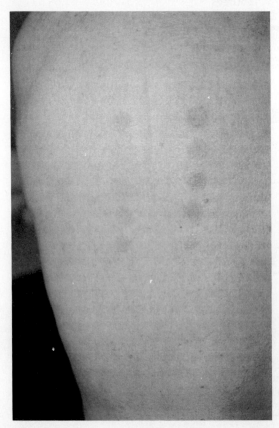

FIG. 37–4. Aluminum reaction to Finn chambers. All chambers caused a ringed eruption where contact occurred. (See color Plate 30.)

BERYLLIUM

Beryllium is used in alloys for electrical equipment, in pottery, and in dental metals to refine the granular structure.[29] It is also used to lower the casting temperature in the casting of metals.[30] It has been used in manufacture of grenz ray tubes and fluorescent lamps as well as microwave equipment.

Beryllium in the maximization test is a grade 4 (strong) sensitizer.[31] Acute reactions to beryllium include papules, pustules and vesicles, conjunctivitis, rhinitis, pharyngitis, and bronchitis. The insoluble form causes granulomas, while the soluble salts can cause contact sensitization,[30] but both seem to be forms of delayed hypersensitivity.[32]

There are reports of both gingivitis[30] and stomatitis from dental metals and hand eczema in a dental technician.[29] Contact sensitization was also reported to follow an orthopedic implant, but a causal relationship was not proved.[29]

Patch testing is often done in either a metals series or a dental series using 1% aqueous[30] or in petrolatum.[29]

CADMIUM

Cadmium is used as a corrosion inhibitor, plastics stabilizer, in certain batteries, as a neutron brake in atomic piles, in dye production, and in photochemistry.[33] Rudzki et al.[34] found no reactors in two plants examined, although a number of the workers were allergic to other allergens. Reactions to patch testing at a 2% concentration are likely to be irritant and patch tests to 1% concentration are seldom positive.[34] Wahlberg and Boman[35] found no relevant history in 25 patients who reacted to a 2% (aqueous) concentration. Only one also responded to the 1% concentration. Kaaber et al.[35a] found a number of reactors at a 2% concentration, but such reactions were likely irritant, as only one reacted at 1% concentration and the 2% reactions were difficult to reproduce on retesting. Cadmium chloride is a weak sensitizer in the guinea pig maximization test.[36]

Raith et al.[37] found a locksmith who reacted to cadmium as low as 0.5% concentration, and he had been exposed to a zinc alloy which contained cadmium. He was not zinc-allergic, but he was allergic to epoxy. It may have been a concomitant reaction.

Cadmium sulfide produces a bright yellow tattoo pigment which Björnberg[38] investigated in Swedish sailors. The yellow color was found in the Swedish flag, butterflies, and flowers and it tended to cause a phototoxic reaction in the tropics. The wavelength responsible was 380 to 450 nm. Cadmium sulfide is sometimes added to mercuric sulfide in red tattoos to increase the brightness of the (red) color, and this substance can cause a photoallergic reaction.[39,40]

COPPER

Copper is perhaps best known for its tendency to turn blond hair green in swimming pools.[41] It is found in tap water from copper pipes,[42] spectacles,[43,44] a copper-contaminated natural hair dye,[45] and brass (copper and zinc) manufacture.[46] It may produce reactions following tap water exposure and permanent waving.[47] It may also cause nail pigmentation.[48] Sensitization may occur in the ceramics industry,[33] but it is perhaps best known in dental amalgams,[49] where it is one cause of oral lichen planus[50] (see

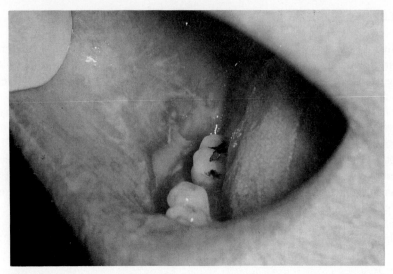

FIG. 37–5. Erosive oral lichen planus in a patient allergic to copper in his dental amalgams. (See color Plate 31.)

Figs. 37-5 and 37-6). Romaguera and Grimalt[51] and Barranco[52] reported what was probably systemic contact dermatitis and pruritus from copper sensitivity induced by an intrauterine contraceptive device.

Karlberg et al.[53] found copper to be a weak sensitizer. Because copper sulfate 2% in petrolatum can be irritant and because the responses seemed not to be relevant, they recommended that positive reactions be confirmed by testing to dilutions, 2%, 1%, 0.5%, 0.25%, and 0.125%. The metal itself is not suitable for patch testing because it is poorly released by sweat.[54]

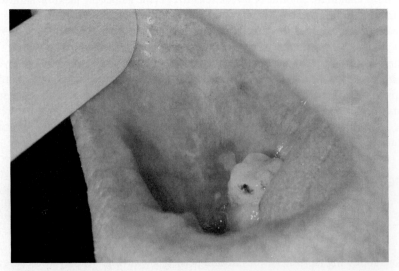

FIG. 37–6. Clearing of the erosive lichen planus following removal of the copper-containing dental metals.

GOLD

The number of reported cases of allergic contact dermatitis to gold is low.[12-17] Gold is an inert metal and relatively insoluble but must be considered as a possible allergen in ACD to jewelry. A concomitant or primary nickel dermatitis should be investigated, since allergy to nickel occurs in over 50 percent of patients with gold allergy. Even expensive gold jewelry may contain some nickel. A dermatitis under a gold ring may also be due to primary irritation from trauma, accumulation of detergents, or the corrosive action of salts.[15] Oral stomatitis has also been reported to gold dental materials.[12] A DMG spot test is again helpful in this situation. If patch testing is done, gold salts should be used, since testing with metallic gold may produce a false-negative result.[12] Since most investigators do not patch test to gold routinely, the actual incidence of gold allergy is uncertain. It occurs often enough in persons exposed, however, to suggest that patch testing with gold should be done more often.[17a]

Gold dermatitis may also resemble pityriasis rosea,[18] lichen planus,[19] or irritant dermatitis.[20] It sometimes causes a chronic papular eruption[21] (Fig. 37-7) or a granuloma.[15] Histologically it may cause a pseudolymphomatous picture.[22]

Nonallergic reactions to gold include black dermographisms, where a black deposit is left by small particles of the softer metal following abrasion with a harder substance such as talc or titanium dioxide. In gold smudging, the metal abrasion is often supplemented by corrosion caused by prolonged contact with sulfur compounds, amino acids, or cyanide produced by certain plants.[23] Gold potassium cyanide can cause nail discoloration, onycholysis, and sterile pustules of the dorsal fingers and crusting and erosions of the lower lip.[20]

Reactions are typically to jewelry (Figs. 37-7 and 37-8)[24,25] and to dental metals in the mouth.[26,27] Sometimes those with stomatitis will tolerate jewelry on the skin. Allergic contact dermatitis to gold may present as an eczematous reaction or even as persistent nodules. Nodules on earlobes resembling lymphocytoma cutis have been reported.[17]

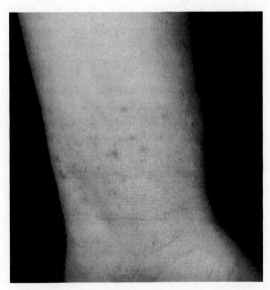

FIG. 37-7. Papular gold dermatitis. (See color Plate 32.)

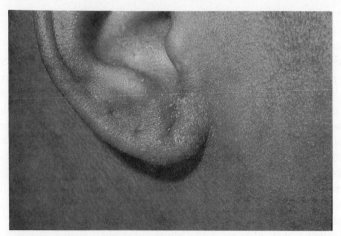

FIG. 37–8. Contact allergy to gold earrings.

Occupational exposure to gold may occur in the electronics and gold-plating industries and among photographers using gold in their work.

Patch testing is done to gold sodium thiomalate 0.5% to 2% in petrolatum or gold sodium thiosulfate 0.5% in petrolatum. Gold trichloride tends to be irritant and may cause pseudolymphomatous infiltrates and persistent patch-test responses. Gold leaf is unreliable for patch testing.[28]

MERCURY

Mercury sensitivity occurs to several different antigens including elemental mercury, but most individuals are patch-test positive to ammoniated mercury.[73] The eruption may take many forms, from an obvious eczematous contact dermatitis to erosive stomatitis with a lichen planus picture[74] to a reaction in the red part of a tattoo[75] to systemic contact dermatitis. The classic description of systemic contact dermatitis was that of Nakayama.[76] Sensitization was often to merthiolate and the precipitating exposure was typically to either the vapor of elemental mercury following a broken fever thermometer or to a recent dental amalgam. Morphologically, one sees a widespread erythema or erythematopapular eruption (sometimes with pustules) typically involving the perineum, antecubital and popliteal areas, axillae, trunk, and inner thighs. Similar eruptions have been reported by others as well.[77–80] An erythema multiforme–like eruption occurred from systemic contact to mercury from cleaning up a broken fever thermometer.[81]

Contact reactions may be to Mercurochrome,[82] to freckle creams,[83] medications, cosmetics, disinfectants, soap and detergents, dental amalgams, vaccinations, weed killers, contact lens solution, and massage oils.[84]

Oral lichen planus opposite dental amalgams can be from mercury sensitivity,[85,86] and a facial dermatitis in one mercury-allergic patient was unresponsive until the dental amalgams were removed.[87] Much of this is caused by exposure at home, but sensitivity[88,89] and elicitation[90] can occur from occupational exposure. Dentists and dental personnel sometimes demonstrate eczema of the hands and other areas from handling the metal.[89,91]

Most patch testing is done with ammoniated mercury, although it is not easily available except as a commercial patch-test antigen. Both 1% ammoniated mercury and thimerosal 0.5% have been considered suitable screening antigens for mercury sensitivity, and pulverized amalgam in a 20% concentration detects reactors to that alloy. A 5% concentration detected 10 of 13 sensitive patients.[92] Metallic mercury has also been used, but the homogeneity varies with the antigen. Because the metal tends to collect and settle, storage of syringes in the horizontal position is recommended.[93,94]

Patch testing to mercury using aluminum chambers can be a problem, as corrosion occurs to aqueous solutions, accompanied by irritation and false-positive responses. It is less likely with petrolatum as a vehicle and with nonmetallic chambers or coverings.[95,96]

PALLADIUM

Palladium reactions are usually associated with allergy to nickel,[59–62] although this is not universal.[63] Reactions to the pure metal are usually negative in persons allergic to palladium chloride,[62] although three persons in one series reacted to a metal disk of palladium but not to palladium chloride.[64] Palladium is used in jewelry and in dental metals, but the latter release very few metal ions because the alloys are so corrosionproof.[65]

The significance of positive reactions to palladium chloride are in some question, as they are commonly associated with sensitivity to nickel and tests to the pure metal as foil or disk are negative in most cases. Stomatitis can occur, however, which is associated with a positive patch test[66] and which clears following removal of the metal from contact with the mucosa.[67,68]

The explanation for sensitivity to both nickel and palladium is probably not contamination in most cases. Both are in group VII of the periodic table, and some feel that this makes cross reactivity likely. The lack of a response to metal foil and disks may be due to the difficulty in releasing sufficient metal ion from the pure metal.

Patch testing is usually done with 1% to 2% palladium chloride in petrolatum, but some recommend using a disk of the pure metal. Cross-reactivity with nickel is a problem. Interestingly, Wahlberg and Bomas[69] sensitized guinea pigs to both metals, and those sensitized to palladium reacted to both nickel and palladium while those sensitized to nickel were allergic only to nickel. At present, reactors should be carefully evaluated for relevance.

PLATINUM

Delayed hypersensitivity to platinum is a very rare event, probably because of the insolubility of the metal in sweat.[71] Sheard[71a] reported a patient allergic to two rings containing platinum as well as "pure" metallic platinum. Most industrial cases are skin and respiratory reactions to complex platinum salts; this has been termed platinosis. Levene[72] regarded these as a form of immediate hypersensitivity which on repeated skin testing could cause an Arthus-like picture. Scratch or intradermal testing could in some cases prove to be dangerous and is not recommended as a routine test.

SILVER

Allergic contact dermatitis to silver is said to be rare today but was less so when silver nitrate was used more often therapeutically. Gaul and Underwood[55] reported a postal clerk with fingertip and palmar eczema from handling silver coins. A photographic worker exposed to silver-containing photographic film developed an eczema under her watch.[56] Heyl[57] described a refinery clerk who reacted to "silver coat" silver cyanide with a positive patch test but who had no response to the metal. Itching, irritant, and allergic contact dermatitis was caused by silver fulminate encountered by workers in an explosives plant. Patch tests were allergic in some, irritant in some, and negative in others.[58]

Patch testing is done to 1% silver nitrate (aqueous).

TIN

Tin may be an overlooked contact allergen. Menne et al.[70] reported seven persons who reacted to the metal. Six were allergic to nickel also, and one was allergic to spectacle frames. Tin is a component of dental amalgams, so it probably deserves closer scrutiny. It has perhaps been understudied. The allergen is available from Chemotechnique as 50% in petrolatum.

REFERENCES

1. Fowler JF: Allergic contact dermatitis to metals. *Am J Contact Dermatitis* 1:212, 1990.
2. Christensen OB: Nickel dermatitis. *Dermatol Clin* 8:37, 1990.
3. Larsson-Stymne B, Widstrom L: Ear piercing—a cause of nickel allergy in schoolgirls? *Contact Dermatitis* 13:289, 1985.
4. Christopherson J, Menne T, Taughos P, et al: Clinical patch test data evaluated by multivariate analysis. *Contact Dermatitis* 21:291, 1989.
5. Massone L, Anonide A, Borghi S, Isola V: Positive patch test reactions to nickel, cobalt and potassium dichromate in a series of 576 patients. *Cutis* 47:119, 1991.
6. Fischer AA: *Contact Dermatitis,* 3d ed. Philadelphia, Lea & Febiger, 1986, pp 710–761.
7. Moller H: Intradermal testing in doubtful cases of contact allergy to metals. *Contact Dermatitis* 20:120, 1989.
8. Gawkrodger DJ, Cook SW, Fell GS, Hunter JAA: Nickel dermatitis: The reaction to oral nickel challenge. *Br J Dermatol* 115:33, 1986.
9. Veien NK, Hattel T, Justensen O, Norholm A: Oral challenge with nickel and cobalt in patients with positive patch tests to nickel and/or cobalt. *Acta Derm Venereol (Stokh)* 67:321, 1987.
10. Santucci B, Cristando A, Cannistraci C, Picardo M: Nickel sensitivity: Effects of prolonged oral intake of the element. *Contact Dermatitis* 19:202, 1988.
11. Schubert H, Berova N, Czernielewski A, et al: Epidemiology of nickel allergy. *Contact Dermatitis* 16:122, 1987.
12. Elgart ML, Higdon RS: Allergic contact dermatitis to gold. *Arch Dermatol* 103:649, 1971.
13. Fischer AA: Ear piercing and sensitivity to nickel and gold. *J Am Acad Dermatol* 17:853, 1987.
14. Fox JM, Kennedy R, Rostenberg A: Eczematous contact-sensitivity to gold. *Arch Dermatol* 83:956, 1961.
15. Comaish S: A case of contact hypersensitivity to metallic gold. *Arch Dermatol* 99:720, 1969.
16. Fowler JF: Allergic contact dermatitis to gold. *Arch Dermatol* 124:181, 1988.

17. Iwatsuki K, Yamada M, Takigawa M, et al: Benign lymphoplasia of the earlobes induced by gold earrings: Immunohistologic study on the cellular infitrates. *J Am Acad Dermatol* 16:83, 1987.

17a. Bruze M, Edman B, Björkner B, Möller H: Clinical relevance of contact allergy to gold sodium thiosulfate. *J Am Acad Dermatol* 31:579–583, 1994.

18. Wile UI, Courville CJ: Pityriasis rosea-like dermatitis following gold therapy. *Arch Dermatol Syphilol* 42:1105, 1940.

19. McKenna WB: Lichenoid dermatitis following gold therapy. *Br J Dermatol* 69:61, 1957.

20. Budden MG, Wilkinson DS: Skin and nail lesions from gold potassium cyanide (letter). *Contact Dermatitis* 4:172, 1978.

21. Shelley WB, Epstein E: Contact sensitivity to gold as a chronic papular eruption. *Arch Dermatol* 87:388, 1063.

22. Monti M, Berti E, Cavicchini S, Sala F: Unusual cutaneous reaction after a gold chloride patch test. *Contact Dermatitis* 9:150, 1983.

23. Rapson WS: Skin contact with gold and gold alloys (review). *Contact Dermatitis* 13:56, 1985.

24. Roeleveld CG, van Ketel WG: Contact eczema caused by a gold wedding ring? *Contact Dermatitis* 1:333, 1975.

25. Silvennoinen-Kassinen S, Niinimaki A: Gold sensitivity blast transformation. *Contact Dermatitis* 11:156, 1984.

26. Fregert S, Kollander M, Poulsen J: Allergic contact stomatitis from gold dentures. *Contact Dermatitis* 5:63, 1979.

27. Klaschka F: Contact allergy to gold. *Contact Dermatitis* 1:264, 1975.

28. Fowler JF Jr: Selection of patch test materials for gold allergy. *Contact Dermatitis* 17:23, 1987.

29. Vilaplana J, Romaguera C, Grimalt F: Occupational and non-occupational allergic contact dermatitis from beryllium. *Contact Dermatitis* 26:295, 1992.

30. Haberman AL, Pratt M, Storrs FJ: Contact dermatitis from beryllium in dental alloys. *Contact Dermatitis* 28:157, 1993.

31. Kligman AM: The identification of contact allergens by human assay. *J Invest Dermatol* 47:393, 1966.

32. Henderson WR, Fukuyama K, Epstein WL, Spitler LE: In vitro demonstration of delayed hypersensitivity in patients with berylliosis. *J Invest Dermatol* 58:5, 1972.

33. Motolese A, Truzzi M, Giannini A, Seidenari S: Contact dermatitis and contact sensitization among enamellers and decorators in the ceramics industry. *Contact Dermatitis* 28:59, 1993.

34. Rudzki E, Rebandel P, Stroinski J, Parapura K: Reactions to cadmium. *Contact Dermatitis* 18:183, 1988.

35. Wahlberg JE: Routine patch testing with cadmium chloride. *Contact Dermatitis* 3:293, 1977.

35a. Kaaber S, Cramers M, Jepsen FL: The role of cadmium as a skin sensitizing agent in denture and non-denture wearers. *Contact Dermatitis* 8(5):308, 1982.

36. Wahlberg JE, Boman A: Guinea pig maximization test method—cadmium chloride. *Contact Dermatitis* 5:405, 1979.

37. Raith L, Schubert H, Goring HD: Contact dermatitis from cadmium chloride? *Contact Dermatitis* 8:267, 1982.

38. Björnberg A: Reactions to light in yellow tattoos from cadmium sulfide. *Arch Dermatol* 88:267, 1963.

39. Clemons DE: Reactions in tattoos (letter). *J Dermatol Surg Oncol* 10:20, 1984.

40. Goldstein N: Mercury-cadmium sensitivity in tattoos: a photoallergic reaction in red pigment. *Ann Intern Med* 67:984–989, 1967.

41. Goette DK: Swimmer's green hair (letter). *Arch Dermatol* 114:127–8, 1978.

42. Nordlund JJ, Hartley C, Fister J: On the cause of green hair. *Arch Dermatol* 113:1700, 1977.

43. Verbov J: Green hair due to copper in spectacle metal (letter). *Clin Exp Dermatol* 15:234, 1990.

44. Verbov J: Green hair due to copper in spectacle metal (letter). *Clin Exp Dermatol* 15:467, 1990.

45. Tosti A, Mattioli D, Misciali C: Green hair caused by copper present in cosmetic plant extracts (letter). *Dermatologica* 182:204, 1991.

46. Wright S, Auger DW: Rumbler operator's green hair. *Contact Dermatitis* 19:310, 1988.

47. Gould D, Slater DN, Durrant TE: A case of green hair—A consequence of exogenous copper deposition and permanent waving. *Clin Exp Dermatol* 9:545, 1984.

48. Wolf R, Perluk C, Krakowski A: Nail pigmentation resulting from selenium sulfide and copper (letter). *Int J Dermatol* 28:556, 1989.

49. Nordlind K, Liden S: Patch test reactions to metal salts in patients with oral mucosal lesions associated with amalgam restorations. *Contact Dermatitis* 27:157, 1992.

50. Mobacken H, Hersle K, Sloberg K, Thilander H: Oral lichen planus: Hypersensitivity to dental restoration material. *Contact Dermatitis* 10:11, 1984.
51. Romaguera C, Grimalt F: Contact dermatitis from a copper-containing intrauterine contraceptive device. *Contact Dermatitis* 7:163, 1981.
52. Barranco VP: Eczematous dermatitis caused by internal exposure to copper. *Arch Dermatol* 106:386, 1972.
53. Karlberg AT, Boman A, Wahlberg JE: Copper—A rare sensitizer. *Contact Dermatitis* 9:134, 1983.
54. Boman A, Karlberg AT, Einarsson O, Wahlberg JE: Dissolving of copper by synthetic sweat. *Contact Dermatitis* 9:159, 1983.
55. Gaul LE, Underwood BG: The effect of aging a solution of silver nitrate on its cutaneous reaction. *J Invest Dermatol* 11:7, 1948.
56. Marks R: Contact dermatitis due to silver. *Br J Dermatol* 78:606, 1966.
57. Heyl T: Contact dermatitis from silver coat. *Contact Dermatitis* 5:197, 1979.
58. White IR, Rycroft RJ: Contact dermatitis from silver fulminate-fulminate itch. *Contact Dermatitis* 8:159, 1982.
59. Camarasa JG, Serra-Baldrich E, Lluch M, et al: Recent unexplained patch test reactions to palladium. *Contact Dermatitis* 20:388, 1989.
60. van Joost T, Roesyanto-Mahadi ID: Combined sensitization to palladium and nickel (review). *Contact Dermatitis* 22:227, 1990.
61. Rebandel P, Rudzki E: Allergy to palladium. *Contact Dermatitis* 232:121, 1990.
62. Todd DJ, Burrows D: Patch testing with pure palladium metal in patients with sensitivity to palladium chloride. *Contact Dermatitis* 26:327, 1992.
63. Camarasa JG, Burrows D, Menne T, et al: Palladium contact sensitivity. *Contact Dermatitis* 24:370, 1991.
64. de Fine Olivarius F, Menne T: Contact dermatitis from metallic palladium in patients reacting to palladium chloride. *Contact Dermatitis* 27:71, 1992.
65. van Loon LA, van Elsas PW, van Joostl T, Davidson CL: Contact stomatitis and dermatitis to nickel and palladium. *Contact Dermatitis* 11:294, 1984.
66. Castelain PY, Castelain M: Contact dermatitis to palladium. *Contact Dermatitis* 16:46, 1987.
67. Downey D: Contact mucositis due to palladium. *Contact Dermatitis* 21:54, 1989.
68. van Ketel WG, Niebber C: Allergy to palladium in dental alloys. *Contact Dermatitis* 7:331, 1981.
69. Wahlberg JE, Boman AS: Cross-reactivity to palladium and nickel studied in the guinea pig. *Acta Derm Venereol* 72:95, 1992.
70. Menne T, Andersen KE, Kaaber K, et al: Tin: An overlooked contact sensitizer? *Contact Dermatitis* 16:9, 1987.
71. Hjorth N, Wilkinson DS: Contact dermatitis. 3 (review). *Br J Dermatol* 80:482, 1968.
71a. Sheard C: Contact dermatitis from platinum and related metals. *Arch Dermatol* 71:357, 1955.
72. Levene GM: Platinum sensitivity (review). *Br J Dermatol* 85:590, 1971.
73. Nebenfuhrer L, Korossy S, Vincze E, Gozony M: Mercury allergy in Budapest. *Contact Dermatitis* 10:121, 1984.
74. Mobacken H, Hersle K, Sloberg K, Thilander H: Oral lichen planus: Hypersensitivity to dental restoration material. *Contact Dermatitis* 10:11, 1984.
75. Fregert S: Sensitization to mercury in kerosene and exacerbation from red tattoo. *Contact Dermatitis* 1:255, 1975.
76. Nakayama H, Niki F, Shono M, Hada S: Mercury exanthem. *Contact Dermatitis* 9:411, 1983.
77. Faria A, de Freitas C: Systemic contact dermatitis due to mercury. *Contact Dermatitis* 27:110, 1992.
78. Bartolo E, Brandao FM: Mercury exanthem. *Contact Dermatitis* 18:172, 1988.
79. Pambor M, Timmel A: Mercury dermatitis. *Contact Dermatitis* 20:157, 1989.
80. Andersen KE, Hjorth N, Menne T: The baboon syndrome: Systemically induced allergic contact dermatitis. *Contact Dermatitis* 10:97, 1984.
81. Vermeiden I, Oranje AP, Vuzevski VD, Stolz E: Mercury exanthem as occupational dermatitis. *Contact Dermatitis* 6:88, 1980.
82. van Ketel WG: Sensitization to mercury from Mercurochrome. *Contact Dermatitis* 6:499, 1980.
83. Sun CC: Allergic contact dermatitis of the face from contact with nickel and ammoniated mercury in spectacle frames and skin-lightening creams. *Contact Dermatitis.* 17:306, 1987.
84. Wekkeli M, Hippmann G, Rosenkranz AR, et al: Mercury as a contact allergen. *Contact Dermatitis* 22:295, 1990.

85. Mobacken H, Hersle K, Sloberg K, Thilander H: Oral lichen planus: Hypersensitivity to dental restoration material. *Contact Dermatitis* 10:11, 1984.
86. Nordlind K, Liden S: Patch test reactions to metal salts in patients with oral mucosal lesions associated with amalgam restorations. *Contact Dermatitis* 27:157, 1992.
87. Feuerman E: Dermatitis due to mercury in amalgam dental fillings. *Contact Dermatitis* 1:191, 1975.
88. Goh CL, Ng SK: Occupational allergic contact dermatitis from metallic mercury. *Contact Dermatitis.* 19:232, 1988.
89. Kanerva L, Komulainen M, Estlander T, Jolanki R: Occupational allergic contact dermatitis from mercury. *Contact Dermatitis* 28:26, 1993.
90. Swinyer LJ: Allergic contact dermatitis from metallic mercury. *Contact Dermatitis* 6:226, 1980.
91. Ancona A, Ramos M, Suarez R, Macotela E: Mercury sensitivity in a dentist. *Contact Dermatitis* 8:218, 1982.
92. von Mayenburg J, Rakoski J, Szliska C: Patch testing with amalgam at various concentrations. *Contact Dermatitis* 24:266, 1991.
93. Mellstrom GA, Sommar K, Wahlberg JE: Patch test preparations of metallic mercury under the microscope. *Contact Dermatitis* 26:64, 1992.
94. Mellstrom GA, Wahlberg JE: Patch test preparations of mercury ammonium chloride under the microscope. *Contact Dermatitis* 27:193, 1992.
95. Kubo Y, Anan S, Nonaka S, Yoshida H: Does patch testing with ammoniated mercury in a Finn chamber give a false positive reaction? *Contact Dermatitis* 27:118, 1992.
96. Kalveram KJ, Rapp-Frick C, Sorck G: Misleading patch test results with aluminum Finn chambers and mercury salts. *Contact Dermatitis* 6:507, 1980.
97. Clemmensen O, Knudsen HE: Contact sensitivity to aluminum in a patient hyposensitized with aluminum precipitated grass pollen. *Contact Dermatitis* 6:303, 1980.
98. Fischer T, Rystedt I: A case of contact sensitivity to aluminum. *Contact Dermatitis* 8:343, 1982.
99. Kotovirta ML, Salo OP, Visa-Tolvanen K: Contact sensitivity to aluminum. *Contact Dermatitis.* 11:135, 1984.
100. Meding B, Augustsson A, Hansson C: Patch test reactions to aluminum. *Contact Dermatitis* 10:107, 1984.

38

PLANT DERMATITIS

Jere D. Guin

Contact dermatitis to plants can mimic almost any other form of contact dermatitis, but most cases are easily recognized because poison ivy and its relatives are the leading cause of plant dermatitis. With experience, one can also recognize most cases of weed dermatitis caused by the Compositae and other sesquiterpene lactone-containing plants. Primula, a house plant becoming more commonly grown, causes severe contact dermatitis, especially in exposed areas. Irritant reactions may range from a mild to severe urticaria (e.g., nettles or *Urtica*) to a blistering or blinding dermatitis (e.g., manchineel). Such reactions are common only locally and would be more easily suspected where these plants are likely to be contacted. Almost any plant could rarely be the cause of some type of reaction without having reported problems with specific plants, so we shall cover the more prominent causes. A number of comprehensive publications are available,[1-4] so our emphasis is on the more common and prominent reactions one might expect to see clinically in North America.

The severity of plant-induced contact dermatitis is not only dependent on the plant's irritant or allergic potential but also the degree of exposure and the sensitivity of the individual. Even plants which rarely cause contact dermatitis may produce severe eruptions in highly allergic patients. Phytophotodermatitis can cause poison ivy–like streaks in light-exposed areas, followed by hyperpigmentation if psoralens are present. An irritant effect can also resemble allergic contact dermatitis. Recognition depends on one's index of suspicion as well as some knowledge of the patterns usually seen. Therefore, we shall discuss several of the more important causes of plant dermatitis, the patterns they present, how to confirm the diagnosis, and the approach to treatment.

TOXICODENDRON DERMATITIS

RECOGNITION

The typical pattern in most patients with poison ivy or oak dermatitis is caused by a transfer of the antigen [pentadec(en)yl or heptadec(en)yl catechols][5] from the hands or fingers to the affected area.[6] Consequently, one sees streaks from finger transfer, broader localized involvement of areas from rubbing, and sometimes even handprints in a mitten pattern. The eruption may be an almost flat erythema, but usually it is prominently raised and vesicular, often weeping, oozing, and crusting when acute. It is *severely* pruritic. The most prominent areas of involvement are usually in exposed sites where the hands can reach. Areas such as the midline of the back, which are hard to reach, are usually spared. The scalp also is not involved in most cases. The palms (which may spread the antigen) and soles are usually not involved but may be, especially if the skin is broken. Poison ivy dermatitis of the hands may typically occur in the finger webs or as streaks on the backs of the hands or fingers.

The eruption may seem to spread after its initial appearance, and this is true apparently without any additional exposure. The face may be the first area involved[7]; if so, it is usually the first area to clear spontaneously. This is probably based on the propensity to absorb the antigen as much as the opportunity for exposure.

There are regional differences in the rate of absorption,[7,8] with the face being involved early while the forearms may take several days to break out; this takes longer in areas where the skin is thicker.[7] Many patients feel that the reason for this is reexposure or a failure on the part of their treatment. Again, it is probably based on exposure and the rate of absorption through the skin in different parts of the body.

In endemic areas, poison ivy dermatitis should be suspected in any individual with a severe contact dermatitis. When this condition is sudden in onset in the summer months, this diagnosis is presumptive until it is disproved, especially if the eruption is characterized by streaks, finger marks, and hand prints. However, persons treating warts with immunotherapy using dinitrochlorobenzene (DNCB) or squaric acid dibutyl ester can develop a similar eruption with hand transfer. One also sees streaks with *Primula, Phacelia*,[9] English ivy, and phytophotodermatitis. *Phacelia* dermatitis seems to occur in botanists who know the source. *Primula* reactions often include the fingertips and occur in older women. Phytophotodermatitis is usually followed by hyperpigmentation.

To confirm the diagnosis of *Toxicodendron* dermatitis, one should look at the pattern of the eruption and place the patient's hand over this to see how it might have been transferred from the hand.[6] Then, by taking a history, one can usually elicit an opportunity for exposure. For an acute eruption of the face, this may have taken place the same day as the eruption. For other parts of the body, it may require 1 or 2 days or sometimes much longer.[10] Rarely, it may take 2 weeks or more even in a person who is already allergic.[7] One should ask the patient about outdoor activity and in particular being in the woods or working in the yard. If this is negative, look for exposure to animals which had been outdoors, clothing worn by others who have worked outdoors, exposure to topsoil or potting soil, and a history of handling firewood. Ask about previous episodes of dermatitis from poison ivy (or poison oak on the Pacific Coast). Persons who are unusually sensitive require much less exposure.[10]

SOURCES OF THE ANTIGENS

The antigenic component of poison ivy, poison oak, and poison sumac, called *urushiol*, is found within secretory canals located in the leaves, the roots, and the plant's phloem, which is just below the bark.[11] In the case of poison ivy, exposure may occur to the tiny brown rootlets which attach the vine to the tree or post on which it climbs. More commonly, exposure occurs when the leaf surface is broken, so that the sap containing the oleoresin is released. Brushing against the plant seldom causes a problem. Exposure to the injured plant when pulling weeds, trimming hedges, or cleaning grass clippings from a lawnmower bag is a powerful source of the allergenic oleoresin.

ANTIGEN TRANSFER

The allergen may also be transferred from the fur of animals (who usually do not break out), from fomites[10] such as clothing or garden tools, or from one member of the family to another (connubial contact dermatitis or filial contact dermatitis).[12] Poison ivy dermatitis can be caused by a family's house cat whose avocation is climbing trees to which poison ivy vines are attached. The antigen can be transferred from the animals' fur to a favorite chair or couch, which becomes the source of exposure. Family members may transfer the antigen not only to themselves but also to other family members. Poison ivy may also be transferred as particles in smoke, as the antigen seems to be relatively heat-tolerant; but this is largely limited to individuals who are especially allergic, as the levels of antigen are relatively low.

The eruption does not occur through pollen (air) transfer. In fact, one often sees honeybees gathering nectar from the flowers of poison ivy and I have personally never seen anyone break out from exposure to honey. Another common myth is the putative spread from the blister fluid.[13] This simply does not happen. The antigen is not located within blister fluid and even highly sensitive individuals will not break out when exposed to blister fluid. The notion that scratching the lesion tends to spread the eruption apparently comes from the tendency for poison ivy dermatitis to get worse for several days after it first appears. This is apparently due to the irregular absorption of the antigen through uneven exposure and the differences in the rate of absorption in different parts of the skin surface. Under experimental control, one also does not see transfer from the exposed area of the skin to new sites for much longer than 3 days experimentally.[10] Naturally, the time that it takes to dissipate the oleoresin from the contaminated surface is probably much shorter, because antigen is removed by washing and tends to be inactivated by water.[10] However, it is so rapidly absorbed that, by the time one sees the eruption, it is no longer a problem to others.

PLANT RECOGNITION

Poison ivy, poison oak, and poison sumac belong to the genus *Toxicodendron*[11,14,15] (formerly classed as *Rhus*, a benign genus). In the United States, there are two species of poison ivy, two of poison oak, and one of poison sumac. In addition, plants in tropical areas may cross-react or produce a similar or even more severe eruption. Poison ivy and poison oak have many features in common, which should alert the weekend gardener or hiker. While leaves of both of these plants have three leaflets (Figs. 38-1 and 38-2), leaflets vary greatly in their shape, so it is relatively easy to overlook these plants. There are some key features which help, and with practice almost anyone can become proficient.

One recognizable characteristic of *Toxicodendron radicans* is the enlargement of the structure holding the leaf as it is attached to the branch. This is illustrated in Fig.

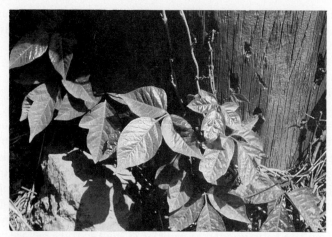

FIG. 38–1. Poison ivy, *Toxicodendron radicans* spp. *negundo.* (See color Plate 33.)

38-3*A* (#2). This structure is also grooved on the distal side in the enlarged portion. The groove allows the flowers and fruit to grow out between the leaf and branch (Fig. 38-3*A*, #2). When the leaf falls off in winter, the grooved leaf stalk attachment leaves a scar which is V- or U-shaped rather than circular (Fig. 38-3*B* #3). This feature is prominent summer and winter in poison sumac and oak as well as poison ivy.

On larger female plants, one may see the empty fruit stalk (Fig. 38-3*B*, #8), even in winter. Sometimes the fruit is present, but if not, the empty stems (which resemble empty grape stems) will be seen attached even when birds have eaten the fruits. The fruits (labeled 6 and 7 in Fig. 38-3*B*) are off-white or ivory in color in the fall and early winter, but this layer peels away during the winter (Fig. 38-3*B*, #6), exposing a chalk-white layer beneath. In the deeper chalk-white layer, there are black lines resem-

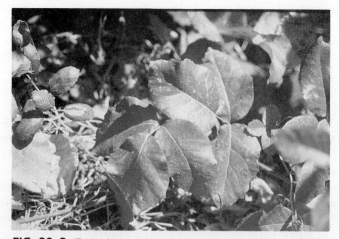

FIG. 38–2. *Toxicodendron diversilobum*, or western poison oak. This is a much larger plant than the eastern species, which does not climb trees. Both have three leaflets per leaf. (See color Plate 34.)

bling the marks on orange slices, which are the tiny canals containing the poisonous oleoresin (Fig. 38-3*B*, #7). This feature is typically present in winter, but only in mature female clones.

The wood on the stem of all *Toxicodendron* plants has many tiny holes, which give a characteristic texture to the surface of the woody part of the plant (Fig. 38-3*B*, #9). These also aid recognition in all seasons. In the growing part of the branch, when the plant is still green, these are often a bright orange color, but they turn into a permanent gray-brown color during the first winter.

Poison ivy (*T. radicans*) tends to climb trees, but poison ivy in much of the northern and western states (*Toxicodendron rydbergii*) is a nonclimbing shrub which is so small that it has often been mistaken for eastern poison oak. This plant grows along the ground in waste areas, and it shares many of the characteristic features of poison ivy mentioned above. Leaflets tend to be cup-shaped, and the stems holding the leaves tend to be quite long. Branches usually divide within a foot or so off the ground and can often be seen protruding through the snow during the winter months. This plant is much smaller than the climbing poison ivy *T. radicans*, but it can still be a very real problem for susceptible persons. This species of poison ivy can also be found in Canada, the Rocky Mountains, and the states of Washington and Oregon.

Poison oak in the eastern United States (*Toxicodendron toxicarium*) is a small shrub that grows in sandy soil along with pine, scrub oak, sassafras, and bunch grasses. It is especially prominent in the coastal sands region of the Southeast and in the ridge and valley areas where sandstone outcroppings occur along with the plants mentioned. This plant is not nearly as common as poison ivy and is much more demanding in its soil requirements, so that it is not found everywhere, although it can be dense in specific geographic areas. Eastern poison oak may be relatively small, but it can produce a brisk reaction with adequate exposure. The leaflets on poison oak are more stiff or leatherlike (coriaceous), and they usually have rounded lobes. In some parts of the southeast, leaflets that closely resemble the leaves of white oak (*Quercus alba*) can fool even an experienced botanist who does not look closely when grabbing a "white oak" sapling. Eastern poison oak does not climb trees and does not have aerial rootlets.[11,14]

Western poison oak (*Toxicodendron diversilobum*), unlike the eastern variety, is often a very large plant. It can grow as a standing shrub or a climbing vine and tends to be found in abundance in canyons and valleys where there is enough moisture to support its growth. Also, unlike eastern poison oak, it is not nearly so particular about its soil requirements. Poison oak leaflets tend to have rounded lobes and are often quite dainty in their appearance (Fig. 38-2). The branches of this plant tend to be much straighter and more reddish-brown in color than those of its eastern relatives. The fruit on female plants tends to hang down rather being borne erect on a stiff stem, and the average leaflet size is smaller.

POISON OAK AND IVY TURN COLOR EARLY

Poison ivy and poison oak tend to turn color earlier in the year than many of the domesticated plants. This can be useful, as it is often possible in the fall to pick out poison ivy and poison oak hidden in a hedge or similar structure, as these toxicodendrons

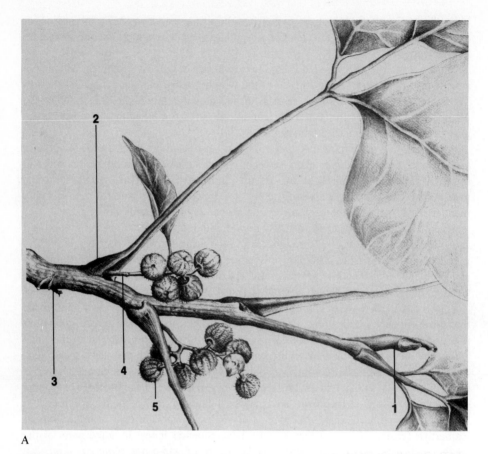

A

FIG. 38–3. *A* and *B*. Nonleaf characteristics of poison ivy used in field recognition. (From Guin JD and Beaman JH,[15] reproduced by permission.)

will turn yellow or red much earlier in the fall than the domesticated plants in the area. Certain other weedy plants (e.g., Virginia creeper) turn color earlier, so this finding is used to suspect poison ivy, not prove its identity. In winter, *T. radicaus* on fence posts is easily distinguished from Virginia creeper by its "medusa head" silhouette (Fig. 38-4).

THE BLACK SPOT

Sometimes a black material resembling black enamel paint can be seen at the sites of injury on poison ivy, poison oak, and poison sumac. This is the toxic sap which has hardened on the surface of the plant. It is not as irritating as the liquid sap, but it is still very allergenic. Following heavy exposure to the plant, one occasionally sees black spots on the skin in the areas of the dermatitis. This is referred to as black-spot poison ivy dermatitis.[16] The tendency for the sap to turn black can be used in the field to confirm the identification of poison ivy, poison oak, and poison sumac.[17] The directions for doing this are given in Table 38-1.

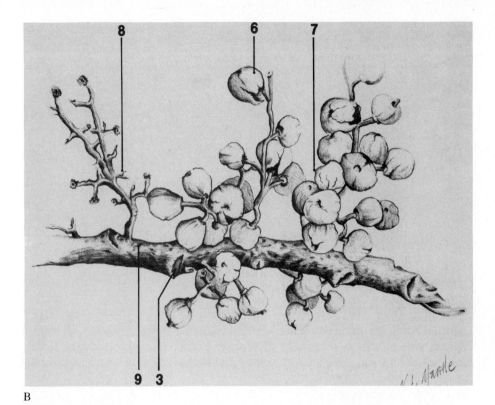

FIG. 38–3. (*Continued*)

PATHOPHYSIOLOGY

Poison ivy and its relatives contain varying amounts of alk(en)yl catechols, which are highly antigenic.[5] Generally, poison ivy has mostly pentadec(en)yl catechols, while poison oak has mostly heptadec(en)yl catechols. The two-carbon difference in the lengths of the two side chains is of relatively minor importance. However, the number of double bonds in the side chain may be more significant, as those molecules with two and three double bonds in this side chain seem to cause a much higher percentage of positive patch-test reactions in individuals allergic to poison ivy and poison oak.[18] The lipophilic side chain of this molecule probably binds to the cell membrane, while the hydroxyl groups in the one and two positions are said to oxidize to quinones[19] and bind with nucleophiles (e.g., S-H, NH_2) on the surface of Langerhans cells.[20]

Because those cells contain DR and other class II antigens, the immune system tends to regard this as an altered self antigen and consequently mounts an attack against the altered cell. The Langerhans cell binds a T lymphocyte to its surface and releases interleukin-1, which activates the T lymphocyte. The T lymphocytes, in turn, produce a number of lymphokines, including interleukin-2 (T-cell growth factor) and gamma interferon, which causes an increase in the number of class II antigens on the surface of the same Langerhans cells. The process, therefore, would be expected to keep going, except that a number of T-suppressor cells are also produced, and these are felt to be

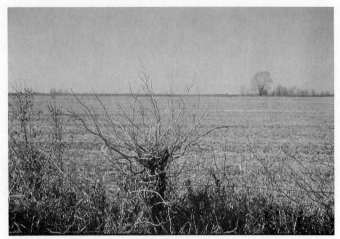

FIG. 38–4. Winter picture of poison ivy on a fence row. The branches grow in a different direction each season which produces the outline of a "Medusa head" recognizable from a moving automobile.

associated with the resolution process.[21] This extremely potent antigen is oil-soluble and has a strong affinity for protein. The former characteristic allows it to be rapidly absorbed and the latter characteristic causes it to bind avidly to the cell surface of the Langerhans cells.

PROPHYLAXIS

Avoidance of the plant is obviously the most effective way to prevent contact dermatitis to poison ivy. This depends in large measure on plant recognition in all four seasons. The methods used for identification of poison ivy, poison oak, and poison sumac are outlined in Table 38-1.

The allergenic component of the plant is so rapidly absorbed through the skin that highly sensitive people must remove the antigen within a few minutes of exposure. Usually, soap and water are used for this, but any organic solvent would be beneficial if it is done immediately. More moderately sensitive people have 30 min or so to try to remove the antigen with soap and water or one of the organic solvents.[10] If none of these is available, water tends to have an inhibitory effect on the eruption.[10,22] Protective clothing can also be a factor, since the eruption is usually found in exposed areas. Plastic or vinyl gloves tend to prevent spread of the eruption by interrupting transfer to the hands. Rubber gloves however, are said to allow penetration of the antigen. Clothing which has been exposed can be laundered or, in severe cases, dry-cleaned to remove any antigens remaining.

Patients with poison ivy dermatitis are frequently concerned with the possibility of spread of the eruption from contaminated fomites. This indeed can occur with animal fur, garden tools, and even clothing. Most often, one only has to wash clothing with soap and water. Heavily contaminated things can be dry-cleaned. Bathing with a

TABLE 38–1. How to Recognize Poison Ivy and Poison Oak

1. Both poison ivy (Fig. 38-1) and poison oak (Fig. 38-2) have three leaflets.
2. The "stem" holding the three leaflets is grooved and enlarged where it is attached to the branch (#2, Fig. 38-3A).
3. Leaf scars on the branches and trunk are U- or V-shaped (#3, Fig. 38-3A and B).
4. Tiny "pores" in the bark give the surface a characteristic texture (#9, Fig. 38-3B).
5. Flowers and (on female plants) fruit (#5, #6, #7, Fig. 38-3A and B) are borne on branched stalks in clusters. During winter, the stalks are often bare, resembling empty grape stems (#8, Fig. 38-3B).
6. On mature female plants, the tiny seedlike fruits are green in summer (Fig. 38-3A), turning off-white in the fall. The outer layer peels in winter (#6, Fig. 38-3B) leaving a chalk-white surface with dark or black lines (#7, Fig. 38-3B).
7. Branches of poison ivy are often gnarled because the bud from which new growth comes is not centered (#1, Fig. 38-3A), therefore, the branch grows out in a different direction each season. In winter, when leaves are absent, the collection of gnarled branches on fence posts resembles the head of Medusa, the mythological creature who had snakes for hair (Fig. 38-4).

The Black Spot Test

The black-spot test is used to confirm that a suspected plant is poison ivy/oak/sumac. It is usually used when one has a plant with many features of poison ivy/oak but still can't be sure.

1. Using a vinyl glove or multiple folded sheets of white paper, grasp several leaves where they are attached to the branch and remove them, keeping them safely inside the paper. There is usually a slight bulge in the "stem" of the leaf where it is attached.
2. Gather the bulges of the stems together and, with the paper folded, crush the stems so that a wet spot is left. The test does not work if there is not enough sap released to wet the paper.
3. Taking care to avoid contact, dispose of the leaves in a safe place.
4. The clear wet sap turns brown in less than 10 min. It takes about 24 h to turn the spot on the paper black, but the test can be read in 10 min or less.

contaminated hand can be a problem, so that individuals with known prominent exposure would do well to avoid such deliberate exposure.

Another method of preventing poison ivy dermatitis is to use a barrier substance such as Stokogard cream[23] or, when available, Ivy Block.[24,25] Stokogard contains a number of amino groups to bind the antigen on the surface, ostensibly preventing absorption.[23] This should be applied before exposure and washed off within a few hours. Ivy Block, an organo-clay mixture, causes surface binding and impressively reduces experimental patch-test reactions. Ivy Shield has activity also, but at a lower level than the other two products.[26]

HYPOSENSITIZATION

For extremely sensitive individuals who cannot prevent exposure, it is sometimes possible to induce a temporary tolerance by administering the causative antigen orally over a period of many months.[27,28] The reduction in sensitivity, while mild, can be somewhat useful. In the older literature, when more aggressive treatment programs were used and side effects were seemingly less important, more prominent reduction in sensitivity was achieved.[29] Interestingly, individuals who work with these antigens every day often develop from chronic exposure a form of tolerance called *hardening*.

This phenomenon has been reported in oriental woodworkers[30] or in individuals who have been repeatedly exposed deliberately through patch testing or other means. This same phenomenon tends to occur after prolonged treatment with other strong allergens in persons with alopecia areata.[31]

TREATMENT OF *TOXICODENDRON* DERMATITIS

Oral corticosteroid therapy must be given in adequate dosage (usually starting at 30 to 60 mg of prednisone daily) over a period of 14 to 21 days.[6] Normally, treatment is continued until at least 14 days after initial exposure. Injectable (IM) corticosteroids can be used, but I know of no advantage. For milder cases, a topical corticosteroid can be used with 24-h occlusion. Category II to V topical steroids should be applied in quantity for at least two 24-h applications. The absorption curve is better for a 1- to 3-day application than for a period less than 24 h.[32] One should be wary of applying potential allergens to any prolonged allergic contact dermatitis without withdrawal from exposure as, at least theoretically, one could facilitate development of allergy to one or more component(s) of the medication. Many commonly asked questions are answered in the patient handout (Table 38-2).

RAGWEED (COMPOSITAE) DERMATITIS

Weed dermatitis can be both a dramatic clinical picture (Fig. 38-5) and a severe problem for those afflicted. The problem is easily missed because it can look so much like light sensitivity,[33] atopic eczema,[34] hand eczema,[34,35] or even poison ivy dermatitis.[36] Patch-test data suggests that in Europe, about 1.5% of those tested are allergic to the screening sesquiterpene lactone (SQTL) mixture, and many would have been missed had the screening test not been included.[35] There are five known patterns of eczema from sesquiterpene lactone–containing plants (Table 38-3).

PATTERN I: PSEUDOPHOTODERMATITIS

The typical patient is an older white male, often a farmer. The classic eruption is commonly misdiagnosed as photosensitivity, although the upper and lower eyelids are often involved. The submental and postauricular sites are also usually involved. However, the eruption is so prominent in exposed sites and the cutoff is so sharp at the collar and sleeve (Fig. 38-6) that one almost instantly suspects light as the cause. In fact, photosensitivty and Compositae allergy seem to go together,[37] as about 45.6 percent of photosensitive persons also have weed dermatitis.[38] Therefore, those suspected either of Compositae allergy or photosensitivity should be both patch tested for Compositae allergy and phototested for the minimum erythema dose (MED) for both UVB and UVA.[38] One should also do photopatch testing to rule out photocontact dermatitis, especially to atranorin and other light-absorbing chemicals in lichens.

The diagnosis can be suspected immediately when the picture is typical, as illustrated in Fig. 38-5. The patient, most often with opportunity for outdoor exposure, presents with severe eczema of the face, hands, and arms with prominent involvement of the

TABLE 38–2. Poison Ivy/Oak Dermatitis

What causes poison ivy dermatitis? The rash caused by poison ivy/oak exposure is an allergic reaction to a chemical in the plant's sap. It is carried in tiny canals beneath the skin of the leaf or just below the bark. Just brushing against the leaves does not cause the rash because the sap is not released unless the leaf surface is broken.

How long does it take to become allergic? On first exposure, we are not allergic. It takes from at least 5 to 7 days or more, probably 10 to 14 days, to become allergic. If enough of the toxic agent stays in the skin when sensitization occurs, the rash will appear. Otherwise, it is not seen until the next exposure.

How do I know it is poison ivy/oak dermatitis? The rash from poison ivy/oak is characteristically in streaks because the poisonous sap is deposited in handprints and finger marks. It may appear as early as 5½ h to as long as 15 days after exposure, but it usually occurs after 24 to 36 h. Sometimes, when a large quantity of the poison is left on the skin, it turns black, resembling black enamel paint. This is called black-spot poison ivy/oak dermatitis.

Can one spread poison ivy from blister fluid? No. This has been tried many times. The rash that appears later is caused by slow absorption or reexposure and not from the blister fluid.

Is it contagious? No, it does not spread from the rash. However, when it is still on the hands, one can spread it over oneself or to others touched.

How can I safely and effectively kill the plant? Herbicides are effective. If the plant is growing in your lawn, use *repeated* applications of a 2-4D herbicide, as this kills broad-leaf weeds but not the grass. Round Up, properly applied, will kill poison ivy with one application. It has the added advantage of becoming inactive when it contacts the earth, so it is less likely to run onto and kill nearby plants. The concentration is important, so read the directions.

What is the best way to prevent the rash? The best protection is from recognizing the plant and avoiding it. Once you are exposed, washing with soap and water is helpful if done within a few minutes to a half hour. Even applying plain water immediately tends to reduce the severity. Exposed clothing can be treated by washing or, after severe exposure, dry-cleaned. Dark black spots left on a garment are indelible and retain the capacity to cause allergy.

Several commercial products applied before exposure may delay or reduce absorption. These are Stokogard cream, Ivy Block (not yet available in late 1994), and, to a lesser degree, Ivy Shield. These are applied to high-risk areas before exposure and washed off later. Vinyl (but not rubber) gloves provide excellent protection for the hands, and covering an area with clothing helps prevent exposure.

How is the rash best treated? Treatment usually means a visit to the doctor as the more effective remedies require a prescription. Oral cortisone-like medications are used for most cases, given after breakfast in a single daily dose. Treatment should continue until at least 2 weeks after the exposure. For persons who cannot take systemic cortisone, one can apply a thick layer of a moderately potent cortisone salve, cover it with plastic (like Saran), and snugly wrap the site with an elastic bandage. This is left in place (or reapplied) for 24 h. Two 24-h applications, one day apart, are usually necessary.

eyelids and thickening of the facial skin, which may even result in leonine facies. There is a sharp cutoff at the (short) sleeve length, often sparing the inner arms, as one might expect with light allergy (Fig. 38-6). This would be typical of bitterweed allergy.

PATTERN 2: THE ATOPIC ECZEMA–LIKE PATTERN

Another typical presentation, especially for ragweed dermatitis, mimics atopic eczema[34] (Fig. 38-7). Sesquiterpene lactone (weed) dermatitis, however, not unlike persistent

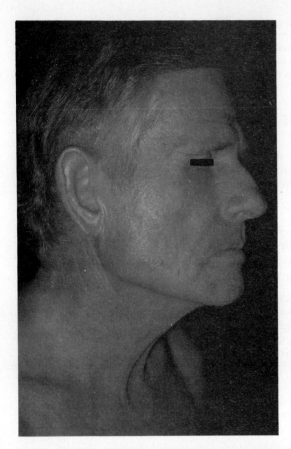

FIG. 38–5. Compositae dermatitis of the face in a horticulturist. The morphology is similar to photodermatitis but typically some light-protected sites are involved. This patient and many other such patients are both Compositae allergic and photosensitive.

light reactions, begins in adult life, tends to spare the feet, and is worse during the summer.[34] The atopic pattern may overlap with the photosensitivity pattern, causing a mixed clinical presentation.[33] This form has even been reported in childhood.[34] However, weed dermatitis in general is rarely reported in children and is less common in women. In adults, the incidence is 20:1 greater in males.[39]

PATTERN 3: EXFOLIATIVE DERMATITIS

Severe cases may cause exfoliative erythroderma, especially in persons allergic to *Parthenium hysterophorus.*[40] This plant has been transported to India in contaminated seed wheat, where it has caused weed dermatitis in epidemic numbers. Over half the adult male workers employed to pull this weed become allergic to it, and many persons become incapacitated by the magnitude of the eruptions. The principal allergen in this plant is parthenin, a water-soluble sesquiterpene lactone.[41]

PATTERN 4: HAND ECZEMA

Routine testing to related chemicals in patch-test screening of patients with contact dermatitis may uncover any of the above patterns or even hand eczema.[35] I have seen

TABLE 38-3. Weed Dermatitis

1. Older males are typically affected.
2. Exposed sites in five patterns:
   a. Photodermatitis-like pattern (but involving the eyelids as well as submental and postauricular sites)
   b. Atopic eczema-like onset is in later life; the rash is better in winter and the feet are likely to be spared.
   c. Hand eczema. The pattern may suggest contact or it may be picked up on routine patch-test screening.
   d. Exfoliative erythroderma which mimics a photoallergic dermatitis (persistent light reaction) or actinic reticuloid.
   e. Localized pattern:
      • Acute—localized patch(es) of an acute eczema similar to the pattern seen in allergy to topical medications or even to that of poison ivy dermatitis.
      • Chronic—lichen simplex–like reaction has been reported with magnolia sensitivity.
3. Outdoor exposure is typical.
4. Occupation or hobbies may be a factor. Farmers, florist, gardeners, woodcutters, and hunters are especially at risk.
5. Summer aggravation is typical.
6. Reduced minimum erythema dose (MED) on phototesting is common and may be a source of confusion.

hand involvement with ragweed allergy[34] and especially with bitterweed dermatitis, and these probably depend upon an opportunity for direct exposure. This pattern is found by patch-test screening of patients in Europe, where those plants are absent,[35] so multiple species can cause this pattern. In the latter group, the diagnosis was not suspected before the positive patch test was found.

PATTERN 5: LOCALIZED DERMATITIS

A fifth pattern is a strong acute eczematous eruption in localized areas.[36,42] Cocklebur dermatitis, often is more localized and spotty.[1-4] It may also be less chronic and consistently present. A more acute eruption may even resemble poison ivy dermatitis.[36] One should be wary of patch-test responses to mayweed, as it often causes an irritant reaction that is sometimes difficult to distinguish from contact allergy. Hausen sent me a slide of a patient who had a local reaction to an extract of arnica, and many other causes are likely to be found later.

THE ANTIGENIC SOURCE(S)

The cause of (allergic) weed dermatitis is delayed hypersensitivity to one or more chemicals called sesquiterpene lactones.[43] These may occur in more than one plant, so a positive reaction, although proving allergy, does not necessarily mean *that* plant is the cause of the patient's problem. The causative chemicals are found in small glands in trichomes, tiny hairlike structures on the plant surface.[44] Although the pollen in a few of these plants may contain antigens, this does not seem to be the case for most.[36] The eruption typically begins as a summertime eczema in exposed sites, extending in subsequent years to later in the fall, until it becomes "perennial," being present through-

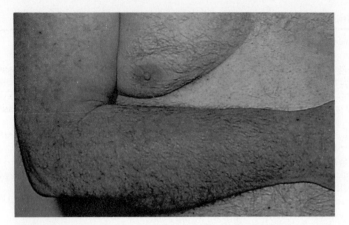

FIG. 38–6. Compositae dermatitis resembling photodermatitis.

out the year. It clears on total removal from the environment, and farmers who move to the city tend to clear in spite of high pollen content in the air.[45–47] Dust from hay may, however, contain the antigen,[48] and in such cases the antigen clearly could be airborne. For the most part, however, it seems to be spread by hand transfer.

Plants from some other plant families (e.g., *Frullania, Magnolia*, and *Laurus*) may

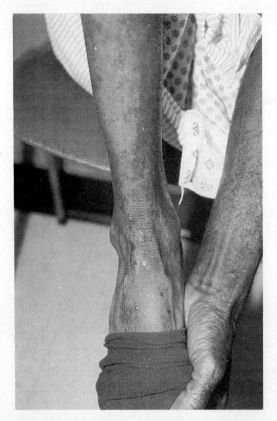

FIG. 38–7. Compositae dermatitis resembling atopic eczema. (See color Plate 35.)

cross-react.[36,42] Patients may also react to Compositae plants to which they have never been exposed, as the same SQTL may be found in multiple species.[43]

PATCH TESTING

To supplement commercially available sesquiterpene lactone mix, one can collect a few of the causative (local) plants and preserve them in a labeled plastic bag in the freezer. A small piece can be cut out for patch testing when needed. Shelmire cautioned against leaving such tests on longer than 1 to 2 h because of irritancy, so if they are left on longer to elicit a positive test, one should run controls. Suggested plants one might collect are as follows:

Bitterweed* (*Helenium amarum*) in the southeastern United States.
Chrysanthemum (*Dendranthema* X cultivar) or the florist's chrysanthemum (one should always test to the actual plants the patient contacts if the history is positive).
Cocklebur* (*Xanthium spinosum*).
Feverfew (*Tanacetum parthenium*), often grown as an herb.
Narrow-leaf marsh elder* (*Iva angustifolia*) where it is local.
Sagebrush (*Artemisia tridentata*) in western states.
Short ragweed* (*Ambrosia artemisiifolia*).
Sunflower (*Helianthus annuus*).
Tansy in western states (*Tanacetum vulgare*).
Wild feverfew* (*Parthenium hysterophorus*) in Texas and other areas where it grows.

Chrysanthemum is a special case, as one must test patients to the plants to which they have been exposed. I have seen one variety produce a prominent reaction, while other varieties of the same species are negative. "Alantalactone," available as helenin from Sigma (as a mixture of alantolactone and isoalantolactone)[49] and other chemical companies, is tested in a 0.1% concentration in petrolatum.[50] It has been used to screen for allergy (to *Frullania*, a liverwort) in woodcutters of the Pacific Northwest.[50] It is irregularly positive in Compositae dermatitis.[51] Mitchell suggests application of leaf, flower head, stalk, and petal, using controls to rule out irritancy.[52] Laurel is freely available as bay leaves in the spice rack at a grocery store, but it may not produce a positive response in sensitive persons.[53] In warmer latitudes of the United States, one can harvest magnolia leaves in the neighborhood at any time they are needed for patch testing, as that tree is an evergreen. Patch testing to plants is summarized in Table 38-4.

TREATMENT

Treatment of chronic dermatitis to Compositae has traditionally been considered to be difficult. Several approaches are indicated: Obviously one should educate the patient as to the cause and how to avoid such plants and minimize exposure. This may even require an occupational change or a move to town. Psoralens and longware ultraviolet light (UVA) therapy can be beneficial,[54] used much the same way one treats photocontact

---

*These comprise the screening series Shelmire used to challenge Texas patients suspected of having some form of Compositae dermatitis, according to J. B. Richardson.

TABLE 38–4. Patch Testing to Plants

1. Primin, the antigen in *Primula*, is available in 0.01% concentration in the ICDRG series from Chemotechnique and Trolab.
2. Alpha-methylene gamma butyrolactone, the antigen in tulip and *Alstromeria*, is available from Chemotechnique.
3. Helenin, 0.1% in petrolatum, is available from Chemotechnique and Trolab; it will detect most but not all *Frullania* reactors.
4. Lichen acids and fumaric acid from Chemotechnique along with usnic acid and Atranorin available from Trolab and Chemotechnique can be used to screen for lichen allergy. Oak moss absolute, which is one of eight components of the perfume mix in the standard series, is also derived from a lichen.
5. Turpentine and colophony in the standard series can indicate allergy to several conifers. Wood tars are available from Trolab and Chemotechnique. Balsams of pine and spruce are available from Trolab. Pine wood, pine tar, and beech tar can be purchased from Chemotechnique.
6. Compositae plants can be tested as leaf, stem, and flower head as is. Magnolia leaf should be excoriated before applying. Bay leaf may produce false-negatives and should be tested as oil of laurel if available.
7. A screening antigen, sesquiterpene-lactone mix, is available commercially from European suppliers. The sensitivity and specificity of this test are not known.
8. Unknown plants can be tested (as is) *if not* irritating, but controls are in order.
   a. Save one specimen to identify botanically.
   b. Save one specimen in a plastic bag in the freezer.
   c. Apply the unknown specimen as leaf, stem, and flower, using controls. Shelmire recommended a 1-h application. For 24- to 48-h application, controls must be used. Irritancy should be excluded using a standard reference.[1-4]
9. Woods are usually tested as sawdust:
   a. Sawdust is taken from a single species, placed in a plastic bag, and labeled with the name.
   b. 10% sawdust in petrolatum is tested originally.
   c. If negative, dry sawdust can be applied.
   d. Wet sawdust can be tried, with controls, if dry sawdust is negative.
10. Nonirritant bulbs can be applied "as is" after removing the outer layer. Onion and garlic are tested as 25% in petrolatum, using controls.

dermatitis. For resistant cases, oral azathioprine has been recommended.[55,56] This provides considerable relief from the pruritus and improves about half such patients markedly. The others are better but retain noticeable dermatitis.

Formerly, oral hyposensitization kits were available, but they no longer are. Biological agents are difficult to standardize and expensive to market in the United States. They can be effective, perhaps based on the development of anti-idiotypic antibodies.[55] Trying this without a commercial product is not recommended.

ALSTROEMERIA AND TULIP

Persons working in retail and wholesale floristry are at risk to become allergic to *Alstroemeria* spp. (Peruvian lily or Inca lily)[57,58] and *Tulipa* (tulip).[59] The acute eruption is typically seen in the grip area of the fingers of retail florists, especially the thumb, index, and middle fingers. Fissures commonly occur within a hyperkeratotic eczema which starts at the free edge of the nail and progresses to the fingertips and proximally to the periungual area.[60] The allergen alpha-methylene gamma-butyrolactone (Tulipalin

A) is derived from tulipsoide A in the plants.[61] Contact to tulip is often from handling the bulbs, but it can also occur from exposure to other parts.[60] The allergen in *Alstroemeria* is especially concentrated in the petals.[61] The same antigen is also found in dog's tooth violet, *Erythronium dens canis* and *Erythronium americanum*.[60]

PATCH TESTING

The antigen, alpha-methylene-gamma-butyrolactone, is commercially available from Chemotechnique as a "various allergen." Testing can also be done with either *Alstroemeria* or *Tulipa*, but because of the high concentration in the petals of *Alstroemeria* especially, there is some risk of both false-positive irritant reactions and active sensitization.[62]

Patch testing can be done with an extract of tulip bulb (Apeldoorn variety is suitable) by shaking in 80% acetone (in water) for 90 min, evaporated dry, and resuspended in a 1% concentration in alcohol 70%.[60] The bulb surface is also satisfactory after the brown outside layer is removed. Controls are recommended.

PREVENTION

The *Alstroemeria* allergen goes through ordinary latex and vinyl gloves, so an impervious glove should be used. Marks[62] and Adams et al.[58] recommend nitrile gloves [Solvex; 15 mils, catalogue number 37-155 or 37-175 (flock-lined); Edmond-Becton Dickinson 1300 Walnut Street Coshocton, OH 43812], but the latter group warn that incidental contact caused by antigen transfer from the counter and fomites may make avoidance impossible without a job change.[58]

PRIMULA DERMATITIS

When you see an older woman with a dermatitis of the fingertips and streaks and patchy eczema on the hands, face, and arms, look for *primula obconica* as a likely cause of the rash.[62a] This plant is such a common contact allergen in Europe that about 1.0 to 1.8 percent of persons routinely patch tested react to the causative allergen, primin, 0.01% in petrolatum as part of the European screening series.[62b,c] The eruption often is not suspected until the positive patch test appears,[62b] and the nondescript pattern may suggest an endogenous cause.[62a]

The allergy is said to be caused when one growing the houseplant pinches off dying blooms to encourage the plant to bloom again. However the allergen is present in shorter "hairs" on the plant surface and more concentrated in smaller leaves, so contact is extremely easy.[62d] Primin is such a strong antigen and is in such variable concentration in the plant that it is better to patch test to the chemical, now commercially available in 0.01% concentration in petrolatum. Unfortunately, however, primin 0.01% does not detect every reactor.[62e] Photodermatitis to primula has been reported,[62f] and phototesting may be indicated in some patients. Delayed readings up to 7 days are important.[61,62]

In warmer climates (e.g., frost-free areas in California), one may see this plant growing outdoors, and it seems to be regularly available in nurseries, at least in San Francisco.[58] Of the some 400 other species of primula grown outdoors or indoors,[63] none seem to cross-react and only a few produce dermatitis, usually irritant in nature.[62] Avoidance is easy once the problem is identified, and a primin-free strain of *Primula obconica* is now available as seed from Thompson and Morgan, although this genus can be difficult to germinate.

PHYTOPHOTODERMATITIS

Streaks of vesicles and bullae in light-exposed sites may be caused by photocontact dermatitis, especially when the acute eruption is followed by pigmentation. Phytophotodermatitis can be due to multiple mechanisms, but most cases are caused by plants containing furanocoumarins or psoralens. Many plants of the Umbelliferae and Rutaceae (citrus), which contain psoralens, cause berloque dermatitis following light exposure.[64] The sensitizer is probably more often spread with the hands, but sometimes the light sensitizer is thrown onto the skin when weeds are being cut with a string trimmer such as the Weed Eater.[65] Of course, it is necessary to have adequate sunlight exposure in addition to contact with the plant.

Photodermatitis in celery harvesters has been said to be more common from plants infected with the pink-rot fungus *Sclerotinia sclerotiorum*.[66] The variety is important in determining psoralen content, and the content may be adequate for a number of varieties when the subject is exposed to large quantities of UVA, as in a tanning salon. Grocery workers have developed photodermatitis from the cut surfaces of uninfected celery if followed by intense sunbathing or a visit to a tanning salon.[67]

Typical plants causing phytophotodermatitis include Persian limes (*Citrus aurantium*), fig trees (*Ficus carica*), gas plants (*Dictamnus albus*), giant hogweed (*Heracleum mantegazzianum*), common rue (*Ruta graveolens*), bishop's weed (*Ammi majus*), wild parsnip (*Pastinaca sativa*), angelica (*Angelica archangelica*), fig (*Ficus carica*), and the scurf pea (*Psoralea corylifolia*).[64] A number of other plants have been reported to produce phytophotodermatitis, including some which are photoallergenic. For example, light-absorbing chemicals in lichens or oak moss (from a lichen) may cause photoallergic dermatitis,[68,69] although this is not experimentally reproducible with atranorin and lichen mix.[70] Several grasses, buckwheat, and others reportedly can cause photoreactions in domesticated animals.[64]

Many other plants which do not contain psoralen reportedly cause photosensitivity, including St. John's wort (*Hypericum perforatum*). The subject has been reviewed recently by Pathak.[64]

IRRITANT REACTIONS

The term *irritant* is used for any nonallergic response which, in the case of plants, covers a multitude of causes. Irritant reactions tend to occur within a few minutes rather than after 2 days and they are more likely to burn rather than itch. These also occur on first exposure and are dose-related. Allergic reactions do not occur on first exposure, and even small amounts of antigen can cause a prominent reaction in highly sensitive subjects. The mechanisms for nonallergic reactions are also greatly variable, from mechanical injury from various species of cactus to urticaria from nettles to strong vesiculation from Euphorbiaceae.

Mechanical injury may occur from thorns of plants, from roses and blackberry to Hawthorn and *Euphorbia* species[71,72] Some grains (e.g., barley) have prominent awns which can produce injury. Many of the Cactaceae also produce mechanical injury. The list of such plants is long, but one can easily make the diagnosis.

Sabra dermatitis from *Opuntia ficus-indica* can simulate scabies.[73] The bunny ears cactus, *Opuntia microdasys*, a commonly grown ornamental, also has collections of tiny spines called *glochidia,* which are the source of immediate irritation, sometimes leading to granuloma formation.[74]

A common source of plant irritation is calcium oxalate, which is found in a number of irritant plants including dumbcane (*Dieffenbachia*), daffodils, *Hyacinth, Arisaema,* lily, pineapple, and other species.[71] The chemical contained in intracellular crystals, called raphides, is ejected from the cell on contact with water. Typically, when leaves of dumbcane are chewed, a burning sensation occurs almost immediately, followed by salivation and perhaps a dermatitis.[75] Mustards (including radish, horseradish, etc.) contain sinigrins which become irritating when they are enzymatically converted into isocyanates. Buttercup (*Ranunculus* species) contain protoanemonin, as do columbine (*Aquilegia*), marsh marigold (*Caltha*), *Clematis, Delphinium,* and *Anemone.*[71]

Some spurges (*Euphorbiaceae*) are not only strong vesicants but contain phorbol esters in the latex that are cocarcinogens as well.[72] Many are tropical plants, such as the infamous manchineel tree. However, equally toxic latex may be found in related houseplants, such as the candelabra cactus. Croton oil is obtained from *Croton tiglium.*[72]

REFERENCES

1. Mitchell J, Rook A: *Botanical Dermatology: Plants and Plant Products Injurious to the Skin.* Vancouver, Canada, Greengrass, 1979.
2. Kingsbury JM: *Poisonous Plants of the United States and Canada.* Englewood Cliffs, N.J., Prentice-Hall, 1964.
3. Lampe KF, McCann MA: *AMA Handook of Poisonous and Injurious Plants.* Chicago, American Medical Association, 1985.
4. Guin JD, Beaman JH: Plant dermatitis. *Clin Dermatol* 4:137, 1986.
5. Baer H: Chemistry and immunochemistry of poisonous Anacardiaceae. *Clin Dermatol* 4:152, 186.
6. Resnick SD: Poison-ivy and Poison-oak dermatitis. *Clin Dermatol* 4:208, 1986.
7. Guin JD: Reaction time in experimental poison ivy dermatitis (abstract). *Contact Dermatitis* 6:289, 1980.
8. Feldmann RJ, Maibach HI: Regional variation in percutaneous penetration of ^{14}C cortisol in man. *J Invest Dermatol* 48:181, 1967.
9. Reynolds G, Epstein W, Terry D, et al: A potent contact allergen *Phacelia* (Hydrophyllaceae). *Contact Dermatitis* 6:272, 1980.
10. Kligman AM: Poison ivy (Rhus) dermatitis. *Arch Dermatol* 77:149, 1958.
11. Guin JD: Poison ivy (Rhus) dermatitis. *J Indiana State Med Assoc* 72:774, 1978.
12. Guin, JD: Poison ivy dermatitis in winter with an example of filial contact dermatitis. *J Indiana State Med Assoc* 76:184, 1983.
13. Sulzberger MB, Katz JH: The absence of skin irritants in the contents of vesicles. *US Naval Med Bull* 41:1258, 1943.
14. Guin JD, Gillis WT, Beaman JH: Recognizing the toxicodendrons (poison ivy, poison oak, and poison sumac). *J Am Acad Dermatol* 4:99, 1981.

15. Guin JD, Beaman JH: Toxicodendrons of the United States. *Clin Dermatol* 4:137, 1986.

16. Mallory SB, Hurwitz RM: Black-spot poison-ivy dermatitis. *Clin Dermatol* 4:149, 1986.

17. Guin JD: The black spot test for recognizing poison ivy and related species. *J Am Acad Dermatol* 2:332, 1980.

18. Johnson RA, Baer H, Kirkpatrick CH, et al: Comparison of the contact allergenicity of the four pentadecyl catechols derived from poison ivy urushiol in human subjects. *J Allergy Clin Immunol* 49:27, 1972.

19. Hausen BM: *Woods Injurious to Human Health—A Manual.* Berlin, de Gruyter, 1981.

20. Breathnach SM: Immunologic aspects of contact dermatitis. *Clin Dermatol* 4:5, 1986.

21. Kalish RS: The use of human T-lymphocyte clones to study T-cell function in allergic contact dermatitis to urushiol. *J Invest Derm* 94:108S, 1990.

22. Guin JD, Reynolds R: Jewelweed treatment of poison ivy dermatitis. *Contact Dermatitis* 6:287, 1980.

23. Orchard S, Fellman JH, Storrs FJ: Poison ivy/oak dermatitis. *Arch Dermatol* 122:783, 1986.

24. Oltman J, Hensler R: Poison oak/ivy and forestry workers. *Clin Dermatol* 4:213, 1986.

25. Epstein WL: Topical prevention of poison ivy/oak dermatitis. *Arch Dermatol* 125:499, 1989.

26. Murrell D: *Advances in the Prevention of Poison Ivy.* Sixteenth Hawaii Dermatology Seminar, Maui, Hawaii, February 9, 1992.

27. Epstein WL, Byers VS, Frankart W: Induction of antigen-specific hyposensitization to poison oak in sensitized adults. *Arch Dermatol* 118:630, 1982.

28. Watson ES: Toxicodendron hyposensitization programs. *Clin Dermatol* 4:160, 1986.

29. Shelmire B: Hyposensitization to poison ivy. *Arch Dermatol Syph* 44:983, 1941.

30. Kawai Ke, Nakagawa M, Kawai Ky, et al: Hyposensitization to urushiol among Japanese lacquer craftsmen: Results of patch tests on students learning the art of lacquerware. *Contact Dermatitis* 25:290, 1991.

31. van der Steen PHM, van Baar HMJ, Perret CM, Happle R: Treatment of alopecia areata with diphenyl-cyclopropenone. *J Am Acad Dermatol* 24:253, 1991.

32. Webster RC, Noonan PK, Maibach HI: Percutaneous absorption of hydrocortisone increases with long-term administration. *Arch Dermatol* 116:186, 1980.

33. Schmidt RJ: Compositae. *Clin Dermatol* 4:46, 1986.

34. Guin JD, Skidmore G: Compositae dermatitis in childhood. *Arch Dermatol* 123:500, 1987.

35. Ducombs G, Benezra C, Talaga P, et al: Patch testing with the "sesquiterpene lactone mix": A marker for contact allergy to Compositae and other sesquiterpene-lactone-containing plants. *Contact Dermatitis* 22:249, 1990.

36. Guin JD: Sesquiterpene-lactone dermatitis. *Immunol Allergy Clin North Am* 9:447, 1989.

37. Frain-Bell W: Photosensitivity and Compositae dermatitis. *Clin Dermatol* 4:122, 1986.

38. Wrangsjo K, Ros AM, Wahlberg JE: Contact allergy to Compositae plants in patients with summer-exacerbated dermatitis. *Contact Dermatitis* 22:148, 1990.

39. Mitchell JC, Fisher AA: Dermatitis due to plants and spices, in *Contact Dermatitis.* Philadelphia, Lea & Febiger, 1986.

40. Mitchell JC, Calnan CD: Scourge of India. *Parthenium* dermatitis. *Int J Dermatol* 17:303, 1978.

41. Lonkar A, Mitchell JC, Calnan CD: Contact dermatitis from *Parthenium hysterophorus. Trans St John's Hosp Dermatol Soc* 60:43, 1974.

42. Guin JD, Schosser RH, Rosenberg EW: *Magnolia grandiflora* dermatitis. *Dermatol Clin* 8:81, 1990.

43. Mitchell JC, Dupuis G: Allergic contact dermatitis from sesquiterpenoids of the Compositae family of plants. *Br J Derm* 84:139, 1971.

44. Rodrigues E, Dillon MO, Mabry TJ, et al: Dermatologically active sesquiterpene lactones in trichomes of *Parthenium hysterophorus* L. *Experientia* 32:236, 1976.

45. Shelmire B: Contact dermatitis from vegetation. *South Med J* 33:337, 1940.

46. Howell JB: Sensitivity to common weeds. *Contact Dermatitis Newsletter* 10:230, 1971.

47. Howell JB: Contact dermatitis from weeds: Facts and fallacies (letters). *Contact Dermatitis* 4:365, 1978.

48. Epstein S: Sensitivity to common weeds. *Contact Dermatitis Newsletter* 11:305, 1972.

49. Stampf J, Benezra C, Klecak G, et al: The sensitizing capacity of helenin and of two of its main constituents, the sesquiterpene lactones alantolactone and isoalantolactone: A comparison of epicutaneous and intradermal sensitizing methods in different strains of guinea pig. *Contact Dermatitis* 8:16, 1982.

50. Mitchell JC: Frullania (liverwort) phytodermatitis (woodcutter's eczema). *Clin Dermatol* 4:62, 1986.

51. De Corres LF: Contact dermatitis from frullania, Compositae and other plants. *Contact Dermatitis* 11:74, 1984.
52. Mitchell JC: Patch testing to plants. *Clin Derm* 4:77, 1986.
53. Farkas J: Perioral dermatitis from marjoram, bay leaf and cinnamon. *Contact Dermatitis* 7:121, 1981.
54. Guin JD, Baker GF, Mitchell JC: Persistent open patch test reaction. *Contact Dermatitis* 6:289, 1980.
55. Stampf J, Castagnoli N, Epstein W, et al: Suppression of urushiol-induced delayed-type hypersensitivity responses in mice with serum IgG immunoglobulin from human hyposensitized donors. *J Invest Dermatol* 95:363, 1990.
56. Baadsgaard O: Circulating and in situ lymphocyte subsets and Langerhans cells in patients with compositae oleoresin dermatitis and increased ultraviolet A sensitivity during treatment with azathioprine. *J Am Acad Dermatol* 14:577, 1986.
57. Thiboutot DM, Hamory BH, Marks JG: Dermatoses among floral workers. *J Am Acad Dermatol* 22:54, 1990.
58. Adams RM, Daily AD, Brancaccio R, et al: *Alstroemeria:* A new and potent allergen for florists. *Dermatol Clin* 8:73, 1990.
59. Gette MT, Marks JE: Tulip fingers. *Arch Dermatol* 126:203, 1990.
60. Hjorth N, Wilkinson DS: Contact dermatitis in IV: Tulip fingers, hyacinth itch and lily rash. *Br J Dermatol* 80:696, 1968.
61. Hausen BM, Prater E, Schubert H: The sensitizing capacity of *Alstroemeria* cultivars in man and guinea pig. *Contact Dermatitis* 9:46, 1983.
62. Marks JG Jr: Allergic contact dermatitis to *Alstroemeria. Arch Dermatol* 124:914, 1988.
62a. Epstein E: Primula contact dermatitis: An easily overlooked diagnosis. *Cutis* 45:411, 1990.
62b. Logan RA, White IR: Primula dermatitis: Prevalence, detection and outcome. *Contact Dermatitis* 19:68, 1988.
62c. Ingber A, Mennet: Primin standard patch testing: 5 years experience. *Contact Dermatitis* 23:15, 1990.
62d. Hjorth N: Primula dermatitis, in Mitchell J, Rook A (eds): *Botanical Dermatology,* Vancouver, Greengrass 1979, pp 554–565.
62e. Dooms-Goossens A, Biesemans G, Vandaele M, Degreaf H: Primula dermatitis: More than one allergen? *Contact Dermatitis* 21:122, 1989.
62f. Ingber A: Primula photodermatitis in Israel. *Contact Dermatitis* 25:265, 1991.
63. Bailey LH, Bailey EZ: *Hortus Third.* New York, Macmillan, 1976, pp 907–912.
64. Pathak MA: Phytophotodermatitis. *Clin Dermatol* 4:102–121, 1990.
65. Freeman K, Hubbard HC, Warin AP: Strimmer rash. *Contact Dermatitis* 10:117, 1984.
66. Birmingham DJ, Key MM, Tublich GE, et al: Phototoxic bullae among celery harvesters. *Arch Dermatol* 83:73, 1961.
67. Seligman PJ, Mathias CG, O'Malley MA, et al: Phytophotodermatitis from celery among grocery store workers. *Arch Dermatol* 123:1478, 1987.
68. Guin JD, Jackson DB: Oakmoss photosensitivity in a ragweed-allergic patient. *Contact Dermatitis* 18:240, 1988.
69. Thune PO, Solberg YJ: Photosensitivity and allergy to aromatic lichen acids, Compositae oleoresins and other plant substances. *Contact Dermatitis* 6:81, 1980.
70. Sandberg M, Thune P: The sensitizing capacity of atranorin. *Contact Dermatitis* 11:168, 1984.
71. Stoner JG: Miscellaneous dermatitis-inducing plants. *Clin Dermatol* 4:94, 1986.
72. Webster G: Irritant plants in the spurge family (Euphorbiaceae). *Clin Dermatol* 4:36, 1986.
73. Shannon J, Sagher F: Sabra dermatitis: An occupational dermatitis due to prickly pear handling simulating scabies. *Arch Dermatol* 74:269, 1956.
74. Snyder RA, Schwartz RA: Cactus bristle implantation. *Arch Dermatol* 119:152, 1983.
75. Lampe KF, McCann MA: *AMA Handbook of Poisonous and Injurious Plants.* Chicago, American Medical Association, 1985, pp 72–73.

39

FOODS

Jose G. Camarasa

Adverse reactions to foods may range from mild dyspepsia to botulism. Cutaneous responses are also quite varied, including such diverse conditions as vasculitis,[1] erythema multifore minor,[2] Stevens-Johnson syndrome,[3] pseudoscleroderma,[4] perioral dermatitis,[5] and shiitake dermatitis,[6] to name a few.

Contact problems from foods include irritant and allergic contact dermatitis, contact urticaria, phototoxic and photoallergic dermatitis, and protein contact dermatitis (Figs. 39-1 to 39-7). All of these and more can be caused not only by the natural foods but also by a multitude of chemical additives such as antioxidants, biocides and other preservatives, flavoring, coloring, pesticides, bleaching agents, emulsifiers, and so on. The possibilities of change from the original product are increased with each step in the processing. Cutaneous problems from food occur in those who grow it, process it, handle it, transport it, sell it, and prepare it—even in those of us who consume it. Many of these are occupational areas, and chefs seem to be more at risk. However even a housewife or anyone preparing his or her own food is at some risk. Despite the ubiquitous exposure, the number of such cases is not as great as one might suspect. However, it may be that only the dramatic or illustrative cases are considered suitable for publication.

The usual patient may present several possible pictures. According to Adams,[7] most reactions are irritant, as this seems to be what most dermatologists see in the office even in a referral practice. However, in some reported series, this is not the case, perhaps because of patient selection. Irritant dermatitis may be more prevalent in patients with an atopic background. Soaps and detergents are leading causes of irritation in patients with nonspecific hand eczema, but certain foods—such as onion, garlic, and raw meat can be very irritating to eczematous skin. Consequently, most dermatologists advise their patients with hand eczema to avoid contact with these foods.

Allergic contact dermatitis sometimes causes a recognizable pattern e.g., garlic dermatitis (Fig. 39-1). This in many ways resembles tulip finger and *Alstroemeria* dermatitis, which are caused by plants containing a different but similar chemical. In other cases the cause is multifactorial, and the diagnosis requires suspicion and investigation, especially patch testing, as relevant positive patch-test responses in allergic contact dermatitis provide critically important information. Some patients with

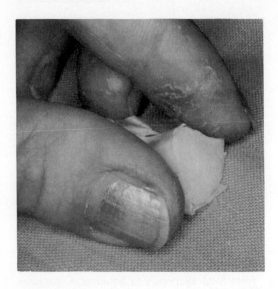

FIG. 39–1. Garlic dermatitis in the area where garlic was held. (Courtesy Dr. Luis Conde-Salazar and Dr. Robert Adams). (See color Plate 36.)

contact urticaria also have positive patch tests, in which case two allergic mechanisms are operating.

A type 1 mechanism is confirmed by scratch, prick, and other tests for immediate sensitivity. Many of these patients have a history of atopy and especially food-induced urticaria, which should make one suspicious. Persons who had childhood eczema should be asked about specific allergies, as most know the foods which cause a problem.

Nonspecific hand eczema such as one sees in adults who formerly had atopic eczema may flare following exposure to anything causing sudden itching, including contact urticaria. There one may see rapid aggravation of an eczema based on an underlying contact urticaria.

An immediate type of hand eczema can occur in chefs and other salad makers with positive prick tests and pompholyx type lesions, which develops within minutes after exposure. In addition, all these clinical aspects can have their origin in the foods themselves or in other substances that are added to them (artificial additives).

Reports of such cases seem to be a product of modern times, with perhaps the classic model being that reported in 1948, involving an itching, papular contact dermatitis of the hands, suffered by a group of workers in a Danish factory that preserved mussels. Some of the workers also complained of urticaria and asthma, with positive intradermal testing and passive transfer.[8]

The combination of type I allergy in eczema patients was mentioned in publications by Malten[9] and by Hjorth and Weismann[10] in kitchen personnel suffering allergic contact hand eczema from certain foods. As a consequence of that, a large patch-testing series of foods was organized to study suspected food-induced dermatitis in chefs and other kitchen personnel who handle such foods as artichokes, wild asparagus, carrots, radish, chicory, lettuce, onions, garlic, lemons and other citrus fruits, cucumber, fish and shellfish, meats, and cheeses.[11-13] The concept of protein contact dermatitis evolved from the data obtained in this study.

There are also some unusual cutaneous reactions to foods which do not fit the usual list of mechanisms. One of these, protein contact dermatitis, is discussed below. Another is shiitake dermatitis.

In Japan and certain other countries, a characteristic eruption follows consumption an edible mushroom, *Lentinus edodes*,[14] if it is uncooked. This begins some 1 to 2 days after the mushrooms are consumed with an erythematous, papular rash in lines suggestive of finger marks. Externally, it fits a hand-transfer pattern, but it is best known as an eruption following ingestion. Histologically one sees spongiosis with dermal edema and a perivascular lymphocytic infiltrate. This does not occur from cooked mushrooms. It may have multiple underlying mechanisms, as both patch tests for delayed hypersensitivity and prick tests for immediate hypersensitivity are positive. Sometimes a generalized toxic erythema is seen.[15] Symptomatology is not limited to cutaneous problems, as respiratory symptoms sometimes occur in persons who work in commercial production.

OCCUPATIONAL EXPOSURE

Obviously one cannot always predict every type or cause of occupational contact dermatitis. However, there are several occupations in which exposure to food is worth mentioning specifically.

GENERAL ASPECTS

Cutaneous reactions to foods comprise irritant and allergic contact dermatitis, immunologic and nonimmunologic contact urticaria, phototoxic and photoallergic dermatitis, and a number of other conditions that are not so easily explained.

Certainly irritant eczemas are a problem, especially in those with an atopic background. Some irritant reactions can parallel certain reactions found in workers in slaughterhouses, fish processing, and chicken processing, where raw meat is handled. This is time- and temperature-dependent to some extent, as the mechanism seems to be enzymatic (due to muscle proteolytic enzymes and contamination from intestinal contents).

Contact urticaria is most often due to fish and other seafood, meats, and occasionally, vegetables, especially onions.

In food service workers, the chief source of allergic contact dermatitis is garlic[16] (Fig. 39-1); this condition seems to be due to diallyldisulfide sensitivity. Most but not all who are allergic to garlic will also react to fresh onion.[12] Most food service workers who have a personal or family history of atopy have positive scratch tests, but most patients with positive scratch tests in the definitive study were not atopic.[12] In Hjorth's series of 33 chefs and sandwich makers referred for a putative occupational problem, 25 had positive scratch tests but only 7 had a personal or family history of atopy. Of the 7, 6 had positive patch tests.[12]

One of the most confusing conditions seen following chronic food exposure is protein contact dermatitis (Fig. 39-2). This, according to Tosti, was originally described in 1952 by Seeberg,[17] when four cases were reported. The definitive paper was probably written by Hjorth and Roed-Petersen[12] when they reported 33 food handlers with four

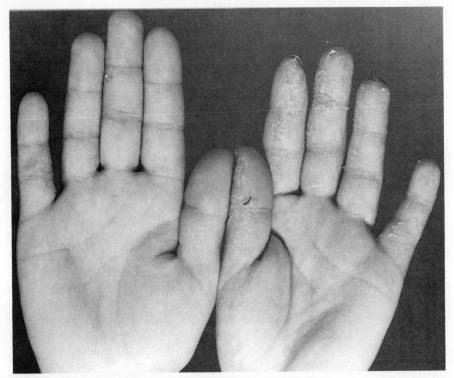

FIG. 39–2. Food handler dermatitis caused by onion in a food handler who held it in her left hand to slice it. (From Niinimäki A: Scratch-chamber tests in food handler dermatitis. *Contact Dermatitis* 16:11–20, 1987; © 1987 by Munksgaard International Publishers Ltd., Copenhagen, Denmark. Reprinted with permission.)

different types of contact dermatitis: (1) irritant and (2) allergic contact dermatitis; (3) a combination of allergic contact dermatitis with positive scratch tests, and (4) an eczematous eruption and positive scratch tests. They named the last of these "protein contact dermatitis." This entity does not fit the traditional concept of the mechanism of eczema and is regarded as contact urticaria by some. However, there are several features of this condition which make that assumption untenable.

Hjorth and Roed-Petersen[12] found that their patients with protein contact dermatitis not only developed pompholyx-like vesiculation on local exposure to specific foods but that they did so after only 20 min. This sounds like an irritant reaction, but—as we shall see—there are close ties with immunologic changes. The foods usually associated are fish and other (seafood) meats and less often certain vegetables, especially onion.

Testing with foods is not always done in the traditional way. Cronin[16] used both prick and patch tests to investigate hand eczema in caterers, including foods brought by patients, and a standard series plus onion and garlic. The last two must be diluted to avoid irritation; if the concentration is too low, however, one sees many false-negative responses. Cronin used 50 percent garlic in arachis oil and 50 percent onion in arachis oil. Prick tests are used to test for immediate reaction to foods. A thin slice of the food in question is applied to the upper back and the skin is pricked through the food sample, using a sterile stylet or hypodermic needle. Histamine 1:100,000 solution was used as a positive control, using the same prick test through it. Of 47 persons, 20 had totally negative tests, but 9 reacted to prick tests, 8 to patch tests, and 2 to both. Cautions about prick testing can be found in Chap. 19.

Niinimäki reported a similar series using the scratch-chamber method.[18] A scratch 5 mm long is made in the skin and the material to be tested is applied inside a chamber for 20 min initially. Then the chamber is removed and the test read. It is then reapplied and left on for 24 h to check for delayed sensitivity. When testing with dried material, Niinimäki applied the test material with wet blotting paper. A 1% histamine phosphate solution was used as a positive control. To be positive, the test response must have been at least half the size of the control. Niinimäki also patch tested persons in his group to a standard series and usually with food additives.

Another technique for urticarial responses is the rub test. This is done by rubbing the crushed foodstuff on and in an area of the hand or finger, usually where there had been a breakout. This sort of open testing is often used for persons with contact urticaria as a first step before doing closed applications.[19] Reactions are seen in Figs. 39-3 to 39-5.

The mechanism of protein contact dermatitis has been studied by Tosti et al.,[20] who found spongiotic epidermal change with parakeratosis in the apparently normal skin. There was also a collection of dermal lymphocytes with helper predominance as well

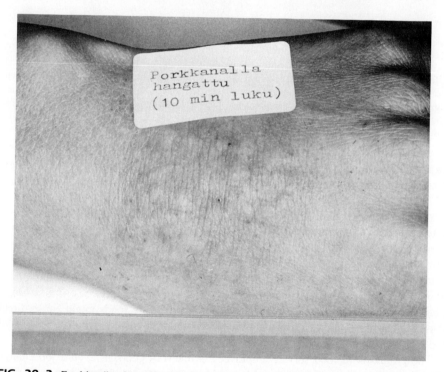

FIG. 39–3. Food handler dermatitis: positive rub test to carrot. (From Niinimäki A: Scratch-chamber tests in food handler dermatitis. *Contact Dermatitis* 16:11–20, 1987; © 1987 by Munksgaard International Publishers Ltd., Copenhagen, Denmark. Reprinted with permission.)

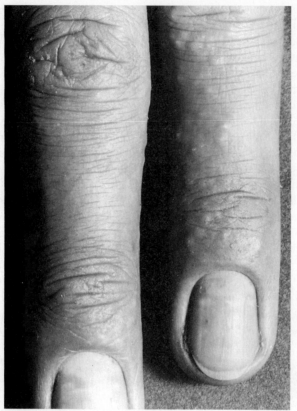

FIG. 39–4. Food handler dermatitis: a positive immediate rub test to tomato. (From Niinimäki A: Scratch-chamber tests in food handler dermatitis. *Contact Dermatitis* 16:11–20, 1987; © 1987 by Munksgaard International Publishers Ltd., Copenhagen, Denmark. Reprinted with permission.)

as an increase in cells with interleukin 2 receptor activity, suggesting an immunologic mechanism. This cannot be explained on the basis of contact urticaria alone because of the spongiotic and parakeratotic epidermal changes and the clinical picture of eczematous vesiculation. It does not fit delayed hypersensitivity because it can be reproduced in 20 min and patch testing is normal. It is not irritant because of the association with positive prick tests and the specificity of the reactants. The answer remains to be elucidated. In the workup, Hjorth and Roed-Petersen recommend using prick tests or a similar procedure to find the allergic urticarial response these patients show. Whether or not it is causally related (and it might seem to be), it is a useful marker. Tosti et al.[20] postulated that mediators liberated by foods might cause direct damage. The association with contact urticaria is unlikely to be fortuitous, because of the specificity and the normal response in controls.

The prognosis in food service employees is not very good, as even a job change does not permanently relieve the problem.[16] Most seem to at least initially benefit from avoidance. The likelihood of exposure to sources other than food is a possibility to be explored.

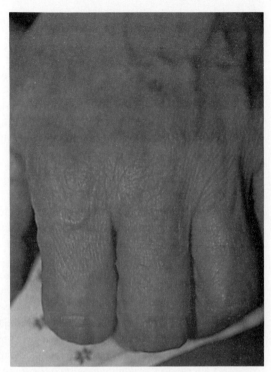

FIG. 39–5. Immediate positive rub test to shrimp. This was seen in a waitress with hand eczema regularly precipitated by the handling of shrimp. (See color Plate 37.)

It is difficult to know the mechanism for this condition based on the data available. Probably nonimmunologic factors have value as well as truly immunologic factors for inducing the lesions. The production of an immediate eczematous eruption by contact of protein-type foods is very interesting, as it does not fit into one of the usual categories of allergy. For more on a proposed mechanism for the eczematous change following IgE-mediated urticaria, a good discussion can be found in Chap. 47 on allergy to the house-dust mite.

DAIRY LABORATORIES

Judging from the number of reports from milk testing laboratories, allergic contact dermatitis to the preservatives that are used to preserve milk samples must be a relatively common problem. Potassium dichromate, bronopol, and Kathon CG are sometimes added to samples to be examined for their protein and lipid composition, and the sensitization index to them seems to be high.[21–24]

BAKERY AND PASTRY

Bakers who handle flour may be at special risk to develop irritant contact dermatitis. This is caused by the wet nature of the job plus the need to use soap and detergents in cleaning. Type I reactions may occur. Candidiasis is also a problem.

For those suspected of having allergic contact dermatitis, the standard patch-test allergens include the following:

1. Flavors: eugenol, isoeugenol, vanillin, cinnamic aldehyde, cinnamic alcohol, anethol, and limonene. Menthol imparts a medical odor or flavor, along with some pharmacologic properties.
2. Antioxidants and preservatives: BHA, BHT, sodium benzoate, sorbic acid, benzoic acid, propionic acid, and octyl, propyl, and dodecyl gallates.
3. Bleaching agents: including ammonium persulfate and benzoyl peroxide.

Allergic contact dermatitis from persulfate bleaching agents in flour[25,26] used to be a problem, but these have been largely eliminated from flour in most countries.[27] One should also consider spices and flavors as well as lotions, rubber chemicals, and so on which are applied to the hands to treat or prevent irritation. Dodecyl and propyl gallate are used as antioxidants of fats and in the manufacture of croissants.[28,29] Sodium metabisulfite is sometimes used in biscuits, salad from salad bars, and other foods to preserve their fresh look.[30]

Spices are discussed earlier in the chapter. Here, too, patients with hand eczema and patch-test reactions to fragrance, balsam of Peru, colophony, and wood tar should probably be evaluated for allergy to kitchen spices. Vanilla can be tested as itself and also with isoeugenol or balsam of Peru.[31,32] The major sensitizer in cinnamon is cinnamic aldehyde (Figs. 39-6 and 39-7). Eugenol is probably responsible for contact allergy to cloves. Cardamom essence at 2% and limonene at 2% in petrolatum are often related to contact allergy to *Cardamomum officinale* (cardamom) often used in pastry.[33] When testing to spices, it is helpful to have the patient bring everything with which he or she works.

MEAT AND FISH PROCESSING

Slaughterhouse workers may develop the same occupational skin disease mentioned in the introduction. Allergic contact dermatitis is less of a problem, perhaps, but reports of occupational contact are sporadic, ranging from dermatitis to the rosewood handle of a butcher knife[34] to contact urticaria from penicillin contamination in a meat product.[35] Slaughterhouse workers develop "gut eczema" from evisceration, especially when the mesenteric fat is removed.[36] The condition tends to occur on the finger webs, extending to the fingers. It is intermittent but work-related and not seen in many other types closely related work in the slaughterhouse. Its duration is usually brief and avoidance results in prompt clearing. Type I reactions are not associated with this condition in one report[36] and were found in less than half in another,[37] which seems to have included patients with more than one type of problem. Protein contact dermatitis is associated with positive tests for immediate hypersensitivity and an immediate eczema. It is also specific.

Butchers, fish handlers, and meat packers often experience an eczematous eruption which is probably irritant, as the patch tests are usually negative. In a fish processing plant, the severity is temperature-dependent and caused by high-molecular-weight compounds.[38,39]

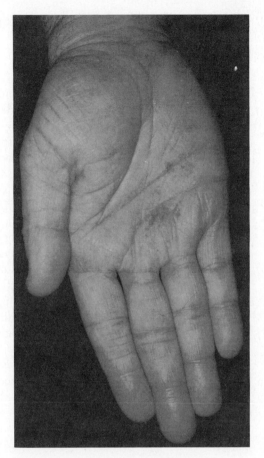

FIG. 39–6. Hand dermatitis due to ingestion of cinnamon.

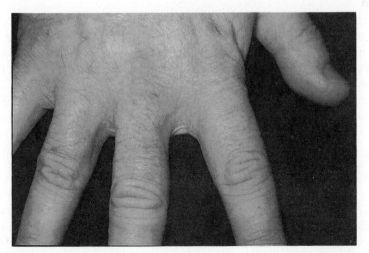

FIG. 39–7. Same patient as in Fig. 39-6 This patient improved on avoiding contact with cinnamon.

FRUITS AND VEGETABLES AS CAUSES

CRUCIFERAE AND COMPOSITAE

The mustard (Cruciferae) and Compositae families contain ragweed and both are natural sources of allergic contact dermatitis. Allergic contact eczema to certain compositae like artichokes (*Cynara scolymus*) is caused by sensitivity to the sesquiterpene lactone cynaropicrina. Bay leaves, a common kitchen spice, are actually leaves of laurel (*Laurus nobilis*), an ornamental commonly seen in yards. The usual allergen, laurenobiolide, can cross-react with similar chemicals in the Compositae family and with magnolia. Contact dermatitis can also be produced by chicory (*Chicorum endiva*) and lettuce (*Lactuca lactucopicrine*). Testing for sesquiterpene lactone allergy has been a problem, as commercial antigens were not available for many years. Now a screening antigen, a sesquiterpene lactone mix, has been developed by Ducombs et al.[40] It is composed of alantolactone, costunolide, and dehydrocostuslactone—at 0.1% each—in petrolatum. This will uncover many unsuspected sources of sesquiterpene lactone sensitivity, but how many are missed is not yet known. This and several other Compositae antigens are available commercially from Chemotechnique, but they are probably not adequate for dermatologists seeing Compositae dermatitis in North America. Another method is to test with the materials in question. Details of patch testing to the plant material can be found in Chap. 38, on plant dermatitis.

Mustard (*Brassica nigra*) and radish (*Raphanus satinus*)—Cruciferae—are strong irritants which can also sensitize. Allyl isothiocyanate is an allergen common to both plants.[41] This substance is also principal ingredient of mustard oil and is widely used as a kitchen condiment. For patch testing, use concentrations in petrolatum from 0.05% to 0.1%.

GARLIC

Garlic is an important allergen in some cultures, especially in Europe.[42] The dramatic picture of a dry, fissured, keratotic, pruritic, chronic eczema on the fingertips of the first, second, and third fingers of the left hand is almost diagnostic (Fig. 39-1). Exposure occurs in this location from holding the garlic to be sliced by the knife that is held in the right hand. The reverse occurs in left-handed persons. Responsible allergens are diallyl sulfur, allyl-propyl sulfur, and allicine.[43-45]

ONIONS

Onions, like garlic, are Amaryllidaceae. One commonly sees contact allergy to onions and garlic in the same patient, although they apparently do not cross-react. However persons allergic to onion may break out to tulips and hyacinth as well.[46] Onion is an irritant, so it must be diluted before patch testing.

CITRUS

Limonene, a terpene, is often responsible for the contact allergy to orange peel and lemon peel. Persons allergic to limonene can also react with fragrance materials containing oil of Bergamot, as both are found in certain citrus fruits.[47] In any event, patch testing with clean peel of oranges or lemons can be helpful. Because the peel of some fruit is irritant, patients should be warned to remove the test should irritation occur. As with other possible irritants, controls are indicated. Limonene is usually tested at 1% in petrolatum.

CARROTS

Carrots (*Daucus carota*) can produce contact cheilitis, irritant[48,49] and allergic contact dermatitis, and—according to some[50]—phototoxic reactions. Cross-reactivity may occur from parsnip (*Pastinaca sativa*), a member of the Umbelliferae, and celery (*Apium graveolens*).[51] Carrots contain pinene, limonene, and other terpenes. Patch tests with the peel or with the pulp are relevant, but the cut surface gives stronger patch-test results.[51]

LETTUCE

Contact dermatitis to lettuce can occur not only in gardeners[52] and cooks[53] but also in anyone who has eaten a salad.[54] The sensitizing sesquiterpene lactones are lactucrin and lactucopicrin. Because light may cause degradation of the antigenic material, fresh lettuce should be used for patch testing.[55] Angioedema in the oropharynx has occurred in persons eating lettuce.[56,57]

MANGO AND PINEAPPLE

The peel of mango fruit is a well-known sensitizer, especially for those already allergic to poison ivy.[58] Patients allergic to mango suffer contact cheilitis and circumoral contact dermatitis from eating the fruit without removing the skin.[58] Persons raised in the Caribbean are less at risk than those from continental North America.[58] There is some suggestion that exposure early in life from mother's milk may be the reason for this,[58] but it is not understood completely. Ingestion can also produce an anaphylactic reaction.[59]

Pineapple juice is an irritant, causing both irritant contact dermatitis and wheals of nonimmunologic contact urticaria, probably from calcium oxalate and the enzymatic activity of bromelin.[60] The sharp "spears" on the fruit can cause mechanical injury, and even its sugar content may have an adverse osmotic effect. Pineapple is a bromeliad. The maya fruit (*Bromelia pinguin*) can cause similar injury.[61]

Contact cheilitis and contact urticaria can occur from kiwi fruit.[62,63]

POTATOES (*Solanum tuberosum*)

Many housewives, especially those with hand eczema, complain of irritation of the skin of the hands from handling sliced raw potatoes.[64] Usually they will have had an irritant or nonspecific dermatitis of the hands, with contact often aggravating an already present eczema. Rarely, one sees allergic contact dermatitis[65] or urticaria[66,67] to potatoes, the latter sometimes with respiratory symptoms. Most persons, however, are able to eat cooked potatoes, although atopic eczema may be aggravated in sensitive individuals. In animals, an eczema of the lower limbs can be seen when inordinate amounts of the whole plants are eaten.[68]

COFFEE

Allergic contact dermatitis to roasted coffee must be rare, although it has been reported. Contact dermatitis to green (unroasted) coffee beans[69] is reported to be due to contamination with castor beans (*Ricinus communis*).[70] The component allergen in the rare cases of coffee allergy is unknown. In the cited case of allergic contact dermatitis of the hands, the patient, who worked in a coffee bar, was allergic not only to ground, roasted coffee, but also to the prepared beverage.[71]

SPICES

ALLERGENS

Kitchen spices tend either to spare antigens or to cross-react with fragrance and flavoring materials. Such reactions seem to be more common than perhaps previously thought, as there are several recent reports.[72-75] Delayed-type allergy to spices is commonly associated with reactions to balsam of Peru, fragrance mix, wood tars, and colophony. Allergic contact dermatitis is not the only problem, as type I reactions are also seen. Immediate reactions from kitchen spices sometimes also involve other organ systems, such as the respiratory mucosa and the gastrointestinal tract,[75] and symptoms can follow inhalation and ingestion. Testing for them is not so easily done, as the method seems often to depend upon the spice material in question.[76] Balsam of Peru, cinnamic aldehyde, limonene, vanillin, and thymol, among others, are the most sensitizing allergens. For patch-test considerations and vehicles see Table 39-1.

PLANTS

The plants that mainly produce these allergens are cayenne pepper (*Capsicum annuum*), cinnamon (*Cinnamomum cassia* and *Cinnamomum zeylanicum*), cloves (*Eugenia caryophyllata*), laurel (*Laurus nobilis*), nutmeg (*Myristica fragrans*), and vanilla (*Vanilla planifolia*). Cardamom (*Elettaria cardamomum*) and curcuma (*Curcuma longa*), present in the manufacture of curry, can also be sensitizers.[77]

**TABLE 39–1. Patch-Test Substances
Related to Foods**

Cardamom essence	2% pet
Cinnamaldehyde	1% pet
Clove oil	2% pet
Eugenol	1% pet
Garlic (fresh)	As is
Isothiocyanate allyl	0.05% pet
Diallyl disulfide	2% pet
Lactone mix (alantolactone, costunolide, dihydrocostunolide)	0.1% each pet
Laurel oil	2% pet
Limonene oil	1% pet
Orange oil	2% pet
Propylene glycol	20% aq
Thymol	1% pet
Vanillin	10% pet
Spices	As is

TESTING FOR ALLERGY TO SPICES

One can suspect sensitivity in persons with hand eczema who are known to be allergic to fragrance mix, balsam of Peru, colophony, or wood tar. The first three are present in standard screening series except the North American series, which lacks fragrance mix. Most kitchen spices are usually tested as is, but onion and garlic are too irritating at 100% concentration and too weak to be reliable at 25% concentration. Many use a 50% concentration, but in any test not done routinely, one might be well advised to run controls.[78]

Fragrance mix and balsam of Peru will detect many sensitivities to clove, nutmeg, cinnamon, and cayenne pepper.[73] The allergens responsible for these reactions could well be different and may even disappear if the spices are added in cooking. Most spices can be tested as is—mainly when there is a suggestive clinical history and the routine allergens are negative. Notable exceptions are onion and garlic. Controls should be run when testing to unknown spices.[78]

FOOD ADDITIVES AS CAUSES

ANTIOXIDANTS

Preserving the fresh look of food may require the avoidance of exposure to air, as oxidation can cause a change in the color and odor of foods. Perhaps the classic change is the darkening of a banana. Flavor change due to oxidation ranges from loss of taste intensity to a rancid odor or flavor. To avoid spoilage of food, antioxidants are added. Most of these chemicals are also used in the preservation of medicaments or cosmetics. Many of the antioxidants employed in the preserving of foods are well-known contact allergens. Allergic contact dermatitis to food is mostly occupational in persons who work in food manufacture or preparation. Some reactions occur in kitchen personnel and housewives as well. There are a few patients, proved to be allergic by patch testing, who flare or develop a disseminated vesicular reaction after ingesting food containing the allergen. The more commonly used agents are given in Table 39-2. All of them have the capacity to cause both irritant and allergic reactions.[79-82]

Parabens are almost ubiquitous in today's world, as they can be found not only in pharmaceutical and cosmetic products but also in edibles. They are used in marmalades, soft drinks, juices, and any type of packed or wrapped food. Sensitivity to parabens became a source of anxiety for industry when cases of contact allergy were first reported, but the overreaction which followed has largely subsided. The ingestion of parabens does not seem to be a particular problem, even in those known to be contact-allergic.[83]

The case of *sorbic acid* is a bit different, as it produces nonimmunologic contact dermatitis in 5 percent of the normal population and allergic contact dermatitis occasionally. Immediate erythema, edema, and general symptoms such as nausea and dizziness can occur from just licking an ice cream containing sorbic acid. In the majority of these patients, it is hard to know whether or not the reaction is immunologically mediated.[84,85]

BIOCIDES

Quaternary ammonium salts are widely used for disinfection in hospitals and business offices, cold storage plants, and so on. Some quaternary ammonium salts are strong sensitizers,[86-89] while others are not. Benzalkonium chloride is irritant in higher concentration and can sensitize,[90,91] but it seldom does.[92] Contact in persons handling food is possible and would have to be evaluated on a case-by-case basis. Because of the irritant nature of many of these products, it may be necessary to do usage testing to prove contact allergy.[93]

Other cases of allergic contact dermatitis caused by TEGO Diocto 5, an ampholytic, surface-active biocide containing diocto-trioctyl-diethyltenetriamine (based on dodecyl-di(aminoethyl)glycine) has caused contact sensitivity from exposure to disinfectants in several occupations and products.[94] One worker in the food processing industry

TABLE 39-2. Additives in Food

Food Additives	Patch Test, % pet
Ammonium persulfate	2 pet
Benzoyl peroxide	1 pet
Butyl hydroxyanisole (BHA)	2 pet
Butyl hydroxytoluene (BHT)	2 pet
Dodecyl, octyl, and propyl gallate	1 pet
Ethyl, methyl, and propyl parahydroxybenzoate	3 pet
Hexamethylenetetramine	1 pet
Nordihydroguaiaretic acid (NDGA)	2 pet
Sodium metabisulfite	10 pet
Sorbic acid	2.5 pet
Tocopherols	10 pet

became allergic from exposure to dodecyldi(aminoethyl)glycine (DDEG) by handling eggs transported for packing through a conveyor belt which had been sprayed with that chemical.[95,96]

Some insecticides (such as potassium persulfate and tetramethylthiuram disulfide, or TMTD), used in spraying bananas and other fruits, can produce contact allergy. The former, a bleaching agent in flour, may also be an allergen in hairdressers. Of course, thiurams, common accelerators in rubber manufacture, are often associated with allergy to latex gloves.

EMULSIFIERS

Some prepared salads and salad dressings contain propylene glycol, which is added as emulsifier. Contact sensitivity may be more common from cosmetics and medications, as propylene glycol is often used in them as a suspending agent, emulsifier, and preservative as well as to solubilize the corticosteroid component of topical corticosteroids. Persons who are patch-test positive can also develop an exanthem following ingestion of a test dose of propylene glycol; such patients would be advised to avoid foods prepared with it.[97,98]

BLEACHING AGENTS

Ammonium persulfate and benzoyl peroxide are bleaching agents used in flours. The former is especially likely to be used in Europe. Both are known sources of allergic contact dermatitis. Sometimes the substitution of potassium bromate will help to avoid the problem.

WAXES AND GUMS

Beeswax, propolis, carnauba, tragacanth, and karaya are used in soups, ice cream, salads, dressings, and cheese. Sensitivity is more likely to be seen in persons who are allergic to balsam of Peru.

FOODS PRODUCING PHOTOTOXIC DERMATITIS

CELERY

Celery (*Apium graveolens*), parsnips (*Pastinaca sativa*; the *wild* parsnip is worse), and parsley (*Petroselinum hortense*) are edible plants which can produce phototoxic dermatitis. These plants contain furocoumarins. Celery phototoxicity is due to 5-methoxypsoralen (5-MOP), also known as bergapten. While the bergapten content of celery is often higher in plants contaminated by the pink rot fungus,[99] *Sclerotinia sclerotiorum*,[100] it can occur prominently in some varieties of ordinary celery purchased in the produce department of a grocery store provided that the UVA exposure is sufficiently intense. Grocery workers have been known to develop "berlock" dermatitis from contact followed by intense sunbathing or tanning-salon exposure.[101,102]

Perhaps the principal cause of berlock dermatitis in the United States is the Persian lime *Citrus aurantifolia*, which seems to be a problem in warmer areas such as south Florida. The cause again is 5-MOP or bergapten, and the phototoxic vesiculobullous eruption is followed by hyperpigmentation. The causative chemical is located in the rind, and a typical history is presented by someone who has squeezed the juice into a mixed drink while being exposed to the sun. There is no convenient way to wipe the wet fingers, so they are wiped on an exposed area of skin to avoid messiness. The phototoxic eruption can be expected in 48 h, more or less.

PARSNIPS

Parsnips, like celery, belong to the Umbelliferae family and contain 5-MOP and 8-MOP, from which phototoxic activity can develop. In some areas of the midwestern United States, the wild variety of this plant, with its yellow blooms, can be seen covering an entire field or vacant lot. Patients who develop the phototoxic eruption break out in exposed sites. Initially there is a vesiculobullous eruption, often presenting with a strong erythema, or vesiculobullous dermatitis in streaks which can closely resemble poison ivy dermatitis. Later, when pigmentation supervenes, the diagnosis of berlock dermatitis becomes obvious. Most patients are persons who work among these plants, such as farmers or gardeners.

REFERENCES

1. Veien NK, Krogdahl A: Cutaneous vasculitis induced by food additives. *Acta Derm Venereol* 71:73–74, 1991.
2. Ashkenazi S, Metzker A, Rachmel A, Nitzan M: Erythema multiforme as a single manifestation of cow's milk intolerance (letter). *Acta Paediatr* 81:729–730, 1992.
3. Steiner GC, Arnold RW, Roth RR, Ice JS: Stevens-Johnson syndrome secondary to ingestion of salmon berries. *Alaska Med* 33:57–59, 1991.
4. Iglesias Diez J, DeMoragas J: The cutaneous lesions of the Spanish oil syndrome. *J Am Acad Dermatol* 9:159–601, 1983.
5. Satyawan I, Oranje AP, van Joost T: Perioral dermatitis in a child due to rosin in chewing gum. *Contact Dermatitis* 22:182–183, 1990.
6. Nakamura T: Shiitake (*Lentinus edodes*) dermatitis. *Contact Dermatitis* 27:65–70, 1992.
7. Adams RM: Dermatitis in food service workers. *Allergy Proceedings* 11:123–4, 1990.
8. Bonnevie P: Some experiences of war-time industrial dermatoses. *Acta Derm Venereol* 28:231, 1948.
9. Malten KE: The occurrence of hybrids between contact allergic eczema and atopic dermatitis (and vice versa) and their significance. *Dermatologica* 136:404, 1968.
10. Hjorth N, Weismann K: Occupational dermatitis in chefs and sandwich-makers. *Contact Dermatitis Newsletter* 11:301, 1972.
11. Hjorth N: Battery for testing of chefs and other kitchen workers. *Contact Dermatitis* 1:63, 1975.
12. Hjorth N, Roed-Petersen J: Occupational protein contact dermatitis in food handlers. *Contact Dermatitis* 2:28–42, 1976.
13. Niinimäki A: Scratch chamber tests in food handler dermatitis. *Contact Dermatitis* 16:20, 1987.
14. Nakamura T: Shiitake (*Lentinus edodes*) dermatitis. *Contact Dermatitis* 27:65–70, 1992.
15. Rantanen T: Allergy and toxicodermia from shiitake mushrooms. *J Am Acad Dermatol* 24:64–66, 1991.

16. Cronin E: Dermatitis of the hands in caterers. *Contact Dermatitis* 17:265–269, 1987.
17. Seeberg G: Eczematous dermatitis from contact with, or ingestion of, beef, pork, or mutton (4 case reports). *Acta Derm Venereol Suppl* 29:320–322, 1952.
18. Niinimäki A: Scratch-chamber tests in food handler dermatitis. *Contact Dermatitis* 16:11–20, 1987.
19. von Krogh G, Maibach HI: The contact urticaria syndrome–An updated review. *J Am Acad Dermatol* 5:328–342, 1981.
20. Tosti A, Fanti PA, Guerra L, et al: Morphological and immunohistochemical study of immediate contact dermatitis of the hands due to foods. *Contact Dermatitis* 22:81–85, 1990.
21. Rogers S, Burrows D: Contact dermatitis to chrome in milk testers. *Contact Dermatitis* 1:378–379, 1975.
22. Rudzki E, Czerwinska-Dihnz I: Sensitivity to dichromate in milk testers. *Contact Dermatitis* 3:107–108, 1977.
23. Herzog J, Dunne I, Claver M, Marks JG: Milk tester's dermatitis. *J Am Acad Dermatol* 19:503–508, 1988.
24. Grattan CEM, Harman RRM, Tan RSH: Milk recorder dermatitis. *Contact Dermatitis* 14:217–220, 1986.
25. Cronin E: *Contact Dermatitis*. Edinburgh, Scotland, Churchill Livingstone, 1980.
26. Fisher AA: *Contact Dermatitis*, 3d ed. Philadelphia, Lea & Febiger, 1986.
27. Adams RM: *Occupational Skin Disease*. New York, Grune & Stratton, 1983, pp 386–387.
28. Brun R: Kontakeczema und Laurylgallat und phydroxybenzoesaure-ester *Berufsdermatosen* 12:281–284, 1964.
29. Bojs G, Nicklasson B, Svensson A: Allergic contact dermatitis to propyl gallate. *Contact Dermatitis* 17:294–298, 1987.
30. Apetato M, Marques MSJ: Contact dermatitis caused by sodium metabisulfite. *Contact Dermatitis* 14:194–195, 1986.
31. Hjorth N: *Eczematous Allergy to Balsams*. Copenhagen, Munksgaard, 1961.
32. Spencer LV, Fowler JF: Thin mint cookie dermatitis. *Contact Dermatitis* 18:185–186, 1988.
33. Fregert S: Allergic contact dermatitis from cardamom. *Contact Dermatitis* 1:175–176, 1975.
34. Fancalanci S, Giorgini S, Gola M, Sertoli A: Occupational dermatitis in a butcher. *Contact Dermatitis* 11:320–321, 1984.
35. de Boer EM, van Ketel WG: Occupational dermatitis caused by snackbar meat products. *Contact Dermatitis* 11:322, 1984.
36. Hjorth N: Gut eczema in slaughterhouse workers. *Contact Dermatitis* 4:49–52, 1978.
37. Hansen KS, Petersen HO: Protein contact dermatitis in slaughterhouse workers. *Contact Dermatitis* 21:221–224, 1989.
38. Halkier-Sorensen L, Heickendorff L, Dalsgaard I, Thestrup-Pedersen K: Skin symptoms among workers in the fish processing industry are caused by high molecular weight compounds. *Contact Dermatitis* 24:94–100, 1991.
39. Halkier-Sorensen L, Thestrup-Pedersen K: Skin temperature and skin symptoms among workers in the fish processing industry. *Contact Dermatitis* 19:206–209, 1988.
40. Ducombs G, Benezra Cl, Talaga P, et al: Patchtesting with the sesquiterpene lactone mix. *Contact Dermatitis* 22:249–252, 1990.
41. Mitchell JC, Jordan WP: Allergic contact dermatitis from the radish (*Raphanus sativus*). *Br J Dermatol* 91:183–189, 1974.
42. Dannaker CJ, White IR: Cutaneous allergy to mustard in a salad maker. *Contact Dermatitis* 16:212–214, 1987.
43. Brandao FM: Dermatite de contacto pelo alho. *Trab Soc Port Derm Venereol* 35:27–28, 1977.
44. Papageorgiu C, Corbet JP, Brandao FM, et al: Allergic contact dermatitis to garlic (*Allium sativum*): Identification of the allergens: The role of mono-di-tri sulfides present in garlic: A comparative study in man and animal (guinea pigs). *Arch Dermatol Res* 275:229–234, 1983.
45. Lembo G, Balato N, Patruno C, et al: Allergic contact dermatitis due to garlic (*Allium sativum*). *Contact Dermatitis* 25:330–331, 1991.
46. Burks JW: Classic aspects of onion and garlic dermatitis in housewives. *Ann Allergy* 12:592–594, 1954.
47. Puglisi V: Dermatoses caused by lemon. *G Ital Dermatol* 92:237, 1951.
48. Peck SM, Spolyar LW, Mason HS: Dermatitis from carrots. *Arch Dermatol Syphilol* 49:266, 1944.
49. Vickers HR: The carrot as a cause of dermatitis. *Br J Dermatol* 53:52, 1941.
50. Pathak MA: Phytophotodermatitis. *Clin Dermatol* 4:102–121, 1986.
51. Klauder JV, Kimmich JM: Sensitization dermatitis to carrots. *Arch Dermatol* 75:149, 1956.
52. Helander I: Contact dermatitis to lettuce. *Contact Dermatitis* 11:249, 1984.

53. Mitchell D, Beck MH, Hausen BM: Contact sensitivity to lettuce in a chef. *Contact Dermatitis* 20:398–399, 1989.
54. Oliwiecki S, Beck MH, Hausen BM: Compositae dermatitis aggravated by eating lettuce. *Contact Dermatitis* 24:318–319, 1991.
55. Hausen BM, Andersen KE, Helander I, Gensch KH: Lettuce allergy: Sensitizing potency of allergens. *Contact Dermatitis* 15:246–249, 1986.
56. Rinkel HJ, Balyeat RM: Occupational dermatitis due to lettuce. *JAMA* 98:137, 1932.
57. Krook G: Occupational dermatitis from *Latuca sativa* and *Chichorium* (endive): Simultaneous occurrence of immediate and delayed allergy as a cause of contact dermatitis. *Contact Dermatitis* 3:27–36, 1977.
58. Lampe KF: Dermatitis producing Anacardiaceae of the Caribbean area. *Clin Dermatol* 4:171–182, 1986.
59. Dang RW, Bell DB: Anaphylactic reaction to the ingestion of mango. *Hawaii Med J* 27:149, 1967.
60. Polunin I: Pineapple dermatoses. *Br J Dermatol* 63:441, 1951.
61. Mitchell JC, Rook AR: *Botanical Dermatology*, Vancouver, Greengrass, 1979, pp 142–143.
62. Veraldi S, Schianchi-Veraldi R: Contact urticaria from kiwi fruit. *Contact Dermatitis* 22:224, 1990.
63. Garcia BE, de la Cuesta CG, Santos F, Cordoba H: A rare case of food allergy: Monosensitivity to kiwi (*Actinida chinensis*). *Allergol Immunopathol (Madr)* 17:217–218, 1989.
64. Bruce RS: Potato sensitivity an occupational allergy in housewives. *Acta Allergol* 21:507, 1986.
65. Carmichael AJ, Foulds IS, Tan CY: Allergic contact dermatitis from potato flesh. *Contact Dermatitis* 20:64–65, 1989.
66. Larko O, Lindstedt G, Lundberg PA, Mobacken H: Biochemical and clinical studies in a case of contact urticaria to potato. *Contact Dermatitis* 9:108–114, 1983.
67. Nater JP, Zwartz JA: Atopic allergic reactions due to raw potato. *J Allergy* 40:202, 1967.
68. Watt JM, Breyer-Brandwijk MG: *The Medicinal and Poisonous Plants of Southern Africa*, 2d ed. Edinburgh, Scotland, Livingstone, 1962.
69. Piraccini BM, Bardazzi F, Vincenzi C, Tardio MP: Occupational contact dermatitis due to coffee. *Contact Dermatitis* 23:114, 1990.
70. Patussi V, De Zotti R, Riva G: Allergic manifestations due to castor beans: An undue risk for the dock workers handling green coffee beans. *Med Lav* 81:301–307, 1990.
71. Piraccini BM, Bardazzi F, Vincenzi C, Tardio MP: Occupational contact dermatitis due to coffee. *Contact Dermatitis* 23:114, 1990.
72. van den Akker TW, Roesyanto-Mahadi ID, van Toorenenbergen AW, van Joost T: Contact allergy to spices. *Contact Dermatitis* 22:267–272, 1990.
73. van den Akker TW, van Toorenenbergen AW, van Joost T: Analysis of delayed-type immunological responses to spices by patch testing. *Curr Probl Dermatol* 20:232–236, 1991.
74. Dooms-Goossens A, Dubelloy R, Degreef H: Contact and systemic contact-type dermatitis to spices. *Dermatol Clin* 8:89–93, 1990.
75. Niinimäki A: Delayed-type allergy to spices. *Contact Dermatitis* 11:34–40, 1984.
76. Niinimäki A, Bjorksten F, Puukka M, et al: Spice allergy: Results of skin prick tests and RAST with spice extracts. *Allergy* 44:60–65, 1989.
77. Goh CL, Ng SK: Allergic contact dermatitis to curcuma lenga (turmeric). *Contact Dermatitis* 17:186–187, 1987.
78. Bruynzeel DP, Prevoo RL: Patch tests with some spices. *Dermatol Clin* 8:85–87, 1990.
79. De Groot AC, Gerkens F: Occupational air borne contact dermatitis from octyl gallate. *Contact Dermatitis* 23:184–186, 1990.
80. Foussereau J: Guide de dermato-allergologic professionelle. Paris, Masson, 1991, pp 92–95.
81. Roed-Petersen J, Hjorth N: Contact dermatitis from antioxidants: Hidden sensitizers in topical medicaments and foods. *Br J Dermatol* 94:233, 1976.
82. Van der Meeren HCM: Dodecyl gallate, permitted in food, is a strong sensitizer. *Contact Dermatitis* 16:260–262, 1987.
83. Fisher AA: *Contact Dermatitis*, 3d ed. Philadelphia, Lea & Febiger, 1986, pp 585–586.
84. Camarasa JG: Acute contact urticaria. *Contact Dermatitis* 8:347, 1982.
85. Fisher AA: Cutaneous reactions to sorbic acid and potassium sorbate. *Cutis* 25:350, 1980.
86. Schallreuter KU, Wood JM: The allergenicity of complex cations. *Biochem Biophys Res Commun* 135:221–227, 1986.

87. Schallreuter KU, Schulz KH: A comparative study of the allergenicity of quaternary ammonium compounds in guinea-pigs. *Clin Exp Dermatol* 11:460–466, 1986.
88. Lachapelle JM, Huriez C, Lefebvre MM, Martin P: 3H-thymidine labelling of the dermal infiltrate in two positive patch test reactions to a quaternary ammonium compound: Cethexonium bromide. *Contact Dermatitis* 1:259, 1975.
89. Estlander T, Jolanki R, Kanerva L: Occupational dermatitis to 2,3-epoxypropyl trimethyl ammonium chloride. *Contact Dermatitis* 14:49–52, 1986.
90. Garcia-Perez A, Moran M: Dermatitis from quaternary ammonium compounds. *Contact Dermatitis* 1:316–17, 1975.
91. Shmunes E, Levy EJ: Quaternary ammonium compound contact dermatitis from a deodorant. *Arch Dermatol* 105:91–93, 1972.
92. Fisher AA: *Contact Dermatitis*, 3d ed. Philadelphia, Lea & Febiger, 1986, pp 190–191.
93. Klein GF, Sepp N, Fritsch P: Allergic reactions to benzalkonium chloride? Do the use test. *Contact Dermatitis* 25:269–270, 1991.
94. Valsechi R, Leghissa P, Piazzolla S: Tego allergy in the food industry. *Contact Dermatitis* 23:188–189, 1990.
95. Wilkinson J, Schouten P, English JSC: Allergic contact dermatitis from Tego-51. *Contact Dermatitis* 24:74–75, 1991.
96. Sinclair S, Hindson C: Allergic contact dermatitis from dodecylaminoathylglycine. *Contact Dermatitis* 18:320–321, 1988.
97. Hannuksela M, Forstrom L: Reactions to peroral propylene glycol. *Contact Dermatitis* 4:41, 1978.
98. Fisher AA: The management of propylene glycol sensitive patients. *Cutis* 25:24, 1980.
99. Birmingham DJ, Key HM, Jobich GE, Perone VB: Phototoxic bullae among celery harversters. *Arch Dermatol Syph* 83:73–87, 1961.
100. Birmingham DJ, Key MM, Tublich GE, et al: Phototoxic bullae among celery harvesters. *Arch Dermatol* 83:73–77, 1961.
101. Seligman PJ, Mathias CG, O'Malley MA, et al: Phytophotodermatitis from celery among grocery store workers. *Arch Dermatol* 123:1478–1482, 1987.
102. Felming D: Dermatitis in grocery workers associated with high natural concentrations of furanocoumarins in celery. *Allergy Proc* 11:125–127, 1990.

40

PRESERVATIVES

Anthony F. Fransway

There are numerous notable circumstances where important and indeed vital biophysiologic mechanisms produce related undesirable effects. An excellent in vivo case in point is that of human autoimmunity. Saprophytic organisms, particularly bacteria and fungi, perform the all-important function of degradation of waste products, debris, and nonvital tissues into potentially reusable by-products and basic elements. These same organisms are responsible for the spoilage of human necessities and conveniences, including food, cosmetic products, and occupational exposures where an aqueous compartment is inherently necessary. It has been the goal of grocers, pharmaceutical and cosmetic companies, employers, and occupational safety personnel to identify chemicals and substances that act to delay, retard, forestall, or negate this undesired and costly bioactivity.

The challenge is simply enough stated: identify an appropriate preservative substance that is nontoxic, nonirritating, completely or generally nonsensitizing, and capable of the destruction or inhibition of those microorganisms that cause such spoilage. Many biocides have been identified that, at adequate concentration, completely inhibit the growth of a number of troublesome saprophytes; however, at such concentrations, irritation or sensitization is often the result. The nonsensitizing biocide has not been identified. From this ideal goal a working hypothesis is formed: identify the substance with acceptable efficacy and a reasonable safety profile that adequately preserves the product. There are a number of preservatives available that fulfill these requirements, although the list is remarkably short in light of the attention given to identifying acceptable substances.

Preservatives have been identified as among the most important causes of allergic contact dermatitis in patients suspected of cosmetic sensitivity; only the fragrance group is believed to be more frequently allergenic.[1-6] Before coming to market, the manufacturer of a specific preservative must provide consequential data attesting to their biocide's efficacy and reasonable safety with respect to sensitization risk. Human and guinea pig maximization testing is often performed, with the major stated objection being that the human in vivo use experience is not reproduced. Additionally, in the grand spectrum of cosmetic biocide use, even the most frequently sensitizing preservatives on

539

the market cause only an inordinately small percentage of individuals to react, thus leaving in-house testing of a limited number of volunteers decreasingly significant. It is unfortunate that only when millions of "volunteers" (through their home use of the product) become exposed does the problem of sensitization surface. Irritancy, on the other hand, develops in the majority of subjects exposed to an adequate concentration of the capable agent and thus may be more appropriately assessed through premarketing techniques. Final to consider logistically is the experience of opening a cosmetic product or food item with intent to consume it only to find that spoilage has occurred; it is fortunate that a vast majority of these products are consumed rapidly, prior to biocide failure.

PRESERVATION STRATEGIES

The cosmetic chemist has several approaches to choose from in preserving a given product, with the technique utilized often being quite dependent upon the nature of the formulation, the probability of rapid consumption, water content, and additional modifying factors such as other ingredients that affect spoilage by microbes. Four basic preservation approaches exist: (1) Utilize the single superior biocide with broad bacterial, yeast, and fungistatic or fungicidal activity in final formulation; quaternium-15, bromonitropropane diol, and methylchloroisothiazolinone/methylisothiazolinone are notable examples. (2) Deploy a small number of biocides in combination (usually two) that act synergistically in the suppression of a broader spectrum of microorganisms; the use of paraben esters with a formaldehyde-releasing biocide such as imidazolidinyl urea is the most frequent combination. (3) Utilize one of the above two approaches, adding other agents that have antimicrobial activity to the final formula. These "preservation potentiators" include aromatic ingredients such as essential oils and fragrances, medium-chain fatty acids and esters, nonionic emulsifiers, and chelating agents.[7] Other agents with preservation function not necessarily related to inhibition of microbes, such as antioxidants and UV absorbers, often find inclusion in the cauldron. Variables within the control of the cosmetic chemist that have ramifications on shelf life include pH, adsorption and/or complexation factors, solubility factors, phase distribution, light sensitivity, oxygen lability, and volatility.[8] Even the container the final product is marketed in may be of importance.[9] (4) A new and as yet not broadly applied possibility is the use of five, six, or even higher numbers of biocides at very low concentrations whose synergistic activity against spoilage microorganisms can be optimized. Few if any cosmetics or pharmaceutical manufacturers have utilized this technique to date.

THE TARGET OF PRESERVATION

The enemy is not unknown: preservation activity can be measured against specific health hazards to normal and diseased skin. These include *Pseudomonas* (both *aeruginosa* and other species); *Proteus; Staphylococcus aureus; Streptococcus; Serratia marcescens; Klebsiella;* several species of *Clostridium;* and the yeasts and molds *Penicillium, Aspergillus,* and *Candida.*[10] Certain cosmetics are more susceptible to particular microbial assault, such as shampoo invasion by gram-negative bacteria and fungal and *Pseudomonas* contamination of mascara and eyeliner.[11]

CLASSIFICATION OF PRESERVATIVES

Although many different classification systems may be used, based either upon functional or structural similarity, a scheme that utilizes both structural similarity and allergenic cross-reactivity seems most applicable (Table 40-1).[12] Only those preservatives reported as allergenic are included in this brief tabulation.

FREQUENCY OF USE OF BIOCIDES IN COSMETICS

Cosmetic manufacturers may voluntarily register their product formulations with the Food and Drug Administration in accordance with the regulations codified in title 21, the code of federal regulation, part 720. The manufacturers of over 20,000 cosmetic formulations reported use of nearly 100 chemicals with preservative function, representing a minute fraction of all available cosmetics and toiletries. Nonetheless, trends in cosmetic preservation over time may be studied, an indication of biocide popularity and efficacy as well as occasionally a reflection of physician and patient perception

TABLE 40–1. A Working Classification of Preservatives

Formaldehyde donors	Isothiazolinones
Formaldehyde	Methylchloroisothiazolinone
Glutaraldehyde	(MCI/MI)
Quaternium-15	Methylisothiazolinone
Bromonitrodioxane	(MCI/MI)
Bromonitropropane diol	Benzisothiazolinone
Imidazolidinyl urea	Octylisothiazolinone
Diazolidinyl urea	Quaternary ammonium compounds
MDM hydantoin	Benzalkonium chloride
DMDM hydantoin	Cetrimonium bromide
Non-formaldehyde donors	Benzethonium chloride
Paraben esters	Miscellaneous
Parabens	Chloroacetamide
Sodium benzoate	Methyldibromoglutaronitrile
Phenolics	(Euxyl K-400)
Chloroxylenol	Sorbic acid
Chlorocresol	Chlorhexidine digluconate
o-Phenyl phenol	Captan
Alcohols	Antioxidants
Benzyl alcohol	Butylated hydroxyanisole
Propylene glycol	Butylated hydroxytoluene
Phenoxyethanol (Euxyl K-400)	Propyl gallate
Chlorobutanol	Vitamin E (tocopherol)
Mercurials	UV absorbers
Phenylmercuric acetate	Benzophenones
Thimerosal	Cinnamates

of biocide safety[13] (Fig. 40-1). Examining these data, it is apparent that certain preservatives have enjoyed increasing popularity over the last 10 years, including the paraben esters, imidazolidinyl urea, and methylchloroisothiazolinone/methylisothiazolinone, while others—such as DMDM hydantoin and diazolidinyl urea—are relatively new biocides, increasingly employed as they establish market share. Conversely, quaternium-15, bromonitropropane diol, and formaldehyde are exhibiting decreased frequency of utilization, perhaps secondary to the scrutiny these biocides have undergone; such scrutiny may be in part the result of available allergenicity data.

The more important of these allergens are examined individually, with discussion of those factors specifically related to usage trends. For more detailed information regarding particular antigens, rationale for use, and industry and consumer perception, the interested reader is referred to one of several recent detailed review articles.[14,15]

THE INDIVIDUAL ALLERGENS

FORMALDEHYDE

Formaldehyde exists as a colorless substance with characteristic odor in solid (paraformaldehyde), liquid (formalin, 37 percent formaldehyde), and gaseous (methanol) phases (Fig. 40-2A). In the environment, contact generally occurs in the form of free formaldehyde, formaldehyde donated from a formaldehyde-releasing preservative, and amino and phenolic formaldehyde resins. The issue of formaldehyde is covered in depth in Chap. 20, and the reader interested in greater toxicity and sensitivity detail is referred to the excellent work of Feinman.[16]

Although ubiquitous, common sources of formaldehyde in the environment include cosmetic products preserved with formaldehyde or formaldehyde donors; industrial biocides in metalworking fluids; formaldehyde released from resins used as treatment for textiles, furs, and leather; paper products treated with formaldehyde resins or utilizing inks and dyes containing formaldehyde; and direct occupational contacts (e.g., medical and dental technicians and embalmers). Formaldehyde is broadly accepted to be a strong sensitizer as assessed through guinea pig and human maximization testing,[17–19] with the threshold of allergic reactivity showing remarkable interpersonal variation; a dose-response relationship may be demonstrated.[20] Patients with exquisite formaldehyde sensitivity are often troubled by exposure to garments treated with amino formaldehyde resins,[21] although formaldehyde sensitivity does not appear to be a necessary condition to formaldehyde resin sensitivity, as previously believed.[22]

Far and away the most common scenario of formaldehyde sensitization is that of the individual sensitized through cosmetic products in which free formaldehyde may be found, with patch testing also revealing one or several other coreactive formaldehyde-releasing biocides. Nearly half of all cases of formaldehyde sensitivity are seen in combination with alternative formaldehyde-releasing biocide allergy,[23] and conversely between one-third and one-half of patients with formaldehyde-releasing biocide allergy also show a positive patch test to formaldehyde.[23,24] When assessed at 1 to 2% concentration in screening fashion as part of a standard patch-test tray, formaldehyde positivity frequency ranges from 1 to 9 percent, with a mean of between 4 and 5 percent in 30 larger studies.[14] Although many patients sensitized to formaldehyde appear to have

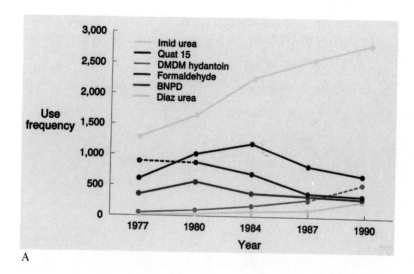

A

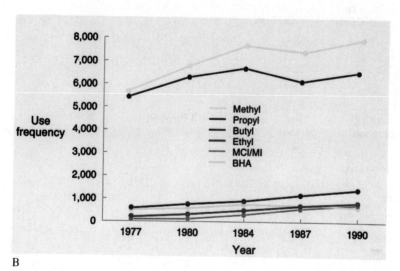

B

FIG. 40–1. *A.* Trends in preservative use: the formaldehyde-releasing biocides. *B.* Trends in preservative use: biocides acting independently from formaldehyde release.

become so through cosmetic exposures, nine major studies of patients with dermatitis due to cosmetic products also demonstrate this same formaldehyde sensitivity prevalence of roughly 4 percent.[14]

The significance of the positive responses to formaldehyde tested at 1 to 2% aqueous concentration has traditionally been questioned; between two-thirds and three-fourths appear to be relevant.[23,25] Cronin[26] has also found formaldehyde positivity to be of relevance in at least 50 percent of men and in the majority of women, particularly in association with hand eczema.

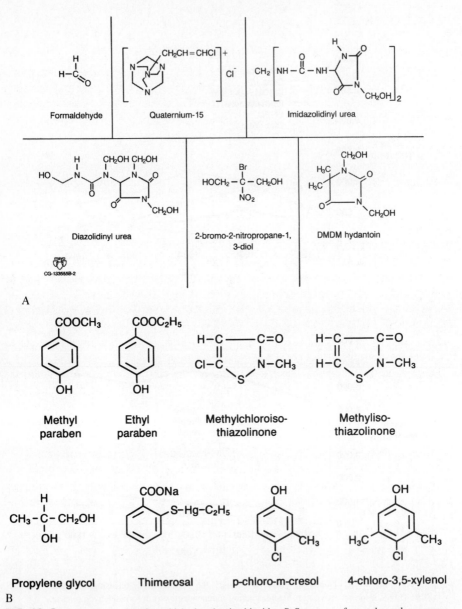

FIG. 40–2. *A.* Structures of the formaldehyde-releasing biocides. *B.* Structures of several popular preservatives acting independently from formaldehyde release.

Patch testing to formaldehyde is performed at 1% aqueous concentration, with occasional irritancy, but less so than the significant false-positivity rate found at 2%; the possibility that a percentage of patients sensitive to formaldehyde are not detected at the 1% aqueous concentration has not been excluded.[27]

QUATERNIUM-15

This odorless, colorless, highly water-soluble formaldehyde-donating biocide is discussed in greater detail in Chap. 23; it provides effective and indeed superior antimicrobial activity against bacteria, yeasts, and molds at low concentration and may therefore be used in sole fashion. Quaternium-15 is one of a group of quaternary ammonium compounds, many of which also have preservative function but none of which release free formaldehyde or cross-react with quaternium-15 (Fig. 40-2A). Marketed under the trade name Dowicil 200,* quaternium-15 was determined to be potentially sensitizing in the mid-1970s and showed prevalence rates in screening series ranging from 0 to 5 percent by geographic location (mean, 3.3 percent) in a total of 11 studies recently reviewed.[14] Perhaps of more concern are data provided by the North American Contact Dermatitis Group, which demonstrates that quaternium-15 sensitivity is increasing over the course of time; 2.3 percent of patients in 1975 reacted, with a corresponding prevalence of 6.7 percent in 1985. A figure of 9.1 percent was obtained during their prospective 5-year study of patients specifically believed to have allergy to cosmetic products.[3] This trend toward increasing prevalence of sensitivity has served to focus attention on the safety of quaternium-15, particularly in light of its theoretical sensitizing potential. The use of this particular biocide has diminished in cosmetic products over the last decade, perhaps reflexive to this greater sensitization trend (Fig. 40-1A). The reason for increasing sensitization to quaternium-15 is not known but may relate to its use in several widely popular moisturizing lotions.

Quaternium-15 represents the most potent of the frequently used formaldehyde-donating biocides, releasing 100 ppm formaldehyde into a 0.1% aqueous solution[20]; several groups of investigators have confirmed this significant potential for formaldehyde release, with the majority of patients exhibiting quaternium-15 sensitivity also being responsive to formaldehyde. Other formaldehyde-releasing biocides such as imidazolidinyl urea, diazolidinyl urea, DMDM hydantoin, and bromonitropropane diol may also react; when a significant number of these biocides react together, it may be advisable for the patient to avoid the entire class of formaldehyde donors.[23,24,28] Although exposure to quaternium-15 is frequent in certain occupations, reports of contact sensitization in the workplace are rare.

Quaternium-15 is best tested at 2% concentration in petrolatum, as a large number of cases are missed with the aqueous vehicle.[28]

IMIDAZOLIDINYL UREA

This biocide is also discussed in greater detail in Chap. 14. Imidazolidinyl urea (Germall 115)[†] is a water-soluble, colorless, odorless, and tasteless preservative that has good bacterial inhibition activity and lesser activity against yeasts, molds, and fungi (Fig. 40-2A). It is synergistic against these and other microorganisms when used in conjunction with a different class of preservative, such as the paraben esters. Imidazolidinyl urea, although a formaldehyde donor, is not a potent one, and many patients with

*Dow Chemical USA; Midland, Michigan.

†Sutton Laboratories Inc.; Chatham, New Jersey.

formaldehyde and/or quaternium-15 allergy tolerate exposure to this biocide. For this reason, a large number of "hypoallergenic" cosmetic formulations contain imidazolidinyl urea. The opinion that imidazolidinyl urea is a safe and relatively nonsensitizing biocide is reflected in its frequency of usage in cosmetic products, increasing to the point where currently it is second in popularity only to the paraben ester group[13] (Fig. 40-1A).

Frequency of sensitization in screening series is low compared to those of the other formaldehyde-releasing biocides, ranging from 0.1 to 2.2 percent in nine major studies (mean, 1.7 percent).[14] As one might suspect, the incidence may be slightly higher in patients specifically sensitized to cosmetics, although Broeckx et al.[5] and DeGroot et al.[6] found no sensitivity in their patients tested in the late 1980s. The two prospective landmark studies over 5 years by the North American Contact Dermatitis Group demonstrated a 3 percent positive response rate in patients with dermatitis due to cosmetic products.[3]

The optimum testing conditions for imidazolidinyl urea are still the subject of debate. Although several investigators still utilize a water-based formulation, 2% imidazolidinyl urea in petrolatum appears to be more sensitive, with a high false-negativity rate found at 2% aqueous concentration.[29,30] The North American Contact Dermatitis Group currently tests with both 2% aqueous and petrolatum formulations. As unpublished data would suggest, concurrent positivity of both forms is unusual and the use of only one vehicle may miss relevant cases of allergy.

BROMONITROPROPANE DIOL

This substituted aliphatic diol is highly soluble in water, insoluble in oils, stable for prolonged periods (with alkaline pH or heating decreasing the time required for decomposition), and is marketed under the commercial and cosmetic trade names of Myacide BT and Bronopol (Fig. 40-2A). Bromonitropropane diol (BNPD) shows strong inhibition of both gram-positive and gram-negative bacteria, particularly *Pseudomonas aeruginosa,* with measurable activity to a lesser degree against spoilage yeast and fungi. Although BNPD is a recognized superior biocide, its frequency of use has declined over the past 6 years, perhaps in part due to the attention it has received as a formaldehyde donor and potential sensitizer (Fig. 40-1A).[23,24,31,32]

The frequency of sensitization to BNPD is highly variable between studies, which may be due in part to its inherent irritancy when tested at concentrations of 0.5% or greater and/or may stem from regional or geographic exposural differences. European studies have generally shown sensitivity rates under 1 percent; the North American Contact Dermatitis Group data suggests prevalence of sensitivity to be between 2 and 3 percent when screened in the standard tray; and at the Mayo Clinic we have seen positivity rates of 4 to 5 percent over the past 10 years. A number of these positive cases also coreact to formaldehyde, and BNPD is known to be a moderately potent formaldehyde donor.[14,20] The incidence of sensitivity appears to be no greater in patients believed to have cosmetic product allergy.[14]

Coreaction to formaldehyde appears to be less frequent than for quaternium-15. Only 6 of Ford and Beck's[24] 20 BNPD-sensitive subjects coreacted with formaldehyde, while just over 20 percent of 244 BNPD-positive patients reported by the Mayo Clinic showed concomitant formaldehyde allergy.[23] It is correctly surmised that in cases of BNPD positivity where irritation is unlikely (patch-test concentration of 0.5% or less with allergic patch test response morphology), BNPD is most frequently a sensitizer sui generis and not positive on the basis of its ability to liberate formaldehyde. In their definitive work screening over 8100 patients with a standard tray, the European Experimental Contact Dermatitis Research Group (EECDRG) found a low rate of irritancy of 0.12 to 0.5 percent BNPD tested in petrolatum and a similarly low 0.47 percent allergenicity rate; in only 17 cases (0.2 percent) was BNPD deemed of current or past clinical relevance.

Several clinical settings have been associated with increased frequency of BNPD sensitivity; Storrs and Bell[31] reported 7 patients sensitized to BNPD from the use of a hydrophilic ointment, while Peters and colleagues[32] stated that the prolonged use of bronopol-containing lubricants in a referral population of patients with chronic severe extensive dermatitis appeared to be predisposing conditions.

The currently recommended patch-test concentration for BNPD is 0.5% in petrolatum with the recognition of mild irritant reaction potential. Aqueous vehicle has not been utilized in 12 major studies and does not appear to increase sensitivity with specificity; irritant responses in aqueous formulation may increase the false-positivity rate.[29]

DIAZOLIDINYL UREA

This preservative, a 1982 introduction to the market under the trade name Germall II,* is present in cosmetic products at concentrations of 0.1 to 0.5% (Fig. 40-2A). Its popularity, although increasing, has not reached plateau, as it is yet to achieve its market share potential (Fig. 40-1A). A member of the imidazolidinyl urea group, diazolidinyl urea exhibits excellent antibacterial activity; although its antifungal properties are superior to those of the related imidazolidinyl urea, an additional biocide is added for fungal inhibition. Parabens are often the agents selected for use with diazolidinyl urea.

Initial guinea-pig studies failed to show any sensitization responses, and diazolidinyl urea was not believed to be a potent irritant.[33] The first case of allergic contact dermatitis was reported in 1985 by Kantor and colleagues,[34] with four more reported by DeGroot and his associates[35] 3 years later. Both groups of investigators, utilizing diazolidinyl urea in a screening tray, detected no other cases of relevant allergic sensitization. At the Mayo Clinic, we have identified 58 patients who screened positively to aqueous 1% diazolidinyl urea, 81 percent of whom also concomitantly responded to formaldehyde.[27] A mere 10 percent of these cases were deemed relevant, confirmed with a traceable environmental antigen source identified as proximal cause and/or with positive use test. Most frequently, the diazolidinyl urea response was determined to be due to formaldehyde liberation and therefore based upon formaldehyde sensitivity.[36] The ability of diazolidinyl urea to be both sensitizer and formaldehyde donor is well recognized, although the actual sensitization risk is yet to be determined.[36,37]

The optimal conditions for testing diazolidinyl urea are undefined, although the 1% aqueous formulation may be the more sensitive of the vehicles.[38] Previous investigators

*Sutton Laboratories Inc.; Chatham, New Jersey.

have utilized 1 to 2% aqueous concentration. Irritancy is not believed to occur at this concentration range.[29]

DIMETHYLOLDIMETHYL HYDANTOIN

This preservative goes under a number of generic (DMDMH, DMDM hydantoin, dimethyloldimethyl hydantoin) and trade (Glydant, Dantoin DMDMH-55)* names. It is a stable, colorless, odorless biocide that is employed in cosmetic products at 0.2 to 0.4% concentration and is active against a variety of gram-negative and gram-positive bacteria as well as molds and fungi.[39,40] Products in which it is utilized and where DMDM hydantoin's antimicrobial activity has been demonstrated include creams, pastes, liquid shampoos, hair conditioners, cream rinse conditioners, facial makeups, antiperspirants, body lotions, liquid soft soaps, and bubble bath products. Its popularity has slowly increased since its introduction to the market as Glydant in 1978, although it has yet to establish its actual market share[13] (Fig. 40-1A).

DMDM hydantoin has remarkable formaldehyde donor potential and is believed to act at least partially if not primarily on the basis of this formaldehyde liberation; in solution, an equilibrium exists between DMDM hydantoin and formaldehyde, with 2% formaldehyde concentration identified by assay. Over 17 percent of combined formaldehyde is identifiable by weight. From this information it would be suspected that patients who are formaldehyde-sensitive would frequently react to DMDM hydantoin, both in cosmetic products and when assessed by epicutaneous patch testing. Such appears to be the case, with coreactivity and cross-reactivity with the other formaldehyde-releasing biocides quite common; 57 percent of one small series of formaldehyde-sensitive subjects reacted to DMDM hydantoin, with 33 percent reacting to the related transitional compound methyloldimethyl hydantoin (which has half the formaldehyde-releasing potential of the larger dimethylol moiety).[41] Two series of over 500 patients have been described, both of which found prevalence of sensitivity between 1 and 2 percent; one of these two studies suggested that an aqueous formulation was the more sensitive vehicle in testing.[38,42,43] We have found DMDM hydantoin to be frequently positive in patients with formaldehyde and other formaldehyde-releasing biocide sensitivity, with positive response deemed relevant but environmental sources infrequently identified.[44]

Further study regarding the frequency of sensitivity to this particular biocide is required before its true potential as a sensitizer is defined; until that time, close observation is warranted. Patch testing may be performed in both aqueous vehicle and in petrolatum, although the aqueous formulation at 2% concentration may be the single best choice for screening; again, further study is warranted.[29,38]

NON-FORMALDEHYDE-RELEASING BIOCIDES

PARABENS

The alkyl esters of parahydroxybenzoic acid are the most widely used preservative class in the cosmetic industry (Fig. 40-1B). Seventy years of experience with this class

*Lonza, Inc.; Fairlawn, New Jersey.

of biocides has demonstrated not only their efficacy against fungi and gram-positive bacteria (with lesser efficacy against gram-negative bacteria) but also their general overall safety. Many paraben esters exist and only certain parabens have reached the market (including benzyl paraben); four major parabens (methyl, ethyl, propyl, and butyl) are widely used, with the methyl and ethyl parabens being by far the most popular (Fig. 40-2B). As a group, parabens are nontoxic, nonirritating, colorless, odorless, stable, and effective over a rather wide pH range. Their relative insolubility in water limits efficacy against *P. aeruginosa*. Methyl and ethyl parabens are used more frequently due to their lower molecular weight and superior water-solubility characteristics. Parabens find use in pharmaceutical products, cosmetics, foods, and industrial products, with antimicrobial activity potentiated by and synergistic with other biocides including the formaldehyde-releasing biocides, phenylethanol, ethylenediamine tetraacetic acid, and propylene glycol. Nonionic surfactants such as Tween 80 inactivate parabens.[45,46]

Although relatively safe as biocides, paraben esters are capable of inducing a broad spectrum of immunologic and allergic responses. In 38 recently chronicled studies reporting prevalence of allergy to parabens,[15] all but 6[47-52] reported prevalence rates of 3 percent or less; in light of the parabens' rather ubiquitous nature, their extensive use in cosmetic and pharmaceutical products, the intensive scrutiny that they have undergone in the past 15 years, and the routine use of paraben mix as a screening assay for paraben sensitivity by most if not all investigators, such low sensitivity rates confirm their safety. The frequency in patients suspected of having cosmetic allergy appears no higher; critical analysis of data also fails to identify a differential response between European and North American studies. In addition to allergic contact dermatitis (Figs. 40-3 and 40-4), paraben esters have been reported capable of inducing angioedema,[53] contact urticaria,[54] bronchospasm,[55] pruritus,[56] and systemic contact dermatitis in the form of a generalized eczematous reaction from ingestion of parabens.[57,58] Such reactions are believed to be rare.

The "paraben paradox" proposed by Fisher[53] is characterized by dermatitis when paraben-containing topical agents are applied to altered skin while being simultaneously well tolerated on comparably normal skin. The increase of paraben sensitivity in chronic eczematous conditions such as atopic dermatitis and stasis eczema that has been reported[59] would appear to be analogous to that seen for other preservatives, including methylchloroisothiazolinone/methylisothiazolinone.[60] Many factors may enter into this unusual phenomenon, including penetration; preexistent inflammatory responsiveness; occlusion; concentration of paraben used; and concentration, form, and vehicle of patch-test application.

Despite their inclusion in the group of para-amino compounds—including para-aminobenzoic acid, local anesthetics, and paraphenylenediamine—there does not appear to be any cross-reaction between parabens and the other members of this group, and paraben-sensitive patients generally tolerate paraphenylenediamine and other related compounds well.

Patch testing has traditionally been performed to a mixture of four to five paraben esters at 3% concentration each in order to increase sensitivity of testing while decreasing the number of test sites needed. Menne and Hjorth[61] have questioned this recently, showing a differential response between the individual paraben esters in patients reactive to the mix itself; these authors question whether or not higher concentration of individual components may actually be both more accurate and more sensitive on assay.

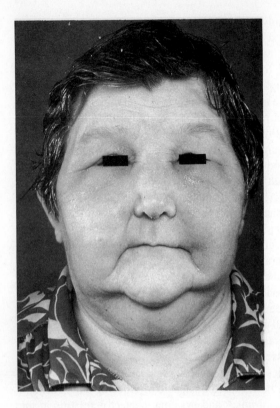

FIG. 40-3. Allergic contact dermatitis of face, sensitive to parabens in topical antibacterial silver sulfadiazine cream applied to foot abrasion and inadvertently spread to face. (See color Plate 38.)

METHYLCHLOROISOTHIAZOLINONE/METHYLISOTHIAZOLINONE (MCI/MI)

This biocide was introduced into the market in 1980 under the trade name Kathon CG* (CG standing for cosmetic grade, one of a number of isothiazolinone grades and derivatives used in both industry and cosmetics and pharmaceutical manufacture). This odorless, colorless biocide exhibits superior microbicidal activity against fungi, yeast, gram-positive bacteria, and gram-negative bacteria, comparing favorably to both formaldehyde-releasing and non-formaldehyde-releasing biocides (Fig. 40-2B). MCI/MI finds cosmetic applications in creams, hair tonics, balsams, wash softeners, makeups, and tissue papers. Industrial uses include metalworking fluids, paper and pulp manufacture, telecommunications industry, and film processing; industrial chemists, painters, laboratory technicians, and workers in the plastics industry may also be exposed. Out of the group of isothiazolinone family members, other less frequent sensitizers identified include octyl-isothiazolinone and benzisothiazolinone.[62-64]

MCI/MI has undergone intense scrutiny with respect to its sensitizing potential over the past 8 years, being the subject of over 100 original investigative articles and publications. Despite this scrutiny and the narrow escape of MCI/MI from deletion in the U.S. market, its popularity as a cosmetic preservative has continued to rise over the period in question[13] (Fig. 40-1B). MCI/MI is presently the sixth most popular preservative used in the United States (behind the four parabens and imidazolidinyl

*Rohm and Haas Company, Inc.; Philadelphia, Pennsylvania.

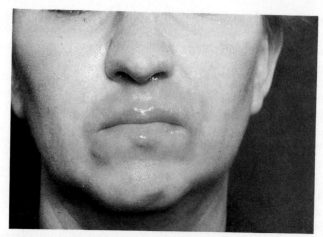

FIG. 40-4. Erosive perioral dermatitis due to paraben-containing lip balm; irritant and secondary monilial invasion factors complicate this situation. (See color Plate 39.)

urea), with most of these applications being in hair care products, but MCI/MI is also found in several frequently used topical moisturizing creams and lotions (Fig. 40-5).

Initial statements of concern regarding MCI/MI as a potential sensitizer came from Europe, where concentrations in the range of 15 to 30 ppm or more were regularly utilized in cosmetic products that did not require and therefore had no labeling of

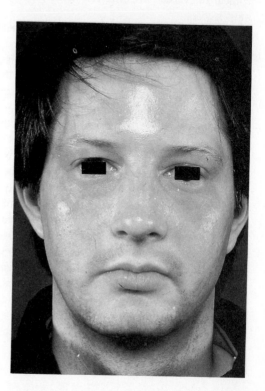

FIG. 40-5. Allergic contact dermatitis of face from MCI/MI in shampoo; positive patch test to MCI/MI, positive use test and resolution of dermatitis with change of shampoo confirm relevance. (See color Plate 40.)

ingredients on the package container. Finland, Sweden, The Netherlands, Italy, and West Germany all were among those reporting high rates of positivity in the early 1980s.[65-69] Factors potentially affecting these high rates include not only use at concentrations above those currently recommended by the manufacturer but also the variability of patch-test concentrations and geographic variations of exposure and reactivity. Over the past 7 years, additional experience has been gained, with the frequency of patch-test reactivity in 20 major series reviewed recently ranging from 0.2 to 7.0 percent at 100 to 200 ppm test concentration.[15] The variable European experience is most apparent in the EECDRG report of 1991 (including 22 European contact dermatitis clinics), with positivity rates from a low 0.4 percent in England to the highest 11.1 percent in Italy at 100 ppm MCI/MI patch-test concentration.[70] Their 3 percent overall positivity rate is deemed relevant in light of response frequencies to formaldehyde (2.6 percent) and to the parabens (1.1 percent). Both European and U.S. investigators recommend standard series location for MCI/MI.[15,70]

Since the initial Mayo Clinic report of a 3.6 percent MCI/MI allergy prevalence in 365 patients in 1988, additional U.S. experience would suggest that MCI/MI at recommended use concentration is a safe biocide.[60] Two studies by the North American Contact Dermatitis Group have documented prevalence rates of 1.7 to 2.6 percent,[71,72] a rate commensurate to that of 1.9 percent for the most recent 2000-plus patients assessed at the Mayo Clinic. The reason for decrease of sensitivity in our population over time is unknown but may involve testing, exposural, or selection variability.

The relevance of the positive response to MCI/MI has also been questioned, with provocative use testing recommended in any positive patch-test response of questionable clinical relevance. MCI/MI relevance rates from 50 to 75 percent are common in most studies.

The cosmetic ingredients review (CIR) panel of the Food and Drug Administration has issued the definitive statement regarding the use of this biocide in the United States, allowing 15 ppm MCI/MI in rinse-off products and 7.5 ppm in leave-on formulations. From available efficacy and sensitivity data, these levels should allow continued use of this excellent biocide in concentrations adequate for antimicrobial activity while minimizing risk of sensitization.

Although a degree of interfamily cross-reactivity is believed to exist, MCI/MI is not known to cross-react with any other allergens in the standard tray.

Optimal patch-test concentration and technique has long been an issue regarding MCI/MI, with concentrations under 100 ppm believed inadequate to detect the majority of cases of sensitivity; concentrations over 100 ppm are believed to be (at least by most investigators) potentially irritant in nature. An aqueous concentration of 100 ppm is globally the most widely accepted patch test condition, while the North American Contact Dermatitis Group utilizes 100 ppm MCI/MI in both aqueous and petrolatum vehicles (with at least some cases believed to go undiagnosed using aqueous medium alone). Of the two vehicles available, the aqueous form is believed to be the more sensitive patch-test indicator. Certain authors, pointing to problematic factors—including the morphology of test reaction and the difficulty in tracing allergens in Europe—continue to recommend 200 ppm as a more sensitive initial patch test concentration to utilize; serial dilutions are recommended as well as use tests in cases of positivity.[73]

PROPYLENE GLYCOL

Propylene glycol is a widely used, colorless, odorless, synthetic polyol which is soluble in a variety of aqueous and/or organic solvents (Fig. 40-2B). Documented antibacterial activity is seen against gram-positive and gram-negative organisms (including *Pseudomonas* species) as well as certain fungal and yeast microorganisms. Propylene glycol finds use as a food and drug additive, as a solvent in dyes and flavoring agents, and as a humectant/softening agent that has been useful in dermatologic diseases such as asteatosis, psoriasis, and atopic dermatitis.

Propylene glycol as an allergen is incompletely understood. Because of its irritant potential, high incidences of positivity for patch tests were reported at concentrations of 10 to 20%; lower prevalences found at concentrations of 2 to 10% aqueous solution have been questioned with respect to adequacy for threshold determination. Most series screening propylene glycol find 0.5 to 2.0 percent of cases reactive,[15] while a prevalence of 4 to 5 percent has been reported in the United States for patients suspected of cosmetic allergy.[2,3] We have detected 50 cases of allergy in over 4000 patients, 1.1 percent of our population, half of whom have been sensitized to topical corticosteroids and/or moisturizing products popular in the Rochester area.[74] Other potential exposures which may be relevant sources of sensitization include antifreeze, varnishes, synthetic resins, baking and candy production, shampoos, conditioners, contraceptive gels, shaving creams, antiperspirants, and pharmaceutical preparations. The interested reader is referred to an excellent recent review.[75]

Because of the issues regarding the threshold of sensitivity response and the frequency of irritant response, the optimum concentration for patch testing to propylene glycol is still the subject of much debate. A 10% aqueous concentration is currently recommended, with lower concentrations likely to miss a significant percentage of relevant positives. Several authors recommend a higher concentration of 20% aqueous solution, with awareness of irritant response potential.[76,77]

CHLOROCRESOL, CHLOROXYLENOL

These two phenolic biocides are used extensively in pharmaceutical products, adhesives, glues, inks, varnishes, paints, metalworking fluids, and occasionally textile finishes. Pharmaceutical products such as topical corticosteroids may also be so preserved. Both of these biocides are odorless, soluble in oil and water, and active against gram-positive and gram-negative bacteria; the pair have been shown to be potential irritants as well, chlorocresol more so than chloroxylenol. Positivity rates in screening series of 0.2 to 2.0 percent are common, with the majority of series showing positivity in under 1 percent of patients.[15] Although variable, cross-reactivity between chloroxylenol and chlorocresol is frequently seen. Guinea pig maximization testing has suggested chloroxylenol to be a potent sensitizer; this is believed to be an overestimate of the sensitizing potential, the authors indicating their belief that both chloroxylenol and chlorocresol are rather weak contact sensitizers.[78]

THIMEROSAL (See also Chap. 45)

Thimerosal, or sodium ethylmercurithiosalicylate, is another mercurial exhibiting good antibacterial activity with little or no fungal or yeast inhibition (Fig. 40-2B). Thimerosal finds its broadest application in ophthalmologic and otic preparations as well as biologic products such as vaccines and desensitization solutions. All of these have proven to be potential sources of sensitization, with the use of thimerosal in heat-killing vaccines in all probability the most consequential of these. Screening series have demonstrated positivity to thimerosal in the range of 1.6 to 15.3 percent, with a mean of 4.5 percent calculated for 11 series studying over 17,000 patients[15]; the vast majority of these patients are not believed to have been exposed to Merthiolate or topical mercurial-based disinfectant products in childhood, although a percentage of patients may be so sensitized.[79] High rates of positivity in population subgroups that have broadly been vaccinated support exposure to heat-killed vaccines as a primary mode of sensitization.[80] Although subsequent injection with thimerosal-preserved vaccines may induce localized edema, erythema, or even generalized reaction, the majority of patients so vaccinated fail to show measurable response.[81] The decision as to whether vaccination should be performed in this population depends upon history of response (generalized dermatitis, systemic illness versus mild or no localized reaction) and the need for vaccination (for example, hepatitis B vaccination in health care personnel). Most investigators have found vaccination safe in this population.[82]

Antigen extracts,[83] ophthalmologic contact,[84] and cosmetic exposure are other potential sources of sensitization, although these are believed to be much less frequent than that of vaccination.

Other than the subcomponents of mercury and thiosalicylic acid, no other cosensitization or cross-reaction is believed to occur from other allergens on the standard tray. There have, however, been multiple reports of thimerosal-allergic contact sensitivity and photosensitivity in relation to piroxicam photosensitivity. This particular nonsteroidal anti-inflammatory agent should be avoided in patients sensitive to thimerosal.[85]

Thimerosal is tested in the standard series at 0.1% in petrolatum.[29] Occasional irritation may be seen at this concentration.

BENZALKONIUM CHLORIDE

Benzalkonium chloride is a quaternary ammonium compound that acts as surfactant, disinfectant, and preservative in ophthalmologic, nasal, cosmetic, hair, and other proprietary products. Sensitization through these sources is quite infrequent albeit not rare, with sensitivity prevalence ranging from 0.2 to 2.5 percent in various series reported.[15] Isolated series of cases sensitized through topical application of medicaments containing benzalkonium chloride have also been documented.[86] Benzalkonium chloride, like related nonsensitizing quaternary ammonium salts, is a recognized contact irritant and is therefore tested at 0.01 to 0.1% aqueous concentration.

METHYLDIBROMOGLUTARONITRILE/PHENOXYETHANOL

This combination biocide, marketed under the trade name Euxyl K400,* shows broad synergistic activity against bacteria and fungi alike and has been found nonirritating and nonsensitizing by guinea pig maximization testing. First introduced to the European market in 1985, reports of sensitization began to surface in 1991 with Tosti's series of 11 cases, and subsequent cases having been reported from other European locations.[87,88] Patch testing is presently best performed to both phenoxyethanol and to the combination biocide. Although incorporation into cosmetics in the United States is still extremely limited, isolated cases of sensitivity have been noted by the North American Contact Dermatitis Group; the true incidence of sensitivity needs to be determined, with time required for the development of a steady-state plateau.

SUMMARY

Preservatives are among the most frequent causes of allergic contact dermatitis. Awareness of biocides capable of inducing such responses and the clinical presentations seen is essential in the management of such cases. The preceding is intended to provide the essentials of preservative use and discuss preservatives on the standard tray, with an overview of other biocides that occasionally mandate but generally merit assessment as well.

REFERENCES

1. Romaguera C, Camarasa JMG, Alomar A, et al: Patch tests with allergens related to cosmetics. *Contact Dermatitis* 6:167–168, 1983.
2. Eiermann HJ, Larsen W, Maibach HI, et al: Prospective study of cosmetic reactions: 1977–1980. *J Am Acad Dermatol* 6:909–917, 1982.
3. Adams RM, Maibach HI, Clendenning WE, et al: A five-year study of cosmetic reactions. *J Am Acad Dermatol* 13:1062–1069, 1985.
4. DeGroot AC, Liem DH, Nater JP, et al: Patch tests with fragrance materials and preservatives. *Contact Dermatitis* 12:87–92, 1985.
5. Broeckx W, Blondeel A, Dooms-Goossens A, et al: Cosmetic intolerance. *Contact Dermatitis* 16:189–194, 1987.
6. DeGroot AC, Beverdam EGA, Ayong CT, et al: The role of contact allergy in the spectrum of adverse effects caused by cosmetics and toiletries. *Contact Dermatitis* 19:195–201, 1988.
7. Kabara JJ (ed): *Cosmetic and Drug Preservation: Principles and Practice.* New York, Dekker, 1984, pp 237–338.
8. McCarthy TJ: Formulated factors affecting the activity of preservatives, in Kabara JJ (ed): *Cosmetic and Drug Preservation: Principles and Practice.* New York, Dekker, 1984, pp 359–388.
9. McCarthy TJ: Interaction between aqueous preservative solutions and their plastic containers: I. *Pharm Weekly* 105:557–563, 1970.
10. Bruch CW: Objectionable microorganisms in nonsterile drugs and cosmetics. *Drug Cosmet Ind* 110:32, 116, 1972.
11. Cowen RA, Steiger B: Why a preservative system must be tailored to a specific product. *Cosmet Toilet* 92:16–20, 1977.
12. Cosmetic preservatives encyclopedia. *Cosmet Toilet* 102:25–40, 1987.

*Calgon Corporation, Tuscola, Illinois; Schulke & Mayr GMBH, West Germany.

13. Frequency of preservative use in cosmetic formulas as disclosed to FDA, 1990. *Cosmet Toilet* 105:45–47, 1990.

14. Fransway AF: The problem of preservation in the 1990s: I. Statement of the problem, solution(s) of the industry, and the current use of formaldehyde and formaldehyde-releasing biocides. *Am J Contact Dermatitis* 2:6–23, 1991.

15. Fransway AF: The problem of preservation in the 1990s: III. Agents with preservative function independent of formaldehyde release. *Am J Contact Dermatitis* 2:145–174, 1991.

16. Feinman SE (ed): *Formaldehyde Sensitivity and Toxicity.* Boca Raton, Fla, CRC Press, 1988.

17. Magnusson B, Kligman AM: The identification of contact allergens by animal assay: The guinea pig maximization test. *J Invest Dermatol* 52:268–276, 1969.

18. Anderson KE, Boman A, Hamann K, et al: Guinea pig maximization tests with formaldehyde releasers: Results from two laboratories. *Contact Dermatitis* 10:257–266, 1984.

19. Marzulli FN, Maibach HI: The use of graded concentrations in studying skin sensitizers: Experimental contact sensitization in man. *Food Cosmet Toxicol* 12:219, 1974.

20. Jordan WP, Sherman WT, King SE: Threshold responses in formaldehyde-sensitive subjects. *J Am Acad Dermatol* 1:44–48, 1979.

21. Anderson KE, Hamann K: Cost benefit of patch testing with textile finish resins. *Contact Dermatitis* 8:64–67, 1982.

22. Fowler JF Jr, Skinner SM, Belsito DV: Allergic contact dermatitis from formaldehyde resins in permanent press clothing: An underdiagnosed cause of generalized dermatitis. *J Am Acad Dermatol* 27:962–968, 1992.

23. Fransway AF, Schmitz NA: The problem of preservation in the 1990s: II. Formaldehyde and formaldehyde-releasing biocides: Incidences of cross-reactivity and the significance of the positive response to formaldehyde. *Am J Contact Dermatitis* 2:78–88, 1991.

24. Ford GP, Beck MH: Reactions to quaternium-15, bronopol, and Germall 115 in a standard series. *Contact Dermatitis* 14:271–274, 1986.

25. Epstein E, Maibach HI: Formaldehyde allergy: Incidence and patch test problems. *Arch Dermatol* 94:186–190, 1966.

26. Cronin E: Formaldehyde is a significant allergen in women with hand eczema. *Contact Dermatitis* 25:276–282, 1991.

27. Hectorne K, Fransway AF: Diazolidinyl urea sensitivity: Incidence of sensitivity and relevance. *Contact Dermatitis* 30:16–19, 1994.

28. Parker LV, Taylor JS: A five-year study of contact allergy to quaternium-15. *Am J Contact Dermatitis* 2:231–234, 1991.

29. Andersen KE, Rycroft RJG: Recommended patch test concentrations for preservatives, biocides, and antimicrobials. *Contact Dermatitis* 25:1–18, 1991.

30. DeGroot AC, Weyland JW: Hidden contact allergy to formaldehyde in imidazolidinyl urea. *Contact Dermatitis* 17:124–125, 1987.

31. Storrs FJ, Bell DE: Allergic contact dermatitis to 2-bromo-2-nitropropane-1,3-diol in a hydrophilic ointment. *J Am Acad Dermatol* 8:157–170, 1983.

32. Peters MS, Connolly SM, Schroeter AL: Bronopol allergic contact dermatitis. *Contact Dermatitis* 9:397–401, 1983.

33. Wallhauser KH: Antimicrobial preservatives used by the cosmetics industry, in Kabara JJ (ed): *Cosmetic and Drug Preservative: Principles and Practice.* New York, Dekker, 1984, pp 657–659.

34. Kantor GR, Taylor JS, Ratz JL, et al: Acute allergic contact dermatitis from diazolidinyl urea (Germall II) in a hair gel. *J Am Acad Dermatol* 13:116–119, 1985.

35. DeGroot AC, Bruynzeel DP, Jagtman BA, et al: Contact allergy to diazolidinyl urea. *Contact Dermatitis* 18:202–205, 1988.

36. Jordan WP: Human studies that determine the sensitivity potentials of haptens: Experimental allergic contact dermatitis. *Dermatol Clin* 2:533–538, 1984.

37. Stephens TJ, Drake KD, Drotman RB: Experimental delayed contact sensitization to diazolidinyl urea (Germall II) in guinea pigs. *Contact Dermatitis* 16:164–168, 1987.

38. Storrs FJ, Rosenthal LE, Adams RM, et al: Prevalence and relevance of allergic reactions in patients patch tested in North America: 1984 to 1985. *J Am Acad Dermatol* 20:1038–1045, 1989.

39. Schanno RJ, Westlund JR, Foelsch PH: Evaluation of 1,3 dimethylol-5,5-dimethylhydantoin as a cosmetic preservative. *J Soc Cosmet Chem* 31:85–96, 1980.

40. Rosen M: Glydant and MDMH as cosmetic preservatives, in Kabara JJ (ed): *Cosmetic and Drug Preservation: Principles and Practice.* New York, Dekker, 1984, pp 165–190.
41. DeGroot AC, Van Joost TV, Bos JD, et al: Patch test reactivity to DMDM hydantoin. *Contact Dermatitis* 18:197–201, 1988.
42. DeGroot AC, Bos JD, Jagtman BA, et al: Contact allergy to preservatives (II). *Contact Dermatitis* 15:218–222, 1986.
43. Mitchell JC, Adams RM, Clendenning WE, et al: Results of patch tests with substances abandoned. *Contact Dermatitis* 8:336–337, 1982.
44. Mayo Clinic, unpublished data.
45. Aalto TR, Firman MC, Rigler NE: P-hydroxybenzoic acid esters as preservatives: I. Uses, antibacterial and antifungal studies, properties, and determination. *J Am Pharm Assoc* 42:449–457, 1953.
46. Matthews C, Davidson J, Bauer E, et al: P-hydroxybenzoic acid esters as preservatives: II. Acute and chronic toxicity in dogs, rats, and mice. *J Am Pharm Assoc* 45:260–267, 1956.
47. Rudner EJ, Clendenning WE, Epstein E, et al: The frequency of contact sensitivity in North America: 1972–1974. *Contact Dermatitis* 1:277–280, 1975.
48. Rudner EJ: North American Group results. *Contact Dermatitis* 3:208–209, 1977.
49. Blondeel A, Oleffe J, Achten G: Contact allergy in 830 dermatologic patients. *Contact Dermatitis* 4:270–276, 1978.
50. Vestey JP, Gawkrodger DJ, Wang WK, et al: An analysis of 501 conservative contact clinic consultations. *Contact Dermatitis* 15:119–125, 1986.
51. Hogan DJ, Hill M, Lane PR: Results of routine patch testing of 542 patients in Sasketoon, Canada. *Contact Dermatitis* 19:120–124, 1988.
52. George NP, Srinivas CR, Balachandran C, et al: Sensitivity to various ingredients of topical preparations following prolonged use. *Contact Dermatitis* 23:367–368, 1990.
53. Fisher AA: Alleged localized angioedema of the soft palate and penis due to parabens in Accutane. *Am J Cont Derm* 1:148, 1990.
54. Henry JC, Tschen EH, Becker LE: Contact urticaria to parabens. *Arch Dermatol* 115:1231–1232, 1979.
55. Aldrete JA, Johnson DA: Allergy to local anesthetics. *JAMA* 207:356–357, 1979.
56. Simon RA: Adverse reactions to drug additives. *J Allergy Clin Immunol* 74:623–630, 1984.
57. Aeling JL, Nuss PD: Systemic eczematous "contact-type" dermatitis medicamentosa caused by parabens. *Arch Dermatol* 110:640, 1974.
58. Carradori S, Peluso AM, Faccioli M: Systemic contact dermatitis due to parabens. *Contact Dermatitis* 2:238–239, 1990.
59. Stoltze R: Dermatitis medicamentosa in eczema of the leg. *Acta Derm Venereol* 46:54–64, 1966.
60. Fransway AF: Sensitivity to Kathon CG: Findings in 365 consecutive patients. *Contact Dermatitis* 19:342–347, 1988.
61. Menne T, Hjorth N: Routine patch testing with paraben esters. *Contact Dermatitis* 19:189–191, 1988.
62. DeGroot AC, Weyland JW: Kathon CG: A review. *J Am Acad Dermatol* 18:350–358, 1988.
63. DeGroot AC, Herxheimer A: Isothiazolinone preservative: Cause of a continuing epidemic of cosmetic dermatitis. *Lancet* 2:314–316, 1989.
64. DeGroot AC: Methylisothiazolinone/methylchloroisothiazolinone (Kathon CG) allergy: An updated review. *Am J Contact Dermatitis* 1:151–156, 1990.
65. Hannuksela M: Rapid increase in contact allergy to Kathon CG in Finland. *Contact Dermatitis* 15:211–214, 1986.
66. DeGroot AC: *Skin Allergy News* 18:(5):1, 1987.
67. Bjorkner B, Bruze M, Dahlquist I, et al: Contact allergy to the preservative Kathon CG. *Contact Dermatitis* 14:85–90, 1986.
68. Tosti A, Manuzzi P, De Padova MP: Contact dermatitis to Kathon CG. *Contact Dermatitis* 14:326–327, 1986.
69. Frosch PJ, Schulze-Dirks A: Kontaktallergie auf Kathon CG. *Hautarzt* 38:422–425, 1987.
70. Menne T, Frosch PJ, Veien NK, et al: Contact sensitization to 5-chloro-2-methyl-4-isothiazolin-3-one and 2-methyl-4-isothiazolin-3-one (MCI/MI): A European multicenter study. *Contact Dermatitis* 24:334–341, 1991.
71. Rietschel RL, Nethercott JR, Emmett EA, et al: Methylchloroisothiazolinone/methylisothiazolinone reactions in patients screened for vehicle and preservative sensitivity. *J Am Acad Dermatol* 22:734–738, 1990.

72. Marks JG, Moss JN, Parno JR, et al: Methylchloroisothiazolinone/methylisothiazolinone (Kathon CG) biocide—United States multicenter study of human skin sensitization. *Am J Contact Dermatitis* 1:157–161, 1990.

73. Färm G, Wahlberg JE: Isothiazolinones (MCI/MI): 200 ppm versus 100 ppm in the standard series. *Contact Dermatitis* 25:104–107, 1991.

74. Fransway AF: Propylene glycol sensitivity: Incidence and significance. Presentation at the annual meeting of the American Academy of Dermatology, Washington, D.C. 1988.

75. Catanzaro JM, Smith JG Jr: Propylene glycol dermatitis. *J Am Acad Dermatol* 24:90–95, 1991.

76. Frosch PJ, Pekar V, Enzmann H: Contact allergy to propylene glycol: De we use the appropriate test concentration? *Dermatol Clin* 8:111–113, 1990.

77. Cronin E: *Contact Dermatitis*. New York, Churchill Livingstone, 1980.

78. Andersen KE, Hamann K: How sensitizing is chlorocresol? Allergy test in guinea pigs versus the clinical experience. *Contact Dermatitis* 11:11–20, 1984.

79. Melino M, Antonelli C, Barone M: Contact dermatitis from Merthiolate. *Contact Dermatitis* 14:125, 1986.

80. Hansson J, Möller H: Cutaneous reactions to Merthiolate and their relationship to vaccination with tetanus toxoid. *Acta Allergol* 26:150–156, 1971.

81. Cox NH, Morley WN, Forsyth A: Vaccination reactions and thimerosal. *Br Med J* 294:250, 1987.

82. Aberer W: Vaccination despite thimerosal sensitivity. *Contact Dermatitis* 24:6–10, 1991.

83. Tosti A, Guerra L, Bardazzi F: Hyposensitizing therapy with standard antigenic extracts: An important source of thimerosal sensitization. *Contact Dermatitis* 21:354–355, 1989.

84. Rietschel RL, Wilson LA: Ocular inflammation in patients using soft contact lenses. *Arch Dermatol* 118:147–149, 1982.

85. Cirne DeCastro JL, Freitas JP, Brandao FM, et al: Sensitivity to thimerosal and photosensitivity to piroxicam. *Contact Dermatitis* 24:187–192, 1991.

86. Garcia-Perez A, Moran M: Dermatitis from quaternary ammonium compounds. *Contact Dermatitis* 1:316–317, 1975.

87. Tosti A, Guerra L, Bardazzi F, et al: Euxyl K-400: A new sensitizer in cosmetics. *Contact Dermatitis* 25:89–93, 1991.

88. Torrez V, Soares AP: Contact allergy to dibromodicyanobutane in a cosmetic cream. *Contact Dermatitis* 27:114–115, 1992.

41

MEDICATIONS

Elizabeth Sherertz

In evaluating a patient with possible contact dermatitis, any material that has been in contact with the skin should be suspected. Too often we might overlook topical medications themselves as a potential source of allergic reactions. Certain medications, such as benzocaine and neomycin, are well recognized for their potential to cause contact dermatitis; they are discussed in other chapters. Topical corticosteroids are very frequently prescribed yet probably underrecognized as an occasional cause of worsening dermatitis. This is also discussed in another chapter. Photosensitivity reactions to some systemic or topical medications may occur; these are also considered elsewhere.

The growing market of over-the-counter topical medications; international travel, during which people acquire and use unfamiliar topical products; and gaps in the patient's medication history ("But, Doc, I haven't put *anything* on it . . . well, maybe once or twice") all contribute to the challenge of diagnosing contact dermatitis in response to a topical medication. There are numerous case reports in the literature of irritant, allergic, and urticarial contact reactions to individual medications. Premarketing evaluation of topicals may not reveal the true sensitization potential when a product is more widely used on inflamed skin or mucosa. This chapter provides an overview of how to recognize and evaluate the possibility that a topical medication is the cause of or a contributing factor to a patient's contact dermatitis.

RECOGNIZING MEDICATION-INDUCED CONTACT DERMATITIS

HISTORY

When the patient presents with a suspected contact dermatitis, the first step is to elicit a history of any and all topical medications that have been applied to the site during the entire course (Table 41-1). This is not as easy as it seems, as patients may tell you only what they've used most recently, may forget the chronology of therapy, or may be reluctant to reveal what nonprescription or "shared from a friend or relative" creams

TABLE 41-1. The Clinical Setting for Allergic Contact Dermatitis to Medication

Clinical appearance
    Erythema, papules-vesicles, scale, crust
    Arrangement of lesions—marginated, circular, etc. Corresponding to method of application
    Distribution around ears, eyes, on primary dermatitis site, etc.
    May be patchy if topical is applied unevenly
    May be mixed pattern of underlying skin disease (e.g., psoriasis, wart, acne) and eczematous change
History
    History of what and how products were applied
    Over-the-counter and "borrowed" medications
    Drops, sprays, medicated bandages, transdermal patch, etc.
    Medications given or applied to other members of household (include pets)
Some occupations in which medications are handled
    Nursing
    Pharmaceutical synthesis or manufacture
    Pharmacy
    Home nursing care
    Veterinary medicine
    Animal care
    Medical research lab

or ointments they may have tried. Explain to the patient how and why it is important to have this information. Encourage patients to bring everything they've used on their skin. Try to have the patient reconstruct how the eruption started—was there a traumatic lesion (e.g., scratch, insect bite, sunburn, surgical site) to which something was then applied? Was there another initial dermatologic diagnosis (e.g., acne, stasis dermatitis, tinea pedis, Darier's disease, etc.) which had been treated topically, with subsequent change or worsening in the eruption?

Certain dermatologic diseases and therapy are more often associated with contact dermatitis as a potential complication, especially stasis dermatitis, otitis externa, and leg ulcers.[1-3] Darier's disease,[4] atopic dermatitis,[5] acne,[6] alopecia,[7-8] and many other skin diseases[9-12] have been associated with topical medications which have triggered contact dermatitis. *Thus, be suspicious of contact dermatitis in any dermatology patient in whom the recommended topical therapy (prescribed or over-the-counter) does not improve the condition or produces more eczematous change.*

Consider exposures other than intentional application, such as airborne reactions to a medicated spray, body contact with another person who is using a topical medication (as in connubial contact dermatitis[13]) or applying a topical medication to or handling oral medications for another person, leading to hand eczema.[14] Patients may overlook eyedrops or eardrops as "medications" and should be specifically asked about these. Transdermal devices may cause a patchy eczematous reaction that might not be recognized as related to the patches and should be inquired about.[15]

Ask about occupation, and be attuned to the potential for medication allergy, particularly in individuals who work in health-related fields where they handle medication, such as nursing, pharmacy, pharmaceutical manufacturing, and veterinary medicine.[16,17] With the trend toward home care, also ask about the patient's role in home nursing care.

CLINICAL APPEARANCE

The clinical presentation of a contact dermatitis due to a medication can range from contact urticaria to an acute vesicular eczematous eruption, but typically one sees a spreading (usually acute) eczema where some treatment has been applied (Figs. 41-1 and 41-2). Less inflammatory, subacute to chronic red, scaling eruptions can also occur. If a topical medication had been applied to already inflamed or altered skin (e.g., an underlying dermatitis, dermatosis, or scar) the "typical" features of contact dermatitis might be mixed with those of the primary process, making recognition more difficult. Atypical patterns such as lichenoid contact dermatitis (gentamicin, neomycin), purpura (benzoyl peroxide), or pustular eruptions (e.g., 5-fluorouracil) may occur.

As with other types of contact dermatitis, the *arrangement* and *distribution* are often key clues to the triggering factor. A circular or demarcated area may suggest that a product was rubbed in at a certain location. Periorbital involvement might suggest use of an ophthalmic product applied to the eyes, involvement of the ears and surrounding area of the neck and cheeks suggests eardrops, and more extensive facial involvement would suggest a direct topical or airborne exposure. As mentioned above, any inflamed site to which a topical product has been applied should be evaluated, at least clinically, for the possibility of contact dermatitis. For example, patients with vulvar dermatoses may have contact allergy as a component.[18] If a patient has a generalized papular or vesicular eruption resembling autoeczematization or "id" reaction, look to the primary inflamed site (often on the feet or legs) and evaluate the topical medications that had been used at that site.

Even in hand dermatitis, topical medications should be considered as a potential contributing factor or cause. Topical antibiotics,[19] tar and anthralin preparations, and many other topicals besides topical corticosteroids have been implicated. In occupation-related cases of medication-induced contact dermatitis, the hands are very commonly involved. In the nursing and pharmaceutical trades, handling of *systemic* medications has been associated with hand dermatitis. Hopefully this will be reduced as protective glove use is mandated in health care. In veterinarians, topical antimicrobials have most frequently been implicated.

WHICH TOPICAL MEDICATIONS ARE MORE LIKELY TO CAUSE CONTACT DERMATITIS?

In this discussion, *irritant* contact dermatitis has not been the focus. Many topical products cause transient stinging, burning, or redness with application, which can be considered as mild irritant reactions. We recognize that some products, by their nature or their vehicle (e.g., tretinoin, 5-fluorouracil, anthralin, salicylic acid, propylene glycol, alcohol) may cause irritant reactions if applied to normal or inflamed skin or if over-lapped, and we generally warn patients about this. Choice of vehicle is particularly important in patients with atopic dermatitis to avoid irritant effects of the therapy itself.

Table 41-2 summarizes some of the more common topical medications that have been associated with allergic contact dermatitis, along with suggested patch-test concentrations. Table 41-3 lists agents that have caused contact dermatitis by type of preparation.

(Text continues on page 565)

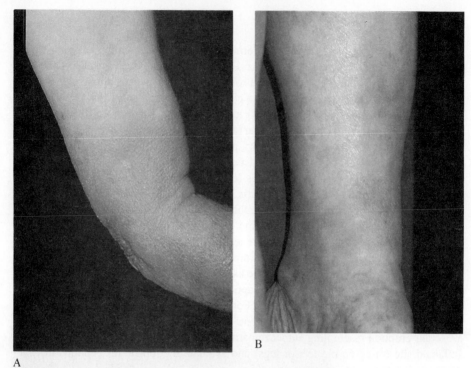

A

B

C

FIG. 41–1. *A.* Typical spreading eczema from allergy to a topical agent. This can be a medication, a home remedy, or a cosmetic lotion used to treat an underlying eczema. *B.* Contact dermatitis to a moisturizer used to treat stasis eczema. The only positive patch test was to the moisturizer itself, and withdrawal cleared the eruption. *C.* Allergic contact dermatitis to mustargen applied to a plaque of cutaneous T-cell lymphoma. The eruption cleared locally in the plaques where the patient had experienced allergic contact dermatitis. (See color Plate 41*A, B,* and *C.*)

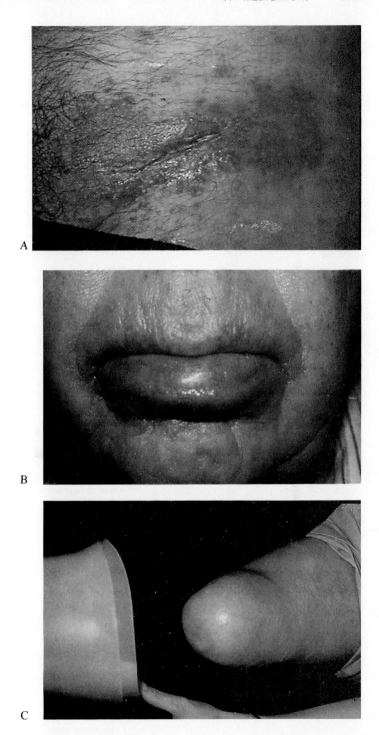

FIG. 41–2. *A*. Contact dermatitis to an antibiotic ointment applied to an infected surgical wound. *B*. Allergic contact dermatitis from topically applied bacitracin ointment. *C*. Allergic contact dermatitis of an amputation stump from an antibiotic ointment. (See color Plate 42.)

TABLE 41–2. Some Topical Medications Associated with Allergic Contact Dermatitis

Medications	Patch-Test Concentration, percent[a]	Source Examples	Cross-Reactions
Acyclovir (Zovirax)	5	Antiviral	
Aluminum acetate (Burow's solution)	1–5 Aq plastic chamber	Eardrops, topical astringent	
Amikacin	20 Aq	Eyedrops, eardrops	Neomycin, Gentamicin, Tobramycin, other aminoglycosides
ε-Aminocaproic acid	0.1–10 Aq	Eyedrops	
Bacitracin	20	Antibiotic—eye, ear	Neomycin
Benzocaine	5	Anesthetic anti-itch cream, first aid spray, hemorrhoidal analgesic	Other ester anesthetics, see Chap. 10
Benzoyl peroxide	1	Acne meds, leg ulcer Rx, industrial use	
Chloramphenicol (Chloromycetin)	5	Eyedrops, eardrops	
Clioquinol (chinoform, Vioform, iodochlorhydroxyquin)	5	Antibiotic creams, veterinary meds	Other quinolines, quinine
Clonidine	9	Transdermal agents	
Coal tar	5	Tar cream, shampoos	
Corticosteroids	See Chap. 42		
Diphenhydramine (Benadryl)	Injectable solution	Anesthetic anti-itch cream, first aid	
Dithranol	0.05	Anthralin preparations	
Dyclonine	1	Anesthetic, throat lozenge or spray	
5-Fluorouracil	1–5	Topical chemotherapy	
Gentamicin sulfate	20	Antibiotic, eyedrops, eardrops, intravenous solution	Neomycin, tobramycin, amikacin, other aminoglycosides
Hydroquinone	1	Bleaching creams	
Idoxuridine	0.5	Antiviral, eyedrops	
Lidocaine HCl	15	Anesthetic	Amide anesthetics
Mechlorethamine (nitrogen mustard)	0.02 Aq	Topical chemotherapy	
Miconazole (or other imidazole antifungals)	1 Petrolatum or ethanol	Antifungal	Other imidazoles
Minoxidil	2 Propylene glycol	Hairgrowth solution	
Neomycin	20	Antibiotic eyedrops, eardrops, first aid creams	Other aminoglycosides
Nitroglycerin	0.2 mg/mL Aq	Transdermal patches	
Nitrofurazone (Furacin)	1	Burn dressing, veterinary meds	
Oleyl polypeptide (Cerumenex)	25–50 ethanol	Eardrops	

TABLE 41–2 (Continued). Some Topical Medications Associated with Allergic Contact Dermatitis

Medications	Patch-Test Concentration, percent[a]	Source Examples	Cross-Reactions
Phenylephrine HCl	1–5 or 10 Aq	Eye, ear, and nose drops	
Procaine HCl	1	Anesthetic	Other ester anesthetics
Promethazine HCl	2	Topical anti-itch (outside U.S.) agent	
Propolis (bee glue)	10	Homeopathic meds, health foods	Balsam of Peru fragrance
Pyridoxine HCl (vitamin B$_6$)	10	Vitamin additive	
Quinoline	See clioquinol		
Resorcinol	2	Acne meds, Castellani's paint	Hexylresorcinol, resorcinol monoacetate
Salicylic acid	0.5	Keratolytic acne meds, wart remover	
Scopolamine	1	Transdermal patch	
Sulfanilamide	5	Burn dressing, veterinary meds	Other sulfonamides
Tetracaine HCl	1	Anesthetic, eyedrops, eardrops	Other ester anesthetics
Thiamine HCl (vitamin B$_1$)	10	Vitamin additive	
Timolol	1	Eyedrops	Other betablockers
Tobramycin	20 Aq	Eardrops, eyedrops	Neomycin, gentamicin, other aminoglycosides
Tocopherol (vitamin E)	10	Vitamin additive	

[a]Percent in petrolatum unless otherwise indicated.

Aq = aqueous.

Topical antibiotics, antivirals, and imidazole antifungals have all been associated with contact allergy.[20–22] Topical antipruritics/anesthetics such as benzocaine and diphenhydramine may cause allergic or even photoallergic contact dermatitis.[23] A number of eyedrops and eardrops have been implicated, and there are isolated case reports of a number of other topical medications.[24–26] In other countries, topical antiinflammatory agents have been reported to cause contact allergy.[27–29] Even herbal or homeopathic medications may be the source.[30,31] The systemic medications frequently implicated in occupational cases are phenothiazines and antibiotics, and these may cause immediate urticarial reactions.[32,33] Please note that Tables 41-2 and 41-3 consider only reactions to the medication itself and do not include products in which a vehicle ingredient is implicated. It is beyond the scope of this text to discuss the individual medications at length. Cross-reactions are noted between chemically similar medications (e.g., imidazole antifungals), and this should be considered in changing therapy.

TABLE 41-3. Types of Preparations and Agents That May Cause Allergic Contact Dermatitis

Antibiotics, antifungals, antivirals
  Acyclovir
  Amikacin
  Bacitracin
  Benzoyl peroxide
  Chloroamphenicol
  Chloroxylenol
  Clioquinol
  Clotrimazole
  Croconazole
  Cyclopyroxoxolamine
  Dibrompropamidine
  Econazole
  Fentichlor
  Gentamicin
  Idoxuridine
  Iodochlorhydroxyquin
  Iodoform
  Isoconazole
  Ketoconazole
  Miconazole
  Neomycin
  Nitrofurazone
  Nystatin
  Oxiconazole
  Parachlorometaxylenol
  Polymyxin B
  Poxidone
  Proflavin
  Quinoline mix
  Ribostamycin
  Rifamycin
  Silver sulfadiazine
  Tetrachlordecaoxide
  Ticonazole
  Tobramycin
  Tolnaftate
  Tromantadine
  Vioform
Topical anesthetics
  Amethocaine
  Benzocaine
  Dyclonine
  Lidocaine
  Procaine
  Propanocaine
  Tetracaine
Topical antihistamines
  Diphenhydramine
  Promethazine
Anti-inflammatory agents
  Benzydamine
  Bufexamac
  Etofenamate
  Ibuprofen
  Ibuproxam

Indomethacin
Ketoprofen
Methyl salicylate
Oxyphenbutazone
Dermatologics, other
  Anthralin
  Benzoin
  Benzoyl peroxide
  Capsacin
  Coal tar
  Colophony (wart remover)
  Corticosteroids
  Crotamiton
  Dinitrochlorobenzene
  Diphencyclopyrone
  Dithranol
  5-Fluorouracil
  Isopropyl alcohol
  Leech extract (Hirucreme)
  Mechlorethamine
  Minoxidil
  Palmitoyl collagenic acid
  Petrolatum
  Propolis
  Resorcinol
  Retinol palmitate (vitamin A)
  Salicylic acid
  Thioxolone
  Vitamin E
  Wood tars
Ophthalmic, otic preparations
  Acyclovir
  Aluminum acetate
  ϵ-Aminocaproic acid
  Atropine
  Benzalkonium chloride
  Chloramphenicol
  Chlorpheniramine
  Corticosteroids
  Metipranolol
  Neomycin
  Oleyl polypetide
  Phenylephrine
  Sisomycin
  Sodium cromoglycolate
  Tetracaine
  Timolol
  Tobramycin
  Tolazoline
  Trifluoridine
Transdermal devices
  Clonidine
  Estradiol
  Nicotine
  Nitroglycerin
  Scopolamine

PATCH TESTING TO DIAGNOSE CONTACT DERMATITIS TO MEDICATIONS

When an allergic contact dermatitis to a medication is suspected, the first "diagnostic" technique is to stop use of the medication. Patch testing can be helpful in clarifying the offending allergen. With regard to medications, it is reasonable to do screening closed patch tests with the medication as is, but caution must be used in interpretation, since some vehicles and medications may produce an irritant reaction under occlusion. A repeated open application or usage test, in which the patient applies the product twice daily to normal skin for several days to reproduce "use," can also be helpful. If either or both of these techniques indicate a probable allergic reaction to a medication, the next step is to obtain individual ingredients for patch testing to distinguish whether the medication or a vehicle or preservative ingredient is the cause. Suggested patch-test concentrations are indicated for some of the medications in Table 41-2. Practically speaking, both the physician and patient must be highly motivated to pursue this time-consuming detective work, as it usually involves communication and cooperation with the manufacturer of the medication as well as repeat visits for patch testing. Manufacturers are usually very helpful, but delivery of the individual ingredients in a medication or components of a transdermal patch takes time. An adverse-reaction report is requested by most companies. This course should be pursued if the medication is needed for ongoing therapy (such as eyedrops for glaucoma), is likely to be encountered again (e.g., an antifungal for recurrent dermatophyte infection), or a substitute medication is not readily available (e.g., topical minoxidil for alopecia). Generally, this extensive ingredient patch testing will clarify the problem. Occasionally, a patient will react to the medication preparation "as is" but not to individual ingredients. This is termed *compound allergy* and is well documented to occur with various topical medications.[34] It may be that the mixture of specific ingredients is necessary for adequate penetration or allergen recognition. (Compound allergy may also be caused by an additive effect of subclinical reactions to two or more ingredients.)

Patch test concentrations can be important, as well as the time of reading. For example, neomycin and bacitracin will give false negatives unless tested in 20% concentration. Furthermore, delayed readings as late as 7 days may be necessary. The concentrations of many antigens are included in Appendix A. A more complete list can be found in de Groot's book.

SYSTEMIC MEDICATIONS AND CONTACT DERMATITIS

There are several clinical settings in which there may be a relationship between contact dermatitis and systemic medications. The first is *direct skin contact* with a systemic medication (pill, intravenous fluid, etc.), as may be seen in a health care worker or pharmacist handling a medication. A careful listing of exposures is necessary to try to clarify the offending agent where multiple medications are being dealt with. Antibiotics (especially penicillin derivatives) and phenothiazines top the list of systemic drugs causing this type of contact dermatitis.[32,33] Table 41-4 lists some of the systemic medications that have been associated with allergic contact dermatitis.

The second type is called *systemic contact dermatitis*.[35] This refers to an eczematous

TABLE 41–4. Some Systemic Medications That Have Been Associated with Allergic Contact Dermatitis

Medications	Suggested Patch-Test Concentration, percent[a]
Aminophylline	Ampoule content
Ampicillin	20
Carbenicillin	20
Cephalexin	1, olive oil
Cephalosporins	20
Chloramphenicol	5
Chloroquine	1
Chlorpheniramine	2
Chlorpromazine	2
Clonidine	9
Cloxacillin	20, or ampoule content
Colistin	1,000,000 Iu/g Aq
Cyanocobelamine (B$_{12}$)	0.5% (Ampoule content)
Cytosine arabinoside	0.1–1
Dimethylsulfoxide (DMSO)	10
Disulfiram	2
Doxycycline	10
Ethambutol	1
Famotidine	
Gentamicin	20
Heparin	Ampoule contents, prick test
Isoniazid	0.05–1
Kanamycin	1
Levopromazine	
Methotrexate	
Mitomycin C	0.01–0.1
Nitroglycerin	0.2 mg/mL Aq
Oxolamine	
Oxytetracycline	10
Penicillin	10,000 Iu/g
Perphenazine	2
Phytomenadione (vitamin K)	10
Piperazine	1, Aq
Piroxicam	10
Procaine	2, Aq
Promazine	2
Pseudoephedrine	0.1–3
Pyribenzamine	2
Quinidine	Saturated, Aq
Quinine sulfate	1
Ranitidine	5
Rifampicin	0.5–10
Scopolamine	1
Spironolactone	1, ethanol
Streptomycin	10, Aq
Sulfathiazole	5
Tetracaine	Ampoule content
Tetracycline	10

[a]Percent in petrolatum unless otherwise indicated.
Iu = international units.

or marginated pattern of an eruption in a patient who has received a systemically administered medication. There are two types: one is a distinctive bright-red eruption often limited to the buttocks and flexural areas and is nicknamed the "baboon syndrome."[35] Examples of medications that may cause this are pseudoephedrine and cough syrup (flavoring).[36] Local instillation of medication (such as mitomycin C) into the bladder has caused a similar reaction.[37] A second type of systemic contact dermatitis is an eczematous pattern occurring at sites of previous skin reaction to a substance that is chemically related to the medication being given systemically. Examples are an eruption in a thiuram-sensitive patient who is given disulfiram (Antabuse) for alcohol abuse or in an ethylenediamine-sensitive patient given parenteral aminophylline.[38] A less common example is thimerosal sensitivity, which may render a patient more susceptible to oral piroxican (Feldene).[39]

A third setting in which a medication given for systemic effect may cause a local skin reaction is the transdermal delivery system. This has been reviewed in recent literature.[15,40] Transdermal clonidine has a fairly high reaction rate, but most other transdermal systems have been well tolerated. It appears that some patients who have cutaneous reactions to transdermal medications (e.g., nitroglycerin, scopolamine) can subsequently tolerate systemic administration of the same medication.[40] Subcutaneous injections of medications such as heparin or vitamin K have rarely been associated with localized eczematous reactions.[42,43] Patch testing with the injectable medication and its components has proven helpful in clarifying these cases. Vaccines have received attention for occasionally causing localized eczematous eruptions or a more generalized "systemic" pattern.[44] The preservatives thimerosal (e.g., in hepatitis vaccine) or neomycin (in measles-mumps-rubella) have most often been the cause.[45] Preservatives in other injectable medications also sometimes cause local reactions.

Is patch testing useful to diagnose a generalized eruption to a systemic drug? This technique is controversial both in how to interpret results and in ethical considerations

---

TABLE 41–5. Patient Education—Medication Allergy

You are allergic to the medication called _____.
The purpose of this medication is to _____ (kill germs, reduce itching, etc.)
Other names for the medication are _____.

It maybe found in these types of products (circle)

- Skin creams, ointments, or sprays
- Throat lozenges, sore throat medicine
- Eardrops
- Eyedrops
- Medicated bandage
- Other

With this allergy, you may also react to the following things. Discuss the pros and cons of using these products with the doctor.
  (List cross-reacting medications, etc.)

You should avoid using this medicine!

- *Read labels* of any similar product.
- Let your doctor and pharmacist know.
- Be suspicious of any similar product that causes a skin reaction.

and has been associated with exacerbations of generalized erythrodermic reactions.[46-48] Patch testing for systemic drug reactions has been done in Europe, particularly with anticonvulsants, but is not standardized or routinely done in the United States.

PATIENT EDUCATION

If a patient is diagnosed as having a contact dermatitis to a topical medication, educational efforts are important for the patient, and the offending agent should be listed with medication allergies. General suggestions for patient education are outlined in Table 41-5. Discontinuance of the topical therapy and treatment of the contact dermatitis are indicated, and this should often be done before substitution of another (possibly allergic) topical medication. In some settings, particularly otitis externa or leg ulcers, *no* topical therapy may improve the clinical appearance! Attention should be paid to possible cross-reactions within a medication class, and substitutions should be made accordingly. Patients should be made aware of potential reactions to future systemic administration of the offending medication if this applies.

REFERENCES

1. Wilson CL, Cameron J, Powell SM, et al: High incidence of contact dermatitis in leg ulcer patients: Implication for management. *Clin Exp Dermatol* 16:250–253, 1991.
2. Lembo G, Nappa P, Balato N, et al: Contact sensitivity in otitis externa. *Contact Dermatitis* 19:64–65, 1988.
3. Beauregard S, Gilchrest BA: A survey of skin problems and skin care regimens in the elderly. *Arch Dermatol* 123:1638–1643, 1987.
4. Remitz A, Lauerma AI, Stubb S, et al: Darier's disease, familial benign chronic pemphigus and contact hypersensitivity. *J Am Acad Dermatol* 22:134, 1990.
5. Rystedt I: Atopy, hand eczema and contact dermatitis: Summary of recent large scale studies. *Semin Dermatol* 5:290–300, 1986.
6. Haustein UF, Tegetmeyer L, Ziegler V: Allergic and irritant potential of benzoyl peroxide. *Contact Dermatitis* 13:252–257, 1987.
7. Tosti A, Bardazzi F, Ghetti P: Unusual complication of sensitizing therapy for alopecia areata. *Contact Dermatitis* 18:322, 1988.
8. Wilson C, Walkden V, Powell S, Shaw S, et al: Contact dermatitis in reaction to 2% topical minoxidil solution. *J Am Acad Dermatol* 24:661–662, 1991.
9. Heidenhiem M, Jemec GBE: Concomitant psoriasis and allergic contact dermatitis: Coexistent interrelated clinical entities. *Am J Contact Dermatitis* 2:175–180, 1991.
10. Cameli N, Vassilopoulou A, Vincenzi C: Contact allergy to colophony in a wart remover. *Contact Dermatitis* 24:315, 1991.
11. Mansell PWA, Liturin MS, Ichinose H, Krementz ET: Delayed hypersensitivity to 5-fluorouracil following topical chemotherapy of cutaneous cancers. *Cancer Res* 35:1288, 1975.
12. Rudzki E, Koslowska A: Sensitivity to salicylic acid. *Contact Dermatitis* 2:178, 1976.
13. Caro I: Connubial contact dermatitis to benzoyl peroxide. *Contact Dermatitis* 2:362, 1976.
14. Fowler JF: Allergic contact dermatitis to quinidine. *Contact Dermatitis* 13:280–281, 1985.
15. Holdiness MR: A review of contact dermatitis associated with transdermal therapeutic systems. *Contact Dermatitis* 20:3–9, 1989.
16. Rudzki E, Rebandel P, Gryzwa Z: Contact allergy in the pharmaceutical industry. *Contact Dermatitis* 21:121–124, 1989.
17. Rudzki E, Rebandel P, Gryzwa Z: Patch tests with occupational contactants in nurses, doctors, and dentists. *Contact Dermatitis* 20:247–250, 1989.

18. Marren P, Wojnarowska F, Powell S: Allergic contact dermatitis and vulvar dermatoses. *Br J Dermatol* 126:52–56, 1992.
19. Fisher AA: Reactions to topical antibiotics, in Fisher AA (ed): *Contact Dermatitis,* 3d ed. Philadelphia, Lea & Febiger, 1986, pp 195–210.
20. Angelini G, Vena GA, Meneghini U: Contact allergy to antiviral agents. *Contact Dermatitis* 15:114–115, 1986.
21. Baes H: Contact sensitivity to miconazole and other imidazoles. *Contact Dermatitis* 24:89–93, 1991.
22. Goh CL: Contact sensitivity to topical antimicrobials. *Contact Dermatitis* 21:166–171, 1989.
23. Coskey RJ: Contact dermatitis caused by diphenhydramine hydrochloride. *J Am Acad Dermatol* 8:204–206, 1983.
24. Sherertz EF, Reed JW, Zanolli MD, Goldsmith SM: Severe allergic kerato conjunctivitis and erythema multiforme following a routine eye exam: Discerning the cause. *Ann Ophthalmol* 23:173–176, 1991.
25. O'Driscoll JB, Beck MB, Kesseler ME, Ford G: Contact sensitivity to aluminum acetate eardrops. *Contact Dermatitis* 24:156–157, 1991.
26. Valsecchi R, Cainelli T: Contact allergy to cerumenex. *Contact Dermatitis* 18:312, 1988.
27. Kubo K, Shirai K, Akaeda T, Oguchi M: Contact dermatitis from ibuprofen piconol. *Contact Dermatitis* 18:188–189, 1988.
28. Perret CM, Happle R: Contact allergy to befexamac. *Contact Dermatitis* 20:307–308, 1989.
29. Vasecchi R, Cainelli T: Contact dermatitis from ibuproxam, a case with cross-reactivity with ketoprofen. *Contact Dermatitis* 22:51, 1990.
30. Boj G, Srensson A: Contact allergy to garlic used for wound dressing. *Contact Dermatitis* 18:179–1810, 1988.
31. van Ulsen J, Stolz E, van Joost T: Chromate dermatitis from a homeopathic drug. *Contact Dermatitis* 18:56, 1988.
32. Johansson G: Contact urticaria from levomepromazine. *Contact Dermatitis* 19:304, 1988.
33. Rudzki E, Rebendel P: Occupational contact urticaria from penicillin. *Contact Dermatitis* 13:192, 1985.
34. Kellett JK, King CM, Beck MH: Compound allergy to medicaments. *Contact Dermatitis* 14:45–48, 1986.
35. Andersen KE, Hjorth N, Menne T: The baboon syndrome: Systemically induced allergic contact dermatitis. *Contact Dermatitis* 10:97–100, 1984.
36. Tomb RR, Lepoitterin JP, Espinassouze F, Heid E, Foussereau J: Systemic contact dermatitis from pseudoephedrine. *Contact Dermatitis* 24:86–88, 1991.
37. Arregui MA, Aguirre A, Gil N, Goday J, Raton JA: Dermatitis due to mitomycin C bladder instillations. *Contact Dermatitis* 24:368, 1991.
38. van Hecke E, Vermander F: Allergic contact dermatitis by oral disulfiram. *Contact Dermatitis* 10:254, 1984.
39. Serrano G, Bonillo J, Aliaga A, Cuadra J, et al: Piroxicam-induced photosensitivity and contact sensitivity to thiosalicylic acid. *J Am Acad Dermatol* 23:479–483,
40. Hogan DJ, Maibach HI: Transdermal drug delivery systems: Adverse reactions—dermatologic overview, in Menne T, Maibach HI (eds): *Exopenous Dermatoses: Environmental Dermatitis.* Boca Raton, FL, CRC Press, 1991, pp 227–234.
42. Sanders MN, Winkelmann RK: Cutaneous reactions to vitamin K. *J Am Acad Dermatol* 19:699–704, 1988.
43. Klein GF, Kofler H, Wolf H, Fritsch PO: Eczema-like, erythematous, infiltrative plaques: A common side effect of subcutaneous heparin therapy. *J Am Acad Dermatol* 21:703–707, 1989.
44. Cox NH, Moss C, Forsyth A: Allergy to non-toxoid constituents of vaccines and implications for patch testing. *Contact Dermatitis* 18:143–146, 1988.
45. Cox NH, Forsyth A: Thimerosal allergy and vaccination reactions. *Contact Dermatitis* 18:229–233, 1988.
46. Romaguera C, Grimalt F, Vilaplana J, Azon A: Erythroderma from carbamazepine. *Contact Dermatitis* 20:304–305, 1989.
47. Vaillant L, Camenen I, Lorette G: Patch testing with carbamazepine: Reinduction of an exfoliative dermatitis. *Arch Dermatol* 125:299, 1989.
48. DeGroot AC, Conemans J: Allergic urticarial rash from oral codeine. *Contact Dermatitis* 14:209–214, 1986.

42

ALLERGY TO TOPICAL CORTICOSTEROIDS

Antti I. Lauerma
Sakari Reitamo
Lars Förström

CORTICOSTEROIDS

Topical (gluco)corticosteroids are the most widely used medicaments in dermatologic practice. They are used in various formulations: ointments, creams, gels, and liquids. The efficacy and the degree of side effects of a topical corticosteroid depend on its bioavailability—that is, its vehicle and the potency of the corticosteroid molecule itself. The potency of corticosteroids varies greatly depending on modulations in their chemical structure.[1]

INDICATIONS

Indications for topical corticosteroid therapy include most dermatoses with inflammatory and/or hyperproliferative features. These include psoriasis, atopic dermatitis, nummular eczema, lichen planus, urticaria, sarcoidosis, discoid lupus erythematosus, lichen sclerosus et atrophicus, pruritus, and sunburn, to name just a few. One of the main indications of topical corticosteroid therapy is contact dermatitis, allergic or irritant.[1] Because mild corticosteroids such as hydrocortisone are available over the counter in most countries, it is likely that they are used in most adverse skin conditions.

ADVERSE EFFECTS

The action of topical or systemic corticosteroids at the subcellular level is not fully understood. However, it seems that it is mediated through an intracellular glucocorticoid receptor, which also mediates its side effects. This fact explains the finding that enhancement of the potency and therapeutic effects of topical corticosteroids results also in increased adverse effects. Topical corticosteroids tend also to lose their efficacy during use and more potent corticosteroids are needed for the same effect. When therapy is discontinued, a rebound syndrome with erythema may be seen. Such erythema is a rebound from the natural vasoconstrictive effects of the corticosteroid.[1] While almost all side effects of topical corticosteroids are mediated through the glucocorticoid receptor, hypersensitivity to corticosteroids probably is not. Hypersensitivity reactions to corticosteroids have been seen after both topical and systemic use.[2]

CLINICAL FEATURES

CLINICAL PICTURE

The clinical picture of contact allergy to topical corticosteroids can range from acute eczematous reactions to inefficacy of the topical corticosteroid product. An eczematous eruption which does not heal as expected seems to be the most common type of clinical picture. Lesions looking like typical contact dermatitis are also often seen. Photocontact dermatitis has also been reported. Sometimes organs other than skin may be exposed to allergenic corticosteroids, which could result, for example, in conjunctivitis or nasal eczema.

It seems likely that, in topical corticosteroid allergy, the pharmacologic action of corticosteroid simultaneously suppresses the allergic reaction, which can result in clinical features that may be difficult to diagnose. Therefore, topical corticosteroid allergy is to be suspected if the skin condition deteriorates despite therapy or if the corticosteroid preparation shows unexplained inefficacy in a particular patient.[2,3]

PATIENTS WITH INCREASED RISK OF CORTICOSTEROID ALLERGY

Corticosteroid contact allergy is often seen in patients who use corticosteroids intensively. These include contact dermatitis and leg ulcer or stasis dermatitis patients, who are also likely to develop other contact allergies to topical medications. Presence of other contact allergies is also a risk factor for corticosteroid contact allergy.[4]

It is advisable to suspect corticosteroid (triamcinolone acetonide) allergy in patients who have previously used Mycolog Cream or its generic equivalents. Also, many steroid-sensitive patients seem to have ethylenediamine contact allergy.[5]

CROSS-REACTION PATTERNS IN CORTICOSTEROID CONTACT ALLERGY

As there are many corticosteroids available for use in the market, it is not possible to patch test to all of them.[5] Therefore it would be useful to know the cross-reaction patterns between corticosteroids causing contact allergy. An attempt has been made to classify different corticosteroids in cross-reactive groups. In this classification, 85 percent of the allergic cross-reactions published so far fall inside four structural corticosteroid "classes" rather than outside them.[6] The differences between these classes were based on structures in the D ring of the steroid molecule. The classes were as follows:

1. *Hydrocortisone type:* Cloprednol, cortisone, cortisone-21-acetate, hydrocortisone, hydrocortisone-21-acetate, fludrocortisone, methylprednisolone, methylpredniso-lone-21-acetate, prednisolone, prednisolone-21-acetate, prednisone, and tixocortol pivalate
2. *Triamcinolone acetonide type:* Amcinonide, budesonide, desonide, fluocinolone acetonide, flucinonide, halcinonide, triamcinolone acetonide, and triamcinolone al-cohol
3. *Betamethasone type:* Betamethasone, betamethasone-21-disodium phosphate, dexa-methasone, dexamethasone-21-disodium phosphate, and fluocortolone
4. *Hydrocortisone-17-butyrate type:* Alclometasone dipropionate, betamethasone-17-valerate, clobetasol-17-propionate, clobetasone-17-butyrate, fluocortolone-21-hexa-noate, fluocortolone-21-pivalate, hydrocortisone-17-butyrate, hydrocortisone-17-valerate

Although this classification has evidential support, reactions between these classes are also frequent. Furthermore, in hydrocortisone allergy, the antigenic structure which is important seems to be in rings A to C and not in the D ring. It may be that local metabolism of corticosteroids affects contact allergy reactions, therefore making conclu-sions from structure unreliable. However, it has been shown that most patients with hydrocortisone contact allergy react to tixocortol pivalate. Also, we have seen that such patients often had allergy to hydrocortisone-17-butyrate.[4,7] In a recent study, hydrocortisone-17-butyrate-allergic patients often reacted to budesonide.[8] At present it is not advisable to conclude that one corticosteroid is not causing contact allergy because a related corticosteroid is not. Rather, a negative patch-test reaction to individual corticosteroids should be seen to make such conclusions.

SYSTEMIC CORTICOSTEROIDS

REACTIONS TO SYSTEMIC CORTICOSTEROIDS IN CONTACT ALLERGY TO CORTICOSTEROIDS

Corticosteroids are also widely used as oral preparations. If a corticosteroid causing contact allergy is administered orally, flareup reactions of earlier contact dermatitis to corticosteroids may occur[9] (Fig. 42-1) or, alternatively, a widespread exanthematous drug reaction may be seen.[2]

ANAPHYLACTOID REACTIONS TO SYSTEMIC CORTICOSTEROIDS

Systemic corticosteroid administration may cause immediate anaphylactoid-type reac-tions, with symptoms ranging from urticaria to laryngospasm. Immediate allergy to systemic corticosteroids seems to be rare, due to the low number of reported patients.[2] At present, immediate reactions have not been associated with contact allergy to topical corticosteroids when the same corticosteroids were given orally. It does not seem very likely, therefore, that contact allergy would cause such potentially fatal reactions. However, there is no experience of intravenous administration of corticosteroids causing

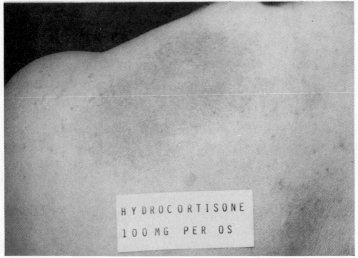

FIG. 42–1. A flare-up reaction to 100-mg oral hydrocortisone on the skin of a shoulder of a patient with hydrocortisone contact allergy.

contact allergy, and great care should be taken when intravenous corticosteroids are given to a patient with contact allergy to corticosteroids.

USE OF SYSTEMIC CORTICOSTEROIDS IN CORTICOSTEROID CONTACT ALLERGY

In patients with corticosteroid contact allergy, only steroids with negative patch-test results should be used. If there is uncertainty about possible corticosteroid allergy and an oral therapy is needed, it is preferable to start with low oral dose and increase it over a few days to the desired level so as to avoid intense skin reactions.

ENDOGENOUS STEROID HORMONES AND CORTICOSTEROID ALLERGY

Because hydrocortisone is also a hormone produced by the human adrenal cortex, it is possible that stimulation of its production may cause allergic skin reactions, as was seen in our study. When four patients with hydrocortisone contact allergy were challenged with 100 to 250 mg hydrocortisone orally, all of them had erythematous flareup reactions on sites where hydrocortisone had earlier caused contact allergy reactions. When one patient was further challenged with an ACTH stimulation test, which causes maximal secretion of the body's own hydrocortisone (cortisol) from the adrenal cortex, similar reactions were seen, showing that endogenous steroids may cause allergic reactions.[9] Interestingly, allergies to other nonglucocorticoid steroid hormones, such as progesterone and testosterone, have been demonstrated in hydrocortisone-allergic patients.[10] The clinical significance of these findings is at present not known and may be negligible.

FREQUENCY

FREQUENCY OF ALLERGY TO TOPICAL CORTICOSTEROIDS

There has been a great increase in the number of reported patients with topical corticosteroid allergy.[3] This may be because dermatologists are now more aware of it. Contact allergy reactions have been reported to more than 50 corticosteroids so far.[2] Reports on corticosteroid contact allergy have mostly been case reports. However, there are a few screening studies which provide evidence on the prevalence of contact allergy to corticosteroids. These studies have been performed as part of standard patch-test series and therefore reflect the occurrence of corticosteroid contact allergy in patients with suspected contact allergy.

HYDROCORTISONE ALCOHOL

In Belgium 17/1150 (1.5 percent)[8] and in Finland 2/521 (0.4 percent) patients[11] had allergic reactions to hydrocortisone alcohol (Fig. 42-2). In Denmark 6/1835 (0.3 percent) patients had allergic patch reactions to a mixture of hydrocortisone alcohol and hydrocortisone acetate.[12] Because hydrocortisone as a hydrophilic compound penetrates the skin poorly, patch testing with it is very difficult. A recent study showed that almost all patients with allergic patch-test reactions to tixocortol pivalate reacted to intradermal injections of hydrocortisone sodium succinate.[13] Later studies have shown that such reactions were due to contact allergy to hydrocortisone structure itself.[14] Because allergic patch reactions to tixocortol pivalate have been very common, hydrocortisone contact allergy is also frequent.

Tixocortol Pivalate

In a multicenter study of 4319 patients in Europe, 0.2 to 3.4 percent reacted to tixocortol pivalate.[15] In later studies, frequencies of 4.8 (24/497), 3.9 (28/727), and 1.1 percent (22/2073) were seen in England,[13] Finland,[11] and Belgium,[8] respectively. Tixocortol

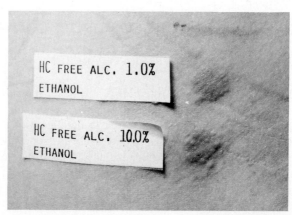

FIG. 42–2. Allergic patch-test reactions to 1% and 10% hydrocortisone in ethanol.

pivalate is marketed as a nasal, eye, ear, or rectal preparation. It is not in use as a dermatologic preparation (such as an ointment) and is not marketed in most countries. It has caused the most positive test reactions in most studies published. Allergic patch-test reactions to tixocortol pivalate are predictive of hydrocortisone contact allergy.[13]

Hydrocortisone-17-Butyrate

Hydrocortisone-17-butyrate caused allergic reactions in 48/8362 patients (0.6 percent).[2,4,7,11,16] Our recent study showed that the prevalence of hydrocortisone-17-butyrate contact allergy increased in patients with suspected contact allergy; it was 0.3 percent in 1985 and 1.4 percent in 1990.[16] This increase may be related to an increase of corticosteroid and/or hydrocortisone-17-butyrate consumption in our patient population.[16] In another study from Belgium, a frequency of 1.0 percent (20/2027) was reported.[8]

Other Corticosteroids

A study from Belgium reported the following frequencies of contact allergy to corticosteroids: amcinonide, 0.5 percent (10/1910); fluocortinbutyl ester, 0.4 percent (8/1960); clobetasol propionate, 0.2 percent (4/1960); triamcinolone acetonide, 0.3 percent (6/1747); budesonide, 3.0 percent (21/710). The last of these had the highest frequency among the eight corticosteroids studied, which also included hydrocortisone alcohol, tixocortol pivalate, and hydrocortisone-17-butyrate.[8]

CLINICAL SIGNIFICANCE OF CORTICOSTEROID CONTACT ALLERGY

The frequency of corticosteroid contact allergy is quite remarkable in view of two recent studies. Corticosteroids were the sixth most common contact allergens in Helsinki, Finland (after nickel sulfate, neomycin sulfate, bacitracin, fragrances, and cobalt chloride),[2] and the seventh most common in Leuven, Belgium,[8] among standard patch-test series patients. Therefore, contact allergy to topical corticosteroids is a common problem.

TESTING FOR CORTICOSTEROID CONTACT ALLERGY

PATCH TESTING WITH PURE PREPARATIONS

Patch testing with corticosteroids (Table 42-1) should be done with pure compounds obtained in powder form and dissolved in petrolatum and/or ethanol. It seems that patch testing with the ethanol vehicle is more sensitive than with the petrolatum vehicle (Fig. 42-3). However, ethanol may cause irritation; therefore an appropriate ethanol vehicle control must always be included. This irritation usually lasts for only about 2 days and vanishes thereafter while an allergic reaction to a corticosteroid is usually at its most intense up to the fourth day after testing. It may also be that corticosteroids

TABLE 42–1. Patch Testing with Corticosteroids

Preparation:	Pure corticosteroid dissolved at therapeutic[a] or 10-fold concentration[b] in ethanol or petrolatum or commercial ointment preparation.
Application:	Small Finn chamber on Scanpor tape is applied on intact skin of the back for 48 h. Filter paper is used with ethanol preparations.
Interpretation:	At 48 h and 72 to 96 h, reaction with erythema and edema or more is considered positive. Erythema at 72 to 96 h is considered suggestive of hypersensitivity, especially if clinical history suggests allergy.
Controls:	Vehicles. Ethanol irritation should begin to vanish after 48 h. Petrolatum should not produce any reactions. Ingredients of commercial vehicles should be tested after a positive reaction with commercial corticosteroid preparation if possible.

[a]Concentration in a commercial corticosteroid preparation.
[b]Hydrocortisone alcohol should be tested at 2.5% when in ethanol.

degrade in storage with ethanol. However, in our experience, storage of corticosteroids in ethanol for a limited time does not alter patch reactions.

The concentrations used in patch testing with corticosteroids vary. We have used both the same concentrations used in topical products and ten-fold higher concentrations.[4] Concentrations up to the saturation point in alcoholic solutions have been suggested; with hydrocortisone alcohol, such a concentration is 2.5%.[3] As corticosteroids also

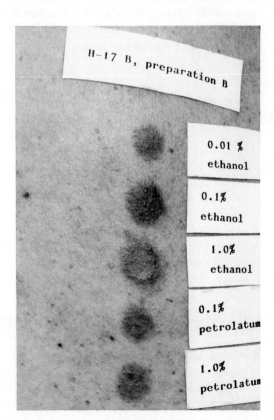

FIG. 42–3. Allergic patch-test reactions to hydrocortisone-17-butyrate in different vehicles. Please note that only 1/10 concentration of hydrocortisone-17-butyrate was needed in an ethanol vehicle when compared to a petrolatum vehicle for similar reactions.

"mask" the patch-test reaction due to their pharmacologic action, a higher concentration might not produce positive test reaction, while the lower concentration might. Also, mild patch reactions (erythema, slight edema) should not be ignored because of these difficulties in testing. A usage test or a trial of efficacy with the respective steroid could follow mild patch reactions to gauge the clinical significance of such reactions.

In patch testing with corticosteroids, late readings (up to the seventh day) have been recommended, because late reactions sometimes occur. Whether these are due to modification of the allergic reaction because of the corticosteroid's anti-inflammatory action or due to active sensitization is not clear. In our experience, such late reactions represent a small minority of all reactions.

PATCH TESTING WITH COMMERCIAL PREPARATIONS

When corticosteriods are not available in pure powder form, the only possibility is to use commercial preparations. In interpreting such reactions, one must, of course, bear in mind that any of the ingredients of a topical corticosteroid preparation, such as lanolin, may cause an allergic patch-test reaction. Commercial preparations, however, are usually designed with improved skin penetration of the corticosteroid in mind; therefore they may be better patch-test materials than petrolatum-based corticosteroid preparations.[3] This applies at least to hydrocortisone-17-butyrate.[17] Finally, as patients in practice are exposed to corticosteroids in commercial preparations, such preparations should always be included in testing, along with the pure compounds.

ROUTINE PATCH TESTING WITH SCREENING MARKERS IN STANDARD SERIES

Recent studies show that the diagnosis of corticosteroid contact allergy is remarkably improved if corticosteroids are included in the standard patch-test series. Because of apparent limitations in testing, only one or two corticosteroids may usually be included in standard series at a time. When available, tixocortol pivalate (as Pivalone nasal spray; Jouveinail Laboratoires, Fresnes, France) is recommended as the test substance. It mainly detects hydrocortisone contact allergy, but other corticosteroid sensitivities may also be found.[10,18] Other corticosteroids which are promising as screening markers are hydrocortisone-17-butyrate[4,7] and budesonide.[8]

TESTING WITH A CORTICOSTEROID PATCH-TEST SERIES

A separate patch-test series for corticosteroids is highly recommended for further testing in patients with suspected corticosteroid sensitivity. Its constitution may vary, but it is recommended that it include those corticosteroids that are commercially most often used in the particular area. Furthermore, the series must, when applicable, contain as controls the constituents of the vehicles of corticosteroids used in testing. Both pure

TABLE 42–2. Intradermal Testing with Corticosteroids

Preparation:	0.1 mL of parenteral 10 mg/mL corticosteroid preparation. If parenteral preparation is not available, 1 mg of corticosteroid is dissolved in 0.1 mL 0.9% NaCl.[19]
Application:	With tuberculin needle to the dermis.
Interpretation:	48 h after injection. Erythema and induration with a diameter of at least 5 mm is considered positive in the absence of a reaction from the vehicle.
Controls:	Vehicle.
Caution:	The patient should not leave facility for 30 min after intradermal testing because of a minor possibility of immediate reactions. A prick test with the same preparation(s) may precede intradermal test(s) for 30 min if there is a higher index of suspicion of such reactions.

compounds, preferably in ethanol, and commercial preparations should be used in such series.

INTRADERMAL TESTING

Because of poor penetration of the compound, contact allergy to hydrocortisone is difficult to diagnose with a patch test. Therefore intradermal testing with hydrocortisone sodium phosphate has been used with successful results.[12] This approach (Table 42-2) is easy to use in practice because many such preparations are readily available. It may be that other corticosteroids also are more easily detected as allergens if intradermal tests are used.[19,20] To avoid any severe anaphylactoid reactions, a prick test with the same preparation should precede the intradermal test, as risk for such reactions is much smaller with prick than with an intradermal test. Intradermal test with vehicle control is very important to avoid false-positive interpretations due to irritation.

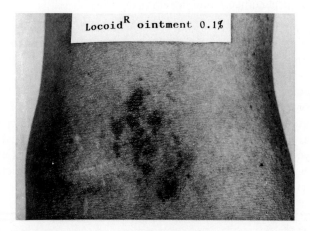

FIG. 42–4. A positive use test reaction on the skin of crook bend of arm due to Locoid (hydrocortisone-17-butyrate) ointment application.

USE TESTING

Use tests or repeated application tests are performed on a marked area on intact skin on the forearm or upper back where the corticosteroid preparation can conveniently be applied by the patient. The application should be done two to three times daily for up to a week. An erythema on the site of testing suggests corticosteroid contact allergy (Fig. 42-4). This test method does not seem to be as sensitive as patch testing.[4,7]

CONCLUSIONS

Contact allergy to corticosteroids is not rare. When a patient does not respond to corticosteroid therapy or should the skin condition deteriorate with treatment, it is

PATIENT INFORMATION SHEET

CONTACT ALLERGY TO TOPICAL CORTICOSTEROIDS

Topical corticosteroids are "cortisone"-related medicaments which are used to treat inflammation and thickening in the skin. They are present in many ointments, creams, lotions, gels, and liquids used for treating the skin. There are many different topical corticosteroids available in the market.

Contact allergy is a condition where a person, through direct skin contact with a substance, has become allergic to it. When the same person is in direct skin contact with the same substance again, an allergic reaction results. This reaction in contact allergy starts after a waiting period of 1 to 2 days and continues for at least 4 days, but it may persist for a longer time depending on further contact with the compound causing the contact allergy.

Contact allergy to topical corticosteroids may cause a rash where topical corticosteroids have been used, or one may see only aggravation or failure to respond to topical corticosteroid therapy.

You have been found to have contact allergy to one or many topical corticosteroids. Your physician will give you the names of the corticosteroids to which you are allergic. You must avoid using them because of your allergy. When you are being treated for your skin diseases or when you purchase topical ointments, creams, lotions, gels, or liquids for your skin, you must ask if they contain corticosteroids or "cortisone." If so, you must check the contents of the preparation. If a corticosteroid you are allergic to is present in the contents of the preparation, you must not use it. Your physician will name the topical corticosteroids that you may use. If you are treated with topical preparations in the future or are given any other medications, you must always tell your physician that you have contact allergy to corticosteroids.

This information is provided to help persons with contact dermatitis in the understanding of their problem. The contents are subject to change as more information becomes available and are not intended as a substitute for medical treatment.

advisable to suspect corticosteroid contact allergy. In that case, corticosteroid therapy should be discontinued and other therapy relieving symptoms of inflammation should be sought—for example, wet dressings and oral antihistamines, if possible.[3] Patch and possibly intradermal testing should be done when the skin condition in the test areas, back, and forearm, allows it. One can also select usable corticosteroids through testing. However, as several problems may be associated with testing, the patient's clinical response to a particular corticosteroid preparation should also be taken into account in choosing the preparation.

REFERENCES

1. Vickers CFH: Topical corticosteroids, in Fitzpatrick TB, Eisen AZ, Wolff K, et al (eds): *Dermatology In General Medicine.* New York, McGraw-Hill, 1987, pp 2540–2545.
2. Lauerma AI: Contact hypersensitivity to glucocorticosteroids. *Am J Contact Dermatitis* 3:1–17, 1992.
3. Dooms-Goossens A: Contact dermatitis to topical corticosteroids: Diagnostic problems, in Menne T, Maibach HI (eds): *Exogenous Dermatoses: Environmental Dermatitis,* Boca Raton, FL, CRC Press, 1991, pp 299–310.
4. Reitamo S, Lauerma AI, Stubb S, et al: Delayed hypersensitivity to topical corticoseroids. *J Am Acad Dermatol* 14:582, 1986.
5. Guin JD: Contact sensitivity to topical corticosteroids. *J Am Acad Dermatol* 10:773, 1986.
6. Coopman S, Degreef H, Dooms-Goossens A: Identification of cross-reaction patterns in allergic contact dermatitis from topical corticosteroids. *Br J Dermatol* 121:27, 1989.
7. Reitamo S, Lauerma AI, Förström L: Detection of contact hypersensitivity to topical corticosteroids with hydrocortisone-17-butyrate. *Contact Dermatitis* 21:159, 1989.
8. Dooms-Goossens A, Morren M: Results of routine patch testing with corticosteroid series in 2073 patients. *Contact Dermatitis* 26:182, 1992.
9. Lauerma AI, Reitamo S, Maibach HI: Systemic hydrocortisone/cortisol induces allergic skin reactions in presensitized subjects. *J Am Acad Dermatol* 24:182, 1991.
10. Schoenmakers A, Vermorken A, Degreef H, et al: Corticosteroid or steroid allergy? *Contact Dermatitis* 26:159, 1992.
11. Lauerma AI: Screening for corticosteroid contact hypersensitivity: Comparison of tixocortol pivalate, hydrocortisone-17-butyrate and hydrocortisone. *Contact Dermatitis* 24:123, 1991.
12. Alani MD, Alani SD: Allergic contact dermatitis to corticosteroids. *Ann Allerg* 30:181, 1972.
13. Wilkinson SM, Cartwright PH, English JSC: Hydrocortisone: An important cutaneous allergen. *Lancet* 337:761, 1991.
14. Wilkinson SM, English JSC: Hydrocortisone sensitivity: An investigation into the nature of the allergen. *Contact Dermatitis* 25:178, 1991.
15. Dooms-Goossens A, Andersen KE, Burrows D, et al: A survey of the results of patch tests with tixocortol pivalate. *Contact Dermatitis* 20:158, 1989.
16. Lauerma AI, Förström L, Reitamo S: Incidence of allergic reactions to hydrocortisone-17-butyrate in standard patch test series. *Arch Dermatol* 128:275, 1992.
17. Reitamo S, Lauerma AI, Förström L: Optimal testing for contact allergy to topical corticosteroids, in Frosch P, Dooms-Goossens A, Lachapelle J, et al (eds): *Current Topics in Contact Dermatitis.* Berlin, Springer-Verlag, 1989, pp 244–247.
18. Dooms-Goossens AE, Degreef HJ, Marien KJC, Coopman SA: Contact allergy to corticosteroids: A frequently missed diagnosis? *J Am Acad Dermatol* 21:538, 1989.
19. Wilkinson SM, English JSC: Patch tests are poor detectors of corticosteroid allergy. *Contact Dermatitis* 26:67–68, 1992.
20. Wilkinson SM, Heagerty AHM, English JSC: A prospective study into the value of patch and intradermal tests in identifying topical corticosteroid allergy. *Br J Dermatol* 127:22–25, 1992.

43

OCCUPATIONAL CONTACT DERMATITIS

Robert M. Adams

Nearly 24 percent of all reported cases of occupational disease are diseases of the skin,[1] and contact dermatitis accounts for nearly 95 percent of these. Two-thirds of the cases arise from manufacturing jobs, but the greatest frequency in relation to numbers of employees occurs in agriculture. Since 1974, the incidence of occupational skin disease has been gradually decreasing in the United States, but many cases are never reported, either because they are unrecognized as work-related by physicians and patients or they are deliberately treated as non-work-related dermatoses. These underreported cases have been estimated to represent more than 20 to 50 times the number that are reported.[2] The annual cost of occupational skin disease in this country has been estimated to be between $222 million and $1 billion per year when lost worker productivity, medical and legal costs, and disability payments are considered.[2] Most, if not all, of this morbidity is preventable, as ideally all occupational skin disease can and should be prevented.[3]

It is convenient to classify occupational contact dermatitis into (1) irritation and (2) allergic groups. Photodermatitis and contact urticaria, both irritant and allergic, are also included.

IRRITANT CONTACT DERMATITIS

Highly irritating chemicals, which will cause a reaction on any individual's skin if given sufficient duration of action and in a high enough concentration, are not considered in this chapter because they cause what are essentially chemical burns. The responsible chemicals include strong alkalis and acids, such as sodium and potassium hydroxides, and nitric and sulfuric acids.

Most instances of irritant dermatitis are less severe and develop slowly, after a relatively long period of exposure and from repeated contact. The substance causing such a reaction could be almost anything; the most common causative agents are soaps and detergents, solvents, mild acids and alkalis, metal salts, and so on. A variety of factors converge to induce this common type of dermatitis. Important are the pH of the chemical, its solubility and detergent action, and also its physical state—whether it is gaseous, liquid, or solid. Individual factors are very important, such as the area of skin affected; the presence of occlusion, sweat, pigmentation, dryness, and sebaceous activity; and concurrent or preexisting skin disease. Environmental factors in the work environment which influence the development of contact dermatitis include the ambient temperature of the workplace; the relative humidity; the presence of repeated friction, pressure, and occlusion (as from gloves, for example); and the existence of concomitant skin disease. The age, sex, race, and genetic background of the patient are also important.

An especially common environmental factor in initiating dermatitis is the existence of low relative humidity in the workplace, especially when it falls below 35 to 40, which is commonly the case in many offices and workplaces, especially during winter.[4] In such an environment, the stratum corneum becomes dry and brittle and small cracks appear, allowing irritants such as soaps, detergents, solvents, and so on to enter the deeper layers of skin. Pruritus is an early symptom, following by redness and scaling. If the irritation continues, the skin becomes thickened from scratching, and the condition enters a chronic phase, which may persist for a long time. Such skin is especially likely to develop allergic contact sensitization. Individuals with ichthyosis and/or an atopic background are likely to develop dermatitis if they work in such an environment.

If the irritant is airborne, the face, neck, anterior chest, and arms are commonly affected. Volatile substances such as solvents, dusts containing irritating substances, and resins which are heated during curing are especially likely to induce airborne irritation.

Special examples of irritants include *hydrofluoric acid,* which is highly irritating even in concentrations of 15 to 25%. However, immediately following contact there may be little or no pain. This appears only several hours later, when the acid has penetrated deep into the skin. An excruciating, throbbing, deep pain then develops. Because the acid has a special affinity for bone, it may cause serious damage and even loss of a digit.[5]

Rough, *irritating fabrics* in clothing are frequent causes of irritant dermatitis. For example, the heavy, thick, bulletproof vests commonly worn today by the police may induce a severe irritant dermatitis in individuals with an atopic background. Contact with *fibrous glass*[6] produces a characteristic and very pruritic contact dermatitis. Glass fibers larger than 3.5 μm in diameter are responsible; they enter the sweat glands and induce severe itching. The symptoms usually subside in a few weeks, and many workers can return to contact with the fibers without recurrence. Atopics, however, usually must change jobs.[6] Rough paper *face masks* frequently produce irritation, as does much *fire-retardant clothing,* especially in atopics.

Ethylene oxide is another special example of a highly irritating substance. The gas is widely used in hospitals to sterilize gowns, sheets, drapes, and instruments. If the sterilizer malfunctions and complete aeration of the contents fails to occur, contact with these sterilized articles (containing traces of ethylene oxide) can result in a severe bullous eruption.[7-9]

Chromic acid and hexavalent chromium salts have been recognized for nearly two centuries as notorious causes of chrome ulcers, perforation of the nasal septum, and an especially severe irritant dermatitis. *Copper dusts* produce folliculitis with a blue-black discoloration of the skin. Other causes of an irritant folliculitis include *arsenic trioxide, glass fibers, oils and greases, tar, asphalt, chlorinated naphthalenes, polyhalogenated biphenyls, and others.*[10]

Miliaria resulting from work in hot environments is especially likely to develop under occlusive clothing and may sometimes be confused with acute contact dermatitis. *Increased pigmentation* may result from an episode of irritant dermatitis, especially in persons with darker skin. Phototoxic agents—such as psoralens from plants, tar, asphalt, and others—are also common causes. Certain metal salts, such as those of mercury, arsenic, bismuth, and gold and also UV, infrared, microwave, and ionizing radiation readily induce increased pigmentation. *Hypopigmentation and depigmentation* of the skin result from contact with a large group of chemicals, especially those phenolic compounds related to hydroquinone. *Contact urticarial reactions* may result from contact with numerous chemicals.[11]

A large number of irritating plants exist, especially those with spines, thorns, or sharp-edged leaves and those containing needlelike crystals of calcium oxalate, as in certain cactuses. Other irritating chemicals present in plants are formic and acetic acids and various proteolytic enzymes. Those families causing the greatest irritation are chiefly *Euphorbiaceae* (in spurges, crotons, poinsettias), *Ranunculaceae* (buttercup) and *Cruciferae,* also called *Brassicaceae* (black mustard).[12]

Farm workers, nursery personnel, florists, and gardeners are at greatest risk for developing *phototoxic* eruptions from plants. The causative chemicals are furocoumarins, usually 5-methoxypsoralen (bergapten). The plant families responsible for most of the reactions are Umbelliferae (carrot, cow parsley, wild chervil, celery, parsnip, fennel, dill), Rutaceae (lime, lemon, bergamot, bitter orange, gas plant, burning bush), Moraceae (fig), Cruciferae (mustard), Ranunculaceae (buttercup), and Compositae (chrysanthemum and many others). The dermatitis is rapid in onset and characterized by redness and bullae at the sites of contact, and exposure to UVA in wavelengths of 300 to 340 nm. Hyperpigmentation follows soon after the eruption.[12]

Celery, especially, is the source of a bullous eruption in grocery clerks following contact with wet celery and exposure to either sunlight or radiation from the scanners at the checkout stands. Much of today's celery has been genetically altered so that it contains large amounts of psoralens, which possess natural insecticide properties. Grocery clerks and baggers today are frequently exposed.[13]

ALLERGIC CONTACT DERMATITIS

Although allergic contact dermatitis (ACD) in the working environment occurs less frequently than irritant dermatitis, the statistics are somewhat misleading, because many cases are not diagnosed, are never reported, or both. In the United States, it has recently become very difficult to obtain the necessary allergens for testing persons with occupational skin disease. This has caused many physicians to lose interest in investigating these cases—which, even with the proper equipment, is a difficult and time-consuming task. In countries where the allergens have been available for years, the reported incidence of ACD is much greater than in the United States.[14]

In the workplace, the development of allergic sensitization can have far-reaching consequences for affected workers. Many must change jobs and learn a new trade, a very difficult undertaking even for younger workers. Those workers who are perhaps 10 years from retirement and develop allergic sensitivity to an allergen of central importance to their jobs, as to epoxy resin in a boat builder, for example, are often unable to find another job and must retire with permanent disability. Sometimes an employer can make changes in the materials used in the job, but this is rarely possible, and only if the exact allergen is known and a suitable substitute can be found.

The mechanism of ACD is fully discussed elsewhere in this book and will not be presented here.

Allergic sensitization is more likely to develop in persons with preexisting irritant contact dermatitis. The frequency of concomitant rubber glove sensitivity is a vivid illustration of this. Atopic persons develop allergic contact sensitivity nearly as often as persons without an atopic family or personal history.[15-17] It appears, however, that when atopic dermatitis is active and widespread areas of skin are involved, there is less likelihood that ACD will develop.[18]

CONTACT URTICARIA

There are four types of contact urticaria: (1) nonallergic (primary urticariogenic); (2) allergic (immunologic); (3) combined allergic, nonallergic, and urticarial; and (4) combined allergic eczematous and urticarial.[19]

In the nonimmunologic type, exposed individuals develop a reaction without previous sensitization. Substances which may induce this type of contact urticaria are shown in Table 43-1. Workers commonly affected include gardeners, cooks, and other kitchen personnel, medical and dental workers, and so on.

Allergic contact urticaria is often reported by food handlers (Table 43-2). Raw potato and fish are common causes, as is meat, especially raw liver.[20] Antibiotics and other medications, epoxy resin hardeners,[21] and woods[22] are frequently found to be causative agents.

Of uncertain mechanism is the rare but very severe reaction to *ammonium persulfate,* used as a "booster" in bleaching hair to obtain a platinum blond effect. This dermatitis, occurring mostly in the clients of hairdressers, is sudden in onset and characterized by erythema, edema, severe itching, urticaria, and occasionally syncope, with wheezing and dyspnea. The reactions appear to be allergic, but the very rapid release of histamine and other vasoactive substances by the persulfate may be nonallergic.[23,24] Hairdressers should be alert to this reaction.

PATCH TESTING

The single most important, indispensable diagnostic tool for the diagnosis of allergic contact dermatitis is the patch test. Not only can it discover the exact cause of the dermatitis, but when all possible allergens have been tested and found negative, it can effectively rule out allergic contact dermatitis as the cause of the condition. In the past, testing was often performed with substances brought to the physician by the patient and tested "as is," without knowledge of their constituents or irritant potential. False-negative as well as false-positive reactions occur, and these are sometimes very severe, leading to misdiagnosis, with long-range serious consequences for the patient (or to severe burns). In recent years, with the availability of the Material Safety Data Sheets (see below) and the Freedom of Information Act, permitting the physician to learn the

TABLE 43–1. Agents That Can Produce Nonallergic Contact Urticaria

Acetic acid
Alcohol
Balsam of Peru
Benzoic acid
Caterpillar hair
Cinnamic acid
Cinnamic aldehyde
Cobalt chloride
Dimethyl sulfoxide
Insect stings
Moth hairs
Sodium benzoate
Sorbic acid
Trafuril (nicotinic acid ester)

Source: Fisher.[11] Reproduced with permission.

exact ingredients of substances previously labeled "trade secrets," knowledge of the allergens responsible for allergic contact dermatitis has become possible. More than 300 allergens for testing are now commercially available in Europe. When used intelligently, these tests can point to the cause of most cases of allergic contact dermatitis. If a suspected chemical is not available, it can often be obtained pure from the manufacturer and mixed in a nonirritating vehicle (usually white petrolatum) at a nonirritating concentration and tested on control subjects to rule out irritancy before testing patients.

When the cause is thought to be a substance causing contact urticaria, prick testing can be done, resulting in a wheal-and-flare reaction within 15 to 30 min if positive. This method is fraught with the possible hazard of an anaphylactic reaction, especially in atopics, and should be done with great care and with the prescribed treatment modalities available should a severe reaction ensue. It is preferable to test by rubbing the suspected material on the skin and covering it with paper tape for 30 min. A single latex finger cot on one finger can be used to screen for latex sensitivity.

TABLE 43–2. Foods That Have Been Reported to Produce Contact Urticaria

Apple	Flour
Bean	Lettuce
Beer	Meat (chicken, lamb, turkey,
Caraway seed	beef, liver, pork)
Carrot	Milk
Egg	Peach
Endive	Potato
Fish	Spices

Source: Fisher.[11] Reproduced by permission.

PANELS OF PATCH-TEST ALLERGENS

The following are several suggested panels of allergens for testing individuals in certain occupations[25]:

MACHINISTS

Balsam of Peru 25% petrolatum (some fragrances in cutting oils)
Benzotriazole 1% petrolatum
Bioban P 1487 1% petrolatum
Bronopol 0.25% petrolatum
Chloroacetamide 0.2% petrolatum
p-Chloro-m-xylenol 1% petrolatum
Chlorocresol 1% petrolatum
Cobalt chloride 1% petrolatum
Dichlorophene 0.5% petrolatum
Fluorescein sodium 1% petrolatum

Grotan BK 1% aqueous
Hydrazine sulfate 1% petrolatum
Kathon CG 0.01% petrolatum
o-Phenylphenol 1% petrolatum
Pine oil 1% olive oil
Phenylmercuric nitrate 0.05% petrolatum
Propylene glycol 10% aqueous
Proxel (1,2-benzisothiazolin-3-one), 0.05% alcohol
Tribromosalicylanilide 1% petrolatum
Triethanolamine 1% petrolatum

COSMETOLOGISTS

p-Aminodiphenylamine 0.25% petrolatum (dyes)
p-Aminophenol 1% petrolatum (dyes)
Balsam of Peru 25% petrolatum (fragrances)
p-Chloro-m-xylenol 1% petrolatum (creams and lotions)
Benzalkonium chloride 0.01% aqueous (germicidal solutions)
BHA 2% petrolatum (antioxidant)
Bronopol 0.25% petrolatum (preservative)
Captan 0.25% petrolatum (shampoos)
Diazolidinyl urea 1% petrolatum (shampoos and skin care products)
DMDM hydantoin 1% aqueous (preservative)
Glyceryl monothioglycolate 1% petrolatum ("acid" perms")
Hydroquinone 1% petrolatum (bleaches)
Kathon CG 0.01% petrolatum (germicide)

Methyl, ethyl, and butyl methacrylates 5% petrolatum (artificial nails)
o-Nitro-p-phenylenediamine 2% petrolatum (semipermanent hair dyes)
Paraben mix 12% petrolatum (preservatives)
m-Phenylenediamine 2% petrolatum (hair dyes)
Propylene glycol 10% aqueous (numerous creams, lotions, etc.)
Pyrogallol 1% petrolatum (hair dyes)
Resorcinol 2% petrolatum (hair dyes)
Sorbic acid 2% petrolatum (creams)
p-Toluenediamine 1% petrolatum (hair dyes)
Triclosan 2% petrolatum (soaps and cosmetics)
Tricresyl phosphate 2% petrolatum (nail polishes)

DENTAL PERSONNEL

Amethocaine (tetracaine) 5% petrolatum (topical anesthetic)

Balsam of Peru 25% petrolatum (medications)

Beeswax 30% petrolatum (impression materials)

Benzalkonium chloride 0.01% aqueous (disinfectants)

Benzocaine 5% petrolatum (anesthetics)

Benzophenone 1% petrolatum (light absorber in plastics)

BIS-GMA 2% petrolatum (plastic)

BIS-MA 2% petrolatum (plastic)

Bronopol 0.25% petrolatum (disinfectant)

Caine mix 8% petrolatum (anesthetic)

Chlorhexidine digluconate 1% aqueous (antiseptic)

p-Chloro-m-xylenol 1% petrolatum (antiseptic)

Chlorothymol 1% petrolatum (medications)

Cinnamon oil 0.5% petrolatum (medications and toothpaste)

Cobalt chloride 1% petrolatum

Copper sulfate 2% aqueous

N,N-Dimethyl-p-toluidine 2% petrolatum (catalyst)

Ethylene glycol dimethacrylate 5% petrolatum (plastic)

Eugenol 4% petrolatum (various)

Glutaraldehyde 0.25% petrolatum (disinfectant)

Gold chloride 0.1%

Hexachlorophene 1% petrolatum (disinfectant)

Hexylresorcinol 1% petrolatum (medications)

Hydroquinone 1% petrolatum (inhibitor in acrylic resin systems)

2-Hydroxy-4-methoxy-benzophenone 2% petrolatum (UV inhibitor)

N-Isopropyl-N'-phenyl-p-phenylenediamine (IPPD), 0.1% petrolatum (rubber)

Menthol 1% petrolatum (medications)

Mercury (metallic) 0.5% petrolatum

Methyl ethyl ketone peroxide 1% petrolatum (catalyst, acrylic resins)

Methyl dichlorobenzene sulfonate 0.5% petrolatum (impression materials, Impregum catalyst)

Methyl methacrylate monomer 1% petrolatum (dental plastic)

Methyl salicylate 2% petrolatum (toothpaste flavor)

Paraben mix 12% petrolatum (medications, toothpastes)

Penicillin 1% petrolatum

Phenylmercuric acetate 0.01% aqueous

Potassium dicyanoaurate 0.001% aqueous

Procaine 1% petrolatum (anesthetics)

Triethyleneglycol dimethacrylate 0.2% petrolatum (plastics)

Urethane dimethacrylate 2% petrolatum

4-Tolyldiethanolamine 2% alcohol (catalyst)

CARPENTERS

Cobalt chloride 2% petrolatum (driers in varnishes)

Pentachlorophenol 1% aqueous (wood preservatives)

Phenol formaldehyde resin 10% petrolatum (resin, adhesives, glues, plywood)

Plants (Toxicodendron, Frullania, Compositae, etc.)

Turpentine 10% olive oil (solvents)

Wood sawdusts 10% petrolatum (pine, "exotic" woods, etc.)

PHOTOGRAPHERS

p-Aminophenol 1% petrolatum
  (developers)
1,2,3-benzotriazole 0.5% aqueous
  (restrainer)
Camphor 10% petrolatum
CD-2 1% petrolatum (color developer)
CD-3 1% petrolatum (color developer)
CD-4 1% petrolatum (color developer)
2,4-Diaminophenol 2% petrolatum
Dichlorophene 1% petrolatum
  (mildewcide)
Dimethylhydantoin-formaldehyde resin
  1% in alcohol
Glutaraldehyde 0.25% aqueous (print
  hardener)
Gold sodium thiosulfate 0.1%
  petrolatum (toner)

Hydrazine sulfate 1% petrolatum
  (developer)
Hydroquinone 1% petrolatum
  (developer)
N-Isopropyl-N'-phenyl-p-
  phenylenediamine (IPPD) 0.1%
  petrolatum (rubber)
Metol 1% petrolatum (developer, black-
  and-white film)
PBA-1 0.1% aqueous (persulfate bleach
  accelerator for motion picture film)
Platinum chloride 1% aqueous
Potassium metabisulfite 1% aqueous
Pyrocatechol 2% petrolatum
  (developers)
Pyrogallol 1% petrolatum (developers)
Resorcinol 2% petrolatum (developers)

MATERIAL SAFETY DATA SHEETS

Material Safety Data Sheets (MSDS) have been required since 1986 in every workplace. They must be provided by all chemical manufacturers, importers, and distributors in the United States for every chemical which is produced, distributed, or used. Furthermore, the OSHA Hazard Communication Standard (29CFR 1910, 1200) mandates that signs or labels must be present on containers and products which contain potentially hazardous chemicals. In addition, all employers are required to provide MSDS information to each employee.

These sheets contain information such as ingredients, their physical data, fire and explosion data, health hazard information, and so on. Unfortunately there is often little detailed information regarding the exact chemicals present. However, a physician can usually obtain this information by using a telephone number on the first sheet of the MSDS.

Unfortunately, the law requires that only those substances in concentration greater than 1 percent be listed on the MSDS. Many preservatives, for example, of which several are well-recognized allergens, are present in concentration under 1 percent. Nevertheless, this information is usually available by telephone.

HISTORY AND PHYSICAL EXAMINATION

Without a thorough history, it is usually impossible to determine with certainty whether a patient with contact dermatitis has developed the condition from exposure in the workplace, at home, or both. The evaluation must provide the following information[26]: (1) determination of the type and location of the dermatitis. Is the condition consistent with contact dermatitis? (2) determination of whether the dermatitis is aggravated by the work if found to be nonoccupational; (3) establishment of a definite relationship between the dermatitis and the work; are there workplace exposures to potential irritants and allergens? (4) Is the anatomic distribution of the dermatitis consistent with the workplace exposure? (5) establishment of the primary etiologic agent(s), especially if the condition is allergic contact dermatitis; (6) evaluation of the predisposing and contributory factors; (7) initiation of a treatment program, considering the possibility of rehabilitation and a job change, if necessary.

To establish a work relationship, the history should bring out that the condition began during a period of occupational exposure. The condition should improve during periods away from work provided there are no major aggravating factors in the non-work environment. If improvement is seen away from work, recurrence should regularly develop on returning to the same job. Occasionally the only evidence for a work relationship is the fact that improvement regularly occurs when the patient is not working and recurrences always develop on returning to work. Most insurance carriers will accept this as evidence of a work relationship, but only when a thorough examination has been done, including patch testing when indicated.

A history and examination form is shown in Fig. 43-1.

PROGNOSIS

In a well-motivated patient, the prognosis for irritant dermatitis is quite good, especially if the condition has been present for only a short period of time. Workers who have had repeated episodes, and those who are older or atopics, have a poorer prognosis for complete recovery. This is especially true for atopics, where repeated episodes of dermatitis are very common. Many atopics must leave work where there is heavy contact with soaps, detergents, food products, cleaning agents, and so on.[27,28]

Patients with ACD often require a change of occupation. Occasionally patients can remain on the job and minimize recurrence by the use of proper skin protection, especially if the allergen is known and the company provides protective measures, which may include engineering controls at the work site.

PERSISTENCE

The most important cause of persistence of occupational dermatitis is incomplete or imprecise diagnosis. An unrecognized irritant or allergen is usually the cause, and/or the presence of aggravating factors during home and/or recreational activities. Inappropriate medication, usually over-the-counter home remedies, may be responsible for failure to improve. It is possible but rather unusual for patients to maintain disease activity by deliberate application of irritants or allergens.

WORKERS' COMPENSATION

The workers' compensation system began in the United States in 1911, and today all 50 states have such systems, although they vary in coverage and benefits. All, however, possess the following basic features[29]:

1. Liability without fault

(*Text continues on page 596*)

Name _____ Date _____
Address _____ Age _____ Sex _____
Home phone _____ Soc. sec. no. _____ Referred by _____
Current employer (name and address) _____
_____ Job title at present _____
Employer at onset of injury (name and address) _____

Date employed _____ Date terminated _____
Job title at onset of injury _____ Date _____
Insurance carrier (name and address) _____

Present Illness

Date of onset _____ Dates of disability _____
Location at onset _____
Patient's description _____
_____
_____
_____

Time off work (incl. vacations)? _____
Effect of return to work? _____
Workers' Compensation claim? _____
Previous job(s)? _____ How long? _____

Previous Treatment

1. Plant dispensary _____
2. Other physician _____
_____
3. Self-treatment _____

Description of Work

_____
_____
_____
_____

Materials contacted _____
_____

Other workers affected?   Yes _____ No _____ No. affected _____
How many workers on this job? _____
Methods of cleaning skin at work (and frequency) _____
_____
Protective creams (names) _____
Protective clothing (incl. gloves) _____

Past History

Previous compensation claims? Yes _____ No _____ Explain _____
_____
Previous skin diseases _____
Relation to occupation? Yes _____ No _____ Place of birth _____
Past health _____
Allergic history: Hay fever _____ Asthma _____ Eczema _____ Allergic to
cosmetics, medications, creams, ointments, jewelry, drugs, perfumes? (circle which)
Describe _____
Family history of atopy or psoriasis? Yes _____ No _____ Second job _____

Hobbies

Contacts at Home

Housework _____ Full-time _____ Part-time _____
Married _____ Single _____ Widow _____ Divorced _____
Children _____ Yes _____ Number _____ Ages _____
Emotional factors _____

FIG. 43–1. Suggested medical forms for recording medical history and physical examination of patients with skin disease suspected to be of occupational origin. (From Freeman S: Diagnosis and differential diagnosis, in Adams RM (ed): *Occupational Skin Disease,* 2d ed. Philadelphia, Saunders, 1990, pp 196–197. Reproduced by permission.)

Physical Examination

General appearance _____

Description of disease _____

Other skin diseases _____

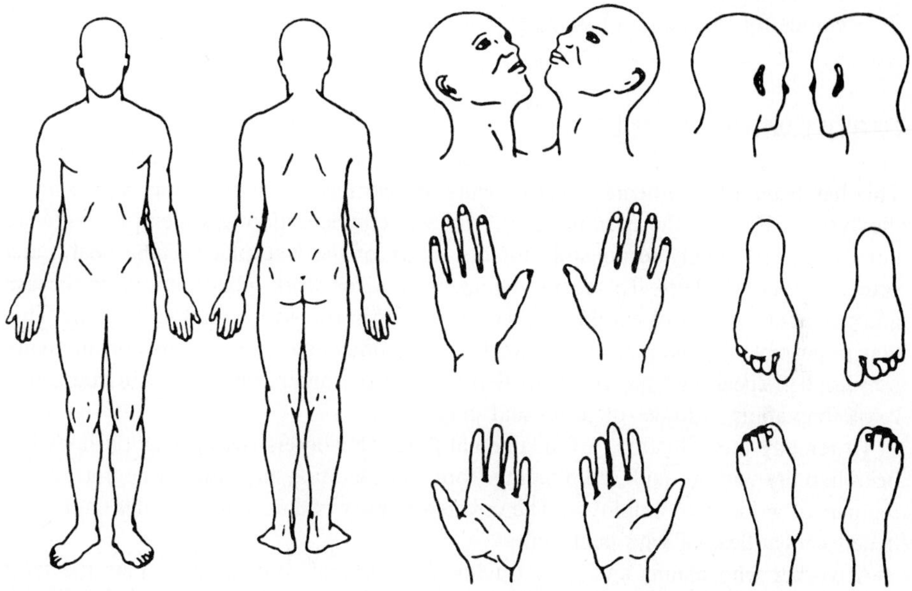

Diagnosis

Eczema	Yes _____	No _____	Different _____
Contact dermatitis	Entirely _____	Partially _____	No _____
Endogenous dermatitis	Atopic _____	Discoid _____	Seborrheic _____
	Hand _____	Foot _____	Asteatotic _____
	Face _____	Stasis _____	Unclassified _____

Pre-Patch Test Diagnosis

Sensitizers	Relevance	
Irritants	Relevance	
Occupational	Yes _____	No _____ Don't know _____

Special Tests

KOH _____ Fungal culture _____ Bacterial culture _____

Biopsy _____

Patch testing (results) Sensitizers _____

Relevance _____

Occupational Yes _____ No _____ Clinical photographs? Yes _____ No _____

Treatment _____

Disability Yes _____ No _____ Occupational Yes _____ No _____

Remarks and Recommendations _____

Post-Patch Test Diagnosis

Sensitizers _____	Relevance _____
Irritants _____	Relevance _____
Occupational _____	Yes _____ No _____

FIG. 43–1. (*Continued*)

2. Compulsory insurance
3. Automatic benefits
4. Medical care provisions
5. Income protection
6. Death benefits
7. Methods for resolution of disputes

LIABILITY WITHOUT FAULT

This has been a fundamental tenet of workers' compensation since the beginning of the system. Prior to the enactment of workers' compensation laws, employers were not considered legally responsible for the safety of the workplace or the health and safety of their workers. To receive compensation for work-related injury or disease and payment for loss of earnings, a worker had to resort to a common-law suit. This was impossible for the majority of workers, and unattainable especially for the many non-English-speaking immigrants of that day. Also workers rarely won in court, due to the prevailing attitudes of juries and judges.

To remedy this situation, a fundamental tenet of workers' compensation laws has been liability without fault, eliminating from consideration any issue of negligence on the part of workers or employer. The covered worker is thus automatically entitled to benefits regardless of who is at fault.

A worker who claims an injury (under the workers' compensation law, the term *injury* includes disease) is entitled to evaluation by physicians and payment of all expenses for that evaluation, regardless of the costs, even if the condition ultimately is adjudicated as not being work-related. In some states, the employer is allowed to choose the physician for the first 30 days after the claimed injury, but afterward, the worker may choose. The worker must also report the injury to the employer, and the latter must file the claim with the industrial compensation bureau of the state.

COMPULSORY INSURANCE

Workers' compensation insurance is financed exclusively by employers' contributions, and the cost is proportional to the risk represented by the class of activity in which an employer is engaged. Rates for office work, for example, are much lower than for construction companies. Compensation may be secured from a private insurance carrier, a state insurance fund, and/or self-insurance. The latter programs are utilized by large corporations with sufficient reserve funds to meet emergencies. Claims adjustments are often provided by contract with private claims adjustment companies.

AUTOMATIC BENEFITS

Compensation benefits must be automatic and prompt. The worker first notifies, if able to do so, the employer as soon as injury or illness is apparent and suspected of being of occupational origin. The employer must then file a report, usually within a certain period of time. If the employer ignores the claim, a fine may be levied. The physician must also file a report ("Doctor's First Report"—see that for California, Fig. 43-2) within a prescribed period of time. The report must include the date of injury or illness; its nature and extent; the method of causation; and finally the diagnosis, treatment, and prognosis, including whether hospitalization was necessary. Physicians may be fined if the reports are not received by the compensation bureau in a timely fashion. Even if the condition is later found to be unrelated to the work, the filing of a claim is required if the worker believes the condition arose from the employment. The physician will be compensated by the insurance carrier for the initial examination and treatment even if the condition proves to be unrelated to the work.

Aggravation of preexisting conditions is also compensable. Dermatologists frequently treat patients with conditions such as psoriasis, dyshidrotic eczema, lichen planus, and so on which are made worse by the work. The aggravation is usually temporary, but in some cases, especially in psoriasis, the aggravation may be permanent.

MEDICAL CARE

In more than 80 percent of the cases, the first and only benefit is medical care. There are no limitations on the care; not only physicians (M.D., D.O.) may provide care but also chiropractors and in some states Christian Science practitioners. The worker must cooperate with the physicians and meet appointments as scheduled. If not, penalties will be leveled and taken from the final award, if any.

The initial medical report and any follow-up reports must be submitted promptly. In more complicated cases, a lengthy report is required. An outline of such a report is shown in Table 43-3.

INCOME PROTECTION

This is a central tenet of the workers' compensation system. It is designed to compensate the worker for lost wages during recovery from injury or illness. The cost is borne by the employer through the insurance carrier unless the employer is self-insured. There are various types of disability: temporary disability, which may be either partial or complete; and permanent disability, partial or total. There is usually a waiting period of a few days for temporary disability, but it begins immediately if the worker is hospitalized. Temporary disability payments consist of a prescribed percentage of the worker's wages to be paid during the period of recovery until the worker is able to return to work. Permanent disability compensation is usually based on the degree of permanent impairment, loss of earning capacity in the labor market, and loss of wages.

SECOND INJURY FUNDS

If an injured worker had a physical impairment prior to sustaining an industrial injury, the combination may result in a greater impairment than either alone. A hairdresser

DOCTOR'S FIRST REPORT OF OCCUPATIONAL INJURY OR ILLNESS

STATE OF CALIFORNIA

Within 5 days of your initial examination, for every occupational injury or illness, send this report to **insurer or employer (only if self-insured).** Failure to file a timely doctor's report may result in assessment of a civil penalty. **In the case of diagnosed or suspected pesticide poisoning,** send one copy of this report directly to the Division of Labor Statistics and Research, P.O. Box 603, San Francisco CA 94101; and notify your local health officer by telephone within 24 hours and by sending a copy of this report within seven days. For a supply of this form, please call (415) 557-1924.

		PLEASE DO NOT USE THIS COLUMN
1. INSURER NAME AND ADDRESS		Case No.
2. EMPLOYER NAME		
3. Address: No. and Street / City / Zip		Industry
4. Nature of business (e.g., food manufacturing, building construction, retailer of women's clothes)		County
5. PATIENT NAME (First name, middle initial, last name)	6. Sex ☐ Male ☐ Female / 7. Date of Birth Mo. Day Yr.	Age
8. Address: No. and Street / City / Zip	9. Telephone number ( )	Hazard
10. Occupation (Specific job title)	11. Social Security Number - -	Disease
12. Injured at: No. and Street / City / County		Hospitalization
13. Date and hour of injury or onset of illness Mo. Day Yr. Hour ___ a.m. ___ p.m.	14. Date last worked Mo. Day Yr.	Occupation
15. Date and hour of first examination or treatment Mo. Day Yr. Hour ___ a.m. ___ p.m.	16. Have you (or your office) previously treated patient? ☐ Yes ☐ No	Return Date/Code

Patient please complete this portion, if able to do so. Otherwise, doctor please complete immediately. Inability or failure of a patient to complete this portion shall not affect his/her rights to workers' compensation under the California Labor Code.

17. DESCRIBE HOW THE ACCIDENT OR EXPOSURE HAPPENED (Give specific object, machinery or chemical. Use reverse side if more space is required.)

18. **SUBJECTIVE COMPLAINTS** (Describe fully. Use reverse side if more space is required.)

19. **OBJECTIVE FINDINGS** (Use reverse side if more space is required.)

   A. Physical examination

   B. X-ray and laboratory results (State if none or pending.)

20. **DIAGNOSIS** (If occupational illness, specify etiologic agent and duration of exposure.) Chemical or toxic compounds involved? ☐ Yes   ☐ No

21. Are your findings and diagnosis consistent with patient's account of injury or onset of illness? ☐ Yes   ☐ No
   If "no", please explain.

22. Is there any other current condition that will impede or delay patient's recovery? ☐ Yes   ☐ No
   If "yes", please explain.

23. **TREATMENT RENDERED** (Use reverse side if more space is required.)

   If further treatment required, specify treatment.

24. If hospitalized as inpatient, give hospital name and location.   Date   Mo.   Day   Yr.   Estimated duration
                                                                     admitted   Estimated stay

25. **WORK STATUS**   Is patient able to perform usual work? ☐ Yes   ☐ No
   If "no", patient can return to: Mo.   Day   Yr.
      Regular work _____
      Modified work _____   Specify restrictions _____

Incomplete information or delay in submitting this report may cause delay in benefits to your patient.

Doctor's Signature _____   Date _____

Doctor Name and Degree (Please Type) _____   CA License Number _____

Address _____   IRS Number _____

                               Telephone Number (____) _____

FORM 5021 (Rev. 3)
1989   89 53614

FIG. 43-2. Physician's report form for occupational injury of illness. (From the State of California Division of Labor Statistics and Research.)

FIG. 43-2. (*Continued*)

599

TABLE 43–3. Outline for Dermatology Examination of Workers' Compensation Patients

1. History	13. Discussion
2. Job description	14. Disability status
3. Current treatment	15. Factors of disability
4. Present complaints	Subjective
5. Past medical history	Objective
6. Family history	16. Apportionment
7. Social history	17. Future medical care
8. Personal data	18. Vocational
9. Medical record review	Rehabilitation
10. Physician examination	Work restrictions
11. Diagnosis	19. Disclosures
12. Support for diagnosis	20. Signature

who develops allergic contact sensitivity to glyceryl monothioglycolate (GMTG) and later becomes allergic to an accelerator in rubber gloves will have greater disability than sensitivity to the GMTG alone, because the percentage of the open labor market from which the worker is excluded because of the rubber sensitivity is greater than if the sensitivity were to GMTG alone. The liability of the employer in such cases varies between states. If the GMTG sensitivity precluded the employment at the hairdresser's present job, the liability would be divided between insurance companies. If the rubber sensitivity preceded the sensitivity to GMTG and arose from a nonoccupational source, there is increased disability because there are two sensitivities. Compensation for these may come from "second injury" funds, which most states provide. Payment for the difference between the industrial disease and the combined disease may be paid from this second injury fund.

DEATH BENEFITS

States vary greatly in their payments for the death of a worker because of a work-related injury, but awards have increased in recent years and almost always include a fixed payment for burial expenses.

METHODS FOR RESOLUTION OF DISPUTES

The most common methods of hearing disputes are (1) in a court-administered system, (2) in a wholly administrative system, and (3) in a combination of both. In more than 90 percent of the cases of work-related dermatitis, the worker either loses no time from work or returns to work after a brief period. There is no dispute, and the claim can be closed without conflict. However, when the claim cannot be closed without some dispute between employer or insurance company on the one hand and the worker on the other, the claim is handled by one of the above methods. For further discussion of these methods, the reader is referred to standard reference books.[30]

TREATMENT

Treatment of occupational skin disease is no different from that of nonoccupational origin. Patients should be told of the specific cause(s) of their disease and, in the case of ACD, they should know the name of the allergen(s), where they may be present in the environment in addition to the workplace, and how to avoid contact, especially whether gloves will provide adequate protection. Sometimes specific tips on avoidance can be provided, such as suggesting the use of only certain brands of rubber gloves. Patients should also be made aware that although the skin appears normal, a degree of hyperirritability may persist for several months after a severe episode of dermatitis. To prevent future recurrence, care should be taken to avoid irritation, especially in daily home activities. The prolonged and/or excessive application of topical corticosteroids may induce atrophy and cause the skin to become even more sensitive than before.

Workers whose cases are litigated require special attention, with thorough reports that are carefully written in language nonmedical readers can understand. The key to a successful outcome, whether in favor or not in favor of the worker, is a clearly written, complete report by a knowledgeable physician. Too often, physicians hedge in making difficult decisions in these cases, which is unfortunate and prolongs the litigation.

PLANT SURVEY

An often neglected part of the evaluation of patients with occupational skin disease is a survey of the plant where the patient works. The focus of such a visit should not be exclusively on the patient's work site but should encompass the entire plant if possible. A convenient time should be arranged, often early in the morning, shortly after the beginning of the shift. The plant person guiding the tour preferably should be someone in authority and also a person with detailed knowledge of the work of the plant. When there have been cases of dermatitis in the past, the causes of these cases should be discussed. The use of protective clothing and the existence of engineering controls such as adequate exhaust, hoods, proper ventilation, and so on; the general neatness of the plant; and the ambient temperature and relative humidity, should be noted. A review of the Material Safety Data Sheets is important; this often reveals critical information. Detailed examination of the patient's work site may reveal previously unrecognized clues as to the cause of the dermatitis. A detailed report is usually necessary on conclusion of the inspection.

REFERENCES

1. U.S. Bureau of Labor Statistics, 1988.
2. Mathias CGT: The cost of occupational skin disease. *Arch Dermatol* 121:332–334, 1985.
3. Emmett EA, Suskind RR: Occupational dermatoses, in Fitzpatrick TB (ed): *Dermatology in General Medicine,* 2d ed. New York, McGraw-Hill, 1979, pp 1007–1016.
4. Rycroft RJG: Low-humidity occupational dermatoses: Symposium on Contact Dermatitis. *Dermatol Clin* 2:553–559, 1984.

5. Vance MV: Hydrofluoric acid (HF) burns, in Adams RM (ed): *Occupational Skin Disease,* 2d ed. Philadelphia, Saunders, 1990 pp 18–21.
6. Adams RM: Dermatitis due to fibrous glass, in Adams RM (ed): *Occupational Skin Disease,* 2d ed. Philadelphia, Saunders, 1990, pp 16–17.
7. Hanifin JM: Ethylene oxide dermatitis. *JAMA* 217:213, 1971.
8. Fisher AA: Post-operative ethylene oxide dermatitis. *Cutis* 12:177, 1973.
9. Taylor JS: Dermatologic hazards from ethylene oxide. *Cutis* 19:189, 1977.
10. Adams RM: *Occupational Skin Disease.* New York, Grune & Stratton, 1983, p 7.
11. Fisher AA: Contact urticaria due to occupational exposures, in Adams RM (ed): *Occupational Skin Disease,* 2d ed. Philadelphia, Saunders, 1990, pp 113–126.
12. Schmidt RJ: Plants, in Adams RM (ed): *Occupational Skin Disease,* 2d ed. Philadelphia, Saunders, 1990, pp 503–524.
13. Seligman PJ, Mathias CGT, O'Malley MA, et al: Phytophotodermatitis from celery among grocery store workers. *Arch Dermatol* 123:1478–1482, 1987.
14. Fregert S: *Manual of Contact Dermatitis,* 2d ed. Copenhagen, Munksgaard, 1981, p 88.
15. Edman B, Möller H: Contact allergy and contact allergens in atopic skin disease. *Am J Contact Dermatitis* 3:27–29, 1992.
16. De Groot AC: The frequency of contact allergy in atopic patients with dermatitis. *Contact Dermatitis* 22:273–277, 1990.
17. Uehara M, Sawai T: A longitudinal study of contact sensitivity in patients with atopic dermatitis. *Arch Dermatol* 125:366–368, 1989.
18. Forsbeck M, Hovmark A, Skog E: Patch testing tuberculin testing and sensitization with dinitrochlorobenzene and nitrosodimethylaniline of patients with atopic dermatitis. *Acta Derm Venereol* 56:135–138, 1976.
19. Fisher AA: Contact urticaria due to occupational exposures, in Adams RM (ed): *Occupational Skin Disease,* 2d ed. Philadelphia, Saunders, 1990, pp 113–126.
20. Hjorth N, Roed-Petersen J: Occupational protein contact dermatitis in food handlers. *Contact Dermatitis* 2:23, 1976.
21. Jolanki R, Estlander T, Kanerva L: Occupational contact dermatitis and contact urticaria caused by epoxy resins. *Acta Derm Venereol (Stockh)* (suppl) 134: 90–94, 1987.
22. Hausen B: *Woods Injurious to Human Health: A Manual.* Berlin, de Gruyter, 1981, pp 7–8.
23. Calnan CD, Shuster S: Reactions to ammonium persulfate. *Arch Dermatol* 88:812, 1968.
24. Fisher AA, Dooms-Goossens A: Persulfate hair bleach reactions. *Arch Dermatol* 112:1407, 1976.
25. Adams RM: Panels of allergens for specific occupations. *J Am Acad Dermatol* 21:869–874, 1989.
26. Mathias CGT: Contact dermatitis and workers' compensation: Criteria for establishing occupational causation and aggravation. *J Am Acad Dermatol* 20:842–848, 1989.
27. Shmunes E, Keil JE: The role of atopy in occupational dermatoses. *Contact Dermatitis* 11:174–178, 1984.
28. Rystedt I: Work related hand eczema in atopics. *Contact Dermatitis* 12:164–171, 1985.
29. Swezey CL: Workers' compensation, in LaDou J (ed): *Occupational Medicine.* San Mateo, Calif, Appleton & Lange, 1989, chap 3.
30. LaDou J: Worker's compensation, in Adams RM (ed): *Occupational Skin Disease,* 2d ed. Philadelphia, Saunders, 1990, pp 280–288.

SUGGESTED READING

Adams RM (ed): *Occupational Skin Disease,* 2d ed. Philadelphia, Saunders, 1990.
American Journal of Contact Dermatitis, published quarterly by Saunders, Philadelphia.
Chemical & Engineering News, published weekly by the American Chemical Society, 1155 16th Street NW, Washington, DC 20036.
Contact Dermatitis, a journal published monthly by Munksgaard, Copenhagen.
Cronin E: *Contact Dermatitis,* Edinburgh, Churchill Livingstone, 1980.
Fisher AA: *Contact Dermatitis,* 3d ed. Philadelphia, Lea & Febiger, 1986.
Marks JG Jr, DeLeo VA: *Contact and Occupational Dermatology,* St Louis, Mosby Year Book, 1992.
Rycroft RJG, Menné T, Frosch PJ, Benezra C (eds), *Textbook of Contact Dermatitis,* New York, Springer-Verlag, 1992.

44

THE PEDIATRIC PATIENT

Susan B. Mallory

Allergic contact dermatitis in children is so common that one wonders why more patch testing is not done. While such noted authorities as Cronin[1] consider contact dermatitis to be uncommon in children, this is certainly not universally accepted. Of children who have been tested, the percentage of positive patch tests varies at least somewhat from country to country. Environmental exposure is obviously important and may account for the discrepancies in the range of positive tests.

Rademaker and Forsythe[2] reported 52 percent of pediatric patients had some positive responses to a standard screening series. Ayala et al.[3] reported 35 percent and Gonçalo et al.[4] 52 percent. In most cases these tests were relevant. However, in contrast, Pambor et al.[5] found that only 11 of 298 children tested were positive. To put this in perspective, contact dermatitis in a pediatric population is probably more common than previously realized, and it is usually relevant when positive patch tests are found.[6]

Recognition of contact dermatitis in the pediatric population is not very different from its recognition in the adult population. It is usually straightforward in most cases of *Toxicodendron* dermatitis, where the streaky pattern gives the diagnosis away. However, contact dermatitis can be difficult to recognize when it presents as another eczematous dermatitis. For example, ethylenediamine has been reported as a cause of nummular eczema in two children[7] and allergy to topical corticosteroid may present as an unresponsive eczema or hand eczema.

The two most important factors in recognizing allergic and irritant contact dermatitis are (1) the artificial nature of the eruption, which in many cases suggests the pattern of exposure which induced it, and (2) the failure of the rash to respond to standard therapies. The pattern of dermatitis may be slightly different in children. For example, an eczematous eruption near the umbilicus of an adolescent girl should make one suspicious of nickel sensitivity, since this is a classic location for nickel dermatitis caused by metal fasteners in blue jeans. Another example would be epoxy resin dermatitis, caused by Tufskin jeans or knee patch adhesives; therefore, knees (where most patches occur) would be the obvious site. A rash on the face from allergy to a teddy bear would also be a source unlikely to be seen in an adult.

CLINICAL PRESENTATION

In evaluating a patient with an eczematous dermatitis, one must consider allergic contact dermatitis (ACD), irritant contact dermatitis, atopic dermatitis, other eczema, or any combination of these. If lesions are localized to a specific area, such as the dorsa of the feet (suggesting shoe dermatitis), then the answer often seems obvious (although after patch testing it may turn out not to be). At other times, the problem is not so simple. Fungal cultures and potassium hydroxide (KOH) preps will help rule out dermatophytosis, and patch testing will help confirm ACD. Psoriasis can also occur in childhood, so when dry, hyperkeratotic eruptions occur, one should perhaps look for other stigmata of psoriasis, such as nail pitting or scalp involvement. Perhaps the most difficult presentation is when two or more conditions are superimposed. Here being both suspicious and diligent helps.

A common type of ACD in pediatric patients is *Toxicodendron* dermatitis, which is characterized by papules, vesicles, erythema, and/or edema (Figs. 44-1 and 44-2A). If the process is early, erythema may be the most obvious sign arising before typical papules and vesicles have had time to form (Fig. 44-2B). Pruritus may vary from mild to severe. Children often have more extensive poison ivy dermatitis (Fig. 44-3) because of their inability to recognize the plant and because they may play in areas where these plants are abundant. The presence of black spots makes the diagnosis even easier (Fig. 44-4). The reason for the pattern is that contact dermatitis caused by poison ivy characteristically demonstrates linear lesions or handprints (Fig. 44-5) where the antigen has been transferred by the fingers.

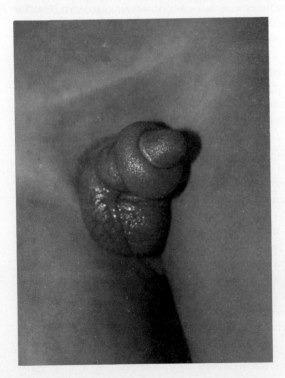

FIG. 44-1. Contact dermatitis causing swelling around the penis.

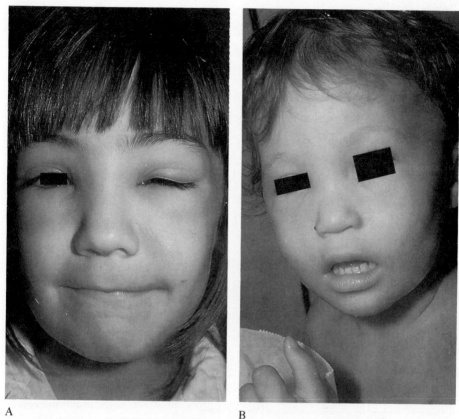

A   B

FIG. 44–2. Edema is often a prominent feature in poison ivy dermatitis around the eyes (*A* and *B*).

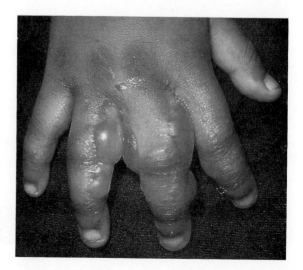

FIG. 44–3. Extensive edema and blistering in a child because of extensive handling of the vine and the inability to recognize the poison ivy plant.

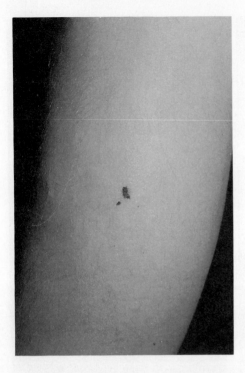

FIG. 44–4. Poison ivy dermatitis. The black spot is evidence of poison ivy oleoresin retained on the skin, causing a "black spot" with surrounding allergic contact dermatitis.

At first the eruption of ACD involves only sites which have been exposed to the allergen. A history of contact will aid the clinician in identifying the provocative agent by correlating exposure to certain allergenic agents. However, as the eruption evolves, it may spread to more distant sites, usually by inadvertent contact with the offending agent, making the identity of the agent more difficult. For other sources of ACD, the pattern and shape of the eruption may furnish clues about what causes to ask about and which agents to include in patch testing.

Certain areas of the body, such as the eyelids and face, have a thinner stratum

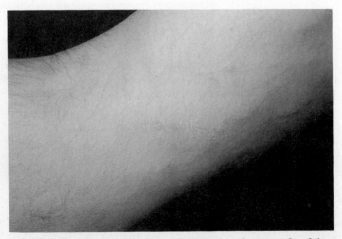

FIG. 44–5. Typical streaky dermatitis from poison ivy caused by finger transfer of the antigen.

corneum and may develop allergenic contact dermatitis to milder antigens more readily than the palms, soles or scalp, which have a thicker stratum corneum. Some cases of ACD of the hands involve the finger webs more than the dorsa, particularly if the offending agent is not washed off totally during hand washing.

Other forms of pruritic dermatoses such as viral toxic erythemas and erythema multiforme occur in children, but the *pattern* of the eruption is the most helpful feature in most cases (Fig. 44-5). A *history* is also extremely valuable. Having the parent fill out a History Sheet (see Appendix B) may help in the search for the correct diagnosis by identifying certain not-so-obvious antigens.

Other eczemas, such as atopic dermatitis, commonly seen in children and young adults have a typical morphology and distribution as well, being characteristically worse in the flexural creases and associated with other atopic stigmata. Some causes of contact dermatitis, such as earring or shoe dermatitis, can be superimposed on the atopic dermatitis and may be confusing. Although Compositae dermatitis is quite rare in children, it can closely mimic the eruption of atopic eczema.

Another eczematous eruption, nummular eczema, appears in coin-shaped plaques and is usually not allergic in nature. However, it is occasionally a form of ACD and therefore the pattern can be deceiving. Even an expert can be fooled.

GENETIC AND PREDISPOSING FACTORS

Although the role of genetic factors in contact allergy has been clearly demonstrated in guinea pigs, little knowledge exists regarding specific genetic factors in humans.[8] Patients with disorders that have accompanying immunologic dysfunction—such as lymphoma, sarcoidosis, and lepromatous leprosy—are known to develop contact-allergic sensitization less often[9] than normal patients.

Whether atopic individuals have an increased or decreased incidence of allergic contact dermatitis has been debated. Although atopic individuals have been thought to have reduced cell-mediated immunity, this concept has recently been challenged. They may react more commonly to certain allergens, particularly nickel. In adults, atopic dermatitis increases the odds for developing hand dermatitis in wet-work occupations (e.g., domestic work, nursing, etc.).[10] Hydrocortisone sensitivity may also be more common in atopic patients.[11]

COMMON SENSITIZERS

The major sensitizers are discussed in detail in other chapters. A brief overview of some of the common sensitizers in a pediatric population would include poison ivy, oak, and sumac; jewelry and other metal objects; nickel; potassium dichromate; paraphenylenediamine; mercaptobenzothiazole (MBT); ethylenediamine; benzocaine; neomycin; fragrance; and thimerosal. More common antigens not found in a standard test series would be PABA and diphenhydramine (which can also photosensitize).

Plant dermatitis is the most common cause of ACD in children[12] (see Chap. 38). Poison ivy, poison oak, and poison sumac (*Toxicodendron* or *Rhus*) are found commonly in the United States. Most people become sensitized by age 13 to 16 years.[13] Exposure

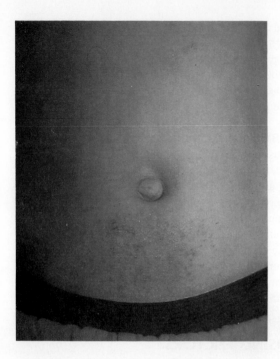

FIG. 44-6. Nickel allergy caused by snaps in jeans typically present around or below the umbilicus.

occurs either by direct contact or by contact with animals which inadvertently carry the antigen on their fur. Other uncommon substances which cross-react with the poison ivy antigen but which should be avoided include cashew nut shell oil, India marking tree, ginkgo "fruit," art objects lacquered with sap from the Japanese lacquer tree, and the peel of the mango fruit.[14]

Information about identifying *Toxicodendron* species can be very helpful in avoiding these plants. Grade-school children can easily learn the phrase "leaflets three, let them be!"

A weeping, oozing dermatitis at the site where the posts of pierced earrings are worn is another give-away diagnosis. *Nickel* is the most common sensitizer here,[14-16] but cobalt and gold can have the same effect. Sweat can extract nickel ions from metal objects that contain nickel, so that the dermatitis is principally in areas of pressure and friction, as underneath a watch, at the waist (where metal fasteners are found in baby clothes), or under snaps on jeans (Fig. 44-6).

Allergic contact dermatitis to *rubber* chemicals often presents as shoe dermatitis.[17] There are five rubber antigens in the standard tray [MBT, mercapto mix, paraphenylene-diamine (PPD) mix, carba mix, and thiuram mix]. The PPD mix is associated with black rubber, thiurams with latex gloves, and carbamates and accelerators with rubber in general. The most common rubber accelerator to cause a problem is MBT, which is also contained in fungicides and flea and tick powder.[18] Other sources of rubber compounds include rubber gloves, adhesives (Fig. 44-7), elastic (Fig. 44-8), and condoms.[19]

Patterns of dermatitis help lead to the diagnosis. The pattern of insole shoe dermatitis sharply outlines the pressure areas on the plantar surface and spares the proximal toes and longitudinal arch of the foot. Waistband dermatitis tends to outline the area where the elastic comes into contact with the skin, and medication sensitivity tends to be a

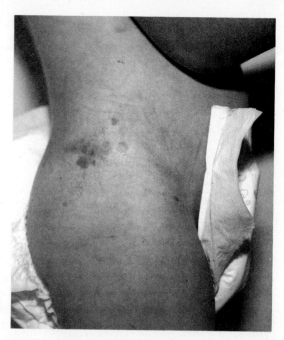

FIG. 44–7. Contact dermatitis to the adhesives in disposable diapers is typically seen over the iliac crests.

dermatitis which spreads from the location of a preexisting rash. Children may present with problems one does not see in an adult, as where the child holds a doll or a rubber toy against the skin or where he or she hugs a puppy. All of these involve a commonsense approach which requires that the clinician know the behavior pattern of the age group involved in order to understand the meaning of what he or she is observing. Table 44-1 lists some of the most common allergens.

Potassium dichromate is used in tanning leather, and sensitivity to it has been documented in children[20] (Fig. 44-9). Leather shoes, particularly the popular leather athletic shoes, are likely to be the source of this sensitization. In adults, however, working with wet cement is the most common source of chromate allergy.

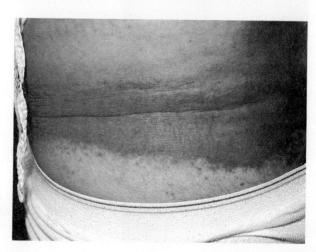

FIG. 44–8. Allergy to elastic in waistbands is usually caused by contact allergic dermatitis to rubber or bleached rubber.

TABLE 44–1. Contact Allergens in Children in Order of Frequency in the United States

Plant dermatitis
Nickel
Rubber chemicals
Formaldehyde
Balsam of Peru
Benzocaine
Tars (coal or wood)
Mercuric bichloride
Paraphenylenediamine (PPD)
Potassium dichromate
Paraminobenzoic acid preservatives

Source: Ref. 26.

Paraphenylenediamine is widely used in permanent hair dyes, fur dyes, some leather dyes, rubber products, and x-ray solutions. Adolescents who are sensitive to PPD often present with a dermatitis at the scalp margins and edema of the eyelids after getting their hair dyed. The scalp itself is more resistant to dermatitis, whereas the face and eyelids are extremely sensitive, and lesions are commonly seen on the surrounding skin of the face. Cross-reactions to PPD can occur with azo and aniline dyes, sulfa drugs, local anesthetics such as benzocaine or procaine, and sunscreens that contain para-aminobenzoic acid (PABA) and its esters.

Contact dermatitis caused by *topical medicaments* may be a problem in children (Fig. 44-10). *Ethylenediamine* hydrochloride, formerly used as a stabilizer in Mycolog

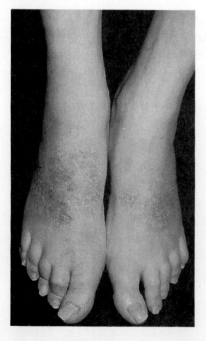

FIG. 44–9. Shoes can cause problems if a patient is allergic to chromates, which are found in leather athletic shoes.

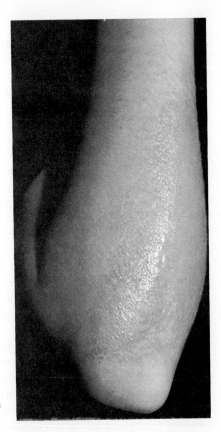

FIG. 44–10. Topical medicaments, in this case bacitracin, are a common cause of allergic contact dermatitis
in childhood.

Cream and its generic equivalents, has been a common sensitizer in the United States
because of its widespread use for diaper dermatitis.[18] For the original product and all
but one generic, the formulation has been changed to eliminate ethylenediamine, but
a number of persons who are allergic still turn up on patch testing. Persons allergic
to ethylenediamine may also have a cross-reaction to aminophylline preparations. If
given intravenous aminophylline, these people have a flare of the original dermatitis
or may even develop a generalized drug reaction. Other sources of ethylenediamine
include ophthalmic solutions (Prefrein-A, Vasocon-A), antihistamine creams (PBZ,
Phenergan), ethylenediamine-related antihistamines (Atarax, Vistaril), insecticides, fungicides, epoxy resin hardeners, and rubber stabilizers.

   Benzocaine is contained in many over-the-counter (OTC) "caine" preparations used
as topical anesthetics,[18] such as poison ivy preparations, toothache medicines, cough
drops, and throat lozenges.[18] Benzocaine is an ethyl ester of PABA and cross-reacts with
injectable local anesthetics based on the PABA structure, such as procaine hydrochloride
(Novocaine) and tetracaine (Pontocaine).

   Topical *diphenhydramine* (Benadryl) is commonly used as a popular OTC treatment
for pruritic rashes. A clue to this sensitivity may be the worsening of the original
dermatitis and spread of lesions. A more generalized eruption may occur if a sensitized
person is given oral diphenhydramine. This agent is often missed by routine patch
testing because it is not in standard patch-test series.

Neomycin is one of the most widely used topical antibiotics in the United States, often being compounded with other antibiotics, e.g., *bacitracin,* which can also be an allergen.[18,21,22] Pruritus and a progressive dermatitis at the site of injury should lead one to suspect these compounds. Cross-reaction to other aminoglycosides such as gentamicin may also occur. Delayed patch-test readings at 1 week may be necessary, as the antigen often is a late reactor.

Formaldehyde dermatitis is a common manifestation of clothing dermatitis (Fig. 44-11). Formaldehyde is found in permanent-press fabric finishes and is added to the clothing for water resistance, moth resistance, and mildew proofing. Other sources of formaldehyde include fungicides, cosmetics, shampoos, fumigants, industrial chemicals, and cosmetic preservatives that release formaldehyde, such as Quaternium-15, Bronopol, and imidazolidinyl urea.[18] Formaldehyde dermatitis often begins in the periaxillary area but spares the axillary vault, as clothing usually does not touch the vault directly. By washing the clothes several times, free formaldehyde can sometimes be greatly reduced. A useful handout can be found in Chap. 20.

Fabric softeners are often suspected in children's clothing dermatitis but are rarely proven to be the culprit. Fabric softeners are more likely to cause an irritant dermatitis rather than a true allergic contact dermatitis. Fragrances in the fabric softeners may be a source of perfume dermatitis. Fortunately, fragrance-free fabric softeners are now readily available.

Common offenders in *cosmetics* are *perfumes,* which are found in soaps, deodorants, sanitary napkins, toilet paper, facial tissue, spray starch, topical medications, and colognes. Perfumes usually contain mixtures of many fragrance chemicals. Some of the most common specific fragrance sensitizers are cinnamic alcohol, cinnamaldehyde, eugenol, isoeugenol, hydroxycitronellal, oakmoss absolute, geraniol, and alpha-amyl cinnamic alcohol. Facial contact dermatitis is commonly caused by perfumes found in cosmetic products applied to the face.

Mercury can cause sensitization in either the organic or inorganic form. The preservative thimerosal (Merthiolate) is found in many topical preparations as well as in germicidals, cosmetics, some immunizations, and dental preparations. Soft contact lens solution used by teenagers often contains thimerosal, which can lead to chronic

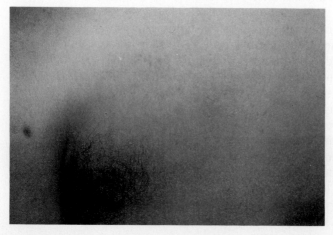

FIG. 44-11. Formaldehyde dermatitis from fabric finishes in clothing. The eruption is accentuated in areas where clothes rub the skin.

conjunctivitis and corneal neovascularization if unrecognized and untreated. Metallic mercury salts are also used in dental amalgams, thermometers, contraceptives, lubricants, weed killers, and preservatives in cosmetics. Some common OTC topical preparations contained mercury compounds at one time.[12] The current contents on these products should be checked, as product ingredients can change overnight.

Para-aminobenzoic acid (PABA), found in many sunscreens, may cause dermatitis in areas of application. However, many sunscreens are now PABA-free. Products which contain the oxybenzone or cinnamate sunscreens do not cross-react with PABA.

An unusual chemical to cause allergic contact dermatitis is *aluminum*. In Denmark, childhood immunizations or vaccines are bound with aluminum. According to one study, 13 children less than 13 years of age were reported to develop excoriated papules at the site of hyposensitization therapy and positive patch tests to aluminum.[23] This should be kept in mind, especially when dermatitis is localized to the area of an injection. For those who do not patch test, there may be difficulty in detecting the cause. For those who do, the diagnosis becomes rather easy, as all of the test sites develop a ringed eruption from contact with the aluminum (Finn) chambers.

PATCH TESTING

The decision to patch test in children should be based on the same criteria as in adults. The patch tests using Finn chambers are mildly uncomfortable when placed on the back and in general are tolerated better in children over 10 years of age. Children do not have as much room on their backs to do extensive testing, so they may have to come back after the skin has had a chance to heal from the first group of tests in order to complete any longer series of tests. Areas such as the abdomen, forearm, and hips are not ideal for patch testing; the back is preferable. Placing only a few pertinent antigens on the upper arm is a more comfortable mode in some patients who, for any reason, would not tolerate a 2-day application of patch tests on the back.

Children may loosen patch tests because of their increased activity, and parents should be advised not to reinforce the tape if the patch tests have come partially off. It is better simply to report the occurrence to the physician. If the tests are negative, they may have to be redone. The use of Mastisol or Hollister adhesive may help to make the Scanpor tape used in patch testing adhere better to the skin.

Some physicians suggest using half-strength patch-test ingredients in children up to 5 years of age.[5] However, many physicians use the adult concentration in their patch tests without any difficulty. Pevny et al.,[24] with 10 years of experience in patch testing from 3 to 16 years of age, concluded that positive patch tests are relatively infrequent but that 90 percent of the positive reactions were relevant. He also found that children can use the same concentrations as adults for patch testing without adverse reactions.

An application called the *use test* may be used for more irritating topical products when the product concentration is not known. The suspected material is rubbed on the normal skin of the upper inner arm, antecubital fossa, or sometimes the face or neck twice daily for 1 to 3 weeks.[25] If an eczematous reaction occurs, the test should be considered positive and the substance avoided, with possible retesting under occlusion at a separate site when the dermatitis clears.

Your child has had a series of patch tests applied to the back or arms.

WHAT EXACTLY IS A PATCH TEST?

When we suspect an allergy to a substance, plant or chemical, we can reproduce the allergy in a limited area in order to prove that the rash is caused by that specific chemical.

WHY DO WE PATCH TEST?

Basically we would like to find the underlying cause of the dermatitis. This is the best way for us to verify the allergy. Knowing exactly what chemical is involved can help us find other sources of the agent with which your child may be coming in contact.

DOES IT HURT?

No, it feels like a Band-Aid on the back and therefore does not hurt. It may cause some mild restriction of motion.

WHAT CAN I TELL MY CHILD?

The nurse will put a small amount of salve in a metal bandage, which then will be attached to the back for 48 hours (2 days). It will feel a little snug, like a watch.

WHAT RESTRICTIONS SHOULD MY CHILD OBSERVE?

Your child should keep the back dry—in other words, no swimming or activities that would cause perspiration. Tub baths are permitted as long as the patch tests don't get wet, but showers are not allowed. This applies until after the next clinic appointment, which is usually at 72 hours (3 days).

ARE ANY PROBLEMS TO BE ANTICIPATED?

If the back itches severely, you should find out which test is causing the problem. You can do so by pressing on each individual disk. The one causing the itching will sting and burn when pressed. Clip that particular disk out of the tape. Wipe the excess patch test material from the site with a damp cloth. You might be instructed to apply a hydrocortisone 1% ointment to that area until you come back for your next visit.

This information is provided to help persons with contact dermatitis in the understanding of their problem. The contents are subject to change as more information becomes available and are not intended as a substitute for medical treatment.

Applying patch tests takes time, and small children can become impatient if the waiting time is too long. It may be helpful to have everything ready before the child is brought into the room. An explanation of everything that is to be done helps to keep the child interested and quiet, while engaging in conversation about school and pets makes the process go more quickly. Some children's books, such as *Where's Waldo?* can help divert their attention also. At our university center, we may even send parent and child to the cafeteria for ice cream while the antigens are being loaded into Finn chambers. The True Test may be helpful here, as it can be applied with very little waiting.

Because the area on a child's back is smaller than on that of an adult, it is important to take accurate measurements, in advance, of the area where the patches are to be placed. This can be done with a panel of empty chambers or a template, using a marking pen to mark the area. Since children are wiggly, and patch tests should be applied when the child is erect and leaning forward to give a little play in the tape.

PREVENTION

Avoidance of the provocative allergen is the most effective therapeutic measure. Handouts on specific antigens are included in Part II (see Chaps. 10 to 29). It is hoped that these will help patients to avoid these substances.

Teaching older children how to recognize poison ivy is helpful. However, if contact with poison ivy is unavoidable, thick protective clothing and the use of a barrier cream such as Stokogard on exposed skin can be helpful. This cream can be left on up to 8 h; it should be washed off with soap and water as soon as possible after plant exposure. If plants must be handled directly, vinyl gloves or plastic baggies can also be worn over the hands to protect the skin.

In order to detect nickel in jewelry or other metallic objects, a nickel detection kit (Allerderm Laboratories, Inc., P.O. Box 931, Mill Valley, CA 94941-0931) can be used. This chemical (dimethylglyoxime) is applied to the metal object and the solution turns pink if free nickel is present. The patient can thus avoid contact with these objects.

Vinyl gloves that do not contain rubber—useful to persons who are sensitive to rubber products—can also be ordered through Allerderm Laboratories.

REFERENCES

1. Cronin E: *Contact Dermatitis.* Edinburgh, Churchill Livingston, 1980, p 20.
2. Rademaker M, Forsythe A: Contact dermatitis in children. *Contact Dermatitis* 20:104–107, 1989.
3. Ayala F, Balato N, Lembro G, Patruno C, et al: A multicentre study of contact sensitization in children. *Contact Dermatitis* 26:307–310, 1992.
4. Gonçalo S, Gonçalo M, Azenha A, et al: Allergic contact dermatitis in children. *Contact Dermatitis* 26:112–115, 1992.
5. Pambor M, Winkler S, Bloch Y: Allergic contact dermatitis in children. *Contact Dermatitis* 24:72–75, 1991.
6. Kuiters GRR, Smitt JHS, Cohen EB, Bos JD: Allergic contact dermatitis in children and young adults. *Arch Dermatol* 125:1531–1533, 1989.
7. Caraffini S, Lisi P: Nummular dermatitis-like eruption from ethylenediamine hydrochloride in 2 children. *Contact Dermatitis* 17:313–314, 1987.

8. Geczy AF, deWeck AL: Molecular basis of T cell dependent genetic control of the immune response in the guinea pig. *Prog Allergy* 22:147–199, 1977.

9. Sharma OP, James DG, Fox RA: A correlation of in vivo delayed-type hypersensitivity with in vitro lymphocyte transformation in sarcoidosis. *Chest* 60:35–37, 1971.

10. Nilsson E, Mikaelsson B, Andersson S: Atopy, occupation and domestic work as risk factors for hand eczema in hospital workers. *Contact Dermatitis* 13:416–423, 1985.

11. Lauerma AI, Reitamo S: Contact allergy to corticosteroids. *J Am Acad Dermatol* 28:618–622, 1993.

12. Fisher AA: *Contact Dermatitis,* 3d ed. Philadelphia, Lea & Febiger, 1986.

13. Epstein WL, Byers VS, Frankart W: Induction of antigen specific hyposensitization to poison oak in sensitized adults. *Arch Dermatol* 118:630–633, 1982.

14. Benezra C, Ducombs G, Sell Y, et al (eds): *Plant Contact Dermatitis.* Toronto, Decker, 1985, pp 68–83.

15. Prystowsky SD, Allen AM, Smith RW, et al: Allergic contact hypersensitivity to nickel, neomycin, ethylenediamine, and benzocaine. *Arch Dermatol* 115:959–962, 1979.

16. Fisher AA: Nickel dermatitis in children. *Cutis* 47:19–21, 1991.

17. Heskel NS: Contact dermatitis in children. *Dermatol Clin* 2:579–584, 1984.

18. Adams RM, Fisher AA: Contact allergen alternatives. *J Am Acad Dermatol* 14:951–969, 1986.

19. Fisher AA: Condom dermatitis in either partner. *Cutis* 39:281–285, 1987.

20. Weston WL, Weston JA, Kinoshita J, et al: Prevalence of positive epicutaneous tests among infants, children, and adolescents. *Pediatrics* 78:1070–1074, 1986.

21. Held JL, Kalb RE, Ruszkowski AM, DeLeo V: Allergic contact dermatitis from bacitracin. *J Am Acad Dermatol* 17:592–594, 1987.

22. Katz BE, Fisher AA: Bacitracin: A unique topical antibiotic sensitizer. *J Am Acad Dermatol* 17:1016–1024, 1987.

23. Veien NK, Hattel T, Justesen O, Norholm A: Aluminum allergy. *Contact Dermatitis* 15:295–297, 1986.

24. Pevny I, Brennenstuhl M, Razinskas G: Patch testing in children. *Contact Dermatitis* 11:201–206, 1984.

25. Epstein WL: The use test for contact hypersensitivity. *Arch Dermtol Res* 272:279–281, 1982.

26. Weston WL, Weston JA: Allergic contact dermatitis in children. *Am J Dis Child* 138:932–936, 1984.

45

THIMEROSAL

Jere D. Guin

WHAT IS THIMEROSAL?

Thimerosal is another name for Merthiolate, the active ingredient in tincture of Merthiolate. Chemically, it is a mercurial derivative of thiosalicylic acid, sodium ethylmercurithiosalicylate,[1] used topically for its antibacterial and antifungal activity. It is widely known as a first aid product available as "tincture of Merthiolate" for home use, but it is also used as a preservative in cosmetics, topical medications, contact lens solutions and eye ointments, topical corticosteroids,[2] antiseptic sprays,[3] tuberculin tests, as a surgical prep, and as a preservative in scratch and intradermal tests,[4] "vaccines" for immunization,[5] and antitoxins.

HOW DOES ONE RECOGNIZE CONTACT ALLERGY TO THIMEROSAL?

The rash associated with thimerosal is so extremely variable that—except for reactions in and around the eyes—it would be difficult to anticipate. Most persons with a positive test do not have a history of an allergic reaction. Thimerosal has been called a "hidden allergen" because most of those who react to it lack a history of relevant exposure.[6] This is thought to be due to sensitization to thimerosal in antigens used in allergy and intradermal testing, in which there is opportunity for sensitization. This theory also explains the predominance of reactors in younger age groups and their large numbers in earlier childhood.[7,8] In some countries, another prominent factor is probably the use of antiseptics and thimerosal-preserved topical agents in the treatment of eczematous eruptions, especially stasis eczema.[9]

When there is a reaction, it may be a blepharitis or follicular conjunctivitis[10]; pompholyx[11]; dermatitis at the site of an immunization (injection)[12]; which may become persistent[13]; aggravation of atopic eczema following an injection[14]; allergy to topical corticosteroids[15]; laryngeal obstruction following use of an antiseptic throat spray[3]; generalized urticaria or exanthematous eruption[16]; cosmetic reactions[17]; eyelid[18] or hand eczema[19] from handling contact lens solution; false-positive skin test intradermal reactions[4]; and photosensitivity to piroxicam (Feldene), where reactors are allergic to thimerosal.[20–22]

This is an extremely relevant allergen in ophthalmology patients,[10] with (in one series) about two-thirds reacting to ophthalmic ointments and a third to contact lens solutions.[10] In fact, the only significant association is in those ophthalmologic problems.[23] In one series of toxic papillary reactions, preservatives (mostly thimerosal) were proved to cause 7.4 percent of problems and another 37 percent were "probable."[24] Thimerosal is also one of the causes of "vehicle" sensitivity.[25]

NATURE OF THE ALLERGY

Many years ago the problem was simple. It was considered an allergy to the thiosalicylic component.[26] Some persons are allergic to that component, some to mercury (both organic and inorganic), and some to both. Some series cited are too small to draw firm conclusions, and one has to use data from numerous studies to see the variation in reactivity which is there.

The lack of a history of a probable sensitizing experience has kept the source a bit of a mystery. Immunization has been suspected,[5] but the incidence following immunization was not high, even where there was a reaction, and the procedure did not cause sensitization experimentally.[9] However, exposure to thimerosal used as a preservative in antigens for immunotherapy,[23] scratch, and intradermal tuberculin testing[9] may be part of the answer. Where tuberculin testing was routine, the incidence of reactions in the normal population in the third decade was high,[9] perhaps because of the putative adjuvant effect of the test material.[9] Other considerations are contamination of the needle used with thimerosal-containing solutions[12] and use of creams and solutions on eczematous skin, especially stasis eczema.[9]

Cross-reactions at one time were said to occur with inorganic mercurials, but not with the organic ones.[27] There are now publications showing that either organic or inorganic mercurials may or may not cause a reaction in these patients,[11–13,28] but the numbers are perhaps not high enough to show all types of reactions in every series, especially the smaller ones. These test series are not in the same population either, as the total number of individuals reacting to thimerosal is greatly different from one to another. For example, cross-reactions with mercury in one series from the United Kingdom were 59 percent (17/29), with an incidence of thimerosal reactivity of 1 percent of those who were patch-tested.[8] In Japan, which seems to have the highest incidence, it was about one-third of the 16.3 percent who were allergic to thimerosal.[5] Ammoniated mercury is more likely to be positive in thimerosal reactors than in nonreactors in larger series.[28] The commonsense solution is to test the patient, as each person may be different, anyway.

Because of its chemical structure, persons allergic to this chemical may be allergic either to the mercury component, to thiosalicylic acid, or to both.[26,29]

CONSIDERATIONS IN PATCH TESTING

The percentage of reactors to thimerosal depends entirely on the group tested. This is one of the few examples of an antigen which is as positive in testing (normal) subjects from the general population as it is in persons suspected of having contact dermatitis.[12] The concentration and vehicle for the test material varies somewhat in published series.

Most groups use 0.1% in petrolatum, but this is a marginal irritant.[30] The concentration used is important, as 0.01% fails to produce reactions in any of those who react at 0.5%.[31]

The choice of vehicle and test patch is also important. An aqueous antigen has also been used, and this has in the past been a satisfactory vehicle for thimerosal. However, there may be a problem in testing with some antigens containing mercury under aluminum, because of the tendency to form an irritant oxide.[32] This was noticed originally when a patient prepped with thimerosal received diathermy with an aluminum electrode, causing a blistering irritant effect.[32] This type irritation also occurs from the interaction of mercury in thimerosal and aluminum in a Finn chamber. Mercury tends to corrode the aluminum chamber, but this is prevented if the chamber is coated with plastic.[33] This seems to be a quality of the aqueous vehicle, and at least one investigator states that this is not a problem with a petrolatum vehicle.[34] Irritant reactions can be prominent, however, if this testing is not done properly. For a long time, we have covered thimerosal patch tests with an adhesive plaster rather than a Finn chamber and have seen fewer 3+ reactions.

Irritation can be a problem anyway, as thimerosal is a marginal irritant in the concentration used.[30,31,35] Most reactions seen are probably allergic, according to Möller, based on a study of responses in identical and fraternal twins.[36]

Tincture of merthiolate may also be used for testing.[28,37] However, reactions to the dyes [D&C Red 22 (fluorescein) and D&C Yellow No. 7 (eosin YS)][28] and sometimes ethylenediamine[28,38] may occur.

The test site should probably be normal skin which has not been treated recently with topical corticosteroids, as even moderately weak topical corticosteroids may prevent a reaction on patch testing.[39]

Photopatch testing is done to piroxicam when photosensitivity to that agent is suspected. Such persons have been reliably allergic to thimerosal by regular patch testing on the basis of similarity of a moiety of piroxicam to thimerosal.[20,21,40-42] Sensitivity is felt to be due to a metabolite of piroxicam, which chemically resembles thimerosal. Guinea pig studies demonstrate that sensitization to thimerosal alone tends to make an animal both allergic and photoallergic to piroxicam.[42]

PREVENTION

It may be possible to immunize some sensitive individuals who are allergic to thimerosal but also must be immunized, without a high incidence of reactions.[43,44] In one series, the only persons with reactions were those given the injection (against the manufacturer's directions) subcutaneously.[44] The needle used should not be contaminated with a Merthiolate-preserved solution.[12] Both patient and physician should be aware of the possibility of both local and systemic reactions which can occur, as any contact with the skin is likely to elicit a reaction.[12]

Normally, the reagents used for immunization as well as intradermal and immunological testing should not contain thimerosal. Use of phenol, which is not very allergenic,[45] as a preservative in scratch-test antigens is supposed to reduce the incidence.

To avoid cross-reactions to products containing mercurials, patch testing or usage testing may have to be done before exposure, as some patients react to mercurials and some do not. Some are not allergic to the thiosalicylate component either,[46] and again, testing depends upon the situation and other positive and negative tests, perhaps in replicate and more than once. Obviously, thimerosal-allergic persons would do well to avoid piroxicam as well as Merthiolate and mercurials.

Irritant reactions to thimerosal are sometimes seen with surgical preps, especially when the agent is allowed to pool with the patient in the lithotomy position. The reaction is supposed to stem from a surplus of Merthiolate, maceration, pressure, and irritation which occur during surgery. The lithotomy position seems to pose a special risk. Leaving the area open and letting it dry before draping reportedly helps to prevent this.[47]

REFERENCES

1. *Merck Index,* 11th ed. Rahway, NJ, Merck & Co, 1989, pp 1467–1468.
2. Wilkinson DS: Thiomersal. *Contact Dermatitis* 5:58–59, 1979.
3. Maibach H: Acute laryngeal obstruction presumed secondary to thiomersal (Merthiolate) delayed hypersensitivity. *Contact Dermatitis* 1:221–222, 1975.
4. Epstein S: Sensitivity to merthiolate: A cause of false delayed intradermal reaction. *J Allergy* 34:225–234, 1963.
5. Osawa J, Kitamura K, Ikezawa Z, Nakajima H: A probable role for vaccines containing thimerosal in thimerosal hypersensitivity. *Contact Dermatitis* 24:178–182, 1991.
6. Wekkeli M, Hippmann G, Rosenkranz AR, et al: Mercury as a contact allergen. *Contact Dermatitis* 22:295–296, 1990.
7. Barros MA, Baptista A, Correia TM, Azevedo F: Patch testing in children: A study of 562 schoolchildren. *Contact Dermatitis* 25:156–159, 1991.
8. Novak M, Kvicalova E, Friedlanderova B: Reactions to Merthiolate in infants. *Contact Dermatitis* 15:309–310, 1986.
9. Möller H: Why thimerosal allergy? *Int J Dermatol* 19:29, 1980.
10. Tosti A, Tosti G: Thimerosal: A hidden allergen in ophthalmology. *Contact Dermatitis* 18:268–273, 1988.
11. Möller H: Merthiolate allergy: A nationwide iatrogenic sensitization. *Acta Derm Venereol* 57:509–517, 1977.
12. Forstrom L, Hannuksela M, Kousa M, Lehmuskallio E: Merthiolate hypersensitivity and vaccination. *Contact Dermatitis* 6:241–245, 1980.
13. Cox NH, Forsyth A: Thimerosal allergy and vaccination reactions. *Contact Dermatitis* 18:229–233, 1988.
14. Cox N, Morley WN: Vaccination reactions and thimerosal. *Br Med J* 294:250, 1987.
15. Coskey RJ: Contact dermatitis due to multiple corticosteroid creams. *Arch Dermatol* 114:115–117, 1978.
16. Tosti A, Melino M, Bardazzi F: Systemic reactions due to thimerosal. *Contact Dermatitis* 15:187–188, 1986.
17. Emmons WW, Marks JG Jr: Immediate and delayed reactions to cosmetic ingredients. *Contact Dermatitis* 13:258–265, 1985.
18. de Groot AC, van Wijnen WG, van Wijnen-Vos M: Occupational contact dermatitis of the eyelids, without ocular involvement, from thimerosal in contact lens fluid. *Contact Dermatitis* 23:195, 1990.
19. Stolman LP, Sands E: Contact-lens hand (letter). *N Engl J Med* 311:1521, 1984.
20. Serrano G, Bonillo J, Aliaga A, et al: Piroxicam-induced photosensitivity and contact sensitivity to thiosalicylic acid. *J Am Acad Dermatol* 23:479–483, 1990.
21. McKerrow KJ, Greig DE: Piroxicam-induced photosensitive dermatitis. *J Am Acad Dermatol* 15:1237–1241, 1986.
22. de la Cuadra J, Pujol C, Aliaga A: Clinical evidence of cross-sensitivity between thiosalicylic acid, a contact allergen, and piroxicam, a photoallergen. *Contact Dermatitis* 21:349–351, 1989.
23. Tosti A, Guerra L, Bardazzi F: Hyposensitizing therapy with standard antigenic extracts: An important source of thimerosal sensitization (see comments). *Contact Dermatitis* 20:173–176, 1989.
24. Wilson FM II: Adverse external ocular effects of topical ophthalmic therapy: An epidemiologic, laboratory, and clinical study. *Trans Am Ophthalmol Soc* 81:854–965, 1983.

25. Hannuksela M, Kousa M, Pirila V: Allergy to ingredients of vehicles. *Contact Dermatitis* 2:105–110, 1976.
26. Ellis FA, Robinson HM: The sensitizing factor in Merthiolate. *J Allergy* 18:212–213, 1947.
27. Fisher AA: Allergic reactions to Merthiolate (thimerosal). *Cutis* 27:580, 582, 587, 1981.
28. Seidenari S, Manzini BM, Modenese M, Danese P: Contact sensitization to thimerosal in healthy subjects [Ita]. *G Ital Dermatolog Venereol* 124:335–339, 1989.
29. Lachapelle JM, Chabeau G, Ducombs G, et al: Multicenter survey related to the frequency of positive patch tests with mercury and thiomersal [Fre]. *Ann Dermatol Venereol* 115:793–796, 1988.
30. Cronin E: *Contact Dermatitis*. Edinburgh, Churchill Livingstone, 1980, pp 689–692.
31. Marzulli FN, Maibach HI: Effects of vehicles and elicitation concentration in contact dermatitis testing: I. Experimental contact sensitization in humans. *Contact Dermatitis* 2:325–329, 1976.
32. Thelwall Jones H: Danger of skin burns from thimerosal. *Br Med J* 2:504–505, 1972.
33. Kalveram KJ, Rapp-Frick C, Sorck G: Misleading patch test results with aluminum Finn chambers and mercury salts. *Contact Dermatitis* 6:507–508, 1980.
34. Lindemayr H, Becerano ST: Interaction of mercury compounds and aluminum. *Contact Dermatitis* 13:274, 1985.
35. Iden DL, Schroeter AL: The vehicle tray revisited: The use of the vehicle tray in assessing allergic contact dermatitis by a 24-hour application method. *Contact Dermatitis* 3:122–126, 1977.
36. Holst R, Moller H: Merthiolate Testing in twins. *Contact Dermatitis* 1:370–372, 1975.
37. Sertoli A, Di Fonzo E, Spallanzani P, Panconesi E: Allergic contact dermatitis from thimerosol in a soft contact lens wearer. *Contact Dermatitis* 6:292–293, 1980.
38. Fisher AA: Cross reactions between ethylenediamine base in merthiolate tincture with ethylenediamine HCl. *Contact Dermatitis* 14:181, 1986.
39. Rietschel RL: Irritant and allergic responses as influenced by triamcinolone in patch test materials. *Arch Dermatol* 121:68–69, 1985.
40. Cirne de Castro JL, Vale E, Martins M: Mechanism of photosensitive reactions induced by piroxicam (letter). *J Am Acad Dermatol* 20:706–707, 1989.
41. de Castro JL, Freitas JP, Brandao FM, Themido R: Sensitivity to thimerosal and photosensitivity to piroxicam. *Contact Dermatitis* 24:187–192, 1991.
42. Kitamura K, Osawa J, Ikezawa Z, Nakajima H: Cross-reactivity between sensitivity to thimerosal and photosensitivity to piroxicam in guinea pigs. *Contact Dermatitis* 25:30–34, 1991.
43. Hansson H, Moller H: Cutaneous reactions to Merthiolate and their relationship to vaccination with tetanus toxoid. *Acta Allergol* 26:150–156, 1971.
44. Aberer W: Vaccination despite thimerosal sensitivity. *Contact Dermatitis* 24:6–10, 1991.
45. Falagiani P: Thimerosal in standard antigenic extracts (letter; comment). *Contact Dermatitis* 21:354, 1989.
46. Hansson H, Moller H: Patch test reactions to Merthiolate in healthy young subjects. *Br J Dermatol* 83:349–356, 1970.
47. Hodgkinson DJ, Irons GB, Williams TJ: Chemical burns and skin preparation solutions. *Surg Gynecol Obstet* 147:534–536, 1978.

46

THE ROLE OF THE HOUSE DUST MITE IN ATOPIC ECZEMA

Hideo Nakayama

ATOPIC ECZEMA IS NOT MONOLITHIC

Atopic dermatitis is a multifactorial disease, and no one underlying cause can explain all of its characteristics. However, various precipitating factors can aggravate the condition. The successful management of atopic dermatitis often requires that these precipitating or trigger factors, often called flare factors, be addressed when one educates the patient or the patient's parents. This helps not only to understand the problem but also to aid in its treatment.

THE ROLE OF THE LOWLY DUST MITE

For a time, allergy as a cause of atopic dermatitis fell from favor with dermatologists, perhaps because immunotherapy was a less than satisfactory method of managing atopic eczema. Recently, however, there has been a renewal of interest in the role of food and respiratory allergens in the aggravation of atopic eczema. This has been especially true for the dust mite. Approximately ten species of such mites are found in sufficient numbers to be clinically relevant. Of these, *Dermatophagoides pteronyssinus, Dermatophagoides farinae, Dermatophagoides microseras,* and *Euroglyphus maynei* are the most important, especially the first two (Fig. 46-1). In 1969, Voorhorst et al.[1] found an association between the house dust mite and allergy to house dust; following that, skin and RAST tests for *D. pteronyssinus* and *D. farinae* were quickly introduced. The antigens for immediate and delayed reactions have traditionally been separated, but now IgE has been found to bind to the Langerhans cell in the epidermis,[2] suggesting that it may be involved in the production of delayed hypersensitivity as well as type I responses. Peripheral blood mononuclear cells bearing the CD4 markers for (helper) activity can be found in patients with skin sensitivity to the house dust mite, *D. pteronyssinus.*[3]

The same antigen has been used to look for both delayed and immediate sensitivity in patients with atopic eczema, and either or both types of reaction may be positive or negative in a given patient. The specific IgE causing immediate reactivity is present in some 20 to 60 percent of persons with atopic eczema,[4,5] and approximately 30 to

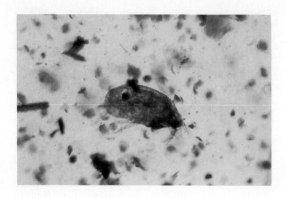

FIG. 46–1. Commonly seen house dust mite *Dermatophagoides,* found in house dust from the home of a patient with atopic dermatitis.

40 percent are patch-test positive.[6–9] The number of persons with immediate reactivity may be greater in patients over 50 years of age,[10] and even a date of birth between May and November is thought by some to influence the likelihood of developing sensitivity.[11]

CAN WE RECOGNIZE THOSE LIKELY TO BE ALLERGIC?

Some studies show an association of disease severity and exposure,[5] but others do not.[12] One report noted an association of increased IgE levels, which was thought to be caused by exposure to mites from scratching.[13]

Imayama et al.[14] described different morphologic presentations of patients with atopic dermatitis according to whether or not they had significant delayed and/or immediate sensitivity to *D. pteronyssinus*. Those with delayed reactivity only are more likely to show a papulovesicular eruption in a flexural location (Fig. 46-2). Patients with immediate sensitivity only tend to develop a diffuse erythematous and edematous eruptions over "every body surface." Those with both types of allergy have erythematous plaques with lichenification and papulovesicular lesions on the face and other areas. Patients who demonstrate neither immediate nor delayed sensitivity to *D. pteronyssinus* were relatively clear.

There are problems with the demonstration of delayed hypersensitivity to the house dust mite, as patch testing to this organism has not been standardized. Van Voorst Vader et al.[6] tried a number of techniques in an effort to optimize the patch test and found that two-thirds of their patients who were positive would have been negative had they not had tape stripping done prior to patch-test application. This is thought to be a function of poor absorption, but immediate reactivity which can exacerbate eczema can be shown to surprisingly low levels when allergens are applied to the surface of normal skin.[13]

Certain technical factors are different from routine patch testing. The tests done with aluminum (Finn) chambers sometimes produce negative responses in an allergic individual, while convex plastic chambers are more likely to be produce positive reactions in the same patient. Other factors that tend to increase the yield include higher concentrations (such as 500 times the amount necessary to cause a positive prick test), 48-h application time, and rigorous tape stripping prior to testing. Nonspecific reactions seem to occur more frequently in patients with more widespread dermatitis.

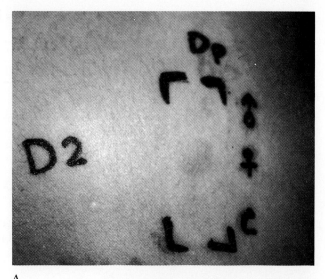

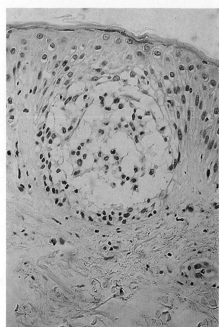

FIG. 46–2. *A*. Strong positive reactions to three crushed *Dermatophagoides* in a patient with atopic dermatitis on day 2 of the patch test. (See color Plate 43.) *B*. Histopathologic examination showed spongiosis of the epidermis, a typical feature of delayed-type contact hypersensitivity.   B

Use of live mites for patch testing is also important. Patch testing is often positive when as few as three live mites are crushed just before the tests are applied, but it is likely to be negative to dead mites in greater quantity (Table 46-1). In one series, 12 of 48 patients were positive to live mites, but no patients reacted to dead mites.[15] The reason may be that certain proteases are present in the live mites. In fact, the antigens found in *D. pteronyssinus* include cysteine proteases and trypsins.[16] The former are subject to denaturization, which may explain the change in antigenicity. In atopic

TABLE 46–1. Comparison of the Results of Patch Tests Using Crushed Live Mites and Dried Dead Mites[15]

Patch-Test Materials	Crushed Live Mites			Dried Dead Mites		
Reaction	Positive[a]	Negative	Total	Positive[a]	Negative	Total
Atopic dermatitis patients	12	36	48	0	24	24
Control patients[b]	0	15	15	0	7	7

[a]More than (+) of ICDRG criteria.

[b]Dermatitis patients other than those with atopic dermatitis, including 14 with contact dermatitis, 1 with corticosteroid dermatosis, and 3 with prurigo vulgaris.

eczema, the antigen seems to be a product of the mite itself rather than the fecal material, which is important in asthma.[17]

The time of reading may vary somewhat, as some tests are positive immediately (with urticarial reactions), some are eczematous at 6 to 8 h, and some at 24 to 48 h.[8] Therefore multiple readings are in order.

WHAT IS THE ASSOCIATION OF ENVIRONMENT WITH ATOPIC ECZEMA?

The number of mites per 0.1 g of dust is higher in the homes of patients with atopic eczema,[18] and it is not caused by scale, as a group of psoriasis patients used as a control group did not show an increase of scale in their environment.[19] Attempts to remove dust from the environment to alleviate the stimulation have met with mixed success. One report denied benefit,[20] while others disagree.[21] It may not even be necessary to stay in a dust-free environment, as patients kept in an experimental environment only 11 h per day were free of itching in 2 to 3 weeks.[22]

Other respiratory antigens can also elicit a positive patch test; in some series, such antigens more commonly lead to positive tests than antigens from the dust mite.[23] The differences are probably as much due to methodology as to patient populations. Until a standard method is available, the result must be interpreted in the light of each patient's situation.

IS THE MECHANISM THE SAME AS IN OTHER TYPES OF CONTACT DERMATITIS?

The initial urticarial response following exposure to respiratory allergens can turn into a type IV response, which can be seen histologically.[9] Positive patch-test reactions tend to show a mild perivascular infiltration of lymphocytes and edema in the papillary dermis at 24 h. At 48 h, the lymphocytic infiltration is more prominent and is mixed with eosinophils. Intercellular edema is present in the epidermis; by 72 h eosinophils and lymphocytes can be found there with spongiotic bullae.[9] Some reports have claimed that the presence of basophils, eosinophils, and mononuclear cells is evidence of cutaneous basophilic hypersensitivity.[24] Repeated application of allergen is followed by an increase in skin mast cells by day 6, the mast cell hyperplasia having replaced the earlier basophilic infiltration.[24]

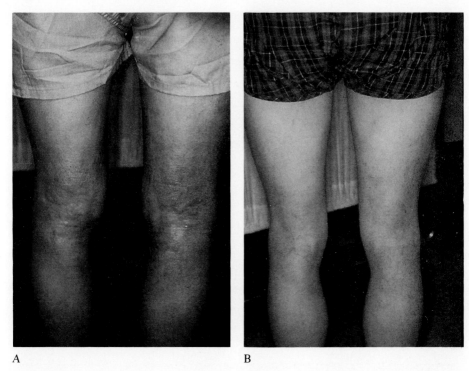

A   B

FIG. 46–3. The dramatic effect of eliminating mites from the home of a patient with atopic dermatitis, a 22-year-old man who was hypersensitive to *Dermatophagoides*. *A*. Characteristic eczema of the popliteal fossa, which could not be cured by any treatment in the previous 5 years, before mite elimination. *B*. The same patient's skin, now normal, exactly 1 year later. (Elimination of mites from the patient's home was completed after the first photograph was taken. Ointments were no longer necessary after removal of mites.) (Photo courtesy Kumei A, M.D.)

WHAT DOES THIS MEAN FOR TREATMENT?

Persons with atopic eczema who do not respond to standard treatment probably have some factor complicating the picture. This may be a contact allergy to a medication such as hydrocortisone, an environmental irritant, or intolerance to some topical medicament. They may also have experienced a break in routine, such as irritation or contact sensitization from textiles, or contact with carpeting or upholstery. They may be bathing too much or be retaining sweat. Sometimes, respiratory and food allergens are worth considering. Sensitivity to the house dust mite is a newcomer to this approach, but it may be an important one (Figs. 46-3 and 46-4). Usually an IgE level or RAST to the mite is obtained and perhaps a prick test is done. If cultured live mites are available, the application of three crushed mites under a convex chamber is advised. If not, vigorous tape stripping may help. Following the establishment of an association, an environment with a greatly reduced dust content is advised even when only a reduced all-night exposure can be worked into the patient's routine. Ventilation and decreased humidity seem to be beneficial.[25]

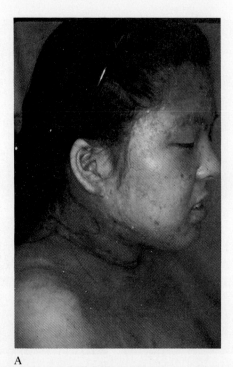

A

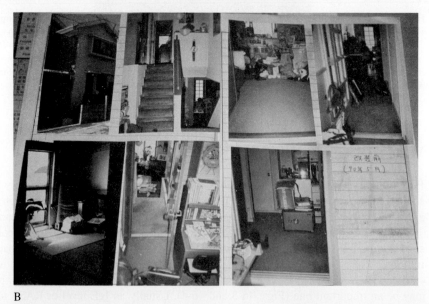

B

FIG. 46–4. Another case of mite elimination. The patient (*A*), a 20-year-old woman, had been suffering from severe atopic dermatitis since childhood. *B*. Based on her hypersensitivity to mites, the mite population in her home was investigated and mites were eliminated. *C*. All carpets, mattresses, bedding, and seating were replaced with mite-resistant types. *D*. The patient's skin exactly 3 months after the first photograph was taken. (Photo courtesy Kumei A, M.D.)

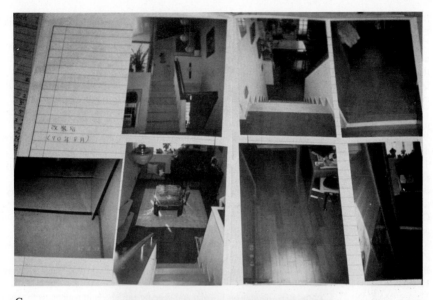

C

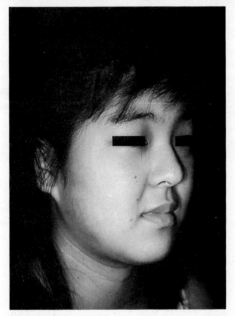

D

FIG. 46–4. *(Continued)*

REFERENCES

1. Voorhorst R, Spieksma FTM, Varekamp H: House dust atopy and the the house dust mite *Dermatophagoides pteronyssinus*. 72:115, 1969.

2. Bruynzeel-Koomen C, Wichen DF, Toonstra J, et al: The presence of IgE molecules on epidermal Langerhans cells in patients with atopic dermatitis. *Arch Dermatol Res* 278:199–205, 1986.
3. Rawle FC, Mitchell EB, Platts-Mills TA: T cell responses to the major allergen from the house dust mite *Dermatophagoides pteronyssinus*—Antigen P1: comparison of patients with asthma, atopic dermatitis, and perennial rhinitis. *J Immunol* 133:195–201, 1984.
4. Seidenari S, Manzini BM, Danese P, Giannetti A: Positive patch tests to whole mite culture and purified mite extracts in patients with atopic dermatitis, asthma, and rhinitis. *Ann Allerg* 69:201–206, 1992.
5. Uehara M, Sawai T: Familial background of respiratory atopy: A factor of type I allergy to house dust mite in patients with atopic dermatitis. *Arch Dermatol* 125:939–943, 1989.
6. Van Voorst Vader PC, Lier JG, Woest TE, et al: Patch tests with house dust mite antigens in atopic dermatitis patients: Methodological problems. *Acta Derm Venereol* 71:301–305, 1991.
7. Tanaka Y, Tanaka M, Anan S, Yoshida H: Immunohistochemical studies on dust mite antigen in positive reaction site of patch test. *Acta Derm Venereol Suppl* 144:93–96, 1989.
8. Bruynzeel-Koomen CA, Van Wichen DF, Spry CJ, et al: Active participation of eosinophils in patch test reactions to inhalant allergens in patients with atopic dermatitis. *Br J Dermatol* 118:229–238, 1988.
9. Gondo A, Saeki N, Tokuda Y: Challenge reactions in atopic dermatitis after percutaneous entry of mite antigen. *Br J Dermatol* 115:485–493, 1986.
10. Kawashima T, Kobayashi S, Miyano M, et al: Senile type atopic dermatitis. *Nippon Hifuka Gakkai Zasshi* 99:1095–1103, 1989.
11. Beck HI, Hagdrup HK: Atopic dermatitis, house dust mite allergy and month of birth. *Acta Derm Venereol* 67:448–451, 1987.
12. Mackie RM, Cobb SJ, Cochran REI, Thompson J: Total and specific IgE levels in patients with atopic dermatitis: The correlation between prick testing, clinical history of allergy, and in vitro quantitation of IgE during clinical exacerbation and remission. *Clin Exp Dermatol* 4:187–195, 1979.
13. Norris PG, Schofield O, Camp RD: A study of the role of house dust mite in atopic dermatitis. *Br J Dermatol* 118:435–440, 988.
14. Imayama S, Hashizume T, Miyahara H, et al: Combination of patch test and IgE for dust mite antigens differentiates 130 patients with atopic dermatitis into four groups. *J Am Acad Dermatol* 27:531–538, 1992.
15. Kumei A, Nakayama H, Sakurai M, et al: Results of patch test using mite components in atopic dermatitis (AD) patients—1st report: "As is patch test" using crushed mites. *Nippon Hifuka Gakkai Zasshi* 100:1127–1134, 1990.
16. Platts-Mills TA, Thomas WR, Aalberse RC, et al: Dust mite allergens and asthma: Report of a second international workshop. *J Allergy Clin Immunol* 89:1046–1060, 1992.
17. Thompson SJ, Whitley HJ, Naysmith JD, Carswell F: IgE antibodies to *D. pteronyssinus* in atopic patients. *Immunology* 64:311–314, 1988.
18. Colloff MJ: Exposure to house dust mites in homes of people with atopic dermatitis. *Br J Dermatol* 127:322–327, 1992.
19. Beck HI, Korsgaard J: Atopic dermatitis and house dust mites. *Br J Dermatol* 120:245–251, 1989.
20. Colloff MJ, Lever RS, McSharry C: A controlled trial of house dust mite eradication using natamycin in homes of patients with atopic dermatitis: Effect on clinical status and mite populations. *Br J Dermatol* 121:199–208, 1989.
21. Vickers CF: A controlled-trial of house dust mite eradication using natamycin in homes of patients with atopic dermatitis (letter, comment). *Br J Dermatol* 122:426, 1990.
22. Fukuda H, Imalyama S, Okada K: The mite-free room (MFR) for the management of atopic dermatitis: Living in the MFR improved first the itch and then the dermatitis. *Jpn J Allergol* 40:626–632, 1991.
23. Reitamo S, Visa K, Kahonen K, et al: Patch test reactions to inhalant allergens in atopic dermatitis. *Acta Derm Venereol Suppl* 144:199–121, 1989.
24. Mitchell EB, Crow J, Williams G, Platts-Mills TA: Increase in skin mast cells following chronic house dust mite exposure. *Br J Dermatol* 114:65–73, 1986.
25. Harving H, Korsgaard J, Dahl R: House-dust mites and associated environmental conditions in Danish homes. *Allergy* 48:106–109, 1993.

47

EYELID DERMATITIS

Hideo Nakayama

A regional distribution of any eczema tends to make the experienced dermatologist consider a group of certain diseases associated with that region. Eyelid dermatitis is a very special case because the eyelids are a region associated with atopic dermatitis, seborrheic dermatitis, rosacea, and irritant and allergic contact dermatitis, to name a few. The condition may be part of a more widespread eczema or it may be found exclusively on the eyelids. Itching of the eyelids may also follow exposure to airborne allergens or contact urticaria. Hand transfer to the eyelid is another common source of eyelid eczema, and it can cause considerable difficulty when the patient's causative allergen is not uncovered with routine testing.

The reason contact dermatitis is a problem on the eyelids is probably related to the high level of percutaneous absorption characteristic of this region, combined with potential for irritation and the ease of hand transfer of allergens because of rubbing. One often expects to differentiate allergic and irritant dermatitis based on morphologic criteria. For example, allergic contact dermatitis typically shows erythema with a papulovesicular eruption and swelling accompanied by itching, while irritant dermatitis may show erythema, dryness, fine scaling, and more burning than itching, or at least less itching than allergic contact dermatitis. However, the combination of these two conditions in many patients and the confusion with eyelid eczema seen in atopic individuals tend to make morphologic differentiation difficult at best and often impossible without testing the patient. A number of published series on eyelid dermatitis have tried to separate the principal causes from the others, and the results vary. In one series, for example, atopic dermatitis was more prevalent than allergic contact dermatitis, although both are common,[1] while the reverse was true in another series.[2] Contact dermatitis of the eyelids, unlike hand eczema, is more often allergic than irritant.[1,3]

WHAT CAUSES ALLERGIC CONTACT DERMATITIS?

Many of the published causes of eyelid dermatitis are listed in Tables 47-1 and 47-2. Obviously, the prevalence depends upon usage in the patient's culture, the concentration used, and the condition of the skin at the time of application. For example, in some

TABLE 47–1. Checklist for Underlying Causes in Eyelid Dermatitis

Atopic dermatitis	Urticaria
Dermatomyositis	Contact
Seborrheic dermatitis	Systemic
Psoriasis	Irritant dermatitis
Rosacea	Bacterial infection
Respiratory	Neurodermatitis
allergy	Airborne contact

countries where Amlexanox is widely used as a noncorticosteroid anti-inflammatory eyedrop, this is perhaps the first consideration in suspected allergic contact dermatitis of the eyelids. Where this product is not marketed, it would not be part of the normal patch-test screen.

Common sources of contact dermatitis of the eyelids are given in Table 47-3. They include the following:

- Eyedrops[4–7]
- Contact lens solutions[8–12]
- Eyelash curlers[13–15]
- Eyelid cosmetics (Fig. 47-1)[16–19]

While chemicals in the workplace,[6,8,20] plants,[22–23] and medications[2,3] also produce contact dermatitis of the eyelids, they frequently involve the face as well.

Nail polish is another cause of allergic contact dermatitis of the eyelids in women. Most commonly, the allergen is *p*-toluene sulfonamide formaldehyde resin (available

TABLE 47–2. Causes of Allergic Contact Dermatitis of the Eyelids

Acrylates[30]	Levobunonol[6]
Artificial nail resins[27]	Nail polish[27]
Artificial nail adhesives[27]	Naphthyl mix[3]
Atropine[7]	Neomycin[2,3]
Balsam of Peru[2,3]	Nickel[2,3]
Benzocaine[3]	Phenylephrine[5]
Black rubber[41]	Pigment (D&C, Red 31, Yellow 11,
Chinoform[3]	phenyl-azo-naphthol, etc.[40]
Chlorhexidine[32]	PPD[3]
Chlorocresol[33]	Prednisolone[31]
Cocamidopropyl betaine[10]	*p-tertiary*-butylphenol formaldehyde
Colophony[3]	resin[3]
Compositae	Thimerosal[2,8]
Diaminodiphenylmethane[2]	Thiuram[3]
Epoxy resin[3,20]	Timolol[4,34]
Ethylenediamine[3]	Toluenesulfonamide formaldehyde resin
Formaldehyde[2]	Toxicodendrons
Fragrance[2,3,40]	Wood tars[3]
Kathon CG[2]	Wool alcohols[3]

**TABLE 47–3. Sources of Allergic
Contact Dermatitis of the Eyelids**

Contact lens solutions[8–11,35]	Makeup removers[39]
Cosmetics[36,40]	Mascara[16,17]
Eyedrops[4–7,31]	Medications
Eyelash curlers[37]	Plants
Eye shadow[17,38]	Sunscreens
Makeup applicators	

from Chemotechnique), although one can (and should) test the patient to individual nail polishes by open application on the upper arm. The reason that items applied to the fingernails can affect the eyelids is that women commonly rub their eyes with the backs of the fingertips. This brings the nail polish into close contact with the thin, readily penetrated eyelid skin. Many companies make nail polish that does not contain the allergen, and proof of safety can easily be determined by patch testing the patient to the product. In fact, in the United States, the patient can patch test herself at the cosmetic counter.

Another source of eyelid dermatitis is hand transfer. This is commonly seen in poison ivy dermatitis, and may be seen in persons handling rubber, metals, and other materials. Typically, photodermatitis spares the eyelids, while Compositae dermatitis may involve the eyelids. The latter is often attributed to "pollen," because the morphology is that of airborne contact, but scientific evidence suggests that it is probably another example of hand transfer in most cases.

Medications used to treat the eyes or eyelids may also be a problem. Reactions to latex or to topical medications, e.g., bacitracin or neomycin, caused by hand transfer can be seen in nurses after treating patients in a hospital or nursing home. Ophthalmic drops and ointments and contact lens solutions are all potential sources of contact dermatitis of the eyelids. Another special and often unsuspected source is sensitivity to topical corticosteroids. It may be necessary to do intradermal testing to totally rule out hydrocortisone as a possibility.

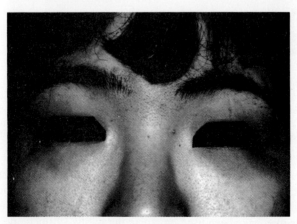

FIG. 47–1. Severe eyelid dermatitis due to contact hypersensitivity to wool alcohols in a 25-year-old woman. It was produced by the usage of eyelid cosmetics containing wool alcohols, and the patch test of 30% wool alcohols in petrolatum was strong positive.

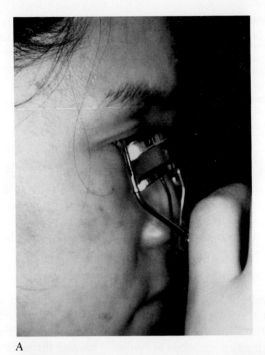

A

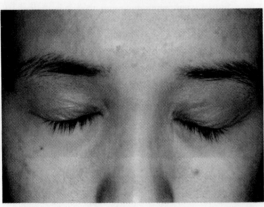

B

FIG. 47–2. Those who are hypersensitive to nickel should refrain from using an ordinary eyelash curler, because nickel is contained at a considerably high percentage. For example, with this case of a 25-year-old woman, the eyelash curler (A) contained nickel at 82.4%, and its occasional usage resulted in the dermatitis of the eyelids demonstrated (B). She showed (+ +) positive reaction to standard nickel sulfate patch-test reagent by ICDRG standards.

A nonallergic contact problem from corticosteroids is a rosacea-like dermatitis or periorbital dermatitis[24] which is a flareup of mild to severe erythema and swelling caused by rebound flare following withdrawal from long-term continuous use of topical corticosteroids. This may have been used on atopic dermatitis, cosmetic dermatitis, or other contact dermatitis of the face. Commonly, the patient will have a recurrent erythematous and papular dermatitis, not only on the eyelids but also on the cheeks and forehead. The patient will usually have a history of using topical corticosteroid preparations on this area for more than a month. Since a number of patients will, for one reason or another, try to hide the previous use of these products, one has to pursue the possibility in typical cases, even with a negative history. Corticosteroids produce many untoward changes in the skin of the face and the eyelids; even hydrocortisone can cause problems,[25] so the experienced dermatologist will seldom use a potent steroid in this region.

Rarely, one can see eyelid dermatitis from respiratory pollen exposure, sometimes complicating allergic conjunctivitis and rhinitis. Pollens responsible for this vary from patient to patient and with the environmental exposure. For example, respiratory problems from apple pollen are seldom seen at any distance from the orchard itself, since the pollen is not carried a great distance in air. But certain other pollens—such as birch, cedar, and ragweed—can be carried great distances. In such cases, eyelid dermatitis tends to be seasonal, when the pollen counts are high.

IRRITANT CONTACT DERMATITIS

Irritant contact dermatitis can be simply defined as an eczematous contact eruption which is not on an allergic basis. Obviously, all these reactions are not caused by the same mechanism. In one review, the irritant reactions were identified simply when patients with negative or nonrelevant patch-test responses gave a history of exposure to known irritants.[2] Sometimes this can be caused by soap or a detergent used to clean the area. Another study found a 15 percent prevalence of irritant dermatitis in patients with eyelid eczema, while eczema without eyelid dermatitis was found to have an irritant etiology in 29 percent of patients.[3] Those authors also found that eyelid dermatitis is less likely to be work-related, a common association with certain other types of irritant dermatitis such as hand eczema.

Patients with irritant reactions more often have burning and stinging rather than itching, and this is more likely to occur rapidly after contact with the offending agent. Patients can usually identify an irritant, but sometimes knowing that a product is irritating does not tell you what component is the causative agent.

In one category of irritant cosmetic reactions, sometimes referred to as *status cosmeticus,* patients are intolerant to cosmetics that are considered to be nonirritating for the great majority of normal individuals. Women are more likely to be susceptible than men, and fair-skinned more than dark-skinned individuals. The use of 5% lactic acid in water has been recommended as a test for individuals susceptible to this.[26] This will detect those susceptible if they are perspiring, but 10% lactic acid may be required when the patient is not sweating.

Identification of the causative agent is not always easy. Ingredients to suspect include propylene glycol, lactic acid, benzoic acid, sorbic acid, urea, quatenary ammonium compounds (such as benzalkonium), and any other surface-active agent.

Generally, the approach recommended to detect nonimmunologic contact urticaria is to apply the preparation directly to a site of previous involvement for 5 min and then to remove it. Sometimes ointment forms require a 30-min exposure. If immunologic contact urticaria is suspected, however, an application to normal skin first may be wise.

A number of products that are normally used around the eye are surprisingly irritating when applied directly to the skin. A good example of this is waterproof mascaras, which will produce a strong 3+ reaction in many patients if a closed patch test with the undiluted product is attempted. Most individuals tolerate a regular application to the eyelashes, but in some a cumulative effect will allow them to become irritated.[27] If patch testing to waterproof mascaras is required, it may be necessary to obtain the ingredients from the manufacturer for testing at the proper concentration.

DIFFERENTIAL DIAGNOSIS

Atopic eczema of the eyelids tends to occur in younger individuals with dry skin and a history of atopy. Such persons tend to show seasonal variations, and they itch when they are sweating. They are more likely to have a personal or family history of allergic rhinitis, irritation from certain textile materials, and eczema of the hands. The many conditions commonly associated with atopy—such as facial pallor, keratosis pilaris, food intolerance, nummular eczema, and nipple eczema—may be present, including pompholyx, ichthyosis, and a Dennie-Morgan fold. For someone with eyelid dermatitis, it is wise to accept a strong history as probably valid, as it usually is.[28] However, before accepting this as the only diagnosis, one has to rule out other diseases, especially irritant and allergic contact dermatitis.

Persons who have had atopic eczema as children may be susceptible to eyelid dermatitis as adults. Often, the typical morphology and distribution are no longer present, but other stigmata can usually be found. The lack of the typical eruption would not invalidate a positive history.

Maibach et al.[27] described eczema of the eyelids which was not on an atopic basis but which was called "endogenous"; they believed it to represent the largest group of patients with upper eyelid dermatitis syndrome. They felt that some of these eruptions might be atopic but that one could not make that diagnosis in the absence of positive findings on physical examination or by history.

Dermatomyositis can produce a heliotrope-like eruption of the upper eyelid with swelling. Frequently, findings are present in other areas, although muscle weakness may not be present at the time the cutaneous eruption appears. The poikilodermatous skin changes are more likely to be found over the joints, and Gottron's papules are characteristic.

Seborrheic dermatitis is usually associated with the same condition in other areas, as is rosacea. Periorbital dermatitis is the eyelid equivalent of perioral dermatitis, and this can be greatly aggravated by, if not secondary to, topical steroid usage.

Psoriasis may be accompanied by a family history. It is frequently seen in isolated plaques, and typical changes of psoriasis may be found in other areas, such as the fingernails, scalp (especially the nuchal area), elbows, and knees.

Staphylococcal infections can also be associated with eczema, and many forms of infection can be associated with inflammation.

The usual diagnostic workup for problem cases is always in order, as swelling of the eyelids can be due to causes as common as irritation and as rare as cavernous sinus thrombosis. With the recent increased prevalence of immunosuppression in the population, whether due to HIV or a kidney or bone marrow transplant, many uncommon infections become much more likely. The morphologic characteristics can be greatly different from those usually seen and a biopsy can be extremely helpful in problem cases.

The diagnosis of allergic contact dermatitis is usually made from physical findings, the history, and patch testing and/or usage testing. According to Svensson and Moller,[1] the incidence is less in atopic individuals, but it tends to occur more commonly in women.[29] Sometimes this is suspected on the basis of routine patch testing, but at other times one has to test patients extensively in order to find the culprit. This is particularly true of cosmetic reactions, which require that the individual be tested to nonirritating cosmetics and often materials which are touched with the hands but are not applied directly to the eyelids. Because the eyelids absorb well and other areas such as the hands may absorb poorly, eyelid dermatitis may be acquired from hand transfer without a concomitant hand dermatitis being present. With the potential for hand transfer, a wide variety of cosmetic preparations are possible causes, so testing the individual to everything in the environment is important. This would include cosmetics, makeup, sunscreen, hand lotions, and other nonirritants handled with the hands. Testing with shampoos, soaps, cleansing creams, and even mascara can be a problem, because the level of irritancy requires such extreme dilution that false-negative tests are likely even in an allergic individual.

THE WORKUP OF THE PATIENT WITH CONTACT DERMATITIS OF THE EYELIDS

The history in patients with suspected contact dermatitis of the eyelids is important. Time can sometimes be saved by having the patient fill out a printed history form. However, this should probably be considered the starting point, as history taking may also require some probing questions directed at causes suspected from the history and physical findings.

The patient should bring in every medication that has been used and every cosmetic product. This would include things to which the patient will obviously not be tested because it gives the physician information on specific ingredients which may be on the labels. Patch testing to cosmetics is an important part of the workup. Even if the primary cause of eyelid dermatitis is another allergen, concomitant sensitivity to a cosmetic product applied to the area may occur and can result in treatment failure even though the original cause is found and eliminated. Patch testing to the routine screening series should be done in almost everyone because the antigens are in optimal concentration and contact allergy of the eyelids can occur from hand transfer when the product ostensibly never comes in contact with the eyelids.

An important area in eyelid dermatitis is ophthalmic medications (e.g., contact lens solutions and over-the-counter eyedrops). Patients with dermatitis at the time of the visit should avoid wearing cosmetics until the condition has cleared. The testing is done to topical medications which are to be used. When 1% hydrocortisone petrolatum is to be used on the eyelids, the patient should have a negative intradermal test to 1 mg of cortisol (done with 0.05 mL of Solucortef diluted to 20 mg/mL). Even then, the ointment has to be applied with the finger in a vinyl or polyethylene glove or wrapped with plastic wrap to avoid hand transfer of an unsuspected antigen. To be absolutely safe, the patient should also be tested to the plastic, since sensitivity to any of these items can be present and aggravation could result from even mild allergy to any of the items used in treatment.

Once the patient has improved by avoiding direct hand contact and has been patch tested, those items which are negative on patch testing can be reinstituted one at a time every 5 to 7 days until the patient's routine has been restored. This is an extremely time-consuming and demanding routine, but eyelid dermatitis can be very difficult to manage if it is not done with discipline.

REFERENCES

1. Svensson A, Moller H: Eyelid dermatitis: The role of atopy and contact allergy. *Contact Dermatitis* 15:178–182, 1986.
2. Valsecchi R, Imberti G, Martino D, Cainelli T: Eyelid dermatitis: An evaluation of 150 patients. *Contact Dermatitis* 27:143–147, 1992.
3. Nethercott JR, Nield G, Holness DL: A review of 79 cases of eyelid dermatitis. *J Am Acad Dermatol* 21:223–230, 1989.
4. Cameli N, Vicenzi C, Tosti A: Allergic contact conjunctivitis due to timolol in eyedrops. *Contact Dermatitis* 25:129–130, 1991.
5. Anibarro B, Barranco P, Ojeda JA: Allergic contact blepharoconjunctivitis caused by phenylephrine eyedrops. *Contact Dermatitis* 25:323–324, 1991.
6. Schultheiss E: Hypersensitivity to levobunolol. *Derm Beruf Umwelt* 37:185–186, 1989.
7. van der Willigen AH, de Graaf YP, van Joost T: Periocular dermatitis from atropine. *Contact Dermatitis* 17:56–57, 1987.
8. de Groot AC, van Wijnen WG, van Wijnen-Vos M: Occupational contact dermatitis of the eyelids, without ocular involvement, from thimerosal in contact lens fluid. *Contact Dermatitis* 23:195, 1990.
9. Vilaplana J, Romaguera C, Grimalt F: Contact dermatitis from nickel and cobalt in a contact lens cleaning solution. *Contact Dermatitis* 24:232–233, 1991.
10. Cameli N, Tosti G, Venturo N, Tosti A: Eyelid dermatitis due to cocamidopropyl betaine in a hard contact lens solution. *Contact Dermatitis* 25:261–262, 1991.
11. Whittington CV: Elicitation of contact lens allergy to thimerosal by eye cream. *Contact Dermatitis* 13:186, 1985.
12. Yorav S, Ronnen M, Suster S: Eyelid contact dermatitis due to Liquifilm wetting solution of hard contact lenses. *Contact Dermatitis* 17:314–315, 1987.
13. Romaguera C, Grimalt F: Dermatitis from nickel eyelash curler. *Contact Dermatitis* 12:174, 1985.
14. Vestey JP, Buxton PK, Savin JA: Eyelash curler dermatitis. *Contact Dermatitis* 13:274–275, 1985.
15. Brandrup F: Nickel eyelid dermatitis from an eyelash curler. *Contact Dermatitis* 25:77, 1991.
16. Karlberg AT, Liden C, Ehrin E: Colophony in mascara as a cause of eyelid dermatitis: Chemical analyses and patch testing. *Acta Derm Venereol* 71:445–447, 1991.
17. Fisher AA: Allergic contact dermatitis due to rosin (colophony) in eyeshadow and mascara. *Cutis* 42:507–508, 1988.
18. Calnan CD: Compound allergy to a cosmetic. *Contact Dermatitis* 1:123, 1975.
19. Fisher AA: Cosmetic dermatitis of the eyelids. *Cutis* 34:216–221, 1984.
20. Hambly EM, Wilkinson DS: Unusual presentation of epoxy resin sensitivity. *Contact Dermatitis* 4:114, 1978.
21. Guin JD, Skidmore G: Compositae dermatitis in childhood. *Arch Dermatol* 123:500–502, 1987.
22. Guin JD: Sesquiterpene-lactone dermatitis. *Immunol Allergy Clin North Am* 9:447–461, 1989.
23. Resnick SD: Poison-ivy and poison-oak dermatitis. *Clin Dermatol* 4:208–212, 1986.
24. Smith EB, Powell RF, Graham JL: Periorbital dermatitis (letter). *Dermatol* 112:563, 1976.
25. Guin JD: Complications of topical hydrocortisone. *J Am Acad Dermatol* 4:417–422, 1981.
26. Frosch PJ, Kligman AM: A method for appraising the stinging capacity of topically applied substances. *J Cosmetic Chemist* 28:197, 1977.
27. Maibach HI, Engasser P, Ostler B: Upper eyelid dermatosis syndrome. *Dermatol Clin* 10:549–554, 1992.

28. Svensson A, Moller H: The role of atopy in contact allergy. *Contact Dermatitis* 15:178–182, 1986.
29. Kaalund-Jorgensen O: Eczema periocular dermatitis of the eyelids. *Acta Derm Venereol* 31:83–90, 1951.
30. Olveti E: Contact dermatitis from an acrylic-metal dental prosthesis. *Contact Dermatitis* 24:57, 1991.
31. Schmoll M, Hausen BM: Allergic contact dermatitis to prednisolone-21-trimethyl acetate. *Zeitschr Hautkrankh* 63:311–313, 1988.
32. van Ketel WG, Melzer-van Riemsdijk FA: Conjunctivitis due to soft lens solution. *Contact Dermatitis* 6:321–324, 1980.
33. Freitas JP, Brandao FM: Contact urticaria to chlorocresol. *Contact Dermatitis* 15:252, 1986.
34. Romaguera C, Grimalt F, Vilaplana J: Contact dermatitis by timolol. *Contact Dermatitis* 14:248, 1986.
35. Yorav S, Ronnen M, Suster S: Eyelid contact dermatitis due to Liquifilm wetting solution of hard contact lenses. *Contact Dermatitis* 17:314–315, 1987.
36. Fisher AA: The management of eyelid dermatitis in patients with "status cosmeticus": The cosmetic intolerance syndrome. *Cutis* 46:199–201, 1990.
37. Calnan CD: Rubber sensitivity presenting as eyelid oedema. *Contact Dermatitis* 1:124–125, 1975.
38. van Ketel WG, Bruynzeel DP: Allergic contact dermatitis from nickel in eyeshadow (letter, comment). *Contact Dermatitis* 21:355, 1989.
39. Ross JS, White IR: Eyelid dermatitis due to cocamidopropyl betaine in an eye make-up remover. *Contact Dermatitis* 25:64, 1991.
40. Nakayama H, Matsuo S, Hayakawa K, et al: Pigmented cosmetic dermatitis. *Internat J Dermatol* 23:299–305, 1984.
41. Hamada T, Horiguchi S: Chronic melanodermatitis due to the rubber peephole of a ship radarscope. *Contact Dermatitis.* 4:245–246, 1978.

48

ECZEMAS OTHER THAN CONTACT DERMATITIS

Jere D. Guin

The terminology used in classifying the eczematous dermatoses is often confusing, as is the definition of the word *eczema*. Some consider dermatitis to be synonymous with eczema, while others define dermatitis as any inflammatory condition of the skin. An eczema is an erythematous, pruritic, and histologically spongiotic skin eruption which in the acute stage is weeping, oozing, crusting, and scaling and in the chronic form shows thickening, hyperkeratosis, and lichenification. A long list of dermatoses can be included under the rubric of eczema. Proper classification is important, as it allows the physician to remove the patient from the cause, speeding comfort and recovery. Treatment of eczematous eruptions is often much easier than advertised provided that an accurate diagnosis is made and the patient can be separated from the underlying causes and aggravating factors. The chapter on treatment addresses the methodology of removal from an unknown cause so that the condition can be improved sufficiently to proceed with the evaluation.

The classification of eczema used here, while not complete, should allow an adequate differential for all but the very unusual. Since the remainder of the book concerns contact dermatitis, that will be mentioned only briefly in this chapter; but it is nevertheless an important component.

STASIS DERMATITIS

This is sometimes called gravitational eczema, although abnormalities of vascular function may have more to do with it than gravity per se. Certain calcium channel blockers may also cause edema, apparently partly or even largely independent of the loss of venous tone, with resultant stasis eczema.[1] The diagnosis is fairly obvious, as one sees swelling of the area, usually the ankle; the area around the medial malleolus is the most common site affected. There may or may not be ulceration or hemosiderin and, with chronic disease, melanin. Ulceration may develop and autoeczematization is common with spread of the eczema locally and to other areas of the body. Perhaps the most important consideration is the tendency for persons with eczema of the lower extremities to become contact allergic, especially to medications applied to treat the condition. The overall incidence of several large series is 61 percent.[2] Patch-test results in patients with ulcers and stasis eczema show an increased incidence of sensitivity to several antigens depending upon the series.[2-7] Some series show sensitivity to germicidal agents and antibiotics to be increased,[2,8] but the percentages vary with the series reported. They range from low values (for antibiotics)[3] of 0 to 1.3 percent to high values of 34 percent of 192 cases (depending upon the agent) in a study of 13 antibiotics.[9] There is also a higher incidence of allergy to corticosteroids[10,11] and to ethylenediamine, which is usually acquired through a topical corticosteroid treatment.[4] Some of the more common antigens are fragrances, antibiotics, benzocaine, and wool alcohols, but the list is very long. Clearing stasis eczema requires the simplest of treatments to avoid sensitization together with correction of any abnormal venous pressure by elevation, elastic stockings, and so on. Care must be taken to avoid exposure to rubber chemicals in any pressure stocking or wrap if the patient is reactive to any of these in the standard tray. Elastic stockings free of rubber include Jobst Fast-Fit and Jobst Ultimate stockings, which are available in 30 mm or greater pressure. One must order the rubber-free products by name, as many of a similar type do contain rubber.

Topical corticosteroids used should comprise only the glucocorticoid and a nonsensitizing base, usually petrolatum. The choice of corticosteroid may also be important, as the prevalence of sensitivity varies,[12] and this may also be true of sensitizing capacity. The safest approach is to use an ointment comprising only a steroid (chemically dissimilar to one previously used) in a petrolatum base. Any corticosteroid can cause sensitivity in areas of chronic stasis eczema, so selecting one to which the patient is negative on patch testing (or for hydrocortisone on intradermal testing) is ideal. Patients should be told to avoid all topical agents not prescribed, especially over-the-counter lotions. Almost anything applied for any length of time is a potential sensitizer, whether it is a home treatment or a prescribed medication.

ATOPIC ECZEMA

The diagnosis of atopic eczema is, in most cases, straightforward and immediately obvious to the experienced clinician. However, there are atypical situations with late onset or localized disease, presentations which are treatment altered, exfoliative dermatitis and superimposed disease such as contact dermatitis or bacterial and viral[13] infection. Perhaps the most difficult area for the inexperienced physician is recognition of the separate components of multiple superimposed dermatologic entities. In atopic eczema, such problems include infection, xerosis, irritation, and even allergic contact dermatitis.

While atopics seem less likely to develop contact allergy to poison ivy,[14] they are, with a slight reduction overall,[15] susceptible to nickel sensitivity,[16,17] and this occurs not uncommonly in infancy.[18] They also react to other metals,[19] fragrance materials, neomycin, and ingredients of topical medications,[20]—especially if the disease remains active and if hand eczema is present,[21]—and to hair dyes, with a pattern similar to that of hand eczema patients in general.[15] Therefore the patch testing of persons with atopic dermatitis and atopic hand eczema can be rewarding, especially in problem cases. One must be wary of irritant reactions, which are especially common in this group.[20]

The condition also has a different pattern in infants and toddlers than in juveniles and adults. In some adults it may be limited to hand eczema, and only careful history taking elicits a prior history of infantile eczema. Recognition is not difficult in typical cases, but, incredibly, some review articles on the subject fail to describe the eruption.

The Hanifin and Lobitz classification, presented in Table 48-1, has been modified from the original by Hanifin and Lobitz.[22,23] The major criteria have been changed to include item 4 as a major or basic feature. The characteristic morphology and distribution in infants involves the face, neck, and extremities especially; in adults the flexural areas of the extremities are typical, but other areas are commonly involved.

INFANTILE ATOPIC DERMATITIS

The eruption in infancy usually starts at 2 to 6 months on the face; the scalp may also be involved, especially with seborrheic dermatitis. The cheeks are typically involved and a weeping of the neck is common. Involvement of the extremities is more likely to be on the extensor surfaces in localized, often weeping, oozing, scaling, pruritic patches or plaques. Sometimes this condition is morphologically the same as nummular eczema. The knees may be involved in those old enough to crawl. The eruption may be so severe that it becomes an erythroderma with dermatopathic lymphadenopathy. While one publication says that the diaper area is commonly affected, the reverse is probably true. Although diaper dermatitis can develop in any child this age, the diaper area is typically spared in infants with widespread atopic dermatitis.

Infants usually respond to local treatment rapidly provided that they avoid all irritants (soaps, washcloths, wool, carpet, propylene glycol in topical lotions and corticosteroids, and so on). The secret is using the weakest corticosteroid which relieves itching, incorporated into a nonirritating vehicle, and switching to weaker but effective ones as symptoms abate. The vehicle used is very important, as hydrocortisone can be quite effective if the parents are given a sufficient quantity and they use it frequently. Teaching patients how to avoid hidden exposure to irritants in clothing, bed coverings, upholstered furniture, and especially topically applied lotions is often an important prerequisite to success. A positive, enthusiastic approach is much more effective, as any pessimism is contagious.

JUVENILE ATOPIC DERMATITIS

After age 2 or 3, the location of lesions on the extremities transfers to the flexural areas. Sometimes nummular and localized lesions are present on the extensor rather than the flexural sites. Hand eczema may also be present.

ADULT ATOPIC DERMATITIS

Adults usually have involvement of the antecubital and popliteal areas as well as the eyelids, neck, and forehead especially. Other flexural areas may be involved; not

TABLE 48–1. *Features of Atopic Dermatitis[a]*

Major Features

Pruritus
Typical morphology and distribution:
   Flexural lichenification or linearity in adults
   Facial and extensor involvement in infants and children
Chronic or chronically relapsing dermatitis
Personal or family history of atopy (asthma, allergic rhinitis, atopic dermatitis)

Minor Features

Xerosis
Ichthyosis/palmar hyperlinearity/keratosis pilaris
Immediate (type I) skin-test reactivity
Elevated serum IgE
Early age of onset
Tendency toward cutaneous infections (esp. *Staph. aureus* and
   herpes simplex)/impaired cell-mediated immunity
Tendency toward nonspecific hand or foot dermatitis
Nipple eczema
Cheilitis
Recurrent conjunctivitis
Dennie-Morgan infraorbital fold
Keratoconus
Anterior subcapsular cataracts
Orbital darkening
Facial pallor/facial erythema
Pityriasis alba
Anterior neck folds
Itch when sweating
Intolerance to wool and lipid solvents
Perifollicular accentuation
Food intolerance
Course influenced by environmental/emotional factors
White dermographism/delayed blanch

[a] Must have 3 or more major (basic) features plus 3 or more minor features.
Source: Hanifin JM: Atopic dermatitis. *J Allerg Clin Immun* 73:211–222, 1984.
Reproduced by permission.

infrequently, popliteal or antecubital involvement is isolated to one or two locations, lacking symmetry. Some persons with childhood eczema have only hand eczema as adults, often presenting with the characteristic nummular pattern. Adult-onset eczema should be evaluated for other causes, as contact dermatitis can be missed for years when it is assumed to be atopic eczema.

DIFFERENTIAL DIAGNOSIS

The differential includes Wiskott-Aldrich syndrome, phenylketonuria, hyperimmuno-globulin E syndrome,[24] DiGeorge's syndrome, selective IgA deficiency, and anhidrotic ectodermal dysplasia.[25] Compositae dermatitis can be almost indistinguishable without patch testing, although summer aggravation, lack of involvement of the feet, and the fact that there is clearing on avoidance of outdoor exposure all help.[26] Other conditions in the differential include ataxia telangiectasia, Swiss-type agammaglobulinemia, and even the Letterer-Siwe type of histiocytosis X.[27] In fact, a long list of immunodeficiency diseases has been associated with a rash resembling atopic eczema, with the archetype being Wiskott-Aldrich syndrome. According to Saurat,[28] these lesions are not very different from the eruption seen in atopic eczema,[28] as they fulfill the (Hanifin and Lobitz) criteria. Following reconstitution of the immune system with a successful bone marrow transplant, patients with Wiskott-Aldrich syndrome tend to clear not only of the rash but of the ichthyosis as well.[28]

PHYSIOLOGIC DIFFERENCES

Persons with atopic eczema have a number of differences in the physiologic and pharmacologic response to stimuli, including white dermographism (replacing the red line when dermatitic skin is stroked)[29] and the delayed blanch response to cholinergic agents[30] rather than the expected axon reflex. Histamine tends to cause flushing in areas where one expects to see the rash,[31] and there is a reduced threshold for histamine release from mast cells.[32] About 84 percent of persons with atopic dermatitis have dry skin,[33] and there is often an ichthyotic change leading to hyperlinearity of the palms and other areas.

There are also a number of immunologic alterations. This subject is complex, but one should be aware of the susceptibility to increased numbers of *Staphylococcus aureus,* with probable aggravation of the disease[34] and cross-infection in a hospital environment.[35] Chronic colonization is apparently related to a reduction in immunologic reactivity to the organism.[36] There is also an increased tendency to develop tinea pedis[37-39] and viral infection.[40,41] The former may be more closely related to respiratory atopy than atopic dermatitis as such.[42] There are numerous immunologic abnormalities, including cell-mediated immune response, decreased chemotaxis of neutrophils and monocytes, and decreased T-cell stimulation of cytotoxic activity.[22] There is also a tendency to overproduce IgE by mononuclear cells, although the explanation is not immediately evident.

There is evidence of contribution from cell-mediated immune mechanisms, as IgE binding on Langerhans cells allows presentation of the allergen to T cells. T cells which produce IL-4 are assumed to be an important part.

The dominant cell is a CD4 + or helper phenotype,[43] and numerous findings suggest an upregulation,[44-46] although it may not be mediated through gamma interferon.[43]

Cooper[47] postulates that a cell with Th-2-type (as in mice) function may be operating. Th-2 cells induce IL-4 and IgE production, whereas the TH-1 cell produces gamma interferon. Certain organisms are less well handled by atopics, and there are lower levels of IL-1,[48] TNF-alpha,[49] and IL-2. A number of cell types may function abnormally,[47] and the feedback mechanisms through IgE and cAMP phosphodiesterase do not function properly.[47]

There is a genetic influence, and both the cause or causes and precipitating factors are multifactorial. A seemingly ever-increasing list of "trigger factors" has evolved; sensitivity to the house dust mite, aggravation by certain foods, local irritation, infection, climatic change, and emotional stress all may play a role.

Atopics in general have a lowered incidence of sensitivity to poison ivy[38] but more susceptibility to certain fungi, bacteria, warts, and molluscum contagiosum. The cellular basis may at least in part be related to the increase in cyclic AMP phosphodiesterase activity, depressing the level of that nucleotide. The increase in basophil histamine release and the elevation of IgE production is linked to abnormally high leukocyte cyclic AMP phosphodiesterase, which keeps the intracellular cyclic AMP levels low.[50]

LICHEN SIMPLEX CHRONICUS

This condition is essentially the chronic form of neurodermatitis, with hyperkeratosis and lichenification or scratch papules from chronic rubbing. The term *neurodermatitis* implies an emotionally induced condition, but this is not infrequently associated with underlying itching rather than stress. The principal difference between lichen simplex chronicus and prurigo nodularis is that the former is caused by rubbing while the latter is due to picking.

Lichen simplex chronicus is not infrequently a secondary phenomenon, occurring from the rubbing of a pruritic primary lesion. Stasis, for example, may be an underlying cause. Since atopics can as a group lichenify more readily, this may be associated with the atopic state; but this is certainly not necessarily true.

Differentiating lichen simplex from contact dermatitis may seem straightforward, but in any case lichen simplex chronicus may be secondary to a low-grade contact and vice versa. Nickel allergy to metal snaps on jeans is not infrequently associated with lichen simplex, and stasis dermatitis may induce itching, with chronic rubbing leading to lichen simplex chronicus.

NUMMULAR ECZEMA

Discoid or nummular eczema is an eczematous eruption with sharply marginated coin-shaped plaques comprising coalescing papulovesicles. According to Bendl,[51] this condition was originally described some 135 years ago, and the cause associated with it seems to change with whatever is in vogue. Nummular lesions are commonly associated with varicosities and autoeczematization,[51] atopic eczema, and xerosis with or without eczema craquelé.[52] The latter may stem as much from edema as from xerosis, however.[53] Autoeczematization from infectious eczematoid dermatitis also seems to be related, and some dermatologists use the terms synonymously. A bacterial etiology is sometimes given.[25]

Nummular eczema is perhaps more often found with irritant contact dermatitis than with allergic contact dermatitis.

SULZBERGER GARBE SYNDROME

Exudative lichenoid and discoid dermatosis of Sulzberger and Garbe or "oid-oid" disease is considered separately from nummular eczema because it involves middle-aged Jewish males; has oval lesions, commonly involves the penis; tends to develop lichenoid and follicular lesions; has flatter, scaly lesions in one stage and raised, exudative lesions in another stage; shows eosinophilia (although this comes and goes in some); and is sometimes accompanied by urticaria.[54]

Of Sulzberger's original 9 cases, 4 were engaged in buying and selling. Kesten[55] once explained that New York physicians believed this to be an entity because they saw it especially in men working in the garment industry, about as stressful an occupation as one can imagine. She also felt that sunbathing in Miami Beach while on vacation was extremely beneficial and numerous others would agree, although Sulzberger's patients did not respond to light and most did not reliably improve with climate change. This issue is discussed at length by Stevens.[56]

The condition is now said to clear spontaneously, but Sulzberger, in 1937, managed the majority of his patients only with hospitalization. Many dermatologists elsewhere would probably call most reported cases a variant of nummular eczema based on the morphologic similarity,[56] and there may be a valid argument. Histologically, one cannot distinguish this condition from dyshidrotic or nummular eczema, contact dermatitis, or id reactions.[56] The present author has seen cases of autoeczematization which look similar to the eruptions in many reported patients with oval, follicular, and lichenoid lesions. However, in Sulzberger's defense, one should examine the illustrations in his original paper before making a firm decision. They are impressive.

CONTACT DERMATITIS WHICH MIMICS NUMMULAR ECZEMA

Nummular eczema is associated with both irritant and sensitization contact dermatitis, including aloe,[57] ethylenediamine,[58] cyanoacrylate,[59] balsam of Peru, and nickel, the last with or without a positive patch test.[60,61] The idea that bacterial antigens are involved is supported by evidence of complement activation.[62] Xerosis and irritation may also lead to eczema with a nummular pattern. A nummular pattern of purpura is seen after the Vietnamese practice of *g,ao gio'*, or coin rubbing.[63]

CHRONIC SUPERFICIAL DERMATITIS

This term is a synonym for small-plaque parapsoriasis (e.g., digitate dermatosis).

ASTEATOTIC ECZEMA

Dry skin is associated with aging, low environmental humidity, overuse of cleansing agents, the atopic state, and other things. The development of tiny annular fissures with pruritus is typical; this may eventuate into nummular eczema with rubbing, washing, and similar stimuli. These stimuli can also be cumulative. Chernosky[63a] described cases of xerosis secondary to overexposure to an air-conditioned environment with resultant low humidity, so that this picture of winter itch (pruritus hiemalis) can be present in the summer months. Perhaps the principal question is whether or not this type eczema should be separated from nummular eczema.

In the differential, allergic contact dermatitis is not so much a problem; irritant contact can cause the picture, especially when soap is the irritant. Also in the differential, one must consider parapsoriasis en plaque and pityriasis rosea which has been over-bathed. Uremic patients have pruritic, dry-looking skin which is often considered xerotic, but the hydration of the stratum corneum is reportedly unimpaired.[64] The dry, atopic skin differs in its increased water loss from asteatotic lesions or winter itch.[65] The skin in psoralen(s) plus UVA (PUVA) therapy can also seem dry in appearance, but its ultrastructure differs from that of the stratum corneum of aging.[66] Some would also consider glucagonoma and zinc deficiency in the differential.[67] Other conditions include bulimia,[68] cimetidine treatment,[69] chloracne,[70] leprosy,[71] Grover's disease,[72] and AIDS-related varicella zoster infection of the skin.[73]

The picture of eczema craquelé is often considered xerotic, but Jillson[53] argues that edema is a major factor in the development of that condition. Certainly that seems often true on the lower extremities.

JUVENILE PLANTAR DERMATOSIS

The eruption of juvenile plantar dermatosis is an eczema of pressure areas on the plantar surface, including the distal toes. It characteristically spares the longitudinal arch and proximal toes, suggesting a contact dermatitis. The etiology has been much debated and many conclude that it is multifactorial. There are almost as many names for this condition as articles on the subject, but the term *juvenile plantar dermatosis*[74] has been most often used recently. It is common, as Verbov[75] collected 189 cases in 15 years. Associations found or presumed include atopy[76,77](and no association with atopy),[76] mechanical trauma, occlusive footwear, and seasonal influence.[78] In some areas the last is worse in summer,[79] and in others most troublesome in winter.[80] This condition has also been related to moisture and bacteria. It occurs more in prepubertals, although adolescents and adults may also be affected.[80] The appearance is that of a shiny, dry, eczematous eruption with a tendency toward fissuring in some patients. The shiny appearance has been described as "similar to the crazed glaze on old porcelain"[81] because of the loss of normal texture of the stratum corneum.

This condition is by definition patch-test negative, but one must do patch testing carefully. I collected a large series of patch-test negative patients at one time only to find the incidence of negative tests greatly reduced when the patch tests were done on the external upper arm, under occlusion (using just enough plastic wrap to cover the shoe-lining sample plus a narrow margin), and with mild pressure (using an elastic bandage). To my chagrin these results were commonly relevant and usually associated with sensitivity to athletic shoes. Romaguera[82] had 6 positive tests in 15 patients with the same morphologic picture.

INFECTIOUS ECZEMATOID DERMATITIS

Infectious eczematoid dermatitis as described classically by Engmann[83] is an eczematous area surrounding (and presumably due to) a draining focus of infection. An eczematous process develops under the purulent drainage. Autoinoculation occurs with peripheral extension, and autoeczematization can induce plaques of eczema at distant sites. The older textbooks describe this condition quite well,[84,85] but it is included in the classification of eczema by some modern texts also.[86] The organisms may be *Staphylococcus, Streptococcus,* or both[87] or even a gram-negative organism such as *Pseudomonas.*[88]

The term *infectious eczematoid dermatitis* is also used for some cases of autosensitization. That condition is very similar, as a localized eczema tends to spread with an id-like reaction at distant sites, comprising papules and papulovesicles which may coalesce into plaques. This distant spread causes a picture not unlike that of infectious eczematoid dermatitis, and the mechanism may be similar. This is essentially an exogenous condition causing endogenous spread. The mechanism is, after so many years, still unclear.

FRICTIONAL LICHENOID DERMATITIS

This eruption was originally described by Sutton[89] in his classic textbook of dermatology as summertime pityriasis of the elbows and knees. The same condition was described by Brunner et al.,[90] again as papular erythema of childhood, in 1962. It was later renamed *frictional lichenoid eruption* in children by Waisman and Sutton.[91] This eruption is distinctive in that it is localized to the knees, elbows, hands, and occasionally elsewhere. It is frequently followed by depigmentation (really hypopigmentation), is seasonal, occurs mostly in prepubertal children[89,91] but occasionally adolescents,[92] and is often associated with atopy.[93,94] The lesions have been described as "pityriasis-like," but we agree with Rasmussen[93] and Menni et al.[95] that they are more prurigo-like papules. These may be discrete, but they often coalesce into plaques. They are regarded by most authors as pruritic, although this is not always prominent.[94,95]

The differential includes sensitivity to rubber (where the elbows are involved),[96] epoxy in knee pads (where the knees are involved),[97] Gianotti-Crosti syndrome, and papulovesicular acrolocated eruption. Patch testing helps in the first two instances, while Gianotti-Crosti is classically associated with hepatitis B, is more erythematous, and generally involves lesions over a wider area.[95] The condition responds well to topical corticosteroid treatment and avoidance of trauma. Some recommend long sleeves.

HAND ECZEMA

Hand eczema is actually a regional form of eczema; it comprises many of the previously mentioned types of eczema. It can also be classified in several ways. The following is one such classification.

POMPHOLYX, OR DYSHIDROTIC ECZEMA

This condition is sometimes erroneously called *dyshidrotic eczema,* based on the original report, but it has nothing to do with sweating.[98] Pompholyx has been assumed to be endogenous because it is usually somewhat symmetrical, the vesicles are individual and deep-seated at the start, and certain systemic allergens are known to cause flares, at least in some cases. Some dermatophytid reactions are indistinguishable, and systemic exposure to certain allergens is reported to exacerbate the condition. Considerable controversy exists over the claim that nickel, topically and systemically,[99] flares the condition, as other metals, including cobalt and chromates, are also reported to do.[100] Aspirin, oral contraceptives, and smoking are also risk factors if not aggravating factors in some.[101] Other underlying causes include local exposure to carbamates,[102] spices,[103] or airborne molds[104]; hereditary factors[105]; and piroxicam photosensitivity.[106] The same or a similar eruption is seen in bullous pemphigoid (which may be purpuric),[107–110] pemphigus,[111] and linear IgA disease.[112] It can also be associated with lichen planus and autoimmune progesterone dermatitis.[113,114]

Treatment involves removal of any underlying cause (if one can be found) and perhaps light therapy. PUVA therapy or UVA[115] reportedly helps problem cases.[116]

According to Schwanitz,[117] pompholyx was classically described by Tilbury Fox in 1873[118] (who called it *dysidrose*) and Hutchison[119] (who used the name *cheiropompholyx*) in 1876. Their criteria were summarized by Muende in 1934[120] as symmetrical individual vesicles of the palms and finger margins, which are tense and pruritic, tend to coalesce, may dry out, and frequently recur.

IRRITANT CONTACT DERMATITIS

This topic is covered in another chapter, but it represents a nonallergic contact dermatitis, often following exposure to soap, detergents, solvents, and other "irritants." Occupational contact dermatitis of the hands is more often irritant.[121] An atopic constitution seems to predispose one to irritation,[20] and certain factors such as wet work, frequent hand washing, exposure to detergents at home, and having to care for small children all seem to increase risk even for hospital workers whose hand eczema is ostensibly occupational.[122] Women are more at risk in certain occupations, probably because such risk factors are more likely to be present and add to the likelihood of irritant dermatitis. While soap and detergent exposure is the expected cause, other irritants are occasionally causative. Atopics are perhaps more at risk.[123] This type eczema causes increased transepidermal water loss, which can be used to quantitate the damage done. In some studies, this diagnosis is made by exclusion.[124]

One of the more common causes of irritant occupational hand eczema is the use of soap and solvents in an attempt to remove particles which are insoluble. This is especially true among automobile mechanics and machinists who are exposed to metal, rubber, or carbon particles. Frequently, removal with a bland cream followed by a mild soap will allow satisfactory cleansing without undue irritation.

ALLERGIC CONTACT DERMATITIS

Allergic contact dermatitis of the hands is caused by delayed hypersensitivity to substances usually contacted externally. This can be found as a primary condition, alone or with irritant contact dermatitis or another eczematous eruption of the hands. The pattern depends upon the causative agent and the pattern of exposure. Classic patterns or distributions are seen in poison ivy dermatitis, (rubber) glove dermatitis, allergy to preservatives in soap[125] or shampoo, tulip finger or alstroemeria dermatitis,[126] reactions to garlic, and glyceryl monothioglycolate dermatitis in beauticians,[127] to name a few. One should look for sensitivity to almost any treatment used on an allergic contact dermatitis of long standing. The diagnosis is often more obvious after patch testing than before, as knowing the underlying sensitivity helps immensely in reconstructing the patterns of exposure. A difficult area is in persons with systemic contact dermatitis, where flares occur after internal exposure. Again, knowing the patch-test results can help in uncovering a source which might ordinarily be impossible to detect or even suspect.

ATOPIC HAND ECZEMA

This can be a confusing term. Schwanitz[117] wrote a book on "atopic palmoplantar eczema," which was primarily a study of dyshidrotic eczema. Meding's[128] main criterion for this category was "a history of previous atopic dermatitis or present atopic dermatitis at other sites of the body." Champion and Parish,[129] however, presented the picture with which the writer is familiar. They regard this as a patchy, somewhat vesicular and lichenified eczema seen as an adult manifestation in persons with a history of childhood atopic eczema. It often has a "discoid" (nummular) pattern which is frequently not distinguishable from hand dermatitis in those with other forms of atopy, such as allergic rhinitis. Persons with persistent atopic eczema in adult life may have diffuse lichenification, depending upon the chronicity and severity of their condition. These individuals are more susceptible to primary irritation and seem to respond better to corticosteroid preparations without propylene glycol.

NUMMULAR ECZEMA

This is classically characterized by coin-shaped plaques which are often weeping, oozing, crusting, and scaling. It may be accompanied by an id reaction on the hands and elsewhere and may be part of a more widespread eruption of the same character.

HYPERKERATOTIC PALMAR DERMATITIS

This category may represent a volar hyperkeratotic dermatitis, often with fissures, and of uncertain cause. However, in such cases one has to rule out, clinically, psoriasis, both primary and secondary. Occasionally lichen planus and other skin diseases in which the Koebner phenomenon occurs may also resemble this type eruption.

UNCLASSIFIED HAND ECZEMA

In her treatise, Meding[117] included in this category cases where a precise diagnosis could not be made at the time of the examination, as when the patient was clear when presenting to the physician. A precise diagnosis can often be made when lesions appear or when adequate data are available.

REFERENCES

1. Salmasi AM, Belcaro G, Nicolaides AN: Impaired venoarteriolar reflex as a possible cause for nifedipine-induced ankle edema. *Int J Cardiol* 30:303–307, 1991.

2. Shupp DL, Winkelmann RK: The role of patch testing in stasis dermatitis. *Cutis* 42:528–530, 1988.
3. Rudzki E, Baranowska E: Contact sensitivity in stasis eczema. *Dermatologica* 148:353–356, 1974.
4. Hogan DJ, Hill M, Lane PR: Results of routine patch testing of 542 patients in Saskatoon, Canada. *Contact Dermatitis* 19:120–124, 1988.
5. Malten KE, Kuiper JP, van der Staak WB: Contact allergic investigations in 100 patients with ulcus cruris. *Dermatologica* 147: 241–254, 1973.
6. Angelini G, Rantuccio F, Menegheni CF: Contact dermatitis in patients with leg ulcers. *Contact Dermatitis* 1:81–87, 1975.
7. Breit R: Allergen change in stasis dermatitis. *Contact Dermatitis* 3:309–311, 1977.
8. Knudsen BB, Avnstorp C: Chlorhexidine gluconate and acetate in patch testing. *Contact Dermatitis* 24:45–49, 1991.
9. Fraki JE, Peltonen L, Hopsu-Havu VK: Allergy to various components of topical preparations in stasis dermatitis and leg ulcers. *Contact Dermatitis* 5:97–100, 1979.
10. Wilkinson M, Cartwright P, English JS: The significance of tixocortol-pivalate-positive patch tests in leg ulcer patients. *Contact Dermatitis* 23:120–121, 1990.
11. Alani MD, Alani SD: Allergic contact dermatitis to corticosteroids. *Ann Allerg* 30:181–185, 1972.
12. Dooms-Goossens A, Morren M: Results of patch testing with corticosteroid series in 2073 patients. *Contact Dermatitis* 26:182–199, 1992.
13. Strannegard O, Strannegard I, Rystedt I: Viral infections in atopic eczema. *Acta Derm Venereol* 65(suppl 114):121–124, 1985.
14. Jones HE, Lewis C, McMarlin SL: Allergic contact sensitivity in atopic dermatitis. *Arch Dermatol* 107:217–222, 1973.
15. Marghescu S: Patch test reactions in atopic patients. *Acta Derm Venereol* 65(suppl 14):113–116, 1985.
16. Caron GA: Nickel sensitivity and atopy. *Br J Dermatol* 76:384–387, 1964.
17. Motolese A, Truzzi M, Seidenari S: Nickel sensitization and atopy. *Contact Dermatitis* 26:274–275, 1992.
18. Ho VC, Johnston MM: Nickel dermatitis in infants. *Contact Dermatitis* 15:270–273, 1986.
19. Fischer T, Rystedt I: False-positive, follicular and irritant patch test reactions to metal salts. *Contact Dermatitis* 12:93–98, 1985.
20. Lammintausta K, Kalimo K, Fagerlund VL: Patch test reactions in atopic patients. *Contact Dermatitis* 26:234–240, 1992.
21. Rystedt I: Contact sensitivity in adults with atopic dermatitis in childhood. *Contact Dermatitis* 13:1–8, 1985.
22. Hanifin JM, Cooper KD, Roth HL: Atopy and atopic dermatitis. *J Am Acad Dermatol* (periodic synopsis) 15:703–706, 1986.
23. Hanifin JM, Lobitz WC Jr: Newer concepts of atopic dermatitis. *Arch Dermatol* 113:663–670, 1977.
24. Hanifin JM: Atopic dermatitis. *J Am Acad Dermatol* 6:1–13, 1982.
25. Braun-Falco O, Plewig G, Winkelman R: Dermatitis and eczema, in *Dermatology:* Berlin, Springer-Verlag, 1990, pp 317–366.
26. Guin JD, Skidmore G: Compositae dermatitis in childhood. *Arch Dermatol* 123:500–502, 1987.
27. Arnold HL, Odom RB, James WD: *Diseases of the Skin.* Philadelphia, Saunders, 1990, pp 68–74.
28. Saurat JH: Eczema in primary immune deficiencies: Clues to the pathogenesis of atopic dermatitis with special reference to the Wiskott-Aldrich syndrome. *Acta Derm Venereol (Suppl)* 114:125–128, 1985.
29. Whitfield A: On the white reaction (white line) in dermatology. *Br J Dermatol* 50:71–82, 1938.
30. Lobitz WC, Campbell CJ: Physiologic studies in atopic dermatitis (disseminated neurodermatitis): The local cutaneous response to intradermally injected acetyl choline and epinephrine. *Arch Dermatol* 67:575–589, 1953.
31. Williams DH: Skin temperature reaction to histamine in atopic dermatitis (disseminated neurodermatitis). *J Invest Dermatol* 1:119–129, 1938.
32. Fantozzi IR, Massini E, Blandina P, Mannaioni PF: Cholinergic histamine release: Evidence of muscarinic receptors in rat mast cells. *Agents Actions* 9:57–58, 1979.
33. Uehara M, Ofuji S: Atopic dermatitis: A discussion concerning its pathogenesis. *J Dermatol* 7:231–238, 1980.
34. Leyden JJ, Marples RR, Kligman AM: *Staphylococcus aureus* in the lesions of atopic dermatitis. *Br J Dermatol* 90:525–530, 1974.
35. Selwyn S, Chalmers D: Dispersal of bacteria from skin lesions: A hospital hazard. *Br J Dermatol* 77:349–356, 1965.

36. Hauser C, Wuethrich B, Matter L, et al: The immune response to *Staph aureus* in atopic dermatitis. *Acta Derm Venereol* 65(suppl 114):125–128, 1985.

37. Svejgaard E, Faergeman J, Jemec G, et al: Recent investigations on the relationship between fungal skin diseases and atopic dermatitis. *Acta Derm Venereol (Suppl)* 144:140–142, 1989.

38. Jones HE, Reinhardt JH, Rinaldi MG: A clinical, mycological, and immunological survey for dermatophytosis. *Arch Dermatol* 108:61–65, 1973.

39. Svejgaard E, Albrectsen B, Baastrup N: The occurrence of tinea of the feet. *Mykosen* 26:450–454, 1983.

40. Currie JM, Wright RC, Miller OW: The frequency of warts in atopic patients. *Cutis* 8:243–244, 1971.

41. Solomon LM, Telner R: Eruptive molluscum contagiosum in atopic dermatitis. *Can Med Assoc J* 95:978–979, 1966.

42. Kaaman T: Skin reactivity in atopic patients with dermatophytosis. *Mycosen* 28:183–190, 1984.

43. Lever R, Turbitt M, Sanderson A, MacKie R: Immunophenotyping of the cutaneous infiltrating and of the mononuclear cells in the peripheral blood in patients with atopic dermatitis. *J Invest Dermatol* 89:4–47, 1987.

44. Van Joost T, Kozel MMA, Tank B, et al: Cyclosporin in atopic dermatitis: Modulation in the expression of immunologic markers in lesional skin. *J Am Acad Dermatol* 27:922–928, 1992.

45. Leung DYM, Coptran RS, Pober JS: Expression of an intracellular adhesion molecule (ELAM-1) in atopic dermatitis and elicited late phase allergic skin reactions (abstract). *Clin Res* 38:448A, 1990.

46. Griffiths CEM, Vorhees JJ, Nickoloff BJ: Characterization of intercellular adhesion molecule-1 and HLA-DR expression in normal and inflamed skin: Modulation by recombinant gamma interferon and tumor necrosis factor. *J Am Acad Dermatol* 20:617–629, 1989.

47. Cooper KD: Atopic dermatitis: Recent trends in pathogenesis and therapy. *Prog Dermatol* 27:1–16, 1993.

48. Resanen L, Reunala T: Langerhans cell antigen presentation and interleukin-1 production in atopic dermatitis. *Acta Derm Venereol (Suppl)* 144:64–66, 1989.

49. Kapp A, Textor A, Krutmann J, Moller A: Immunomodulating cytokines in atopic dermatitis and psoriasis: Production of tumor necrosis factor and lymphotoxin by mononuclear cells in vitro. *Br J Dermatol* 122:587–592, 1990.

50. Hanifin JM: Pharmacologic abnormalities in atopic eczema. *Allergy* 44(suppl 9):41–46, 1989.

51. Bendl BJ: Nummular eczema of stasis origin: The backbone of a morphologic pattern of diverse etiology. *Int J Dermatol* 18:129–135, 1979.

52. Rollins TG: From xerosis to nummular dermatitis: The dehydration dermatosis. *JAMA* 206:637, 1968.

53. Jillson OF: Nummular (orbicular) eczema. *Cutis* 31:131, 134, 137 passim, 1983.

54. Sulzberger MB, Garbe W: Nine cases of a distinctive exudative discoid and lichenoid chronic dermatosis. *Arch Dermatol Syphilol* 36:247–272, 1937.

55. Kesten BM: Personal communication.

56. Stevens DM, Ackerman AB: On the concept of distinctive exudative discoid and lichenoid chronic dermatosis (Sulzberger-Garbe): Is it nummular dermatitis? *Am J Dermatopathol* 6:387–395, 1984.

57. Morrow DM, Rapaport MJ, Strick RA: Hypersensitivity to aloe. *Arch Dermatol* 116:1064–1065, 1980.

58. Caraffini S, Lisi P: Nummular dermatitis-like eruption from ethylenediamine hydrochloride in 2 children. *Contact Dermatitis* 17:313–314, 1987.

59. Belsito DV: Contact dermatitis to ethyl-cyanoacrylate-containing glue. *Contact Dermatitis* 17:234–236, 1987.

60. Veien NK, Hattel T, Justesen O, Nørholm A: Diagnostic procedures for eczema patients. *Contact Dermatitis* 17:35–40, 1987.

61. Veien NK, Hattel T, Justesen O, Nørholm A: Oral challenge with metal salts: II. Various types of eczema. *Contact Dermatitis* 9:407–410, 1983.

62. Parish WE, Welbourn E, Champion RH: Hypersensitivity to bacteria in eczema: IV. Cytotoxic effect of antibacterial antibody on skin cells acquiring bacterial antigens. *Br J Dermatol* 95:493–506, 1976.

63. Primack WA, Person JR: Nummular purpura (letter). *Arch Dermatol* 121:309–310, 1985.

63a. Chernosky ME, Pruritic skin disease and summer air conditioning. *JAMA* 179:1005–1010, 1962.

64. Stahle-Backdahl M: Stratum corneum hydration in patients undergoing maintenance hemodialysis. *Acta Derm Venereol* 68:531–534, 1988.

65. Thune P: Evaluation of the hydration and the water-holding capacity in atopic skin and so-called dry skin. *Acta Derm Venereol (Suppl)* 144:133–135, 1989.

66. Franchimont C: The stratum corneum xerotic from aging and photochemotherapy (PUVA): A study by scanning electron microscopy. *Am J Dermatopathol* 2:295–304, 1980.

67. Binnick AN, Spencer SK, Dennison WL Jr, Horton ES: Glucagonoma syndrome: Report of two cases and literature review. *Arch Dermatol* 113:749–754, 1977.
68. Gupta MA, Gupta AK, Haberman HF: Dermatologic signs in anorexia nervosa and bulimia nervosa. *Arch Dermatol* 123:1386–1390, 1987.
69. Greist MC, Epinette WW: Cimetidine-induced xerosis and asteatotic dermatitis. *Arch Dermatol* 118:253–254, 1982.
70. Zugerman C: Chloracne: Clinical manifestations and etiology. *Derm Clin* 8:209–213, 1990.
71. Pavithran K: Non-pruritic eczemas as presenting manifestation of leprosy. *Indian J Lepr* 62:202–207, 1990.
72. Grover RW, Rosenbaum R: The association of transient acantholytic dermatosis with other skin diseases. *J Am Acad Dermatol* 11:253–256, 1984.
73. Gilson IH, Barnett JH, Conant MA, et al: Disseminated ecthymatous herpes varicella-zoster virus infection in patients with acquired immunodeficiency syndrome. *J Am Acad Dermatol* 20:637–642, 1989.
74. MacKie RM, Husain SL: Juvenile plantar dermatosis: A new entity? *Clin Exp Derm* 1:253–260, 1976.
75. Verbov J: Juvenile plantar dermatosis (JPD). *Acta Derm Venereol (Suppl)* 144:153–154, 1989.
76. Svensson A: Prognosis and atopic background of juvenile plantar dermatosis and gluteo-femoral eczema. *Acta Derm Venereol* 68:336–340, 1988.
77. Moller H: Atopic winter feet in children. *Acta Derm Venereol* 52:401–405, 1972.
78. Lachapelle JM, Tennstedt D: Juvenile plantar dermatosis: A report of 80 cases. *Am J Ind Med* 8:291–295, 1985.
79. Silvers SH, Glickman FS: Atopy and eczema of the feet in children. *Am J Dis Child* 116:400–401, 1968.
80. Enta T: Peridigital dermatitis in children. *Cutis* 10:325–328, 1972.
81. Shrank AB: The etiology of juvenile plantar dermatosis. *Br J Dermatol* 100:641–648, 1979.
82. Romaguera C, Grimalt F, Ferrando J: Dry feet syndrome or juvenile plantar dermatosis. *Contact Dermatitis* 8:219–220, 1982.
83. Engmann MF: An infectious form of an eczematoid dermatitis. *Am Med* 4:769–773, 1902.
84. Sutton RL: *Diseases of the Skin,* 11th ed. St Louis, Mosby, 1956, pp 270–273.
85. Pillsbury DM, Shelley WB, Kligman AM: *Dermatology.* Philadelphia, Saunders, 1956.
86. Burton JL, Rook A, Wilkinson DS: Eczema, lichen simplex, erythroderma, and prurigo, in Rook A, Wilkinson DS, Ebling FJG, et al (eds): *Textbook of Dermatology,* 4th ed. Oxford, Blackwell, 1986, pp 373–375.
87. Weissman K, Hjorth N: Microbial eczema of the feet. *Br J Dermatol* 107:333–337, 1982.
88. Greene SL, Su WP, Muller SA: *Pseudomonas aeruginosa* infections of the skin. *Am Fam Phys* 29:193–200, 1984.
89. Sutton RL: *Diseases of the Skin,* 11th ed. St Louis, Mosby, 1956, p 898.
90. Brunner MJ, Rubin L, Dunlap F: A new papular erythema of childhood. *Arch Dermatol* 85:147–148, 1962.
91. Waisman M, Sutton RL: Frictional lichenoid eruption in children. *Arch Dermatol* 94:592–593, 1966.
92. Goldman L, Kitzmiller KW, Richfield DF: Summer lichenoid dermatitis of the elbows in children. *Cutis* 13:836–838, 1974.
93. Rasmussen JE: Sutton's summer prurigo of the elbows. *Acta Derm Venereol* 58:547–549, 1978.
94. Patrizi A, Di Lernia V, Ricci G, Masi M: Atopic background of a recurrent papular eruption of childhood (frictional lichenoid eruption). *Pediatr Dermatol* 7:111–115, 1990.
95. Menni S, Piccinno R, Baietta S, Pigatto P: Sutton's summer prurigo: A morphologic variant of atopic dermatitis. *Pediatr Dermatol* 4:205–208, 1987.
96. Rietschel R: Forum: Contact dermatitis. American Academy of Dermatology annual meeting, San Antonio, Tex, December 9, 1987.
97. Taylor JS, Bergfeld WF, Guin JD: Contact dermatitis to knee patch adhesive in boys' jeans: A nonoccupational cause of epoxy resin sensitivity. *Cleve Clin Q* 50:123–127, 1983.
98. Kutzner H, Wurzel RM, Wolff HH: Are acrosyringia involved in the pathogenesis of "dyshidrosis"? *Am J Dermatopathol* 8:109–116, 1986.
99. Christensen OB, Moller H: External and internal exposure to the antigen in the hand eczema of nickel allergy. *Contact Dermatitis* 1:136–141, 1975.
100. Kaaber K, Veien NK: The significance of chromate ingestion in patients allergic to chromate. *Acta Derm Venereol* 57:321–323, 1977.
101. Edman B: Palmar eczema: a pathogenetic role for acetylsalicylic acid, contraceptives and smoking? *Acta Derm Venereol* 68:402–407, 1988.

102. Crippa M, Misquith L, Lonati A, Pasolini G: Dyshidrotic eczema and sensitization to dithiocarbamates in a florist. *Contact Dermatitis* 23:203–204, 1990.
103. Niinimaki A: Delayed-type allergy to spices. *Contact Dermatitis* 11:34–40, 1984.
104. Fujisawa S, So Y, Ofuji S: Eczematous dermatitis produced by airborne molds. *Arch Dermatol* 94:413–420, 1966.
105. Curth HO: Familial pompholyx. *Arch Dermatol* 100:520, 1969.
106. Braunstein BL: Dyshidrotic eczema associated with piroxicam photosensitivity. *Cutis* 35:485–486, 1985.
107. Rongioletti F, Parodi A, Rebora A: Dyshidrosiform pemphigoid: Report of an additional case. *Dermatologica* 170:84–85, 1985.
108. Barth JH, Fairris GM, Wojnarowska F, White JE: Haemorrhagic pompholyx is a sign of bullous pemphigoid and an indication for low-dose prednisolone therapy. *Clin Exp Dermatol* 11:409–412, 1986.
109. Barth JH, Venning VA, Wojnarowska F: Palmo-plantar involvement in auto-immune blistering disorders–pemphigoid, linear IgA disease and herpes gestationis. *Clin Exp Dermatol* 13:85–86, 1988.
110. Duhra P, Ryatt KS: Haemorrhagic pompholyx in bullous pemphigoid. *Clin Exp Dermatol* 13:342–343, 1988.
111. Milgraum SS, Friedman DJ, Ellis CN, Waldinger TP: Pemphigus vulgaris masquerading as dyshidrotic eczema. *Cutis* 35:445–446, 1985.
112. Duhra P, Charles-Holmes R: Linear IgA disease with haemorrhagic pompholyx and dapsone-induced neutropenia. *Br J Dermatol* 125:172–174, 1991.
113. Anderson RH: Autoimmune progesterone dermatitis. *Cutis* 33:490–491, 1984.
114. Feuerman EJ, Ingber A, David M, Weissman-Katzenelson V: Lichen ruber planus beginning as a dyshidrosiform eruption. *Cutis* 30:401–404, 1982.
115. Grattan CE, Carmichael AJ, Shuttleworth GJ, Foulds IS: Comparison of topical PUVA with UVA for chronic vesicular hand eczema. *Acta Derm Venereol* 71:118–122, 1991.
116. LeVine MJ, Parrish JA, Fitzpatrick TB: Oral methoxsalen photochemotherapy (PUVA) of dyshidrotic eczema. *Acta Derm Venereol* 61:570–571, 1981.
117. Schwanitz HJ: *Atopic palmoplantar eczema.* Berlin, Springer-Verlag, 1988.
118. Fox T: Clinical lecture on dyshidrosis. *Br Med J* 1:375–376, 1873.
119. Hutchinson J: Cheiro-pompholyx. *Lancet* 1:630–631, 1876.
120. Muende J: Cheiropompholyx. *Br J Dermatol* 46:479–490, 1934.
121. Meding B, Swanbeck G: Consequences of having hand eczema. *Contact Dermatitis* 23:6–14, 1990.
122. Nilsson E, Mikaelsson B, Andersson S: Atopy, occupation, and domestic work as risk factors for hand eczema in hospital workers. *Contact Dermatitis* 13:216–223, 1985.
123. Rystedt I: Work-related hand eczema in atopics. *Contact Dermatitis* 12:164–171, 1985.
124. Meding B: Epidemiology of hand eczema in an industrial city. *Acta Derm Venereol (Suppl)* 153:1–43, 1990.
125. Fowler JF: Para-chloro-meta-xylenol allergy and hand eczema. *Am J Contact Dermatitis* 4:53–54, 1993.
126. Marks JG: Allergic contact dermatitis to *Alstroemeria. Arch Dermatol* 124:914–916, 1988.
127. Storrs FJ: Permanent wave contact dermatitis: Contact allergy to glyceryl monothioglycolate. *J Am Acad Dermatol* 11:74–85, 1984.
128. Meding B, Swanbeck G: Epidemiology of different types of hand eczema in an industrial city. *Acta Derm Venereol (Suppl)* 69:227–233, 1989.
129. Champion RH, Parish WE: in Rook A, Wilkinson DS, Ebling FJG, et al (eds): *Textbook of Dermatology,* 4th ed, vol 1. Oxford, Blackwell, 1986.

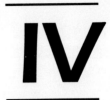

IV

PRACTICAL MANAGEMENT, METHODS, AND SOURCES OF MATERIALS

49

THE PATIENT WITH NEGATIVE PATCH TESTS—WHAT NOW?

Michael H. Beck

The term *idiopathic* can easily be attached to a skin condition in a particular patient and no further thought given to contact allergy. This can be a grave mistake.

When the patch tests have been performed and are negative, this should not by any means be the end of the story. What should be done next? Initially, the answer must be to reassess the patient in full and, furthermore, at each subsequent visit. If such an approach is not taken, there is a continuing danger of overlooking a correctable factor or cause for the individual's skin disorder. If you are satisfied that your patient does not have an allergic contact dermatitis, then you will have to offer guidance in long-term management.

REASSESSMENT OF THE HISTORY

It is important to reassess the primary sites of involvement and the time and mode of onset. A primary distribution involving flexural limbs, especially developing in early childhood (Fig. 49-1), may suggest an atopic cause, particularly if associated with asthma or hay fever. Primary involvement of the scalp, ears (Fig. 49-2), central face, chest, and back, perhaps with intertriginous involvement, may point to a seborrheic dermatitis. A widespread patchy involvement of the skin or a discoid configuration (Fig. 49-3) may suggest a constitutional cause.

The term *constitutional eczema* is used here to mean those eczemas for which we cannot, at our present state of knowledge, determine a cause—although we may be able to state that extrinsic factors do not appear to play a role. The term *endogenous* is also applied to such disorders. These terms are not entirely satisfactory, as environmental factors may still have an influence even if they are not primarily responsible.

An eczematous disorder of the hands and/or feet presenting as visible vesicles or bullae is most likely to be pompholyx. This disorder may be acute, recurrent, or chronic with exacerbations. This pattern and behavior can be a marker of a constitutional disorder. However, there is a major potential pitfall in looking at any apparently

659

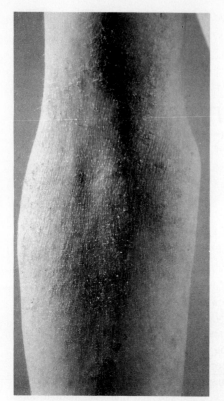

FIG. 49–1. Atopic dermatitis affecting flexural elbow.

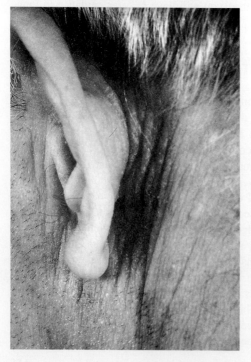

FIG. 49–2. Seborrheic dermatitis affecting the ears.

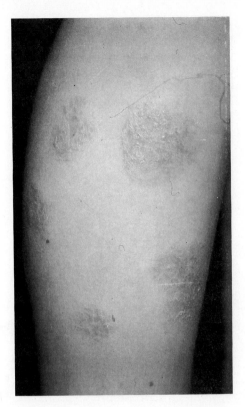

FIG. 49–3. Constitutional discoid eczema.

endogenous pattern of eczema, particularly on the hands, and dismissing contact allergy as a possibility. Never forget that *any* pattern of rash and any constitutional condition may be contributed to or caused by contact allergy, which may also mimic constitutional disorders. Examples of this are shown in Figs. 49-4 through 49-8. Furthermore, a secondary contact dermatitis may develop as a result of irritancy or allergy to topical materials applied to the skin disorder.

A careful occupational reassessment is mandatory. If the individual gives a clear history of deterioration when at work and improvement when away from work, one should again look at the possibility of contact dermatitis. First, one has to consider the distribution of the rash and all the materials handled at work. Next, material safety data sheets should be reexamined. Sometimes one may be able to substantiate a diagnosis of irritant contact dermatitis after these steps have been taken. A fissuring, shiny eruption of the fingertips and possibly the palms may suggest frictional trauma. A more widespread irritation, patchy erythema, and asteatosis of the skin may indicate a low-humidity dermatosis, particularly if others are similarly affected.

If the patient states, on the contrary, that his or her condition is just as bad throughout the year, whether or not at work, then this can be regarded as an indicator of a constitutional condition.

A clear history of exacerbation or development of a dermatitic rash after the use of a topical application—whether it be a medication, moisturizer, or other cosmetic—and negative patch tests are clear reasons to reassess the situation and not to label the

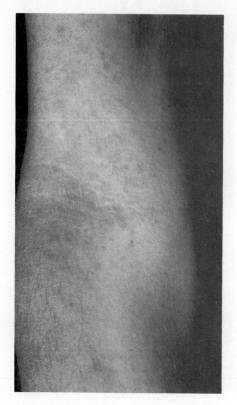

FIG. 49–4. Textile allergy from pilot's uniform, affecting flexural elbow.

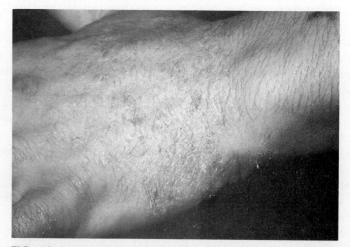

FIG. 49–5. Localized patchy allergic contact dermatitis from chromate in cement.

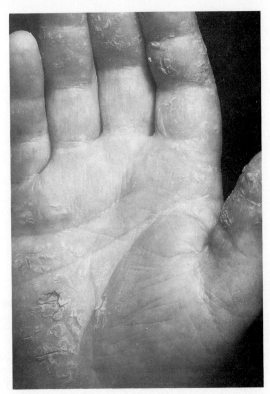

FIG. 49–6. Patchy palmar psoriasiform dermatitis due to allergy from black rubber in tire fitter.

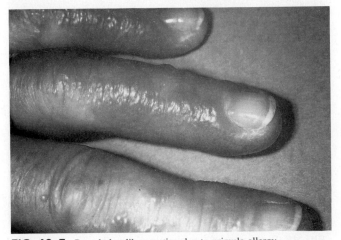

FIG. 49–7. Pompholyx-like eruption due to primula allergy.

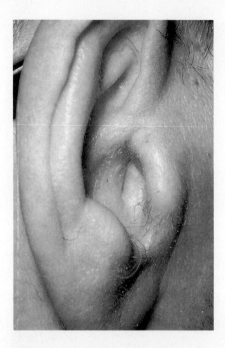

FIG. 49–8. Otitis externa. Allergic to neomycin, framycetin, gentamicin, and quinoline mix.

disorder as being idiopathic. Did the patient give a full history the first time? In this situation, the individual must be asked over and over again what was applied to the area; often he or she will have focused on the wrong product. Remember, makeup has to be applied *and* removed, and it may be the removal which is the cause (Fig. 49-9). Also remember that patients wrongly tend to regard materials with prefixes such as *simple, hypoallergenic,* and *baby* as incapable of inducing allergy. Patients must be

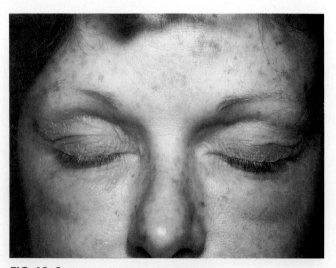

FIG. 49–9. Contact allergy to eye makeup remover.

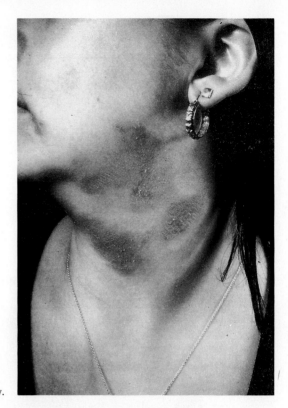

FIG. 49–10. Nail varnish allergy.

encouraged to bring *all* their cosmetics and medicaments for patch testing. All over-the-counter products applied to the skin must be specifically looked for.

While considering cosmetics, I cannot overemphasize the importance of considering allergy to nail products in any person with a persistent rash on the face, neck, and/or chest (Fig. 49-10). In this situation, nail varnishes, varnish remover, false nails and their glues, as well as the components of sculptured nails must be patch tested.

One will need to check again that there is no relationship, in time or place, of the skin condition to exposures in the domestic environment or to hobbies and other spare-time activities. The presence of a plant in the indoor environment is often forgotten. Other factors such as exposure to light, diet, and systemic medications must also be considered.

REASSESSMENT OF THE EXAMINATION

Having ascertained that nothing has been overlooked in the history, one should reexamine the patient's skin *in full*. The distribution of the rash may fall into a well-recognized constitutional pattern. Additional clues may be found, such as a seborrheic dermatitis on the central chest (Fig. 49-11) in an individual with otitis externa or psoriasis on the scalp or in the natal cleft in an individual with a patchy palmar hyperkeratotic "eczema." Indeed, a full examination may alter one's diagnosis from one dermatosis

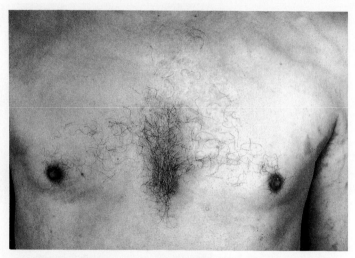

FIG. 49–11. Seborrheic dermatitis affecting central chest.

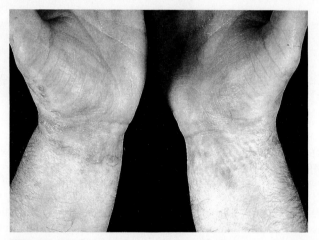

FIG. 49–12. Lichen planus affecting wrist and palm.

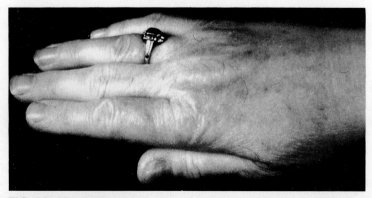

FIG. 49–13. Tinea manuum.

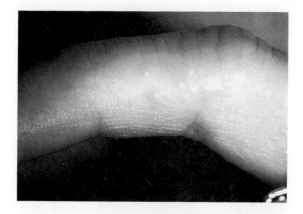

FIG. 49–14. Vesicular id eruption secondary to tinea.

to another. Not only psoriasis but lichen planus (Fig. 49-12) and tinea infections (Fig. 49-13) can cause confusion, particularly when they are confined to the palms and/or soles. Mycological examination of skin scrapings may be necessary. It is particularly important to examine the toe clefts in patients with persistent vesicular foot or hand eczema in order to exclude an id eruption to a dermatophyte (Fig. 49-14). Furthermore, a full examination may bring to light evidence of a missed allergen, such as a rash under the pocket where the allergen is carried (Fig. 49-15) or a severe dermatitis around a varicose ulcer when the dressings are removed (Fig. 49-16).

FURTHER INVESTIGATION

If the history and examination point to a clear exogenous cause that cannot be identified, one is faced with the possibility of a "missed" allergen. In this situation, after the reexamination, a visit to the workplace or domestic environment may be necessary, as important elements may be observed and detected there that were previously missed.

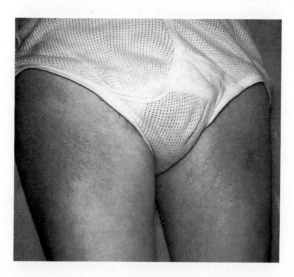

FIG. 49–15. Allergy to "strike any-where" matches carried in pocket.

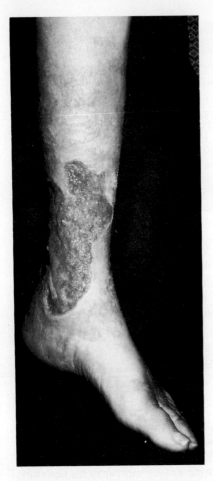

FIG. 49–16. Dermatitis medicamentosa revealed by removal of dressings from varicose ulcer.

A photosensitive rash may require photopatch tests. It is also important to reassess the materials that were patch tested previously, as they may not have been sufficient. Every person must be tested with a standard series. Have all the relevant additional series of allergens been tested? Have all the relevant work materials been tested? When dealing with low-molecular-weight resins, the actual materials handled, including all the hardeners, must be tested, particularly when individuals are in contact with epoxy and phenol formaldehyde resin systems. Have all topical applications, medicaments, and cosmetics been tested? Does the patient use nail cosmetics and have they been tested? Have plants and other materials of relevance in the patient's domestic environment been tested?

Commonly available standard and extra screening series of allergens for testing can be obtained through Chemotechnique and Hermelchemie. One should use a standard series of allergens as a screen for contact allergy, as "aimed" testing will inevitably result in a high rate of failure to detect relevant allergies. The International Contact Dermatitis Research Group (ICDRG) and the North American Contact Dermatitis Group (NACD) give guidance on the content of the standard series (it is not the same), but this can be adapted to one's own circumstances. For instance, in our unit, we have extended the standard series to include phosphorus sesquisulfide and para-chloro-meta-xylenol (PCMX) because, in our geographic area, "strike anywhere" matches are widely used and can cause allergy; also many persons apply PCMX over-the-counter preparations to cuts and rashes and may even wash their clothes and bathe using disinfectants that contain PCMX.

Additionally, we feel that there is a particular problem in identifying corticosteroid allergy. Such allergy, particularly from hydrocortisone, is now recognized as a highly significant cause of "missed" allergy (Fig. 49-17). Tixocortol pivalate is a reliable marker for hydrocortisone allergy, but other corticosteroids used by the patient may need to be tested.

False-negative reactions may take place, not infrequently due to inappropriate storage and infrequent changing of test allergens. These should be changed on an annual basis and kept in the refrigerator, in the dark. It is important to have tested the suspected material at the right concentration and in a vehicle in which it does not degrade. It is most important to do a second reading and perhaps even a third, ideally on days 2, 4, and 7. Certainly a "day 2 only" reading misses a high proportion of positive reactions.

It is strongly advised that the clinician perform the readings personally. An inexperienced assessor, unfamiliar with the patient's specific problems, may miss relevant positive reactions that are weak. Furthermore, it can be confirmed that there has been no loosening or repositioning of the test units, which may account for a false-negative test.

A particular pitfall when patch testing to a cosmetic or medicament is that the finished product may give a false-negative reaction. This was well recognized with

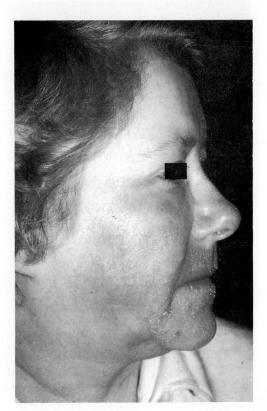

FIG. 49–17. Allergy to hydrocortisone identified by tixocortol pivalate.

neomycin, which must be tested at 20% to confirm allergy, even though it is used at only 0.5% in most topical medicaments. If there is a clear history of a product inducing a contact reaction, it may be necessary to send to the manufacturer for the ingredients and test them individually at appropriate concentrations in order to detect the allergy.

Conversely, compound allergy can be encountered where patch tests are positive to the product but not its ingredients. One should not rely exclusively on screening series but should also test with the finished materials, cosmetics, and medicaments with which the patient has come in contact. Having the patient bring all of these items on the first visit is invaluable.

Usage tests are a helpful adjunctive investigation, particularly if the history and examination suggest a contact reaction despite there being negative patch tests. The suspect material, if nonirritant, can initially be rubbed on an area of normal skin (usually the flexural forearm or the neck) twice daily for 1 week. At the end of this time, the skin is examined for any reaction. Very occasionally, allergic contact dermatitis is site-specific and the previously described usage tests will need to be applied to the affected site in order to confirm this diagnosis.

Prick testing with food should be performed on chefs and other food handlers in view of the observation that immediate reactions to food may progress to a delayed dermatitis in such workers (Fig. 49-18). Prick tests are also required to detect immediate allergy to latex.

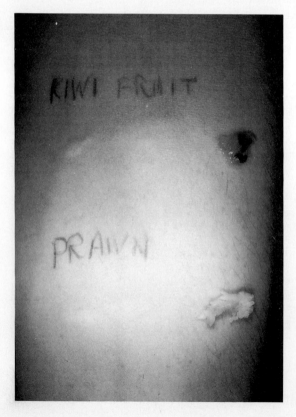

FIG. 49–18. Chef with positive prick tests to food.

CONCLUSION

The message is clear—the labels *endogenous, constitutional,* or *idiopathic* can be dangerous. A reappraisal is required each time the individual is seen. Of course, many persons investigated do have a constitutional disorder to account for their problem, and this must be explained to them. One's discussion with the patient after patch tests should include the caveat that the tests have *only* been for contact *allergy,* as many people are under the misconception that they have been tested for food, respiratory, and drug allergy. It is often useful to give them a guide on the sorts of things which induce contact allergy and what has been tested for (Table 49-1). It may be important to explain that the testing is not for irritants or intolerance.

When patients are informed that their tests are negative (Table 49-2), they may react in very varied ways. Some are pleased, but it is often not clear why they should react this way, particularly as identification of an avoidable cause for their problem might help them. Others are not so pleased, looking down their noses at the investigator who has failed to come up with an answer to their problem. Others are incredulous, indicating that they "know" they are allergic to many things; such individuals often have reactions due to inhalants, irritants, or an intolerance. Fortunately, most are in a frame of mind that can assimilate the explanation that not all skin disorders are due to extrinsic causes and that our knowledge is insufficient to let us explain the roots of their condition. I often say, "I am not clever enough to tell you why you have this condition"—a statement that seems to be accepted much more readily than any other—but I then go on to say, "nor is anybody else," which, one hopes, preempts a requirement for a second opinion!

Management of a constitutional disorder will depend on its nature, its site, and the

---

TABLE 49–1. Common Causes of the "Missed" Allergen

The full history was not taken (or given).
The patient was not completely examined.
Testing to the standard series was not done.
Patch testing with relevant series was not included.
Second patch-test readings (after the initial 2 to 3 days) were not done.
Testing was not done to all relevant materials handled at work.
Relevant materials and cosmetics were omitted, particularly over-the-counter medicaments, makeup removers, moisturizers (including baby lotions), and nail cosmetics.
Domestic materials such as household plants were omitted.
A site visit was not made.
Prick tests to foods were omitted in evaluating salad makers, chefs, and other food handlers.
Corticosteroid screening was not included.
False-negative patch tests occurred because

  Antigens were not stored in the dark and in a refrigerator.
  Antigens were not changed annually.
  Tests were done in inadequate concentration or with an inappropriate vehicle.
  Testing did not include ingredients of cosmetics.
  Finished products were not tested.
  Corticosteroid allergy was not suspected or steroids (systemic or local) caused a negative result.
  There was a rogue negative test result.
  The testing procedure was faulty (fell off, chamber not filled, mismarked sites, etc.).

TABLE 49–2. Information for Patients with Negative Patch Tests

Why have you been patch tested?
The investigation you have undergone, is to establish whether you are allergic to something with which your skin has come into *contact*. The series of tests is undertaken to prove (or disprove) a suspicion of an allergy—but perhaps, more importantly, also to identify a material causing contact allergy that was previously not considered. Unexpected relevant positive patch tests are common and enable your dermatologist to offer advice on avoidance when found.

To what have you been tested?
The test materials selected vary from individual to individual depending upon the case history. More common causes of a contact dermatitis due to allergy include some metals (particularly nickel in costume jewelry and clothing); ingredients of cosmetics, including perfumes; components of medicaments applied to the skin; chemicals in rubber, leather, and cement; plastics and glues; adhesive tapes; preservatives and disinfectants; dyes; and some plants. You will, therefore, have been tested to identify whether you are allergic to these—but, additionally, you may have been tested to other materials relevant to your own situation.

What do negative patch tests mean?
They mean nothing more than that you are unlikely to have a contact allergy to the materials tested.

If my skin develops a rash when it comes into contact with certain soaps, shampoos, and detergents or materials such as solvents or oils, why is the test negative?
What is being described is not necessarily an allergy but a damaging or irritant effect on the skin from the causative material. A careful history identifies such causes; patch tests are inappropriate and unreliable for the recognition of irritants.

If my skin stings when cosmetics are applied to it or if the smell of perfumes makes me sneeze, why are the patch tests negative?
Again, patch tests are not appropriate for such reactions. They are used only to identify the cause of a more persistent rash known as dermatitis.

Do patch tests diagnose drug or ingested food allergy?
The answer is generally no, except in exceptional circumstances.

If I am diagnosed as having a constitutional skin condition following my patch tests, what does this mean?
Not all skin disorders are due to contact allergy or other outside factors. The reason for many skin disorders is not understood well enough for a full explanation to be given about the cause. It is, however, possible in many cases to say that with confidence that no outside cause is responsible, particularly when this opinion is reinforced by the finding of negative patch tests. If a constitutional diagnosis is made, it may be necessary to use treatment on a regular basis with the aim of control rather than cure.

Why are the tests placed on the upper back when the skin problem is elsewhere?
When it comes to contact allergy, the skin behaves in exactly the same way all over the body. The upper back has been shown to be the most convenient site and, normally, a very reliable one for the test.

Could my dermatologist have missed a contact allergy?
No one is perfect and, even in the best of hands, there is always the possibility of a "missed" allergen. If you at a later date have forgotten to mention some material that you think triggers your condition or establishes a link, it is most important to tell your dermatologist, who will be able to run further tests.

---

degree of disability it causes. It is beyond the scope of this chapter to cover management of the different disorders that may have required patch tests which turned out to be negative. Patients' expectations are high, but we must impart realistic advice about their condition and its prognosis, indicating, where appropriate, that regular long-term treatment may be required in place of the cure that is sought. Nevertheless, the message of the chapter is clear—always ask the question, even of those with "idiopathic" dermatoses: Could a missed contact allergy have caused this condition or contributed to it?

50

TREATMENT OF CONTACT DERMATITIS

Jere D. Guin

Treatment of contact dermatitis requires removal from the cause, and when this is not immediately known or strongly suspected, removal from all potential causes by changing the patient's exposure and routine, especially the substances applied in treating and cleaning the skin. The approach to irritant reactions and allergic contact dermatitis is different, but removal of all such patients from potential aggravating factors and sources of (new) allergy is important, as corticosteroid treatment will not likely be effective unless this is done.[1] Because the causes of acute conditions are more likely to be accurately known, management of acute cases of both irritant and allergic contact dermatitis is considered separately.

IRRITANT REACTIONS

AVOIDING ADDITIONAL INJURY

Most acute problems are accidental,[2] so the cause usually is known, and avoidance is possible until the skin has returned to its original state. Chronic irritant dermatitis is another matter; multiple factors can now aggravate the already irritated skin, including lotions, lubricants, and therapeutic agents, which often cause more problems than they cure. The wisdom of "above all else doing no harm" is especially appropriate here.[3,4]

RECOGNITION OF AGGRAVATING FACTORS AT WORK AND HOME

To allow the skin an optimal chance to heal, exposure to all possible sources of irritation—including mechanical factors, chemicals, enzymatic factors, solvents, soaps and detergents, etc.—should be reduced, both at work and at home. Irritancy is reduced where the humidity is about 50 percent and the ambient temperature between 17° and 22°C.[5] A commonsense approach, with diligent care to reduce aggravating factors and protect the already irritated skin, is usually effective.

Even if the patient knows the primary source of contact, he or she is unlikely to suspect additional aggravating factors (e.g., washing the skin or exposure to raw meat or wet vegetables). The method used to clean the skin after work must not be unnecessarily harsh, and this includes the cleaning done at home as well. Many persons with an occupational problem do not realize the added harm that can be done at home. Taking a thorough, directed history not only helps uncover those aggravating factors, but it also provides the opportunity to educate the patient. Sensible improvements in methodology of both household and occupational tasks can result in permanent benefit by helping the patient to work with minimal aggravation.

The principles used in occupational illness[2] can also be applied profitably in the home. A housewife or retiree should also avoid friction (scrubbing with an abrasive cleanser or device—even a washcloth), ultraviolet injury, detergents (including shampoo), acids, alkali, solvents (nail polish remover, paint thinner, etc.), soluble oils, strong oxidizers (bleaches) and reducing agents, organic solvents, and other known irritants (raw meat, fresh vegetables, permanent waving solutions, etc.). At work, checking the pH of a coolant, using a brush to wash dishes, and using a cream to remove carbon and powdered metal all allow the patient to work efficiently without irritating the eczema already present.

PROTECTIVE MEASURES

Where an irritant chemical is contacted, removing it is indicated,[4] but the method used should not be irritating. Protective gloves are essential for certain uses—such as exposure to oven cleaner at home or acids and alkalis at work—but they frequently aggravate nonspecific hand eczema because of the increased sweating, so one must balance the benefit against the harm. In special situations such as handling strong acids or alkalis, protective gloves must meet specifications. Such information often is readily available on the material safety data sheet (MSDS) for that chemical, which is kept in the workplace.

Education of the patient and often the employer takes time and skill in communication, as the message has to be "This is helpful to you because. . . ." In the United States, the employer is often the more difficult to educate, perhaps because of the adversarial legal system.

THE INFORMATIVE HISTORY

An experienced dermatologist can often suspect the precise probable cause from the appearance and location of the eruption. However, snap diagnoses are likely to be neither accurate nor wise in the long run. When one does suspect contact dermatitis, a knowledge of the work and home environments through a careful history is invaluable. This requires time to probe, as the patient is often defensive, especially when there is a question of an occupational cause. Furthermore, most lay persons do not realize the potential for harm which can come from substances and activities considered to be a normal part of their routine. Often such revelations come after a work description is available or becomes known to the physician. Therefore persistent nonconfrontational searching seems to be the best approach. Look for soaps and shampoos which are sometimes used to excess, especially when the skin is already eczematous. Asking mothers with hand eczema how often they shampoo their children's hair can sometimes be more important than learning about their personal use of shampoos. How do you clean after work? Do you apply a moisturizer? Which one? Do you handle food, raw meat, and fresh (wet) vegetables? Do you have babies in diapers? What other household chores do you do? How many children do you have? Do you take care of them alone? What do you apply when your hands are too dry? What medications have you bought? What has been prescribed? What have you found that irritates your skin and what have you done to correct it? Taking a good contact history is not difficult; with a little practice, it soon becomes second nature to those who make the effort.

USING THE MATERIAL SAFETY DATA SHEET

Proper labeling of irritants at work aids worker education. Such information is generally available from the material safety data sheet (MSDS) kept on the premises. The material safety data sheet is an invaluable tool for uncovering the sources of information about the patient's work environment, health hazards, sources of irritation and allergy, and the most effective ways of protecting those who must work with those materials. The document is provided by suppliers of materials used in the work environment and is required to be kept at the place of work. It contains statements on irritancy as well as other health hazards. It also provides a telephone number offering help from a toxicologist familiar with the materials and their potential problems, both irritant and allergic.

Although the forms used are all patterned after the official form from the Department of Labor, every company's forms tend to look, superficially, a bit different from the government form, with the company logo in its distinctive color. However, the material contained is predictably found in the same sections as in the original form. Some sections contain less important data, such as the boiling point or chemical reactivity, which can be critically important to the employer but are not useful to the dermatologist. However, other sections are extremely helpful, providing information not easily obtainable by other means.

Section I contains, among other things, the name of the manufacturer, the chemical name, the common name, and usually the Chemical Abstract Survey registry number. This can help to find allergens and to prepare patch-test materials. Section I also provides the telephone number of a toxicologist near the top of the document. If you suspect a problem with irritancy, the means of protection are usually available on the document in Section VIII or with a telephone call. Also, the types of protective gloves or clothing may be specified. If not, a call usually helps here as well.

For those who are allergic, allergen substitution can save a lifetime of earnings, and this is often possible with help from the manufacturer. For example, an automotive (body shop) mechanic found to be allergic to epoxy by patch testing gives a history of reacting to paint. The only paint product whose MSDS contained epoxy was a rustproof primer. A call to the manufacturer requesting a substitute product without epoxy provided the numbers of their products with acrylic primers used for similar purposes but without epoxy. By examining all MSDS for products used on the job, an adhesive was uncovered which also contained epoxy. A call to the manufacturer provided the name of another product designed for that application which does not contain epoxy. Now the patient has the information to control his environment, thanks to some detective work and the help provided by industry, and everyone profits!

ACUTE ALLERGIC CONTACT DERMATITIS (Table 50-1)

RECOGNIZING AND AVOIDING THE ALLERGEN

The archetype for acute allergic contact dermatitis is poison ivy dermatitis. As with irritants, the patient has to be separated from the cause or all else will fail. As for poison ivy dermatitis, a patient education program is being developed by the American Academy of Dermatology to teach lay people how to recognize the plant. For the standard allergens, recognition of sources of the allergen is made much easier with printed handouts, and such handouts accompany the sections on each allergen. For a cosmetic allergy due to quaternium-15, the patient must learn to read labels to avoid that chemical in all products that contain it.

SYSTEMIC CORTICOSTEROID THERAPY

Acute contact dermatitis is usually treated with a 14-to 21-day course of oral corticosteroids.[6,7] There seem to be as many schedules as there are publications on the subject, but in general the initial dose is about 30 to 50 mg taken once daily after breakfast. This is decreased by 10 mg/day every 2 to 3 days to 20 mg/day and then decreased by 5 mg/day every 2 to 3 days. The initial dose will depend upon the severity, and the length of the course will depend upon the duration of the condition when first seen.

Epstein[8] uses a more aggressive schedule with a very high dose early, administering adrenocorticotropic hormone (ACTH) gel (80 U IM), and the same dose 8 h later, or oral dexamethasone 15 mg (20 tablets) given as 4 tablets five times a day for 3 days and given 20 tablets again after 2 to 3 days if the condition flares.

Acute allergic contact dermatitis can also be treated with (the insoluble) injectable corticosteroids—e.g., triamcinolone acetonide or diacetate, 40 mg IM or methylprednisolone (Depo-Medrol) 40 to 80 mg[9]—but there is less day-to-day control of the systemic level in the event of a problem. Oral therapy must be continued for at least 2 weeks after the original exposure, so the 6-day "Dose-Pak" approach is not advised. Benefit is noted about 2 days after starting treatment, and, if the dose is reduced too rapidly, flares tend to occur about 2 days thereafter.

TABLE 50–1. Treatment of Acute Allergic Contact Dermatitis

Cool wet compresses
Oral corticosteroids (if no contraindication)
Allergen avoidance
Protective gloves, clothing, etc.
Prevention by hyposensitization

LOCAL CORTICOSTEROIDS

During a research project, I had to apply controlled portions of concentrated poison ivy sap to myself, and I took the opportunity to treat some lesions with topical corticosteroids, using occlusion and pressure. It was quite effective compared with the untreated sites. Two 24-h applications of category 2 to category 4 topical corticosteroids with occlusion and mild pressure can also be used with effect. This requires a generous quantity of the therapeutic agent, with reapplication and rewrapping should it be necessary to maintain that level. I have also injected triamconolone acetonide or diacetate 2 mg/mL intradermally under smaller lesions of acute *Toxicodendron* dermatitis, using other untreated lesions as a control. This is very fast treatment, as I have seen lesions disappear in 24 h or less.

HYPOSENSITIZATION (FOR POISON IVY)

For poison ivy dermatitis, prevention with oral hyposensitization is occasionally of some benefit for highly sensitive persons who cannot avoid exposure,[10–14] such as forest workers and firefighters. The injectable preparations do not contain sufficient antigen to predict probable success, but the oral poison ivy/poison oak preparation by Hollistier-Stier may be beneficial provided that it is carried with the contents of more than one kit.[15] Treatment is started after the first frost and must be continued throughout the year. Oral hyposensitization is intended for long-term prevention and is not used when the eruption is present, as it is not beneficial and severe flares can be precipitated. Oral hyposensitization programs have also been used for ragweed[16] and *Parthenium hysterophorus,*[17] but these are no longer commercially available. The mechanism for this methodology may be through formation of anti-idiotypic antibodies.[18] A similar but probably different form of tolerance called "hardening" occurs in most Japanese-lacquer workers following chronic exposure.[19] It is also seen in patients with alopecia areata who have been deliberately treated with a contact allergen to ameliorate the disease.[20] There is no known reliable way to use it therapeutically.

COMPRESSES

Compresses can be used to debride crusts and scales.[6,9] They are less popular today, perhaps because systemic corticosteroids are effective anyway and compresses are not adequate treatment without the corticosteroids. One may use physiologic saline or Burow's solution. The latter is commercially available as USP Burow's (American, Balan, CME-Cons, Denison, Halsey, Humco, Paddock, Rugby) or in the more convenient tablet or powder form (Domeboro, Bluboro). One Domeboro tablet diluted in 12 oz or one packet in 16 oz of water produces (approximately) a 1:40 dilution of modified Burow's solution. Either must be diluted. USP Burow's solution, which is 5% aluminum acetate, is diluted 1:20[9] to 1:40.[21] This is somewhat drying, and the more dilute preparations seem to be less irritating.

Topical antipruritics are available (Sarna, phenolated calamine lotion USP, etc.) and are used by some.[21] Oral antihistamines are sometimes used early, before corticosteroids

TABLE 50–2. Treatment of Chronic Allergic Contact Dermatitis

Removal from all possible causes.
Use of topical agents least likely to sensitize.
Identification of the antigen by history and patch testing.
Removal from exposure to that and related substances.
Short-term systemic corticosteroid therapy.
Topical corticosteroids and occlusion.
For resistant cases (persistent light reactors, Compositae dermatitis) PUVA or immunosuppressive treatment (azathioprine, cyclosporin A).
When clear, reinstitution of exposure to ostensibly safe materials one at a time to uncover unsuspected problems which might arise.

take effect,[9,22] but topical antihistamines (e.g., Benadryl) may sensitize or photosensitize. Plain calamine lotion is drying but otherwise harmless and seems to provide some symptomatic benefit.

CHRONIC CONTACT DERMATITIS

Treatment of chronic contact dermatitis is a very special case as patients are often sensitive to multiple agents to which they have been exposed while in contact with an unrecognized allergen. This commonly includes gloves intended to protect hand eczema and therapeutic agents applied to the original condition. One learns to suspect everything, including topical corticosteroids. To manage such patients, it is necessary to provide an environment with minimal risk of exposure to potential irritants and allergens until the causative factors can be elicited and removed. Treatment of chronic contact dermatitis therefore involves the principles that follow below (see also Table 50-2).

AVOIDANCE OF ALL POSSIBLE CAUSES

The patient must be removed from contact not only with the principal allergen but also with other potential irritants and allergens.

Sometimes the cause of a patient's allergy cannot be determined immediately, as one may not be able to patch test the patient because of an "angry back" or extensive dermatitis. Such patients must be removed from all possible causes. This approach requires total avoidance of all treatments formerly used when success was not obtained. Topical lotions and moisturizers are especially suspect, and topical corticosteroids (and chemically similar products) used before are not especially safe either. For lubrication, either petrolatum (preferably Chesbrough-Ponds Vaseline) or a mixture of Aquaphor and water in equal parts can be used without very much likelihood of causing allergy. A topical corticosteroid which differs in structure from those used previously is selected, usually in a petrolatum vehicle.

IDENTIFICATION OF THE SPECIFIC CAUSE(S) AND AVOIDANCE

An essential part of the history is the search for known or suspected allergies. This will often give the experienced physician some insight into potential cross-reacting chemicals and hidden sources of contact. A patient allergic to benzocaine often will react to other substances with a para-amino benzene structure (e.g., paraphenylenediamine), and many persons with a history of deodorant reactions are perfume-allergic.

The causative allergen can sometimes be suspected from the pattern, but even then it must be confirmed with a positive patch test. It has been widely recommended that patients with suspected contact dermatitis not be patch tested in the presence of a dermatitis because of the risk of aggravation. False-positive reactions may occur especially if one does not recognize the angry back. However, it may be impossible to remove a source if one does not know what it is, but interpretation of positive reactions must be done cautiously when active disease is present. Moreover, positive patch-test results can be enormously helpful in uncovering the underlying cause or causes.

Patch testing, when possible, is used not only to find sensitivity but also to determine what is safe and what is not. One should ask the patient to bring in everything he or she has used. One then tests the patient to all (nonirritating) lotions and therapeutic agents, eliminating the reactors and uncovering the causative ingredient. When corticosteroids are suspected or found to be a cause, a series of steroids of differing chemical structures can be used to find one which can be used safely and effectively. If gloves or a plastic material are used for occlusion, patch testing to the gloves and plastic material should be negative before starting occlusive treatment. When testing to whole products, the ingredient is often in very low concentration in the product, and false-negative patch test results can be obtained.

HAZARDS OF HOME AND OTHER TREATMENT

Sometimes the patient cannot be tested because of the extent or severity of the eruption, so one has to treat the condition before patch testing can be done. Attempting an educated guess as to the probable cause of a new case of chronic allergic contact dermatitis can be a serious mistake. The problem is all too often much broader than suspected, with multiple, unrelated antigens in the case of allergic contact dermatitis and multiple irritants in the case of irritant dermatitis. The patient assumes that the medication or lubricant being used is safe and often does not even remotely consider that it could be a cause. Persons chronically exposed to a contact allergen are prime candidates to develop contact sensitivity to the topical treatments used, including corticosteroids. Therefore the patient must be *totally* isolated from contact with potentially allergenic agents. All therapeutic agents must contain the minimal number of ingredients and the least potential for causing irritation and allergy.

ENVIRONMENTAL CONTROL, ANTIGEN SUBSTITUTION

Once an antigen is identified, the patient must understand how to avoid contact and must make an effort to do so. Printed handouts such as those in this book can be helpful but are not an adequate substitute for communicating with the patient. The concept of ingredients as the actual cause of medication or cosmetic dermatitis may seem automatic to the experienced physician, but it is quite foreign to many lay persons who expect a whole product allergen to be just that and even then by trade name! Such individuals have to be taught to look for the causative ingredient and how to replace it with a less irritating material or a product without that allergen—a procedure commonly called "allergen replacement."[23]

ANTI-INFLAMMATORY AGENTS

Treatment of the eruption can be tried with anti-inflammatory and immunosuppressive measures, carefully using the minimum number of therapeutic agents with the least likelihood of cross-reaction and aggravation.

The most effective medications are mostly glucocorticoids, which may be either systemic or topical. When the cause is known and can be eliminated, oral prednisone is used in one of several treatment schedules over a 10- to 14-day period.[6,7,9] Dosage varies from an initial dose of 30 mg up to 60 mg, tapering to zero after 10 to 14 days. Triamcinolone acetonide or diacetate 40 mg IM is used by some, but day-to-day levels are not as controlled as with the oral route. Systemic therapy is not as desirable in chronic contact dermatitis as in the acute form, because the allergen is usually still there, causing the patient to rebound when the dosage is tapered.

When systemic corticosteroid treatment cannot be used, topical corticosteroid therapy with occlusion can be effective when combined with withdrawal from exposure. Typically a generous quantity of a topical corticosteroid in petrolatum (Synalar ointment is a favorite) is applied and covered with half of a sauna suit (used as either top or bottom and alternating) or a plastic wrap with mild pressure. This is left in place over a period of at least 8 to 24 h, and repetition may be needed. The secrets of success are good occlusion, reapplication of a generous quantity of medication during the 8- to 24-h period, and avoidance of any medication the patient may have used.

PUVA AND IMMUNOSUPPRESSIVE THERAPY

Immunosuppressive therapy with azathioprine and cyclosporin A has been used in a few cases, but this type of treatment assumes that the patient cannot be separated from the causative allergen. Psoralen and ultraviolet A (PUVA) is also an effective treatment for some patients with Compositae dermatitis and photoallergic contact dermatitis. Details of the methods for oral and bath PUVA are given below.

IMMUNOSUPPRESSIVE THERAPY

Azathioprine treatment has been used in a few reported cases of Compositae dermatitis and photoallergic dermatitis. Treatment is given in a dosage of 100 to 200 mg/day[24] or 2.5 mg/kg,[25] with attention to all components of the complete blood count and also to liver function tests. The drug is teratogenic, so pregnancy is, of course, ruled out before starting therapy in female patients of childbearing age and prevented by an effective form of contraception. Drug interactions include allopurinol and medications metabolized by microsomal (liver) enzymes.[26]

Laboratory tests are ordered every 2 weeks during the first 6 months and monthly thereafter. There is an increased risk of malignancy in patients on higher doses of this drug, and hepatic toxicity can be a problem. One should know that on a dose of 100 to 150 mg/day, total control is often not achieved,[27] which is not surprising, because the effect is on the afferent limb rather than the efferent limb of the immune system.[28]

Cyclosporin A has been used for actinic reticuloid in a dosage of 3 to 4 mg/kg/day, maintaining a trough blood drug concentration of 200 to 450 µg/L by radioimmunoassay in one study of two patients,[29] and 100 to 200 µg/L in another case report.[30] However, it had to be stopped in half the patients because of decreased renal function.[29] A reduction in patch-test reactivity was found in 6 persons given 5 mg/kg/day while clearing chronic contact dermatitis within 2 to 3 weeks.[31]

This medication has an adverse effect on renal function and may be associated with hypertension. There also may be an increase in the incidence of non-Hodgkin's lymphoma and cutaneous squamous-cell carcinoma (at least in renal transplant patients).[32]

Topical cyclosporin A has had mixed results, with some reports showing benefit[33,34] and some not.[35,36] Whatever the reason for the conflicting results, this is not yet an accepted methodology and there is no topical preparation commercially available.

PUVA THERAPY

ORAL PSORALENS

Oral 8-methoxy psoralen is given 1 to 6 h (usually 1.5 with new "ultra")[37,38] before light treatment. The traditional dose is 0.6 mg/kg, but 30 mg may be the minimal effective amount according to one study.[39] While doubling the dose may theoretically halve the light required, the plasma level may increase as much as fivefold,[40] so serum levels or redetermination of the minimal phototoxicity dose is perhaps indicated should one increase dose to reduce time in the cabinet.

The optimal dose of UVA (J/cm^2) can be determined by phototesting with incremental doses of UVA on the hip and reading at 48-h and/or 3 days to determine the optimal irradiation. In addition, serum levels of 8-MOP can be measured if available in your local laboratory. However, serum levels of 8-MOP can vary, especially when diet is not controlled.[39] A serum level of 30 to 50 ng/mL is usually necessary to produce an erythematous response, although higher levels are occasionally required.

In case of nausea, the dose can be divided, 30 min apart. For a 2-h dose, it could be given at 1 1/2 and 2 h before light treatment.[38] The greatest absorption is on an empty stomach.[41]

Before starting PUVA treatment, the eyes must be examined to document lens opacities prior to treatment, and yearly thereafter.[42] Sudden appearance of, or increase in, lens opacities is reason to stop PUVA treatment.

During light treatment, the eyes are protected with goggles known to block UV during exposure in the cabinet even with bath therapy (Table 50-3). Following light exposure, the patient must wear a wraparound plastic eye protector which blocks out almost all UV light. (These are available from Noir (313) 769-5565; UV Products Co. (213) 285-3123; and Dioptics (714) 859-7111; among others.[43]) Following exposure, two layers of clothing should be worn in a car or out of doors during daylight hours. We have tested protective clothing by Bullfrog with a light meter and found it to be an excellent block.

TABLE 50–3. PUVA Bath Method

1. Trimethylpsoralen (TMP) 50 mg is dissolved in alcohol and diluted to 150 mL of ethyl alcohol. This is added to 150 gal water in a bath, the temperature of which is tepid to warm (up to 37°C).[50,60] Topical 8-methoxypsoralen can also be used as 30 mL of the 1% solution, which is added to 80 L of bath water.[61]
2. The patient is allowed to soak in the bath water for 10–15 min.
3. Exposure to UVA is given immediately after exiting from the bath (within 10 min.)[50,58]
4. Phototestings can be used to determine the dose, although some start with a dose of 0.28 J/cm^2,[58] which almost all but not *all* tolerate.
5. The eyes are protected, as for oral treatment, and treated skin is protected for 3 days from inadvertent exposure. This is especially true for those treated with 8-methoxypsoralen. Washing the skin after exposure to TMP helps reduce systemic absorption.
6. Trimethylpsoralen solution is not commercially available. It can be compounded by crushing ten 5-mg tablets and dissolving the contents in alcohol. Bioavailability can be proved rather easily with the *Candida albicans* assay, as described by Daniels.[62] The size of the zone produced can also be used to quantitate the amount if a standard is available. The active ingredient is alcohol-soluble, so it can be filtered.

There are multiple treatment schedules published, but two fundamental plans are the basis for most:

1. The American schedule (for psoriasis) is three times weekly at 2-day intervals. Dosage of UVA is increased to maintain a reaction. The pigmentation can make reading of erythema difficult, so application of a small opaque patch at each treatment session (with a predetermined, characteristic shape—e.g., *M* for Monday, *W* for Wednesday, and *F* for Friday—would identify erythema of surrounding skin from the treatment given that day). This is especially helpful when treatment is given by multiple therapists in a unit. The increments for each skin type are given in Table 50-4. However a novel modification can be used by adding a test dose of 1.5, 2.0, and 3.0 J to the hip area every Friday and reading the erythema, if any, on Monday. The dose is increased to obtain minimal erythema. If no erythema is noted, however, an increase in dosage of no more than 3.0 J is used.[44] Some experts usually increase by 0.5 J/cm^2 every other prescription.
2. The European schedule (again for psoriasis) employs UVA four times weekly: Monday, Tuesday, Thursday, and Friday. The minimal phototoxicity dose (MPD) is predetermined on the hips before treatment is started, with erythema read at 2 and/or 3 days. Dosage can be increased as often as twice weekly in increments of 20 to 25 percent, stopping when reaching erythema. This method of treating psoriasis is much faster and requires a lower total dose, but care to maintain all parameters at the same levels is mandatory, as overdose will be given twice before the erythema appears at 48 h or later. Because the second treatment is given at 20 h while erythema does not peak until 48 h, additive phototoxicity can be a problem.

The light source should be a cabinet or one or more banks of UVA lamps. For some applications, the presence of UVB can be helpful, but there are no data to my knowledge for contact dermatitis or photodermatitis. It may even be a negative factor in the latter case, but this is not known. In one psoriasis study, the shorter wavelengths were more effective for the same dosage.[45,46] Dosage determined by UV meters is not uniformly

TABLE 50–4. Initial and Increment UVA Dose by Skin Type

Skin Type[a]	Initial UVA Dose, J/cm^2	Increment Range, J/cm^2
I	1.5	0–0.5
II	2.5	0–0.5
III	3.5	0–1.0
IV	4.5	0–1.0
V	5.5	0–2.0
VI	6.5	0–2.0

[a]Fitzpatrick classification.

the same with all instruments, so one would be well advised to have all instruments calibrated.[47] Duration of treatment will depend upon the result obtained; therefore treatment must be individualized. Immune suppression [decreased reactivity to dinitrochlorobenzene (DNCB)] occurs, but it returns 6 weeks after treatment is stopped.[48]

In some instances, 5-methoxypsoralen (bergapten), the plant chemical which is associated with berloque dermatitis, has also been used successfully in PUVA therapy,[49] but it is only 25 percent as well absorbed as 8-methoxypsoralen and currently is not commercially available in the United States.

Complications include actinic damage, pigmentary changes, and nonmelanoma skin cancer.[50] Immunosuppression, which occurs, is apparently temporary; immune function returns to normal after about 6 weeks.[51] Even contact and/or photocontact dermatitis can occur despite the immunosuppressive activity,[52] much as it does with topical glucocorticosteroids.

TOPICAL PSORALENS

Topical PUVA therapy has been used for vitiligo, psoriasis, mycosis fungoides, and even allergic contact dermatitis. It involves the use of a psoralen applied as a solution, ointment, or bath followed by UVA exposure. Hand and foot eczema is a typical use. Problems arise because the psoralen solution commercially available is in 1% concentration and has to be diluted to be safe. Even then the amount of incidental exposure can be a major problem, as blistering reactions have happened to many, many persons who have received topical 8-methoxypsoralen to be diluted (in alcohol or alcohol and propylene glycol) before using. One study used a dilute concentration in hydrophilic ointment and others have used dilutions of the 1% solution starting with a very dilute product and working up. The cosmetic result is not as reliable as with systemic treatment, so this is not practical for allergic contact dermatitis except perhaps a rare case of localized disease.

PUVA BATH TREATMENT

Psoralens used topically can be spread over the body from the neck down by dissolving the psoralen in alcohol and adding it to a bath.[53] This is very fast, aggressive treatment (mostly of psoriasis), in my experience. When followed by light exposure, the psoralen stays in the skin longer than when it is unexposed, so that the skin remains phototoxic for days.[54] Obviously one has to protect the treated areas until the effect dissipates. There is also some absorption, although perhaps not enough to produce clinical photo-toxicity of the skin. Whether or not the lens can be affected is not known (at least I have not seen such data). Therefore protection of the eyes is probably wise to be completely safe (see Table 50-3).

PUVA bath can be a good alternative in patients with nausea. Total UV dosage is about one-tenth that of oral PUVA therapy with 8-MOP. The stress of cabinet time is also considerably reduced.[55] The temperature is rather important, with 37°C producing an optimal dose.[56] The plasma concentration after a PUVA bath with trioxalen is much below the level obtained with oral administration, but there are individuals with levels as high as 9 ng/mL from trimethypsoralen,[57] and 100 to 200 ng/mL of 8-methoxypso-ralen. This is comparable to oral therapy,[58] so it cannot be universally assumed that the eyes are totally safe until there are data showing that. Using 8-methoxypsoralen, photosensitivity remains for at least 3 days provided that the skin is exposed immediately after psoralen application.[59]

REINSTITUTION

Once clear, reinstitution can be begun of "safe" materials, which are nonirritating and to which the patient is patch-test negative.

Patients who remain clear when treatment has been discontinued are ready to restart exposure to cosmetics, soaps, shampoos, fragrances, etc., provided that patch-test reactions are negative. However, this should be done one at a time for a 5- to 7-day period to rule out a false-negative reaction. In the repeated open application test, a cosmetic or other suspected product is repeatedly applied to an area which absorbs well, such as the face or neck or sometimes the antecubital areas.

REFERENCES

1. van der Valk PG, Maibach HI: Do topical corticosteroids modulate skin irritation in human beings? *J Am Acad Dermatol* 21:519, 1989.
2. Malten KE: Thoughts on irritant contact dermatitis. *Contact Dermatitis* 7:238, 1981.
3. Sulzberger MB, Wolf J, Witten VH, Kopf AW: *Dermatology: Diagnosis and Treatment.* Chicago, Year Book, 1961, pp 166–178.
4. Epstein WL, in Fitzpatrick TB, Eisen AZ, Wolff K, et al (eds): *Dermatology in General Medicine,* 3d ed. New York, McGraw-Hill, 1986, pp 1381–1383.
5. Fischer T: Prevention of irritant dermatitis, in Adams RM, *Occupational Skin Disease.* 2d ed. Philadelphia, Saunders, 1990.
6. Resnick SD: Poison ivy and poison oak dermatitis. *Clin Dermatol* 4:208, 1986.
7. Fisher AA: *Contact Dermatitis,* 3d ed. Philadelphia, Lea & Febiger, 1986.
8. Epstein WL: Contact dermatitis, in Rakel RE, *Current Therapy.* Philadelphia, Saunders, 1986, pp 678–679.
9. Arndt KA: *Manual of Dermatologic Therapeutics,* 3d ed. Boston, Little Brown, 1983, pp 50–53.
10. Epstein WL, Baer H, Dawson CR, et al: Poison oak hyposensitization: Evaluation of hyposensitization. *Arch Dermatol* 109:356, 1974.
11. Shelmire B: Hyposensitization to poison ivy. *Arch Dermatol Syphilol* 44:983, 1941.

12. Guin JD: The case of Dr. Shelmire's nurse: A historical look at the confusion surrounding hyposensitization to toxicodendrons. *Am J Contact Dermatitis* 2:194, 1991.
13. Kligman AM: Hyposensitization against *Rhus. Arch Dermatol* 78:47, 1958.
14. Watson ES: Toxicodendron hyposensitization programs. *Clin Dermatol* 4:160, 1986.
15. Guin JD, Lehman P, Gage D, et al: Evaluation of commercial poison ivy hyposensitization antigens by HPLC/MS analysis (abstract). *J Invest Dermatol* 94:532, 1990.
16. Shelmire B: Contact dermatitis from vegetation, patch testing and treatment with plant oleoresins. *South Med J* 33:337, 1940.
17. Srinivas CR, Krupashankar DS, Singh KK, et al: Oral hyposensitization in Parthenium dermatitis. *Contact Dermatitis* 18:242, 1988.
18. Stampf JL, Castagnoli N, Epstein WL, et al: Suppression of urushiol-induced delayed-type hypersensitivity responses in mice with serum IgG immunoglobulin from human hyposensitized donors. *J Invest Dermatol* 95:363, 1990.
19. Kehchi K, Nakagawa M, Kawai K, et al: Hyposensitization to urushiol among Japanese lacquer craftsmen: Results of patch tests on students learning the art of lacquerware. *Contact Dermatitis* 25:290, 1991.
20. van der Steen PHM, van Baar HMJ, Perret CM, et al: Treatment of alopecia areata with diphenylcyclopropenone. *J Am Acad Dermatol* 24:253–257, 1991.
21. *Drug Evaluations,* 6th ed. Chicago, American Medical Association, 1986, pp 1074–1075.
22. Fisher AA: Contact dermatitis, in Madden S, Brown TH, Lynne-Davies G (eds): *Current Dermatologic Management,* 2d ed, St Louis, Mosby, 1975, pp 110–112.
23. Calnan CD: Studies in contact dermatitis: XXIII. Allergen replacement. *Trans St Johns Dermatol Soc* 56:131, 1970.
24. Leigh IM, Hawk JLM: Treatment of chronic actinic dermatitis with azathioprine. *Brit J Dermatol* 110:691, 1984.
25. August PJ: Azathioprine in the treatment of eczema and actinic reticuloid. *Brit J Dermatol* 107(suppl 22):23, 1982.
27. Roed-Petersen J, Thompsen K: Azathioprine in the treatment of airborne contact dermatitis from Compositae oleoresins and sensitivity to UVA. *Acta Derm Venereol* 60:275, 1980.
28. *AMA Drug Evaluations,* 6th ed. Chicago, American Medical Association, 1986, p 1152.
29. Duschet P, Schwartz T, Oppolzer G, Gschnait F: Persistent light reaction: Successful treatment with cyclosporin A. *Acta Derm Venereol* 68:176, 1988.
30. Norris PG, Camp RDR, Hawk JLM: Actinic reticuloid, response to cyclosporin. *J Am Acad Dermatol* 21:307, 1989.
31. Higgins EM, McClelland J, Friedmann PS, et al: Oral cyclosporin inhibits the expression of contact hypersensitivity in man. *J Dermatol Sci* 2:79, 1991.
32. *Physicians Desk Reference,* 46th ed. Montvale NJ, Medical Economics Company, 1992.
33. Nakagawa S, Oka D, Jinno Y, et al: Topical application of cyclosporin on guinea pig allergic contact dermatitis. *Arch Dermatol* 124:907, 1988.
34. Biren CA, Barr RJ, Ganderup GS, et al: Topical cyclosporin: Effects on allergic contact dermatitis in guinea pigs. *Contact Dermatitis* 20:10, 1989.
35. Cole GW, Shimomaye S, Goodman M: The effect of topical cyclosporin A on the elicitation phase of allergic contact dermatitis. *Contact Dermatitis* 19:129, 1988.
36. De Rie MA, Meinarfi MM, Bos JD: The lack of efficacy of topical cyclosporin A in atopic dermatitis and allergic contact dermatitis. *Acta Derm Venereol* 71:452, 1991.
37. Goldstein DP, Carter DM, Ljuggren B, Burkholder J: Minimal phototoxic doses and 8-MOP serum levels in PUVA patients. *J Invest Dermatol* 78:429, 1982.
38. Stern RS: Oral psoralen photochemotherapy for psoriasis. *Dermatol Clin* 2:421, 1984.
39. McClelland J, Fisher C, Farr PM, et al: The relationship between plasma psoralen concentration and psoralen UVA-erythema. *Br J Dermatol* 124:585, 1991.
40. Walther T, Haustein UF: 8-methoxypsoralen serum levels in poor responders to photochemotherapy. *Int J Dermatol* 30:516, 1991.
41. Herfst MJ, Dewolff FA: Influence on the kinetics of 8-methoxypsoralen photochemotherapy of psoriasis. *Eur J Clin Pharmacol* 28:75, 1982.
42. Farber EM, Epstein JH, Nall L, et al: Current status of oral PUVA therapy for psoriasis. *J Am Acad Dermatol* 6:851, 1982.
43. Gupta AK, Anderson TF: Psoralen photochemotherapy. *J Am Acad Dermatol* 17:703, 1987.

44. Carabott FM, Hawk JL: A modified dosage schedule for increased efficiency in PUVA treatment of psoriasis. *Clin Exp Dermatol* 14:337, 1989.
45. Farr PM, Diffey BL, Higgens EM, Matthews JN: The action spectrum between 320 and 400 nm for clearance of psoriasis by psoralen photochemotherapy. *Brit J Dermatol* 124:443, 1991.
46. Brücke J, Tanew A, Ortel B, Hoenigsmann H: Relative efficacy of 335 and 365 nm radiation in photochemotherapy of psoriasis. *Brit J Dermatol* 124:372, 1991.
47. Diffey BL, Roelandts R: Status of ultraviolet A dosimetry in methoxalen plus ultraviolet A therapy. *J Am Acad Dermatol* 15:1209, 1986.
48. White SI, Friedmann PS, Moss C, Simpson JM: Recovery of cutaneous immune responsiveness after PUVA therapy. *Br J Dermatol* 118:403, 1988.
49. Tanew A, Ortel B, Rappersberger K, Hoenigsmann H: 5-methoxypsoralen (bergapten) for photochemotherapy. *J Am Acad Dermatol* 18:333, 1988.
50. Wolff K: Side-effects of psoralen photochemotherapy (PUVA). *Br J Dermatol* 122(suppl 36):117, 1990.
51. Takashima A, Yamamoto K, Kimura S, et al: Allergic contact and photocontact dermatitis due to psoralens in patients with psoriasis treated with topical PUVA. *Br J Dermatol* 124:37, 1991.
53. Fischer T, Alsins J: Treatment of psoriasis with trioxalen baths and dysprosium lamps. *Acta Derm Venereol* 56:383, 1976.
54. Gange RW, Anderson RR: Topical bathwater PUVA therapy. *J Am Acad Dermatol* 16:401, 1987.
55. Rogers MB: Standard oral versus bath psoralens plus ultraviolet A. *J Am Acad Dermatol* 19:368, 1988.
56. Jansen CT: Water temperature in bath PUVA treatment. *J Am Acad Dermatol* 19:142, 1988.
57. Salo OP, Lassus A, Taskinen J: Trioxalen bath plus UVA treatment of psoriasis. *Acta Derm Venereol* 61:551, 1981.
58. Neild VS, Scott LV: Plasma levels of 8-methoxypsoralen in psoriatic patients receiving topical 8-methoxypsoralen. *Br J Dermatol* 106:199, 1982.
59. Gange RW, Anderson RR: Topical (bathwater) PUVA therapy. *J Am Acad Dermatol* 16:401, 1987.
60. Hannuksela M, Karvonen J: Trioxalen bath plus UVA effective and safe in the treatment of psoriasis. *Br J Dermatol* 99:703, 1978.
61. Lowe NJ, Weingarten D, Bourget T, Moy LS: PUVA therapy for psoriasis: Comparison of oral and bath water delivery of 8-methoxypsoralen. *J Am Acad Dermatol* 14:754, 1986.
62. Daniels F: A simple microbiological method for demonstrating phototoxic compounds. *J Invest Dermatol* 44:259, 1965.

51

MIXING YOUR OWN ANTIGENS

Bo J. Niklasson

WHY MIX YOUR OWN?

A wide variety of patch-test antigens are now available commercially, so why should dermatologists ever mix antigens for themselves? Certainly, using available commercial materials is not only safer and more convenient but probably, in the long run, less expensive. Besides, mixing of antigens must be done carefully. Each antigen has to be matched to the vehicle and in the right concentration, or a false-positive or a false-negative result will occur. However, even with the large number of commercial antigens currently available, one still encounters many potential contactants not found in any standard testing series.

A new patient presumed to have contact dermatitis should bring in all cosmetics and medications which have been used on the skin. Starting with this, a very careful, detailed history is taken. This should include details of the disease development as well as exposure to all potential contact antigens in the home and workplace. It should also include everything that has been applied, and a good starting place would be the items that the patient has brought in, remembering that the average person will not still have on hand everything that has been used. Careful questioning about treatments during the time sequence would normally expand that list. Many people experienced in contact dermatitis supplement this with a printed history form which is mailed out in advance and brought in by the patient. A sample history form can be found in Appendix B.

Most of the time, the standard screening tray is included routinely, as it will detect a majority of allergies to well-known environmental antigens. One can increase the yield by testing with selected series of antigens available from commercial sources, such as Chemotechnique Diagnostics or Hermal Chemie. The selection of antigens to be tested—such as components from cosmetics, plastics, glues, shoes, etc.—should be relevant to the patient's occupation or known exposure. Fortunately, a large number of such series are now commercially available. Yet it is impossible for a standard series to include all possibilities, so one must also test the patient with products relevant to his or her environment. By combining testing to the standard tray, selected series, and the patient's own products—plus the suspicious ingredients in those products— one will have the best chance of finding the cause or causes of allergic contact dermatitis. In medical/legal investigations, it often helps to confirm the cause by finding the reaction to the patient's own product as well as the related antigen in a selected test series. However, positive tests to ingredients (because they are in optimal concentration) with a negative result from the whole product will require some explanation in the report.

One of the biggest caveats in testing to noncommercial antigens is the possibility of an irritant reaction causing a false-positive test. The chances of this can be greatly reduced if control tests are normal on at least 20 other individuals, which would make it unlikely that the material is a primary irritant in that form. In addition, where reactions are positive, serial dilutions can be done until the test is negative, which will help separate an irritant from an allergic reaction.

Misreading a test as allergic when it is not, or reading the result as not allergic when it should be the opposite, is extremely undesirable. While even commercial antigens are not completely free of these problems, one must take special care with nonstandard antigens to safeguard against false-positive and false-negative reactions based on improper testing procedures or irritation. When choosing the patch test unit, it is necessary to use a test chamber that does not interact with the test preparation, to avoid false-positive or false-negative reactions. The effect of reactive test substances attacking the material of the chamber has been described for aluminum chambers, a phenomenon that may result in toxic reactions.[1,2] Aluminum chambers also have the ability to elicit contact allergic reactions in patients already sensitized to this metal. Other undesired effects when using this material are inactivation, modification, and possible absorption of the antigen during contact with the surface of the chamber.[3-5] The basic requirement for a test chamber is therefore that it is made of an inert material such as polyethylene or polypropylene with good occlusion properties. Chambers of these types are Square Chambers (Van der Bend, The Netherlands) and the recently developed IQ Chambers (Chemotechnique Diagnostics, P.O. Box 80, 230 42 Tygelsjö, Malmö, Sweden), a patch test unit that can be made up in advance for efficient testing. The importance of using chambers made of inert plastic material has been pointed out.[2,6]

It is hoped that by following a few simple rules one can make the investigation more accurate. The importance of making a correct diagnosis cannot be overemphasized, especially when patients with a suspected occupational dermatitis are being investigated. The outcome has so much impact on the patient's life that difficult cases should, if possible, be referred to occupationally specialized clinics.

There are some items which are very difficult to test because the level of antigen available from the article itself is quite low. This is especially true for irritants such as soaps or shampoos. Other materials which are available in high concentration have to be tested at the right concentration and in the proper vehicle. The recommended concentration and vehicle can usually be found in one of the references at the end of this chapter or in Appendix A. We shall cover some simple methods of reducing irritancy by buffering, using ultrasound to extract antigen from objects and some of the basic principles of preparing solid and liquid patch-test materials. We shall assume that the products have been brought in by the patient and—for those from the workplace—that material safety data sheets are available.

EVALUATION OF PRODUCTS

First of all, a physical inspection of the product or chemical substance must be made. Check the labeling of the container and find out if the nature of the contents is relevant to what the label tells you. Take precautions with chemical compounds that belong to groups with known high chemical reactivity and compounds that are used in chemical synthesis (e.g., in research laboratories). The testing of such substances can result in patch-test sensitization if the concentration is too high. Therefore, patch-test preparations should match published concentrations and should not exceed 0.1% in concentration of the active component.

Chemical handbooks that give general as well as toxicological information for various compounds will be a valuable source in the evaluation preceding the preparation of patch tests.[7] Products such as detergents, permanent-wave solutions, hair dyes, photographic chemicals, etc., that might be acidic or alkaline should be tested with a pH indicator. By using acid or alkaline buffers as vehicles, these products can be patch tested too.[8] The method of using buffers is important because it often allows one to detect allergy to ingredients (e.g., perfumes and preservatives) that otherwise would have been missed if the products were diluted to the extent that the pH was within an acceptable range. Be careful with products that might contain hydrofluoric acid (stain removers in the graphic industry, cleansers for metals, etc.), which can produce chemical burns, and sniff the product to identify possible solvents that might be irritant to the skin, such as chlorinated solvents, thinners, etc.[9] These types of products should not be tested at all. If material safety data sheets, product ingredient sheets, or recipes are available, check these to find information on toxicity and possible allergenic components. When you strongly suspect products as the cause of a contact dermatitis, get all relevant information from ingredient sheets and material safety data sheets and request the components for patch testing from the manufacturing company.

THE EQUIPMENT FOR MAKING PREPARATIONS

The equipment listed below is needed to make one's own preparations (see Tables 51-1 and 51-2). Such equipment will easily fit on top of an office or laboratory table and can be purchased from companies selling laboratory equipment:

A balance, preferably with a sensitivity to four decimal places
Mortars and pestles
Plastic containers, e.g., 50-mL, to mix the products in
Glass containers, e.g., 100-mL, for mixing and extraction
Vehicles: white petrolatum, distilled or millipore-filtered water, acetone, ethanol, olive oil, methyl ethyl ketone (MEK), acid and alkaline buffers
Wooden stirrers to mix the preparations
An ultrasonic cleaning bath
pH indicators (e.g., Universalindikator pH 0-14, Merck)
Syringes, polypropylene, 5- and 10-mL
Hair dryer
Scissors
Scalpel blades

TABLE 51-1. Composition of Acid Buffer Solution, pH 4.7

Compound	Concentration	Percent of Total Volume
Sodium acetate	0.1 N (8.2 g CH_3COONa/L aqua)	50
Acetic acid	0.1 N (6.0 g CH_3COOH/L aqua)	50

TABLE 51–2. Composition of Alkaline Buffer Solution, pH 9.9

Compound	Concentration	Percent of Total Volume
Sodium carbonate, anhydrous	0.1 M (10.6 g Na_2CO_3/L aqua)	50
Sodium bicarbonate	0.1 M (8.4 g $NaHCO_3$/L aqua)	50

GENERAL NOTES FOR THE PREPARATION OF PRODUCTS

1. If the product is in crystal or powder form, make sure that the material is finely powdered by using a mortar and pestle when necessary.
2. Test all water-based products for pH and determine the appropriate vehicle on the basis of pH. Use water for neutral products, acid buffer for alkaline products, and alkaline buffer for acid products. Dilute the material in buffer if the product is below 4 and above 9 in pH. Buffer solutions greatly widen the range of possible products which can be used for testing. Buffering also allows testing at concentrations 300 to 3000 times those which are tolerated without buffers.
3. Select the most appropriate vehicle depending on the solubility and other characteristics of the product. Petrolatum can be used in many cases. If serial dilutions are to be made, choose the best vehicle depending on solubility characteristics and use liquid vehicles if you intend to make an extensive range of dilutions. Recommendations regarding vehicles and concentrations for various types of products can be found in Table 51-5; for substances, similar recommendations are found in Appendix A, Table A-3.
4. Perform the necessary weighing steps to obtain the desired concentration.
5. Serial dilutions are preferably made by dividing the highest concentration by 3.16 (which is the square root of 10) and continuing in the same order. This gives the most accurate decreasing scale in concentration (e.g., 10%, 3.16%, 1% ...).
6. Mix the product carefully with the vehicle to get a homogeneous preparation.
7. Protect from heat and light until the patch test is performed. Make sure that the vehicle does not evaporate.

HOW TO MAKE PETROLATUM-BASED PATCH-TEST PREPARATIONS

1. If your raw material is solid, grind it thoroughly with a mortar and pestle until you obtain a fine powder.
2. The powder should then be sieved in a fine sieve to reach optimum, controlled small-size particles. Each substance should be sieved in a specific sieve that is not used for any other substance in order to avoid contamination.
3. Perform the weighing steps by applying an appropriate amount of the powder to a weighing paper on an analytical balance (three to four decimals) and a corresponding amount (to the final concentration) of white petrolatum in a plastic container. An easy way of applying the petrolatum is to use 10-mL polypropylene syringes that have been prefilled with the vehicle. If the raw material is a liquid, pour it directly

into the plastic container and add the petrolatum until the desired concentration is reached. If you prepare liquids that might dissolve certain plastic materials, be sure to use either polypropylene or glass containers.
4. After the powder or liquid has been added to the container with petrolatum, mix the material thoroughly for a few minutes by means of a couple of wooden stirrers. Preferably, electrical variable-high-speed homogenizing equipment should be used to mix the material; however, this may not be practical in normal office practice. The use of sieves might also complicate and lengthen the preparation work. For solid materials, a careful grinding procedure using the portion that has the smallest particle size will provide a reasonable quality.
5. Put a label on the container with the name of the substance or product. If you intend to use the preparation later for other patients, transfer the material into a 5-mL polypropylene syringe, make a note of the production date, and store it in a refrigerator.

HOW TO PREPARE PATCH-TEST SOLUTIONS

1. Pour a suitable amount of liquid raw material into a plastic container on an analytical balance and add the corresponding amount of appropriate solvent until the desired concentration has been achieved. If the liquid raw material might dissolve the plastic material, use a glass container instead.
2. If necessary, place the solution in an ultrasonic cleaning bath (UCB) until all raw material is dissolved; otherwise stir or shake the solution for a short time.

ULTRASONIC CLEANING BATH EXTRACTION METHOD

Sometimes it is not possible to elicit allergic reactions by testing with a solid product in its unaltered form because the concentration of the active sensitizer in the product is too low or the sensitizer is bound to the material in such a way that a single application will not elicit a positive reaction. A good method of increasing this concentration of the sensitizer in the patch test is to extract it from the product with a suitable solvent and to use an ultrasonic cleaning bath (UCB) to make the extraction process more efficient.[10]

TABLE 51-3. Materials Suitable for Extraction

Product	Solvent for Extraction
Rubber products	Acetone
Plant materials	Ethanol, acetone, or ether
Paper	Ethanol
Textiles	Ethanol
Plastics	Acetone

**TABLE 51–4. Recommended Concentrations and Vehicles
for Patch Testing Products**

Name	Conc. (w/w) and Vehicle	Comments
Adhesive tape	100%	
After-shave	100%	
Alkyd resins	10% Pet.	
Barrier creams	100%	
Braking fluids	5% o.o.	
Carbamide resins	10% Pet.	
Car brakes	Extract	UCB acetone extract
Car steering wheel and scrapings	Extract	Test with UCB acetone extract
Carbonless paper	Extract	UCB ethanol extract
Color pigments	1% Pet.	
Cooling fluids;		Check pH of both product and working
-concentrates	2–10% Ac.B.	solution
-working solutions	5–20% Ac.B.	If the solution is neutral, dilute with aqua
Cornstarch powder	100%	Scratch-chamber test if contact urticaria is suspected
Cosmetic creams	100%	
Dental composites (tooth fillings, etc.)	10% Pet.	
Dental fluoride protective lacquers	100%	Let the lacquer dry before testing. May contain colophony
Dental impression material	10% Pet.	
Dental restorative methacrylate monomers	2% Pet.	
Deodorants	100%	
Detergents	2–10% Ac.B.	Check pH of both product and preparation
Dishwashing liquids	2–5% Aq.	Check pH of both product and preparation
Eardrops	100%	
Eau de toilette and cologne	100%	
Epoxy glues and lacquers	2% Pet.	
Epoxy glue hardeners	0.5% Pet.	
Eye creams	100%	
Eyedrops	100%	
Eye shadows	100%	
Food dyes	1% Pet.	
Food flavors	2% Pet.	
Food products (vegetables, meat, fish, flour, fruit, etc.)	100%	Test for contact urticaria with scratch chamber or prick test for 20 min and use histamine 1:10,000 in saline as positive control and saline as negative control
Fragrance oils	2% Pet.	
Gasoline dyes	1% Pet.	
Glues, contact for shoes, leather, etc.	10% MEK	
Glues, instant (ethylcyanoacrylate based)	10% Pet.	
Glues, melting type	100%	
Glues, methacrylate-based (Loctite glues, etc.)	2% Pet.	
Greases, various	100%	

TABLE 51–4 *(Continued).* Recommended Concentrations and Vehicles for Patch Testing Products

Name	Conc. (w/w) and Vehicle	Comments
Hair colors	2–10% Ac.B.	Check pH of both product and preparation
Hair conditioners	10% Aq.	Check pH of both product and preparation
Hair shampoo	5% Aq.	Check pH of both product and preparation
Hair spray	100%	
Lacquers, acrylate-based	0.1% Pet.	Concentration is based on the sum of monomers
Latex gloves	100%	Prick test when contact urticaria is suspected Make also UCB saline extract
Leather products (gloves, etc.)	100%	Make scrapings from the material and moisten at test Test also with water extracts
Liquid soap	5% Aq.	Check pH of both product and preparation
Mascaras	10–100% Pet.	
Methacrylate-based adhesives and composite materials	2% Pet.	Concentration is based on the sum of active monomers
Nail lacquers	100%	Allow to dry before test
Oil; drilling, engine, lubricating, mineral, transmission	50% o.o.	
Paint emulsion (water based acrylate)	10% Aq.	
Paints: alkyd based	10% Pet.	Test also with relevant biocides
Paints: latex-, polyacrylate-, or polyvinyl acetate-based	10% Aq.	Test also with relevant biocides
Paper	100%	Test also with UCB ethanol extract
Perfume	10% Alc.	
Permanent fixation fluids	10% Aq.	Check pH of both product and preparation
Permanent-wave fluids	5–10% Ac.B.	Check pH of both product and preparation
Permanent-wave fluids (acid)		
- activator	1–2% Al.B.	Check pH of both product and preparation
- base solution	10% Ac.B.	Check pH of both product and preparation
Pesticides	0.01–0.1% Ac.	
Pharmaceutical ointments	100%	
Phenol resin-based lacquers	5–10% Pet.	
Photographic developers	1–10% Ac.B.	Check pH of both product and preparation
Photographic film	100%	Test also with UCB acetone extract
Photographic fixation fluids	10% Aq.	If the solution has an alkaline or acid pH, use buffers for dilution
Photographic paper	100%	Test also with UCB ethanol extract
Photographic printing plates	Extract	Test with UCB aqua or acetone extract depending on the nature of the plate
Photographic wax	100%	
Plastic color pigments	1% Pet.	
Plastic products	100%	Test also with UCB acetone extract
Plastic UV-protective compounds	1% Pet.	
Polish remover	2–5% Ac.B.	Check pH of both product and preparation
Polyester resin	10% Pet.	
Polyvinyl acetate adhesives	10% Aq.	
Printing inks	10% Pet.	

(Table continues on page 694)

TABLE 51–4 *(Continued).* **Recommended Concentrations and Vehicles for Patch Testing Products**

Name	Conc. (w/w) and Vehicle	Comments
PVC gloves	100%	Test also with UCB acetone extract
Putty	10% Aq.	
Quaternary ammonium compounds	0.1% Aq.	
Rouge	100%	
Rubber products	100%	Test with scrapings or pieces and UCB acetone extracts
Shoes	Extract	Test with UCB MEK extract and pieces or scrapings of the suspected part of the shoe
Shoe polish	10% Pet.	
Skin creams, lotions, and ointments	100%	
Spectacle frames	100%	Test with scrapings and UCB acetone extract
Sunscreens	2% Pet.	
Textile material	100%	Test also with UCB ethanol extract
Textile dyes	1% Pet.	
Tobacco	Extract	Test with UCB ethanol extract and tobacco as is
Topical medicaments; creams, ointments, drops, lotions	100%	Antibacterial, antifungal, antiviral, corticosteroid, and NSAID products—test also with ingredients if suspected
UV-acrylate–based ink and lacquers	0.1% Pet.	Concentration is based on the sum of acrylate monomers
Wax	100%	
Wall-covering glues	10% Aq.	
White spirit	25% o.o.	
Window-cleaning products	10% Aq.	Check pH and if necessary dilute with acid buffer
Wood	Extract	Test with UCB ethanol extract and sawdust
Wood tars	3% Pet.	

Abbreviations: Ac., acetone; Ac.B., acid buffer; Al.B., alkaline buffer; Alc., ethanol 99.5%; MEK, methyl ethyl ketone; o.o., olive oil; Pet., petrolatum; UCB, ultrasonic cleaning bath.

For the extraction of various types of solids like paper, textiles, plastic products, plant materials, rubber products, and so on, use a UCB, according to the steps described below, to extract possible allergenic constituents from the products.

1. Use a small 100- to 250-mL glass container 5 to 7 cm in diameter. Cut the product in small pieces to fit in the bottom of the container, using 5 to 10 g of material.
2. Pour 5 to 10 mL of the appropriate solvent into the container so that the material is completely submerged.
3. Place the container in the ultrasonic cleaning bath and extract for about 5 to 10 min.
4. Remove the product sample and use a simple hair dryer to completely evaporate the solvent.
5. Add 1 mL of the solvent and shake the container so that the residue dissolves

or becomes evenly dispersed in the solvent. Use this extract for patch testing. Preferably a 10-fold dilution of this extract can also be used for the patch test. Make sure that the solvent does not evaporate before the test is performed. The materials listed in Table 51-3 are suitable for extraction.

GENERAL GUIDELINES FOR PREPARING SPECIFIC PRODUCTS

Table 51-4 is designed to provide a basic guide for the dermatologist or assistant to make patch-test preparations of a number of products. Owing to the great number of products and various types of products within a product group, it is difficult to give precise recommendations for each individual product. Some information and recommendations can be found in various textbooks on contact dermatitis.[9,11,12] Treat the information given below as general and use product ingredient sheets, if available, to evaluate the type and concentration of components in the product. Often, testing with two concentrations (e.g., 1% and 10%) of the product will give more information when reading the test results; this is especially valuable when products of uncertain nature are being tested. Whenever possible, use selected test series related to the specific type of product you are testing (e.g., cosmetic series for cosmetic products). Patch tests with the product might not always reveal an allergy, especially when the responsible ingredient is present in a low concentration or appears as a contaminant in the product.

REFERENCES

1. Kubo Y, Nonaka S, Yoshida H: False-positive reaction to patch testing with aqueous mercuric chloride in an aluminum Finn Chamber. *Contact Dermatitis* 26:136–137, 1992.
2. Kubo Y, Anan S, Nonaka S, Yoshida H: Does patch testing with ammoniated mercury in a Finn Chamber give a false-positive reaction? *Contact Dermatitis* 27:118–119, 1992.
3. Björkner B, Niklasson B: Influence of the vehicle on elicitation of contact allergic reactions to acrylic compounds in the guinea pig. *Contact Dermatitis* 11:268–278, 1984.
4. Bruze M, Björkner B, Lepoittevin J-P: Occupational allergic contact dermatitis from ethylcyanoacrylate. *Contact Dermatitis,* 1994, in press.
5. Budavari S: Aluminum and aluminum oxide. The Merck Index, 11th ed. Rahway, NJ, Merck & Co., Inc. 1989.
6. Fisher T: Design considerations for patch testing. *Am J Contact Dermatitis* 5:70–75, 1994.
7. Sax NI, Lewis RJ: *Dangerous Properties of Industrial Materials,* 7th ed. New York, Van Nostrand Reinhold, 1988.
8. Bruze M: Use of buffer solutions for patch testing. *Contact Dermatitis* 10:267–269, 1984.
9. Fregert S: *Manual of Contact Dermatitis,* 2d ed. Copenhagen, Munksgaard, 1981, pp 62–67.
10. Bruze M, Trulson L, Bendsöe N: Patch testing with ultrasonic bath extracts. *Am J Contact Dermatitis* 3:133–137, 1992.
11. Fisher AA: *Contact Dermatitis,* 3d ed. Philadelphia, Lea & Febiger, 1986.
12. de Groot AC: *Patch Testing.* Amsterdam, Elsevier, 1986.

52

HOW TO PATCH TEST
IN A BUSY OFFICE

Arthur D. Daily

For those who have never included patch testing in their office practices, an organized patch test program can be added to the office schedule with surprisingly little difficulty, but it must be done with planning and organization. This includes adjustment in the scheduling of patients so that adequate but not excessive time is allotted. One also needs a well-organized area where material can be stored and easily found and replaced. A work area where patch-test chambers can be loaded and applied to patients can be the same or a different area from that used for storage. With a little planning, patch testing will become an extremely rewarding experience with minimal changes in the normal office routine.

Most of us do not have the luxury of a large number of examining rooms, large storage cabinets, and excessive unused space. However, if you have one consultation room that is quiet and comfortable, well lighted, free of the general office traffic, and which will accommodate a 4- by 8-ft work area, this will more than satisfy the minimum needs. If you have a PUVA cabinet which you plan to use for photopatch testing, locating the room adjacent to this would be ideal for the occasional patient who will require such testing. Otherwise, a small wall-mounted UVA light source can be used for the same purpose.

The former problem of nonavailability of patch-test antigens has been corrected and there are now sources of very sophisticated sets of antigens. Therefore much of the work of assembling the test materials has been done for us. Insurance coverage has also improved, but even self-pay patients appreciate the physician's efforts to investigate their problem thoroughly. For most of us, remuneration is not an impediment.

OFFICE PERSONNEL

Personnel requirements are quite simple; usually one office employee can serve as a patch-test technician on a part-time basis. The ideal individual would be conscientious and diligent, with a calm, nonabrasive personality, who enjoys personal contact and

697

helping others. Most of us select a member of the regular office staff to serve as the patch-test technician. The duties of the technician include the scheduling of patients, preparing mailings to patients, organizing and maintaining patch-test materials, and applying the actual test materials. Most but not all dermatologists read their own tests, but even here, the person who applied the tests can be helpful. The technician also helps with record keeping, including notations in the patient's chart. Obviously, this will require some training.

Training usually starts with good record keeping. Proper design of the record facilitates the recording and retrieving of data. The actual recording of patch-test results may be done in a variety of ways, and you should design a system which best fits into your record-keeping system. Most of us use specific forms for each series or tray, some of which are provided by the manufacturers of antigens. I have even seen doctors use pages photocopied from the Chemotechnique catalog. In any event, it is important to maintain records accurately describing the antigens, since trays are often updated and the number, concentration, and vehicle of antigens may change.

TRAINING PERSONNEL

Training a technician to load and apply patch-test antigens could start with the steps illustrated in Chap. 5. A videotape is available from the American Academy of Dermatology which is extremely helpful in demonstrating the patch testing technique most commonly used. It is also possible to obtain "hands on" training in a facility that regularly performs patch testing. These techniques are covered in certain programs offered at the annual meeting of the American Academy of Dermatology. Another approach is to obtain a listing of members of the American Contact Dermatitis Society in your area and arrange to have your technician attend patch-testing sessions. This type of exposure offers your technician the opportunity to ask the myriad of questions that come up when one first begins patch testing.

SCHEDULING

For the inexperienced, scheduling is at best difficult. The procedure will take less time with practice, and one learns rather quickly how to allocate time. To start, allow an hour at the end of the office day and adjust this. With a little experience, one can safely schedule patients during regular hours. This will require some advanced background information for efficient use of time. For local patients, one can also do initial evaluations and patch testing on separate days.

You do not have to be present in the office at the time the patch tests are applied; in many cases it is preferable to have patch tests applied when office activity is not so hectic, as it is essential that the technician devote his or her undivided attention to the application of the tests. If you utilize the standard trays that are available from commercial sources, you may choose simply to list in your chart the trays, series, or individual tests you wish to have applied. You can also specify any special tests by numbering them, so that your technician will know exactly where they are to be placed.

I personally trace diagrams on the back of the chart to indicate where the tests are to be applied. At times, there may be a portion of the back that is not available for testing due to some active dermatitis. It is then easy to indicate, on the tracing or perhaps stick-ons, where previous tests were applied, if the upper arms were used, and what tests were applied. You should plan to be around at first, however, until your technician gains enough experience to work alone comfortably.

For the reading of the patch tests, I prefer to be in the office. There is still some controversy as to the best time to read tests, but I read at 72 h, with a subsequent reading at either day 4 (96 h) or day 7, if necessary. Since some time is required to discuss with the patient the results of the testing, I schedule these reading appointments at a time when I am not doing surgery and have some extra time to discuss the significance of positive reactions. If the results are complicated, a subsequent visit can be scheduled for this purpose. Since most dermatologists do not work weekends, the patch tests could be applied either on Monday or Tuesday, and the patient could then return on Thursday or Friday for evaluation. I prefer not to have patches on over the weekend, when some patients are physically active and the technician is not available to field questions and problems that may arise. However, others do this commonly. Patch testing can be time-consuming, and many physicians will patch test only two or three patients a week. I find this has worked well in my practice.

THE PATCH-TEST WORK AREA

Unless you do a great deal of patch testing or have extra space in your office, a 4- by 8-foot area in the corner of a room is probably adequate for a patch-test work area, and it can serve more than one purpose. Figures 52-1 and 52-2 illustrate how this can be accomplished. Two such areas in two separate offices are illustrated. A hanging curtain helps ensure privacy should there be any intrusion into the room at the time the patch tests are applied. I also prefer to avoid piped-in music and other distractions in this area, as these might interrupt the technician or distract the patient during the application of the tests. As you will note from the diagrams, at least two or three shelves (or a cabinet) as well as a small, comfortable desk with a hard, washable surface are included. I prefer a Formica surface, as it allows the tape to be easily applied and removed and is easily cleaned to prevent cross-contamination of antigens which inadvertently get on the desk. Such a surface also allows the tests to be laid out and prepared in advance. Many prefer to have the patient wait in a comfortable waiting room, so that the technician is totally undisturbed during preparation of the tests. A good use of this time is to have a preprinted instruction sheet written for patients to review at this time. A refrigerator shown in the diagrams is definitely a convenience although not a necessity. Some patch-test materials need to be refrigerated, and the potency of almost all patch-test materials is lengthened if they are kept refrigerated. You will note from the floor plan that (1) the room is at the end of a corridor and not subject to the noise and distractions of the areas of the office where the traffic pattern is hectic and constant, (2) the patient's privacy is protected by a full-length curtain if anyone else must enter the room during patch testing, (3) if phototesting is necessary, the patient simply has to cross the hall for this to be done and does not have to traverse

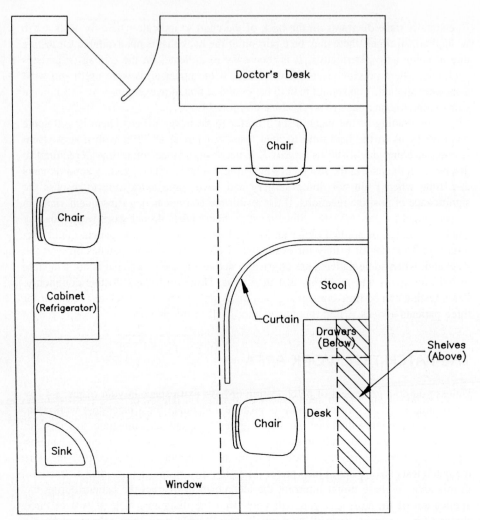

FIG. 52–1. Consultation room.

the rest of the office, (4) adequate lighting in the room is provided by both fluorescent lights and a large, curtained window. Natural light is not necessary, but some prefer it for the reading of certain tests.

Last, the storage area is arranged logically, with a basic simplicity. It is often necessary to temporarily store materials which are brought in by the patient and prepared for testing. However, if this is done, disposable plastic bags or containers should be used, so that the storage drawers are kept clean. The antigens—makeups, medications, and so on—once having been tested, must be discarded or returned to the patient. This not only prevents the patch-test area from becoming cluttered with materials that can confuse the testing but also allows your technician to keep track of special antigens that have been prepared and to note whether or not the results were fruitful and bear future consideration for testing other patients. This storage area should also provide a place in which to keep material safety data sheets for patients during the testing period.

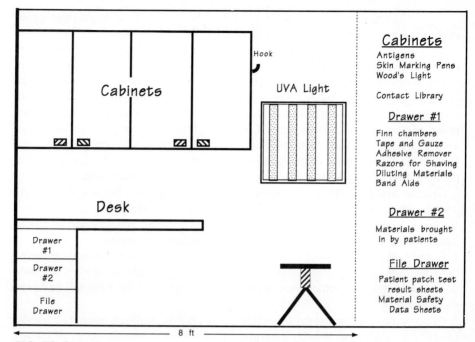

FIG. 52–2. Patch-test area.

Some physicians like to keep these as a permanent portion of the record—I prefer to discard them once the patient has been fully evaluated and appropriate letters have been sent to the referring physician, attorney, or other relevant parties.

Photopatch testing is usually done in or near the same area, and it need not be costly or complicated. Both UVA and UVB fluorescent light bulbs are now available. If obtained in 2-foot lengths, two UVB bulbs are sufficient for performing any UVB or MED testing. Four UVA bulbs, in an appropriate box, are all that is necessary to expose the back in photopatch testing. These may be wall-mounted and provide a simple method of exposure that can be done in your patch-test area. If you have a PUVA cabinet, it can be used nicely with plate glass to accomplish the same purpose.

THE PATCH-TEST LIBRARY

There are a number of essential reference books which one needs to have on hand. Several textbooks are useful, and having more than one is recommended.

Contact Dermatitis (3d ed.) by Alexander Fisher is an excellent textbook with many sources of information. It was published in 1986 and is reasonably priced and informally written in relatively easily understood language for the most part. It also contains many practical suggestions, including numerous useful tests that can be done in the office and an extensive list of suggested patch-test concentrations. A number of chapters in this book are extremely helpful in understanding the significance of a positive patch-test reaction. Sometimes information in the book can be understood by an intelligent patient, but it is written for dermatologists.

Contact Dermatitis by Etain Cronin is another classic. While one might think a 1980 publication would be out of date, it is not. Individual chemicals listed in Material Safety Data Sheets can often be located in this book with explanations of how patients become exposed to them. The chemical nature of the material, sources of exposure, and cross-reactions are often given in the discussion. Details of the chemical structure of many allergens are provided. The sections are organized according to the particular category of allergen, such as foods (including additive), medications, metals, pesticides, plants, photosensitizers, woods, plastics, and so on. Information on patch-test concentrations is given along with each chemical discussed, and the St. John's experience is brought out along with a scholarly discussion of the subject. This book is a must on the bookshelf of anyone who is seriously doing contact dermatitis work.

Occupational Skin Disease by Robert M. Adams is a jewel because it succinctly describes the more common sources of occupational contact dermatitis and the reasons for them. It also contains an excellent list of patch-testing antigens and is another "must" reference book for anyone who sees occupational dermatitis.

Contact and Occupational Dermatology by Marks and Deleo is a well-organized, brief summary of most of the common patch-test antigens that are used. It is a time-saving quick reference which most individuals starting out in this field will find especially helpful.

Occupational and Industrial Dermatology by Howard Maibach contains a number of scholarly articles written by international authorities in various areas of occupational disease.

Botanical Dermatology by John Mitchell and Arthur Rook is an encyclopedic compendium of reactions to plants published through 1979. This book is out of print, but it may be available by writing Dr. Mitchell, who can usually find a copy for you. This book, when published, was an incredible bargain, and it is still an invaluable reference source on plant material. Nothing has ever been published which even comes close to its comprehensive coverage.

Plant Contact Dermatitis by Benezra, Ducombs, Sell & Foussereau is a practical guideline to botanical dermatology problems. Not only does it offer color photographs to help in identification, but it also provides chemical structures of antigens and "how to" patch test information.

The *Merck Index* gives a list of almost every standard industrial chemical and many chemicals obtained in chemical reactions. Structural formulas can be found here as well as solubilities. If someone is mixing patch-test antigens, this is a good place to find compatibilities and solubilities.

The *CTFA International Cosmetic Ingredient Dictionary* (5th ed.), published by the Cosmetic Toiletries and Fragrance Association, contains monographs on many cosmetics ingredients, explaining briefly what many of them do and giving synonyms and CAS numbers for them. Many structural formulas are given and botanical materials often give the botanical name of the source material. The descriptions within this book are very brief. Manufacturers of the particular chemicals are given under the trade names which are synonyms for the approved chemical names listed in the dictionary.

Patch Testing by A. C. de Groot is an invaluable source of concentrations and vehicles for unfamiliar antigens. This book is also taken from published cases and studies and is well referenced.

Two journals are especially helpful. *Contact Dermatitis,* which started publication in 1975, is an invaluable reference source. If you can buy back issues of this, do it and keep your subscription going, because more information on the subject is available in this journal than in any other source!

The American Journal of Contact Dermatitis started publication in 1990 and has included a number of scholarly review articles. Regular subscriptions to this and binding of the volumes is recommended, so that you can look up articles when a patient comes into the office.

A cumulative index is not available for either journal as yet. Looking through 27 or 28 volumes using the brief index in the journal is hardly a satisfactory approach, but one can do this with a computer search.

USING A COMPUTER

Computer searches are available through your medical school library, but you can do them in your office if you have a library card, a computer, and a modem. Many university medical libraries will have a 9600 Baud Modem hookup by telephone. A library search from the office can often bring you whatever information you need on the subject. It does take some practice to learn how to do this, but it is not difficult. Once you know how to do it, you can get an incredible amount of material on line, and you can even limit it to the journals that you have on hand. Silver Platter and Aries both have 5-year data bases on CD ROM. Hopefully, by February 1995 the American Academy of Dermatology will also provide a computer disk with a dermatology data base in the CD ROM format. This will require a CD drive for the computer but will allow almost instantaneous search from the date of the disk back to 1966. The services will search the National Library of Medicine (NLM) Index and provide abstracts on the articles available there. The quality of medicine possible for the physician who has instant availability of the NLM file is nothing short of incredible when one compares the situation today with what it was like in the 1950s. The low cost of effective IBM PC–compatible hardware and the efficiency of the 486, and newer microprocessors have brought main-frame capabilities to Main Street. This technology can tell you where to look in any of the 30 or more volumes of *Contact Dermatitis* for the patch-testing information on N,N'-tetraglycidyl-4,4'-methylene dianiline you would find on a Material Safety Data Sheet. It often becomes much easier than you think, because the MSDS has the CAS number on it and you can search for that specifically! Finding out such information without a computer may be so difficult and time-consuming that few of us would even try.

In summary, it is possible to become very good at diagnosing and treating contact dermatitis. It takes some effort, practice, and motivation, but the improvement in the quality of care is well worth the effort. Besides, contact dermatitis is fun! The experience can be described as Sherlockian, and I find it very positive for both doctor and patient. I have outlined what I consider to be a good starting place. You can improve on it as you work in the area and look for better ways to do things.

APPENDIX A

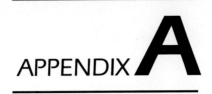

PATCH-TEST CONCENTRATIONS

Bo J. Niklasson

The table of contact antigens provides basic chemical information and literature reference numbers to the Chemical Abstract Service and The Merck Index for a majority of commercially available antigens and for some antigens not available through a commercial source. The table is also designed to give information about general occurrence and areas of exposure for the antigens. To help the dermatologist relate the antigen to the clinical picture as well as to select relevant antigens for patch testing, valuable information is given about airborne contact dermatitis, contact urticaria, cross-reactions, lichen planus, photoallergic and phototoxic reactions, persistent light reactions, pigmentation, depigmentation and discoloration of the skin. The concentrations given in Table A-3 are not specific for a certain type of test chamber and can therefore be used in combination with different brands in the market like aluminum Finn Chambers (Epitest Ltd. Oy, Finland), polyethylene IQ Chambers for filling in advance (Chemotechnique Diagnostics, Sweden), and polypropylene Patch Test Chambers (Van der Bend bv, The Netherlands). However, special attention has to be given to the problem of interaction between aluminum and certain antigens (see Chap. 51).

PATCH TEST CONCENTRATIONS

Bo J. Nilsson

TABLE A-1. Code for Exposure of Antigens

B	= Bakery products, food additives		O	= Oils, cutting fluids
C	= Cosmetic products		OP	= Ophthalmic products
CS	= Corticosteroids		P	= Photographic chemicals
D	= Dental products		PE	= Pesticides
E	= Epoxy products		PL	= Plants, woods
F	= Fragrance products		PG	= Plastics, glues
H	= Hairdressing products		R	= Rubber additives
I	= Isocyanate products		PH	= Photo antigens
ME	= Medicaments, antibiotics		SH	= Shoe chemicals
MA	= Methacrylate-based adhesives		SU	= Sunscreens
MN	= Methacrylate-based artificial nails		TF	= Textile colors and finishes
MP	= Methacrylate-based printing inks		V	= Various exposure

TABLE A-2. Abbreviations in the Table of Contact Antigens

Ac.	= Acetone
Alc.	= Ethyl alcohol
Aq.	= Aqua
CAS	= Chemical Abstract Service (CAS) registry numbers
Cross	= Antigens mentioned are primary sensitizers to which the compound might cross-react
CT	= Chemotechnique Diagnostics, P.O. Box 80, 230 42 Tygelsjö, Malmö, Sweden, Phone/Fax +46 40 466077/466700, Product Catalogue 1992/93
Exp.	= Exposure
FW	= Formula weight
H	= Hermal Kurt Herrmann, D 21462 Reinbek/Hamburg, Federal Republic of Germany, Phone/Fax +49 40 727040/7229296, Product Catalogue 1992
ICU	= Immunologic contact urticaria
MI	= The Merck Index, 11th ed, Rahway, NJ, Merck & Co., Inc., 1989
NICU	= Nonimmunologic contact urticaria
O.O.	= Olive oil
PA	= Compound that may cause photoallergic reactions
Pet.	= Petrolatum
PL	= Compound that may cause persistent light reactions
PT	= Compound that may cause phototoxic reactions
RPC	= Recommended patch test concentration and vehicle
UCU	= Uncertain mechanism type contact urticaria

TABLE A-3. Contact Antigens, Patch Test Concentrations, Exposure, and Other Data[1-13]

Name/Information	Formula	FW	Exp.	RPC	CAS	MI	CT	H
Abietic acid	C20H34	302.46	C,D,O,PG	10% pet	514-10-3	2	x	x
Component in tall oil used as deodorizing agent in cooling fluids. Major component of rosin used in adhesive tapes, glues, inks, sealants, cosmetics, dental impression materials. **Cross: colophony, dihydroabietyl alcohol.**								
Abitol	C20H34O	290.54	C,PG	10% pet	26266-77-3		x	x
Organic alcohol derived from wood rosin. For use in adhesives, mascara, inks, sealants, etc. Plasticizer in plastic materials (hydroabietyl alcohol).								
Achillea millefolium (yarrow)			PL	1.0% pet			x	
Perennial compositae weed with white flowers. Grows in most of Europe and in N. America, New Zealand and southern Australia. Contains the sesquiterpene lactone α-peroxyachifolide. **May cause airborne contact dermatitis.**								
Acid yellow 36	C18H14N3NaO3S	375.38	SH	1.0% pet	587-98-4	5833	x	
Dye used in leather. As indicator (pH) in laboratories. C.I. 13065								
Alantolactone	C15H20O2	232.31	PL	0.1% pet	546-43-0	198	x	x
Sesquiterpene lactone present in, e.g., species of Chrysanthemum plants (Helenin).								
Alclometasone-17,21-dipropionate	C28H37ClO7	526.31	CS	1.0% pet	66734-13-2	213	x	
Topical non-fluorinated corticosteroid with low systemic effects.								
Aluminum	Al	26.98	D,V	100%	7429-90-5	321	x	
As the pure metal or as alloys for utensils, dental materials, aircraft, electrical conductors etc. Occurs also in aluminum paints, analytical agents.								

Aluminum chloride hexahydrate

AlCl3 x 6H2O   241.43   C,D,V   2.0% pet   7784-13-6   338   x

Used in preserving wood, disinfecting stables, etc., in deodorants and antiperspirant preparations. In refining crude oil, dyeing fabrics. In dental ceramics. In topical astringents.

Amerchol L 101

C,ME,O,V   100%   8027-33-6   5231   x

Trade name of product containing **lanolin alcohols** obtained from hydrolysis of lanolin. Emulsifier and emollient in cosmetic and pharmaceutical bases, topical drugs, furniture polish, leather, metal corrosion prevention, paper, inks, textiles, furs, cutting oils, waxes. **UCU.**

4-Amino-azobenzene

C12H11N3   197.24   PG,SH   0.25% pet   60-09-3   430   x

Intermediate in the production of diazo dyes. Pigment in, e.g., plastic materials. Solvent yellow 1.
Cross: para group of compounds.

4-Aminobenzoic acid

C7H7NO2   137.14   C,SU,PH   5.0% pet   150-13-0   434   x

Sun screening agent in cosmetics, moisturizers, shampoos, hair care products, nail polish, lipstick, lip balms, oral vitamin supplements. Used in the production of local anesthetics, folic acid and azo dyes (PABA).
Cross: para group of compounds. PA.

4-Amino-N,N-diethyl-aniline sulfate

C10H18N2.H2SO4   262.33   P   1.0% pet   6056-27-6   x

Color developer and high speed black and aniline sulfate white film developer in photography (TSS, Agfa).
May cause lichen planus.

3-Aminophenol

C6H7NO   109.13   H   1.0% pet   591-27-5   472   x

Coupler for hair dyes. Dye intermediate. In the manufacturing of 4-amino salicylic acid.
Cross: para group of compounds.

TABLE A-3. (*Continued*)

Name/Information	Formula	FW	Exp.	RPC	CAS	MI	CT	H
4-Aminophenol	C6H7NO	109.13	H,P	1.0% pet	123-30-8	472	x	x
Ammonium hexachloro-platinate	Cl6H8N2Pt	443.88	V	0.1% aq	1332-76-9	576	x	x
Ammonium persulfate	H8N2O8S2	228.20	B,H,P	2.5% pet	7727-54-0	569	x	x
Ammonium thioglycolate	C2H7NO2S	109.15	H	2.5% aq	5421-46-5		x	x
Ammonium tetrachloro-platinate	C14H8N2Pt	372.98	P,V	0.25% aq	13820-41-2	577	x	x
Amylcinnam-aldehyde	C14H18O	202.30	F	2.0% pet	122-40-7		x	x

4-Aminophenol
Primary intermediate for hair dyes. Photographic developer. Dye for furs and feathers. **Cross: para group of compounds.**

Ammonium hexachloro-platinate
Precious metal salt. In platinum plating. **ICU.**

Ammonium persulfate
In hair bleaches as oxidizer and bleacher. Decolorizing and deodorizing oils, in electroplating, in making soluble starch. Reducer and retarder in photography. In yeast treatment. In analytical chemistry. **May cause airborne contact dermatitis. UCU.**

Ammonium thioglycolate
Acts as reducing agent in permanent-waving formulations for hair treatment.

Ammonium tetrachloro-platinate
Precious metal salt. In photography. **ICU.**

Amylcinnam-aldehyde
Raw material in the production of perfumes. **Cross: amylcinnamic alcohol.**

Amylocaine hydro-chloride | $C_{14}H_{22}ClNO_2$ | 271.80 | ME | 1.0% pet | 532-59-2 | 650 | x
For use as a topical and local anesthetic agent. **Cross: tetracaine.**

Anethole | $C_{10}H_{12}O$ | 148.21 | B,F,P | 5.0% pet | 4180-23-8 | 675 | x
Flavoring agent in food, dentifrices, etc. In perfumery for soap, etc. In pharmaceuticals as flavor. In photography and in embedding materials in microscopy.

Arnica montana (mountain tobacco) | | | PL | 0.5% pet | | | x   x
Compositae plant that grows on prairies and in mountainous lands in Europe, Asia. Tincture of arnica is used in trauma treatment. Major allergens appear to be helenalin and its esters. **Cross: a number of other Asteraceae plants.**

Atranorin | $C_{19}H_{18}O_8$ | 374.33 | PH,PL | 0.1% pet | 479-20-9 | 885 | x
One of the most common substances found in lichens. Component in extracts of oak moss used as fragrance. **Cross: oakmoss. PA.**

Atropine sulfate | $C_{34}H_{48}N_2O_{10}SxH_2O$ | 694.85 | ME,OP | 1.0% aq | 5908-99-6 | 891
Mydriatic and anticholinergic agent in ophthalmic preparations and preanesthetic medications. Also used as antidote for organophosphous insecticides.

1-Aza-3,7-dioxa-5-ethyl-bicyclo-(3,3,0)-octane | $C_7H_{13}N_2O_2$ | 143.18 | O | 1.0% pet | | | x
Preservative in cooling fluids. Trade name is Bioban CS 1246.

Azodiisobutyro-dinitrile | $C_8H_{12}N_4$ | 164.21 | PG | 1.0% pet | 78-67-1 | 931 | x
Foaming agent and inhibitor in plastic and elastomer materials.

TABLE A-3. (Continued)

Name/Information	Formula	FW	Exp.	RPC	CAS	MI	CT	H
Bacitracin	$C_{66}H_{103}N_{17}O_{16}S$	1421.79	ME	5.0% pet	1405-87-4	948	x	x
Balsam Peru			B,D,F,H,ME	25.0% pet		959	x	x
Balsam Tolu			F,ME	20.0% pet		960	x	x
Basic red 46			TF	1.0% pet			x	
Beech tar			ME,PL,V	3.0% pet			x	x
Befunolol	$C_{16}H_{21}NO_4$	291.36	OP	1.0% aq	39552-01-7	1032	x	x

Bacitracin
Antibiotic agent effective against gram-positive organisms and spirochetes. In products for topical treatment, ear medications, and ophthalmic drugs. Common allergen in leg ulcer treatment. **Cross: polymyxin B sulfate, neomycin sulfate. ICU.**

Balsam Peru
Flavor in tobacco, drinks, pastries, cakes, wines, liquors, spices, etc. Fixative and fragrance in perfumery. In topical medicaments, dentistry, etc. Consists of esters of cinnamic and benzoic acid, vanillin, styracine (Indian balsam, China oil, Black balsam, Honduras balsam, Surinam balsam). **Cross: colophony, balsam Tolu, cinnamates, benzoates, styrax, benzoin, tiger balm, beeswax, benzaldehyde, benzylsalicylate, coniferyl alcohol, coumarin, eugenol, isoeugenol, farnesol, propanidid, propolis, diethylstilbestrol. May produce erythema-multiforme-like eruptions. PT. NICU.**

Balsam Tolu
Resinous material from Myroxylon samum used as perfume fixative, in soap perfumery. Vehicle for cough mixtures, expectorant, antiseptic. **Cross: balsam Peru, benzylbenzoate.**

Basic red 46
Monoazo dye used for acrylic and polyester textiles (sweaters, etc.).

Beech tar
In tar paper and insulation tapes. In topical medicaments.

Befunolol
β-Adrenergic blocker used as antiglaucoma agent in ophthalmic solutions.

Benomyl $C_{14}H_{18}N_4O_3$ 290.32 PE 0.1% pet 17804-35-2 1053 x

Systemic fungicide for vegetables, fruits, bulbs, ornamental plants and lawns. Benlate: [1-[(Butylamino)carbonyl]-1H-benzimidazol-2-yl]carbamic acid methyl ester.

Benzalkonium chloride C,D,ME,OP 0.1% aq 8001-54-5 1066 x x

Topical quaternary ammonium antiseptic agent in ophthalmic preparations, skin disinfectants, cosmetics, deodorants, mouthwashes, dentifries, sterilization solutions, lozenges, and solutions for contact lenses. **Cross: cetrimonium bromide, benzethonium chloride. May cause airborne contact dermatitis.**

1,2-Benzisothiazolin-
3-one C_7HNOS 147.15 O,TF,V 0.05% pet 2634-33-5 x

Preservative in cooling fluids, paints, adhesives paper and in the textile industry (BIT).

Benzocaine $C_9H_{11}NO_2$ 165.19 ME 5.0% pet 94-09-7 3719 x

Local and topical anesthetic used in products such as burn and sunburn remedies, hemorrhoidal creams, suppositories, creams for treatment of poison ivy, oral and gingival products, sore throat sprays/lozenges, astringents, appetite suppressants. (Ethyl-4-amino benzoate). **Cross: para group of compounds, butethamine, procainamide, hydrochlorothiazide, PABA and esters, azo/aniline dyes, PPD, sulfonamides, sulfonylureas, 4-aminosalicylic acid, parabens. PA, UCU.**

Benzoic acid $C_7H_6O_2$ 122.12 B,ME 5.0% pet 65-85-0 1101 x

In preserving foods, fats, fruit juices, etc. For curing tobacco. Antifungal agent in pharmaceutical preparations and cosmetics. **Cross: balsam Peru. ICU.**

1H-Benzotriazole $C_6H_5N_3$ 119.13 O,P,V 1.0% pet 95-14-7 1119 x

Anticorrosive agent in cooling fluids fuels, photographic development, antifreeze, dry cleaning, etc.

Betamethasone-
17-valerate $C_{27}H_{37}FO_6$ 476.26 CS,ME 1.0% pet 2152-44-5 1202 x

Topical and systemic corticosteroid of group C type with a C-16 methyl substitution.

TABLE A-3. (*Continued*)

Name/Information	Formula	FW	Exp.	RPC	CAS	MI	CT	H
Benzoyl peroxide	$C_{14}H_{10}O_4$	242.23	B,PG	1.0% pet	94-36-0	1128	x	x
Benzyl alcohol	C_7H_8O	108.13	C,ME,OP,P	1.0% pet	100-51-6	1138	x	
Benzyl-4-hydroxy-benzoate	$C_{14}H_{12}O_3$	228.26	C,ME,	3.0% pet	94-18-8		x	
Benzyl salicylate	$C_{14}H_{12}O_3$	228.26	C,F	2.0% pet	118-58-1	1160	x	x
Birch tar			ME,PL	3.0% pet		1252	x	x
Bisphenol A	$C_{15}H_{16}O_2$	228.29	E,PG	1.0% pet	80-05-7	1311	x	x

Benzoyl peroxide
Initiator in the polymerization of plastics. Oxidizer in bleaching oils, flour etc. Keratolytic agent in acne medications. **May cause discoloration of the hair and postinflammatory pigmentation and hypopigmentation. May cause airborne contact dermatitis. UCU.**

Benzyl alcohol
Solvent in photography, perfumery and for dyestuffs, inks, pharmaceutical products, etc. Preservative in injectable drugs, ophthalmic solutions, and oral liquids. **Cross: balsam Peru, benzoin tincture. May cause pigmentation of the face. ICU.**

Benzyl-4-hydroxy-benzoate
Preservative in cosmetics and pharmaceutical preparations. (Benzylparaben). **Cross: diethylstilbestrol.**

Benzyl salicylate
Organic solvent for perfumes. Also in tanning creams and lotions. **May cause pigmentation of the face.**

Birch tar
Component in pharmaceutical preparations.

Bisphenol A
Raw material in the production of epoxy and acrylic resins. Component in semisynthetic waxes. (4,4-Isopropylidene diphenol). **Cross: diethylstilbestrol, hydroquinonemonobenzyl ether.**

Bithionol $C_{12}H_6Cl_4O_2S$ 356.07 C,PH 1.0% pet 97-18-7 1316 x x
Antibacterial agent in soaps, cosmetics, agricultural fungicides, veterinary antiseptic and antihelminthic products, industrial cleansers, etc. 2,2-Thiobis(4,6-dichlorophenol). **PA, PL**

2-Bromo-2-nitro-propane-1,3-diol $C_3H_6BrNO_4$ 199.99 C,H,ME,O 0.25% pet 52-51-7 1437 x x
Preservative in cooling fluids, hand & face creams, shampoos, hair dressings, mascaras, cleansing lotions, milk sampling, paints, textiles, humidifiers, pharmaceutical products, washing detergents (Bronopol).

Budesonide $C_{25}H_{34}O_6$ 430.55 CS,ME 0.1% pet 51333-22-3 1455 x
Nonhalogenated corticosteroid for use in topical preparations and for the treatment of rhinitis and asthma. Belongs to the group B (triamcinolone acetonide) type of corticosteroids. Good marker of corticosteroid allergy. **Cross: hydrocortisone butyrate.**

1,4-Butanediol-diacrylate $C_{10}H_{14}O_4$ 198.24 MP,V 0.1% pet 1070-70-8 x
Cross-linking monomer for use in inks, adhesives, textile product modifiers, photo resists, etc. (BUDA).

1,4-Butanediol-dimethacrylate $C_{12}H_{18}O_4$ 226.28 D,MA 2.0% pet 2082-81-7 x
Cross-linking methacrylic monomer for use in dental composite materials, sealants, prostheses, etc. (BUDMA).

n-Butyl acrylate $C_7H_{12}O_2$ 128.17 MN,TF 0.1% pet 141-32-2 1539 x x
Cross-linking acrylic monomer for use in textile and leather finishes, paint formulations, etc. (BA).

4-tert-Butyl-benzoic acid $C_{11}H_{14}O_2$ 178.24 O 1.0% pet 98-73-7 x x
Corrosion inhibitor in cooling fluids.

TABLE A-3. *(Continued)*

Name/Information	Formula	FW	Exp.	RPC	CAS	MI	CT	H
4-tert-Butylcatechol	$C_{10}H_{14}O_2$	166.22	O,PG	0.5% pet	98-29-3		x	x
Antioxidant in polyester resins and as polymerization inhibitor in PVC. Also described as allergen in photocopying paper and as antioxidant in oil. **May cause depigmentation.**								
Butyl-4-hydroxy-benzoate	$C_{11}H_{14}O_3$	194.23	B,C,ME	3.0% pet	94-26-8	1583	x	x
Preservative in foods (salad dressings, mayonnaise, spiced sauces, mustard, frozen dairy products, baked products), cosmetics and pharmaceutical preparations. Butylparaben.								
tert-Butylhydroquinone	$C_{10}H_{14}O_2$	166.22	C	1.0% pet	1948-33-0		x	
Antioxidant in cosmetic products like lipsticks.								
n-Butyl methacrylate	$C_8H_{14}O_2$	142.20	D,MA,MN	2.0% pet	97-88-1		x	
Cross-linking methacrylic monomer for use in dental composite materials, artificial nails, etc.(BMA).								
4-tert-Butyl-4'-methoxy-dibenzoylmethane	$C_{20}H_{22}O_3$	310.20	C,SU	2.0% pet	70356-09-1	1580	x	x
UV-A adsorbing agent in sunscreen cosmetics of the type creams, lotions, lipsticks, sun oils, etc. (Parsol 1789).								
2-tert-Butyl-4-methoxy-phenol	$C_{11}H_{16}O_2$	180.25	B,C,PG	2.0% pet	121-00-6	1547	x	x
Antioxidant in foods (beverages, gum, ice cream, fruits, cereals), cosmetics, topical medications, animal feeds, petroleum products, jet fuels, rubber, plastics, paints, glues. (BHA). **May cause depigmentation.** **May cause airborne contact dermatitis. UCU.**								

4-tert-Butylphenol $C_{10}H_{14}O$ 150.21   PG   1.0%pet   98-54-4   1584   x   x

Intermediate in the production of lacquer and varnish resins. Antioxidant in plastics, adhesives, etc. **May cause depigmentation.**

4-tert-Butylphenol formaldehyde resin   PG,SH,V   1.0%pet   x   x

Resin used in adhesives for shoes and watch straps. Also in do-it-yourself glues, plywood, insulation, automobiles, motor oils, inks, papers, film developers, disinfectants, deodorants. (PTBP). **May cause depigmentation.**

Cadmium chloride $CdCl_2$ 183.32   P,V   1.0%aq   10108-64-2   1615   x

In photography. In the production of cadmium yellow. As fungicide, anticorrosive agent. In pigments for glass, tattoos, and paints.

Camphoroquinone $C_{10}H_{14}O_2$ 166.22   D   1.0%pet   10373-78-1   x

Initiator for visible light cured dental acrylic composite materials.

Cananga oil   F   2.0%pet   10008   x

Fragrance for use in various perfumes. **Cross: benzyl salicylate. May cause pigmentation of the face.**

Captafol $C_{10}H_9O_2NSCl_4$ 349.10   PE   0.1%pet   x

Fungicide for use on vegetables, fruits and seeds. The compound is also used in the lumber and timber industries to reduce losses from wood-rot fungi in logs and wood products. (Difolatan). **May cause airborne contact dermatitis.**

Captan $C_9H_8Cl_3NO_2S$ 300.57   C,H,PE   0.5%pet   133-06-2   1771   x   x

Fungicide for use on vegetables, fruits, and different types of plants. Bacteriostat in soap, shampoos, hair tonics, animal flea and tick sprays. (N-trichloromethylthio-4-cyclohexene-1,2-dicarboximide, Vancide, Dangard, Merpan). **May cause airborne contact dermatitis.**

TABLE A-3. (*Continued*)

Name/Information	Formula	FW	Exp.	RPC	CAS	MI	CT	H
Castor oil				C,H,O,PG,V 100%		1904		
Cetalkonium chloride	$C_{25}H_{46}ClN$	396.12	C,ME,OP,V 0.1% aq		122-18-9	2009		
Cetyl alcohol	$C_{16}H_{34}O$	242.45	C,ME	5.0% pet	36653-82-4	2020	x	
Cetylpyridinium chloride	$C_{21}H_{38}ClN$	339.99	C,ME,R	0.1% aq	123-03-5	2024		
Chamaemelum nobile (Anthemis nobilis).			C,H,PL	1.0% pet			x	
Chloramphenicol	$C_{11}H_{12}Cl_2N_2O_5$	323.14	ME	5.0% pet	56-75-7	2068	x	x

Castor oil

Vehicle in makeup removers, lipstick, and wart removers. Also a basic ingredient in the production of synthetic resins and fibers and as lubricant in metal drawing, machines, hydraulic fluids and engine fuels. Used in the manufacturing of soaps, alkyds, oil based paints, lacquers etc.

Cetalkonium chloride

Quaternary ammonium compound for use as germicide and fungicide in ophthalmic products and cosmetics like deodorants. Used in leather processing, textile dyeing, and as topical anti-infective.

Cetyl alcohol

As emulsifier and emollient in cosmetics and pharmaceutical preparations. UCU.

Cetylpyridinium chloride

Quaternary ammonium compound used as preservative in cosmetics and pharmaceuticals and topical antiinfective and disinfectant. Can also be used on the surface of latex gloves.

Chamaemelum nobile (Anthemis nobilis).

Compositae plant growing in most of Europe, in North Africa, South America, Australia, and New Zealand. A yellow dye is extracted from the dried flowers and is sometimes used in shampoos, hair rinses, and ointments. Anaphylactic reaction following ingestion of chamomile tea has been reported. Kamillosan, containing C. nobile, is used as nappy rash and nipple cream.

Chloramphenicol

Antibiotic and antirickettsial substance produced by Streptomyces venezuelae. Present in eye drops and ointments and for systemic use. As bactericide against the rot of potatoes and other root vegetables. **Cross: azidamfenicol.** ICU.

Chloramine T

$C_7H_7ClNNaO_2S$ 227.67   V   0.05% pet   127-65-1   2066   x

Compound used as sterilizer, antiseptic, disinfectant, and chemical reagent in the medical and pharmaceutical field as well as in the food industry. It can be used to clean wounds and ulcers. (N-chloro-4-toluenesulfonamido)sodium. **ICU.**

Chlorhexidine diacetate

$C_{26}H_{38}Cl_2N_{10}O_4$ 625.56   C,V   0.5% aq   56-95-1   2090   x

Antimicrobial agent in, e.g., cosmetic and disinfection solutions, eye drops, uterine antiseptics, toothpaste, mouthwash, hand and wound cleansers. **PA. ICU.**

Chlorhexidine digluconate

$C_{34}H_{54}Cl_2N_{10}O_{14}$ 897.88   C,PH,V   0.5% aq   18472-51-0   2090   x

Antimicrobial agent in cosmetic and pharmaceutical creams, surgical soaps, anticaries solutions, toothpaste, mouthwash, hand and wound cleansers etc. **PA. ICU.**

2-Chloroacetamide

C_2H_4ClNO 93.51   C,H,O   0.2% pet   79-07-2   2109   x

Preservative in cosmetic and pharmaceutical creams, shampoos, bath lotions, etc. Also as preservative in glues, cooling fluids. **May cause airborne contact dermatitis.**

1-(3-Chloroallyl)-3,5,7-triaza-1-azonia-adamantane chloride

$C_9H_{16}Cl_2N_4$ 251.20   C,H,V   1.0% pet   51229-78-8   2117   x

Formaldehyde-releasing preservative in hand creams, lotions, face creams, shampoos, latex paints, topical medicaments, polishes, metal working fluids, adhesives, inks, etc. (Dowicil 200, Quaternium 15)

4-Chloro-3-cresol

C_7H_7ClO 142.59   C,H,O   1.0% pet   59-50-7   2133   x

Fungicide in creams, topical antiseptics, pharmaceutical products, protein shampoos, baby cosmetics, and cooling fluids. (PCMC). **Cross: 4-chloro-3-xylenol. ICU.**

TABLE A-3. *(Continued)*

Name/Information	Formula	FW	Exp.	RPC	CAS	MI	CT	H
5-Chloro-2-methyl-4-isothiazolin-3-one	C_4H_4ClNOS	149.60	C,H,O,SH	0.01%aq	26172-55-4	x	x	x
4-Chloro-3,5-xylenol	C_8H_9ClO	156.61	C,H,ME,O	0.5%pet	88-04-0	2176		x
Chlorpromazine hydrochloride	$C_{17}H_{20}Cl_2N_2S$	355.35	ME,PH	0.1%pet	69-09-0	2186		x
Chlorquinaldol	$C_{10}H_7Cl_2NO$	228.08	ME	5.0%pet	72-80-0	2191		x

5-Chloro-2-methyl-4-isothiazolin-3-one
The methylchloro isothiazolinone component in Kathon biocides, for use as a preservative in oil and cooling fluids, soaps, latex emulsions, slime control in paper mills, jet fuels, milk sampling, radiography, printing inks, moist toilet paper, detergents, shampoos, hair conditioners, hair & body gels, bubble baths, skin creams & lotions, mascaras, etc. *Kathon CG:* contains also methylisothiazolinone and magnesium salts. The following biocides contain chloro + methyl isothiazolinone: Acticide, Algucid CH 50, Amerstat 250, Euxyl K 100, Fennosan IT 21, GR 856 Izolin, Grotan TK2, Kathon CG, Kathon 886MW, Kathon LX, Kathon WT, Mergal K7, Metatin GT, Mitco CC 31 L, Mitco CC 32 L, Special Mx 323, Parmetol DF 35,-DF 12, -A23,-K50,-K40,-DF 18, P3 Multan D, Piror P109. **May cause airborne contact dermatitis.**

4-Chloro-3,5-xylenol
Preservative in cooling fluids, creams, topical and urinary antiseptics. Also in pharmaceutical products, hair conditioners, toilet and deodorants, soaps, electrocardiogram paste, etc. (PCMX). **Cross: 4-chloro-3-cresol.**

Chlorpromazine hydrochloride
Antiemetic and antipsychotic agent in pills, injections, and suppositories. **Cross: diethazine HCl, promethazine HCl, thiazinamium, ethopropazine HCl. May cause airborne contact dermatitis. PA, PT (systemic).**

Chlorquinaldol
Fungistat and antibacterial agent in topical pharmaceutical preparations. (5,7-dichloro-2-methyl-8-quinolinol, Sterosan). **Cross: clioquinol.**

Chrysanthemum cinerariaefolium (Pyrethrum)

PL   1.0% pet   x

Compositae plant that grows on rocky ground in Europe, Australia, Japan and N.America. Pyrethrum is the main source of the pyrethrum insecticide. Principal allergen is pyrethrosin. **ICU.**

Cinnamic alcohol

$C_9H_{10}O$ 134.18   B.F.   2.0% pet   104-54-1   2305   x   x

Component in perfumed cosmetic products and deodorants. **Cross: balsam Peru, propolis. May cause pigmentation of the face.**

Cinnamic aldehyde

C_9H_8O 132.16   B.F,PH   1.0% pet   104-55-2   2298   x   x

Common ingredient in perfumes for household products like deodorizers, detergents, and soap. Flavor in toothpaste, sweets, ice cream, soft drinks, chewing gums, and cakes. Also present in balsam of Tolu and Peru, hyacinth plant, spices, cinnamon, Ceylon and cassia oil. **Cross: cinnamic alcohol, cinnamon oil. May cause depigmentation. PA. NICU.**

Clioquinol

C_9H_5CIJNO 305.50   C,ME   5.0% pet   130-26-7   4924   x   x

Antiinfective and antiamebic agent in topical pharmaceutical preparations. (5-chloro-7-iodo-8-quinolinol, Chinoform, Vioform). **May cause brown discoloration of the nails and erythema-multiforme-like eruptions. UCU.**

Clobetasol-17-propionate

$C_{25}H_{32}CIFO_5$ 466.73   CS,ME   1.0% pet   25122-46-7   2361   x

Topical corticosteroid belonging to the group D (Hydrocortisone-17-butyrate) type of steroids. **UCU.**

Clove oil

D,V   2% pet   6718   x

Essential oil used in tooth powder, confectionery, microscopy, and as local anesthetic for toothache. Constitutes eugenol, acetyleugenol, caryophyllene, furfural, vanillin, and methyl amyl ketone.

Coal tar

ME,V   5.0% pet   65996-92-1   x   x

By-product in the distillation of coal. Topical antieczematic agent. **PA. PT. PL. May cause postinflammatory hyperpigmentation.**

TABLE A-3. (*Continued*)

Name/Information	Formula	FW	Exp.	RPC	CAS	MI	CT	H
Cobalt(II) chloride-hexahydrate	$CoCl_2.6H_2O$	237.93	D,V	1.0% pet	7791-13-1	2431	x	x

Component in paints for glass and porcelain. As siccative in paints. In various alloys (dental, etc.). **May produce erythema multiforme-like eruptions. May cause airborne contact dermatitis. NICU.**

Cocamidopropyl betaine	R-CONH(CH$_2$)$_3$-N(CH$_3$)$_2$-CH$_2$COO		C,H	1.0% aq	61789-40-0		x	

Surfactant in liquid soaps, shampoos, hair colorants, shower & bath formulations. (Tegobetaine). **Cross: cocobetaine.**

Coconut diethanolamide			C,O	0.5% pet	68603-42-9		x	

Mixture of ethanolamides of coconut acid (cocamide DEA). Component in bath, shower and body cosmetics and in cooling fluids.

Colophony			C,D,O,SH,V	20.0% pet	1065-31-2			x

Yellow resin in the production of varnishes, printing inks, paper, soldering fluxes, cutting fluids, glue tackifiers, adhesives, surface coatings, polish, waxes, cosmetics (mascara, rouge, eye shadow), topical medicaments, violin bow rosin, athletic grip aid, pine oil cleansers. Component in dental impression materials and periodontal packings (rosin, Portuguese origin). **Cross: balsam Peru, dihydroabietyl alcohol. wood tars. May cause airborne contact dermatitis. ICU.**

Copper (I) oxide	Cu_2O	143.08	V	5.0% pet	1317-39-1	2671	x	

Fungicide. Red pigment for glass. In antifouling paints (Cuprous oxide).

Copper sulfate	$CuSO_4$	159.60	D	2.0% pet	7758-98-7	2659	x	x

Fungicide. Pigments in paints. Reagent toner in photography. Copper metal is used in, e.g, dental alloys (Cupric sulfate). ICU.

Costunolide

F.P.L   0.033% pet   x   x

Sesquiterpene lactone isolated from the Compositae plant Saussurea lappa. The oil which is extracted from Saussurea lappa is used in perfumery and in the Orient for all kinds of diseases. Costunolide is present in the plant together with dehydrocostus lactone. **May cause airborne contact dermatitis.**

Cyclohexanone resin

PG   1.0% pet   x

Condensation product from cyclohexanone. Used to enhance the adhesive properties of products like alkyd-, nitro-, and chlorocaoutchouc lacquers. Most often used in floor paints. **May cause airborne contact dermatitis.**

N-Cyclohexyl-2-benzothiazyl sulphenamide

$C_{18}H_{22}N_2$ 264.41   R   1.0% pet   3081-14-9   x   x

Accelerator in natural and styrene-butadienethiazyl sulfenamide rubber (CBS).

N-Cyclohexyl-N-phenyl-4-phenylenediamine

$C_{13}H_{16}N_2S_2$ 266.42   R   1.0% pet   x

Antidegradant in natural rubber, styrene-butadiene and chloroprene rubber (CPPD).

Dehydrocostus lactone

F.P.L   0.033% pet   x   x

Sesquiterpene lactone isolated from the Compositae plant Saussurea lappa. The oil which is extracted from Saussurea lappa is used in perfumery and in the Orient for all kinds of diseases. Dehydrocostus lactone is present in the plant together with costunolide. **May cause airborne contact dermatitis.**

Dexamethasone-21-phosphate disodium salt

$C_{22}H_{28}FNa_2O_8P$ 516.40   CS.ME   1.0% pet   2392-39-4   2922   x

Corticosteroid of the group C (betamethasone) type. Used in eye and ear preparations and in systemic preparations.

Diallyl disulfide

$C_6H_{10}S_2$ 146.28   PL   1.0% pet   2179-57-9   x

One of the three principal low molecular weight allergens of garlic. Allylpropyl disulfide and allicin are the other allergens.

TABLE A-3. (Continued)

Name/Information	Formula	FW	Exp.	RPC	CAS	MI	CT	H
4,4′-Diaminodiphenyl-methane	$C_{13}H_{14}N_2$	198.27	E,I,PG,R,V	0.5% pet	101-77-9	2958	x	x

Curing agent for epoxy resins and urethane elastomers. As corrosion inhibitor. Rubber additive (accelerator, antidegradant, retarder) in tires and heavy rubber products. Also used in adhesives and glues, laminates, paints and inks, PVC products, handbags, eyeglass frames, plastic jewelry, electric encapsulators, surface coatings, spandex clothing, hairnets, eyelash curlers, earphones, balls, shoe soles, face masks. **May produce erythema-multiforme-like eruptions.**

Name/Information	Formula	FW	Exp.	RPC	CAS	MI	CT	H
2,5-Diaminotoluene sulfate	$C_7H_{10}N_2 \cdot H_2SO_4$	220.25	H	1.0% pet	615-50-9		x	x

Primary intermediate in various permanent hair dyes (4-Toluenediamine, PTD).

Name/Information	Formula	FW	Exp.	RPC	CAS	MI	CT	H
2,5-Diazolidinylurea	$C_6H_{14}N_4O_7$	254.10	C,H	2.0% aq	78491-02-8		x	

Preservative used in cosmetic creams, lotions, shampoos, hair gels, etc. (Germall II).
Cross: Imidazolidinylurea [Germall 115 (Sutton)], formaldehyde.

Name/Information	Formula	FW	Exp.	RPC	CAS	MI	CT	H
Dibenzothiazyl disulfide	$C_{14}H_8N_2S_4$	332.50	R	1.0% pet	120-78-5	3377	x	x

Accelerator for natural rubber, nitrile-butadiene, butyl and styrene-butadiene rubber. Retarder for chloroprene rubber. (MBTS).

Name/Information	Formula	FW	Exp.	RPC	CAS	MI	CT	H
1,2-Dibromo-2,4-dicyanobutane	$C_6H_6Br_2N_2$	265.94	C,O,V	0.5% pet*	35691-65-7	3004	x	x

Preservative for metalworking fluids, cosmetics, adhesives, latex emulsions and paints, dispersed pigments and detergents. Active ingredient in Euxyl K 400 and Tektamer 38 (Methyldibromoglutaronitrile). *) Concentration valid for Euxyl K 400.

Dibucaine hydrochloride $C_{20}H_{30}ClN_3O_2$ 379.92   ME   1.0% pet   61-12-1   3016   x   x
As local anesthetic agent (Cinchocaine HCl, Nupercaine HCl, Percaine, Cincaine). **Cross: lidocaine. PA.**

2,6-Di-tert-butyl-4-cresol $C_{15}H_{24}O$ 220.36   B,C,ME,PG 2.0% pet   128-37-0   1548   x   x
Antioxidant in foods (beverages, gum, ice cream, fruits, cereals), cosmetics, topical medications, animal feeds, petroleum products, jet fuels, rubber, plastics, paints, glues (BHT). **Cross: lidocaine. UCU.**

Dibutyl phthalate $C_{16}H_{22}O_4$ 278.35   PG,V   5.0% pet   84-74-2   1586   x
As emollient in aerosol antiperspirants. As insect repeller and as plasticizer in various plastic materials.

Dibutyl thiourea $(C_4H_9NH)_2CS$ 188.37   SH,R   1.0% pet   109-46-6   x   x
Accelerator for mercaptan-modified chloroprene rubber. Activator for ethylene-propylene-diene terpolymers and natural rubber. Antidegradant for natural rubber-latex and thermoplastic styrene-butadiene rubber.

Dichlorophene $C_{13}H_{10}Cl_2O_2$ 269.13   C,O,V   1.0% pet   97-23-4   3059   x
As bactericide, fungicide, and algicide in soaps, cosmetics, shampoos, dentifrices, toothpaste, mouthwashes, deodorants, foot powders, papers, adhesives and bandages, and cooling fluids. **Cross: hexachlorophene.**

Diethyleneglycol diacrylate $C_{10}H_{14}O_5$ 214.21   MP   0.1% pet   4074-88-8   x
Cross-linking acrylate monomer for use in coatings, adhesives, and printing plates of prepolymer type (DEGDA).

Diethylene-triamine $C_4H_{13}N_3$ 103.17   E   1.0% pet   111-40-0   x   x
Hardener for epoxy resins (DETA). **Cross: ethylenediamine dihydrochloride.**

TABLE A-3. (*Continued*)

Name/Information	Formula	FW	Exp.	RPC	CAS	MI	CT	H
Diethyl fumarate	$C_8H_{12}O_4$	172.18	PG, PE	0.1% pet	623-91-6			
Occasionally a contaminant in unsaturated polyester resins due to the reaction between free fumaric acid and ethanol. Unsaturated polyester resins are used in applications such as reinforced glass fiber for boats, piping, bathtubs, roof panels, etc., and as protective coatings, finishes, and lacquers. The compound sometimes occurs as contaminant in the insecticide Malathion. NICU.								
Diethyl maleate	$C_8H_{12}O_4$	172.18	PG	0.1% pet	141-05-9	3113		
Occasionally a contaminant in unsaturated polyester resins due to the reaction between free maleic acid and ethanol. Unsaturated polyester resins are used in applications such as reinforced glass fiber for boats, piping, bathtubs, roof panels, etc., and as protective coatings, finishes, and lacquers.								
N,N-Diethyl-2-methyl-1,4-phenylene-diamine HCl	$C_{11}H_{19}ClN_2$	214.74	P	1.0% pet	2051-79-8		x	x
Color developer for Eastman print and Gevacolor color development baths (CD-2).								
Diethyl thiourea	$(C_2H_5NH)_2CS$	132.25	R, SH	1.0% pet	105-55-5		x	x
Accelerator for mercaptan-modified chloroprene rubber. Antidegradant for natural, nitrile-butadiene, styrene-butadiene, and chloroprene rubbers.								
N,N-Dimethylaminoethyl methacrylate	$C_8H_{15}NO_2$	157.21	D, MA	0.2% pet	2867-42-2		x	
Amine activator in visible light-cured dental acrylic composite materials.								
Dimethylol dihydroxy ethylene urea	$C_5H_{10}N_2O_5$	178.14	TF	4.5% aq			x	
Formaldehyde type of textile resin (Fixapret CPN, 45% active component).								

Dimethylol propylene urea
$C_6H_{12}N_2O_3$ 160.18   TF   5.0% aq   x
Formaldehyde type of textile resin (Fixapret PH, 50% active component).

4,4-Dimethyl-oxazolidine
$C_5H_{11}NO$ 101.15   O,V   1.0% pet*   51200-87-4   x
Preservative for latex paints and emulsions and for cooling fluids (component in Bioban CS 1135, 74.7%). *) Conc. valid for Bioban CS 1135.

N,N-Dimethyl-4-toluidine
$C_9H_{13}N$ 135.21   D   5.0% pet   99-97-8   x   x
Amine accelerator for the polymerization of e.g. dental methacrylic restorative materials.

N,N´-Dimethylthiourea
$C_3H_8N_2S$ 104.18   V   2.0% pet   534-13-4
Antioxidant present in diazo copy paper to prevent yellow discoloration of the paper. **May cause airborne contact dermatitis. PA.**

N,N-Di-β-naphtyl-4-phenylene-diamine
$C_{26}H_{20}N_2$ 360.46   R   1.0% pet   93-46-9   x
Antidegradant for latex, nitrile rubber, styrene-butadiene, and nitrile-butadiene rubber (DBNPD).

Dioctyl phthalate
$C_{24}H_{38}O_4$ 390.57   PG   2.0% pet   117-81-7   1262   x   x
Plasticizer in various plastic materials. Diethylhexyl phthalate (DEHP, DOP).

Dipentamethylenethiuram disulphide
$(C_5H_{10}NCS_2)_2$ 320.60   SH,R   1.0% pet   94-37-1   x   x
Accelerator and vulcanizing agent for latex (gloves) and butyl rubber (PTD).

TABLE A-3. *(Continued)*

Name/Information	Formula	FW	Exp.	RPC	CAS	MI	CT	H
Dipentene	$C_{10}H_{16}$	136.24	B.O.V	1.0% pet	138-86-3	5371	x	x
Pressure stabilizer in oils. Solvent for lacquers, inks, polishes, etc. Commercial dipentene also contains other terpenes (Limonene).								
Diphenhydramine hydrochloride	$C_{17}H_{22}ClNO$	291.82	ME,PH	1.0% pet	147-24-0	3308	x	x
Antihistaminic drug. PA.								
N,N'-Diphenyl-guanidine	$C_{13}H_{13}N_3$	211.27	R,SH	1.0% pet	102-06-7	2235	x	x
Medium accelerator for use with thiazoles and sulfenamides in various rubber products.								
Diphenylmethane-4,4-diisocyanate	$C_{15}H_{10}N_2O_2$	250.26	I,PG,R	2.0% pet	101-68-8		x	x
Diisocyanate in the production of polyurethane lacquers, foam plastics, rubber, and glues (MDI).								
N,N'-Diphenyl-4-phenylene-diamine	$C_{18}H_{16}N_2$	260.34	R	1.0% pet	74-31-7	3331	x	x
Antidegradant for nitrile-butadiene rubber, natural, styrene-butadiene, isoprene, butadiene, and chloroprene rubbers (DPPD).								
N,N'-Diphenyl-thiourea	$C_{13}H_{12}N_2S$	228.32	PG,R,SH	1.0% pet	102-08-9	3337	x	x
Accelerator and activator for chloroprene rubber and ethylene-propylene-diene terpolymers. In sulfur dyes and as heat stabilizer in PVC adhesive tape backing (Thiocarbanilide, DPTU).								

Disperse blue 3 $C_{17}H_{16}N_2O_3$ 296.33   TF   1.0% pet   2475-46-9   x   x
Textile dye of antraquinone type. Dye in nylon , acrylic, polyester and acetate. Stocking dye (C.I. 61505).

Disperse blue 35   296.27   TF   1.0% pet   x
Textile dye of antraquinone type. Dye in nylon, acrylic, polyester, and acetate. **PT.**

Disperse blue 85   TF   1.0% pet   x
Textile dye of azo type.

Disperse blue 106   TF   1.0% pet   x
Monoazo dye used for secondary cellulose fabrics (polyester blouses, garment linings, etc.)

Disperse blue 124 $C_{15}H_{21}N_5O_4S$ 367.47   TF   1.0% pet   x
Azo dye used for secondary cellulose acetate fabrics (stockings, garment linings, etc.)

Disperse blue 153   TF   1.0% pet   x
Textile dye of antraquinone type.

Disperse brown 1 $C_{16}H_{15}Cl_3N_4O_4$ 433.68   TF   1.0% pet   x
Textile dye of azo type.

Disperse orange 1 $C_{18}H_{14}N_4O_2$ 318.34   TF   1.0% pet   2581-69-3   x
Textile dye of azo type. Dye in terylene C.I. 11080.

Disperse orange 3 $C_{12}H_{10}N_4O_2$ 242.24   SH,TF   1.0% pet   730-40-5   x   x
Textile dye of azo type. Dye in acetate, nylon, silk, wool, and cotton. Stocking dye (C.I. 11005).

Disperse orange 13 $C_{22}H_{16}N_4O$ 352.40   TF   1.0% pet   6253-10-7   x
Textile dye of azo type (C.I. 26080).

TABLE A-3. (*Continued*)

Name/Information	Formula	FW	Exp.	RPC	CAS	MI	CT	H
Disperse red 1	$C_{16}H_{18}N_4O_3$	314.35	TF	1.0% pet	2872-52-8		x	x
Textile dye of azo type. Dye in nylon and polyester. Stocking dye (C.I. 11110).								
Disperse red 17	$C_{17}H_{20}N_4O_4$	344.37	TF	1.0% pet	3179-89-3		x	x
Textile dye of azo type. Dye in acetate, silk, wool, and cotton. Stocking dye (C.I. 11210).								
Disperse yellow 3	$C_{15}H_{15}N_3O_2$	269.31	TF	1.0% pet	2832-40-8		x	x
Textile dye of azo type. Dye in acetate and nylon. Stocking dye (C.I. 11855).								
Disperse yellow 9	$C_{12}H_{10}N_4O_4$	274.24	TF	1.0% pet	6373-73-5		x	
Textile dye of nitro type. Dye in terylene (C.I. 10375).								
DMDM hydantoin	$C_7H_{12}N_2O_4$	188.07	C,H,O,P,V	2.0% aq		x		
Functions as a formaldehyde donor and is used as a preservative in cosmetic products and is active against fungi, yeasts, and bacteria. Products preserved are of the type shampoos, skin-care products, hair conditioners, makeup, hair rinses, and cleanliness products. Also used in herbicides, polymers, color photography, latex paints, floor waxes, cutting oils, adhesives, copying paper, inks.								
Dodecyl gallate	$C_{19}H_{30}O_5$	338.45	B,C,ME	0.25% pet	1166-52-5		x	
Antioxidant in cosmetic and pharmaceutical creams and emulsions, various fats, oils, waxes, and foods such as margarine (laurylgallate).								
Dodecyl mercaptan	$C_{12}H_{26}S$	202.41	R,SH	0.1% pet	112-55-0		x	
Polymerization inhibitor added to polyurethane resins and Neoprene glues for use, e.g., in the shoe industry.								

Econazole nitrate

$C_{18}H_{16}ClN_3O_4$ 373.65   ME   1.0% alc   24169-02-6   3476   x

Antifungal agent of the imidazole type used in topical and vaginal preparations to prevent growth of dermatophytes, yeast, and mold. **Cross: miconazole, enilconazole. May produce erythema multiforme like eruptions.**

Epoxy acrylate

500   MP   0.5% pet   x

Acrylate oligomer for use in UV-reactive inks and varnishes.

Epoxy resin

370   E,PG,SH,V   1% pet   x   x

Resin, based on epichlorhydrin and bisphenol A for use in adhesives, surface coatings, electrical insulation, plasticizers, polymer stabilizers, laminates, surface coatings, paints and inks, product finishers, PVC products, vinyl gloves, etc. Also in the building industry, electron microscopy, and sculpture. Oligomers may vary in molecular weight from 340 and higher. The higher the molecular weight, the less sensitizing the compound. **May produce erythema multiforme like eruptions. May cause airborne contact dermatitis. UCU.**

Epoxy resin, cycloaliphatic

370   E   0.5% pet   x

Resin based on diglycidyl ester of hexahydrophthalic acid. Its main use is for the manufacture of electrical insulating components (bushings, apparatus parts, insulators).

Ethoxyquin

$C_{14}H_{19}NO$ 217.30   B,V   0.5% pet   91-53-2   3710   x

Antioxidant in animal feed. Antidegradant in natural rubber and styrene-butadiene rubber. **May cause airborne contact dermatitis.**

Ethyl acrylate

$C_5H_8O_2$ 100.12   MN,MP   0.1% pet   140-88-5   3715   x

Acrylic monomer used in the production of textile and paper coatings, leather finish resins, and adhesives (EA).

Ethyl cyanoacrylate

$C_6H_7NO_2$ 125.10   MN,PG   10.0% pet   7085-85-0

Acrylate compound used in instant glues to mend broken nails and to adhere glue-impregnated silk or linen to the nail plate, which is then filed to shape the nail. Instant glues are also used in medicine to glue tissues and skin cracks. The glue is also used to attach hair and to glue shoes, plastics, and many other materials. **May cause airborne contact dermatitis.**

TABLE A-3. *(Continued)*

Name/Information	Formula	FW	Exp.	RPC	CAS	MI	CT	H
Ethylenediamine dihydrochloride	$C_2H_{10}Cl_2N_2$	133.02	ME,P,O,V	1.0% pet	333-18-6	3752	x	x
Ethylenediamine tetraacetic acid disodium dihydrate	$C_{10}H_{14}N_2\cdot Na_2O_8\cdot 2H_2O$	372.24	C,ME,V	1.0% pet	6381-92-6	3481	x	
Ethyleneglycol dimethacrylate	$C_{10}H_{14}O_4$	198.22	D,MA,P	2.0% pet	97-90-5		x	x
Ethylene urea	$C_3H_6N_2O$	86.10	TF,PG,V	1.0% pet	120-93-4	4830	x	
2-Ethylhexyl acrylate	$C_{11}H_{20}O_2$	184.28	MA,MP	0.1% pet	103-11-7		x	

Ethylenediamine dihydrochloride
Stabilizer in steroid creams and rubber latex. Inhibitor in antifreeze solutions and cooling fluids. May also be present in floor-polish removers. Component in nystatin cream and aminophylline. Epoxy curing agent. Accelerator in color development baths in photography. Used also in veterinary preparations, electroplating and electrophoretic gels, dyes, fungicides, insecticides, synthetic waxes, textile lubricants, eye and nose drops, and as solvent for casein, albumin, shellac (EDA). **Cross: EDTA, antazoline, aminophylline, promethazine HCl, piperazine.** **May produce erythema-multiforme-like eruptions. UCU.**

Ethylenediamine tetraacetic acid disodium dihydrate
As chelating agent for metals and as pharmaceutic aid (chelating agent). As preservative in cosmetic products. Also as anticoagulant (EDTA).

Ethyleneglycol dimethacrylate
Cross-linking methacrylic monomer in dental composites, sealants, prostheses, adhesives, artificial nails, printing inks, etc. (EGDMA). **May cause airborne contact dermatitis.**

Ethylene urea
Finishing agent for textiles and leather. Also used to formulate lacquers, plasticizers and adhesives. Insecticide.

2-Ethylhexyl acrylate
Acrylic monomer for use in UV-curable coatings and inks. Ingredient in some acrylic-based adhesive tapes (EHA).

2-Ethylhexyl-4-dimethyl-aminobenzoate $C_{17}H_{27}NO_2$ 277.41   C,SU   2.0% pet   21245-02-3   x   x
UV-B absorbing agent in sunscreens and cosmetic creams, lotions, lipsticks, sun oils, moisturizers, nail polish, etc. (Eusolex 6007, Escalol 507, Octyldimethyl-PABA).

2-Ethylhexyl-4-methoxy-cinnamate $C_{18}H_{26}O_3$ 290.18   C,SU   2.0% pet   5466-77-3   6687   x   x
UV-B absorbing agent in sunscreens and cosmetic creams, lotions, lipsticks, sun oils, etc. (Parsol MCX, Escalol 557).

Ethyl-4-hydroxy-benzoate $C_9H_{10}O_3$ 166.17   B,C,ME   3.0% pet   120-47-8   3792   x
Preservative in foods (salad dressings, mayonnaise, spiced sauces, mustard, frozen dairy products, baked products), cosmetics, and pharmaceutical preparations (Ethylparaben).

N-Ethyl-N-(2-hydroxyethyl)-2-methyl-1,4-PPD-sulfate, monohydrate $C_{11}H_{20}N_2O_5S \cdot H_2O$ 310.37   P   1.0% pet   25646-77-9   x   x
Color developer for Kodacolor II film identical to Flexicolor or C-41 process (CD-4).

Ethyl methacrylate $C_6H_{10}O_2$ 114.15   D,MN,MP   2.0% pet   97-63-2   x
Methacrylic monomer for use in, e.g., artificial nail products, dentures, hearing aids, printing plates, and bone cement (EMA).

N-Ethyl-N-(2-methane sulfonamidoethyl)-2-methyl-1,4-PPD-sesquisulfate,hydrate $C_{12}H_{21}N_3\text{-}O_2S$ x $1,5\ H_2SO_4$ 436.52   P   1.0% pet   25646-71-3   x   x
Color developer for Eastman color negative film and Ektachrome reversal film (CD-3).

TABLE A-3. *(Continued)*

Name/Information	Formula	FW	Exp.	RPC	CAS	MI	CT	H
4,4-(2-Ethyl-2-nitrotrimethylene) dimorpholine	$C_{13}H_{25}N_3O_4$	287.36	O	0.5% pet*	1854-23-5		x	
N-Ethyl-4-toluene-sulfonamide	$C_9H_{13}NO_2S$	199.27	D,PG	0.1% pet			x	
Eugenol	$C_{10}H_{12}O_2$	164.21	B,D,F,V	2.0% pet	97-53-0	3855	x	x
Euxyl K 400			C,O,V	0.5% pet		3004	x	x
Evernic acid	$C_{17}H_{16}O_7$	332.32	PL,PH	0.1% pet	570-10-5		x	

4,4-(2-Ethyl-2-nitrotrimethylene) dimorpholine
Preservative for use in cooling fluids, crude oil, diesel fuel, heating oil, etc. (20% in Bioban P 1487).
*) Concentration valid for Bioban P 1487.

N-Ethyl-4-toluene-sulfonamide
Resin carrier in dental materials used for isolating cavities below restorations. Plasticizer in PVA lacquers, polyamides, cellulose acetate, etc.

Eugenol
As fragrance in perfumery used as substitute for oil of cloves. Dental analgesic in impression materials and periodontal packings. In the production of vanillin. Insect attractant and component in inhalants and antiseptics.
Cross: balsam of Peru, isoeugenol, benzoin, propanidid. UCU.

Euxyl K 400
Preservative for use in cosmetic products of both leave-on and rinse-off types. The active agent is 1,2-Dibromodicyanobutane (20%), CAS 3591-65-7, also named methyldibromoglutaronitrile, which is present along with 2-Phenoxyethanol (80%). CAS 122-99-6 . MI=7226. Examples of products preserved with Euxyl K 400 are creams, body lotions, shampoos, sun protection lotions. Products preserved with 1,2-Dibromodicyanobutane with the trade name Tektamer 38 include metal working fluids. Adhesives, latex emulsions and paints, dispersed pigments, and detergents.

Evernic acid
Acid present in different lichens. One of the three most common lichen allergens. **Cross: oak moss. PA.**

Fentichlor

$C_{12}H_8Cl_2O_2S$ 287.18   C,H,PH   1.0% pet   97-24-5   3947   x

Fungicide especially used against Monosporium apiospermum. Topical antifungal and antibacterial agent in hairdressings, antifungal creams, and ointments, also used as thermoplastic resin. **Cross (photo): bithionol, hexachlorophene. PA. PT. PL.**

Formaldehyde

CH_2O 30.03   C,D,H,O   1.0% aq   50-00-0   4150   x

Used in the production of urea, phenolic melamine and acetate resins. In textile products. As astringent, disinfectant, preservative in cosmetics, metalworking fluids, shampoos, etc. Other exposure areas include antiperspirant in cosmetics, anticracking agent in dental plastics, anhidrotics, chipboard production, cleaning products, disinfectants and deodorizers, dry-cleaning materials, glues, mineral wool production, paints and coatings, paper industry, phenolic resins and urea plastics in adhesives and footwear, photographic paper and solutions, polishes, printing materials, tanning agents, wart remedies, embalming solutions, fertilizers, wood composites, insulation. *Formaldehyde releasers:* Bakzid P, Biocide DS 5249, Bronopol, Dantoin MDMH, DMDM Hydantoin, Dowicil 200, Germall 115, Germall II, Grotan BK, Hexamethylenetetramine, KM 103, Paraformaldehyde, Parmetol K50, Polyoxymethylene urea, Preventol D1, -D2, -D3. **Cross: aryl-sulfonamide resin, chloroallyl-hexaminium chloride. May cause erythema-multiforme-like eruptions. PA. PT. May cause airborne contact dermatitis. NICU.**

Gentamicin sulfate

$N_5O_7.2.5H_2SO_4$ $C_{19-21}H_{39-43}$ ME,OP   20.0% pet   1405-41-0   4284   x

Topical and systemic broad-spectrum antibiotic with bactericidal action. Also used in ophthalmic drugs. **Cross: neomycin sulfate**

Geraniol

$C_{10}H_{18}O$ 154.25   F   2.0% pet   106-24-1   4298   x

As fragrance in perfumery. As insect attractant.

Geranium oil Bourbon

F,V   2.0% pet   8000-46-2   6732   x

Fragrance for use in various perfumes. Odorant for tooth and dusting powders, ointments, etc.

TABLE A-3. (*Continued*)

Name/Information	Formula	FW	Exp.	RPC	CAS	MI	CT	H
Glutaraldehyde	$C_5H_8O_2$	100.12	P,SH,V	0.2% pet	111-30-8	4366	x	x

In sterilization of endoscopic instruments, dental and barber equipment. Used as embalming fluid, in electron microscopy. Tanning agent for leather. Hardener for photographic gelatin. Pharmacological agent used for hyperhidrosis and antifungal purposes and for treatment of warts and some bullous diseases as well as herpes infections. (glutaral). **May cause airborne contact dermatitis.**

Name/Information	Formula	FW	Exp.	RPC	CAS	MI	CT	H
Glyceryl monothio-glycolate	$C_5H_{10}SO_4$	166.22	H	1.0% pet	30618-84-9		x	x

Component in "acid" permanent waving formulations, mainly for use in hairdressing salons.

Name/Information	Formula	FW	Exp.	RPC	CAS	MI	CT	H
Gold sodium thiosulfate	$AuNa_3(S_2O_3)_2 \cdot 2H_2O$	526.27	D,V	0.5% pet	10233-88-2	4423	x	x

Gold derivative used for screening of contact allergy to dental gold materials.

Name/Information	Formula	FW	Exp.	RPC	CAS	MI	CT	H
Hexachlorophene	$C_{13}H_6Cl_6O_2$	406.91	C,PH	1.0% pet	70-30-4	4602	x	x

Topical antiseptic in germicidal soaps, creams, deodorants, cleansers, shampoos, after-shave creams, pHisoHex surgical cleanser. Cross: bithionol, halogenated salicylanilides. **PA.**

Name/Information	Formula	FW	Exp.	RPC	CAS	MI	CT	H
Hexahydro-1,3,5-tris-(2-hydroxyethyl)triazine	$C_9H_{21}N_3O_3$	219.29	C,O	1.0% aq	4719-04-4		x	

Bactericide in cooling fluids and various cosmetic products, acting as formaldehyde liberator. Active component in **Grotan BK**.

1,6-Hexamethylene-diisocyanate

$C_8H_{12}N_2O_2$ 168.20   I,PG   0.1% pet   822-06-0   x

Isocyanate monomer in polyurethane paints and lacquers (HDI).

Hexamethylene-tetramine

$C_6H_{12}N_4$ 140.19   C,E,R   2.0% pet   100-97-0   5879   x   x

Urinary antiseptic agent. Rubber accelerator and formaldehyde liberator. In the production of phenol-formaldehyde resins. Preservative in cosmetic products. Epoxy curing agent. Corrosion inhibitor for steel (hexamine, methenamine). **May cause airborne contact dermatitis.**

1,6-Hexandiol diacrylate

$C_{12}H_{18}O_4$ 226.28   DMA,-N,-P   0.1% pet   13048-33-4   x

Common acrylic monomer in UV-cured inks, adhesives, coatings, photoresists, castings, artificial nails, etc. (HDDA). Monomer in dental composite materials.

Hydrazine sulfate

$H_6N_2O_4S$ 130.12   O,V   1.0% pet   10034-93-2   4693   x   x

Used as flux for soldering brass, copper, aluminum, and other metals. Pressure stabilizer in cutting oils. **May cause airborne contact dermatitis.**

Hydrocortisone-17-butyrate

$C_{25}H_{36}O_6$ 432.62   CS,ME   1.0% alc   13609-67-1   4710   x

Used as a topical corticosteroid with anti inflammatory properties. Marker for topical corticosteroid allergy.

Hydrogen peroxide

H_2O_2 34.02   H,V   3.0% aq   7722-84-1   4727   x

Component in hair bleaches. Topical antiseptic agent.

Hydroquinone

$C_6H_6O_2$ 110.11   B,H,P,PG   1.0% pet   123-31-9   4738   x

Inhibitor in acrylic monomers. Antioxidant in animal feed. As photographic reducer and developer (HQ). **Cross: resorcinol. May cause depigmentation**

TABLE A-3. (*Continued*)

Name/Information	Formula	FW	Exp.	RPC	CAS	MI	CT	H
Hydroquinone mono-benzylether	$C_{13}H_{12}O_2$	200.23	R,SH	1.0% pet	103-16-2	6159	x	x
Antidegradant added to rubber products. Inhibitor in acrylic resins. **May cause depigmentation.**								
Hydroxycitronellal	$C_{10}H_{18}O_2$	170.25	F	2.0% pet	107-75-5		x	x
Fragrance for use in various perfumes, antiseptics, insecticides and household products. **Cross: citronellal, geranial, methoxycitronellal. May produce hyperpigmentation.**								
2-Hydroxyethyl acrylate	$C_5H_8O_3$	116.12	MA,-N,-P	0.1% pet	818-61-1		x	
Acrylic monomer for use in UV inks, adhesives, lacquers, artificial nails, etc. (HEA).								
2-Hydroxyethyl methacrylate	$C_6H_{10}O_3$	130.15	DMA,-N,-P	2.0% pet	868-77-9		x	
Methacrylic monomer for use in UV inks, adhesives, lacquers, dental materials, artificial nails, etc. (HEMA).								
Hydroxylammonium-chloride	ClH_4NO	69.49	P,V	0.1% aq	5470-11-1	4759	x	
Reducing agent in photography, textiles, chemistry, etc. In floor lacquers and as antioxidant for fatty acids and soaps.								
Hydroxylammonium-sulfate	$H_8N_2O_6S$	164.15	P,V	0.1% aq	10039-54-0	4759	x	
As reducing agent in photography, textiles, chemistry, etc.								

2,2-bis(4-(2-Hydroxy--3-methacryloxypropoxy)phenyl)propane $C_{29}H_{36}O_8$ 512.61   D,MA   2.0% pet   x   x
Common methacrylic monomer in dental composite and sealant materials (**BIS-GMA**).

2-Hydroxy-4-methoxy-benzophenone $C_{14}H_{12}O_3$ 228.24   C,D,H,SU   2.0% pet   131-57-7   6907   x   x
Common UV-adsorber in dental composite materials and other plastic materials. UV-adsorber in topical sunscreens, moisturizers, shampoos, hair care products, lipsticks, lip balms, nail polish, etc. (Eusolex 4360, Escalol 567, Oxybenzone). Cross: **dioxybenzone. PA.**

2-Hydroxy-4-methoxy-benzophenone-5-sulfonic acid $C_{14}H_{12}O_6S$ 308.31   C,PG,SU,TF   5.0% pet   4065-45-6   8963   x
Sunscreen for use in various sunscreen products, moisturizers, nail polish, lipsticks, lip balms, as well as in textiles, plastics, paints and cosmetics. Trade names are Sulisobenzone, Uvinyl MS-40, and Benzophenone 4. **UCU.**

2-Hydroxymethyl-2-nitro-1,3-propanediol $C_4H_9NO_5$ 151.12   O,V   1.0% pet   126-11-4   9667   x
Bactericide and slimicide for use in cooling fluids, paper and pulp industry. As curing agent for certain adhesives (Tris-Nitro).

2-Hydroxy-4-methoxy-4´-methyl-benzophenone $C_{15}H_{14}O_3$ 242.26   C,SU   2.0% pet   1641-17-4   6092   x
UV absorbing agent in sunscreen cosmetics of the type creams, lotions, lipsticks, sun oils, etc. (Mexenone). Cross (photo): **2-hydroxy-4-methoxybenzophenone. PA.**

2(2-Hydroxy-5-methylphenyl)-benzotriazol $C_{11}H_{13}N_3O$ 225.25   C,D,PG   1.0% pet   2440-22-4   x
UV-adsorber for use in plastics, cosmetics, dental materials, acrylic materials, dyes, etc. (**Tinuvin P**).

TABLE A-3. *(Continued)*

Name/Information	Formula	FW	Exp.	RPC	CAS	MI	CT	H
Hydroxypropyl acrylate	$C_6H_{10}O_3$	130.15	MA,MP	0.1%pet				x
Acrylic monomer for use in UV inks, lacquers, adhesives, etc. (2-Hydroxy-1-propylacrylate, 67% + 1-Hydroxy-2-propylacrylate, 33%).								
2-Hydroxypropyl methacrylate	$C_7H_{12}O_3$	144.17	MA,-N,-P	2.0%pet	923-26-2			x
Monofunctional methacrylic monomer in dental composites and sealants, UV-curable resins for inks etc. (HPMA).								
Idoxuridine	$C_9H_{11}IN_2O_5$	354.12	ME,OP	1.0%pet	54-42-2	4819		
Antiviral agent effective against herpes simplex infections. Present in ophthalmic eyedrops as well as ointments and solutions. 2′-Deoxy-5-iodouridine. **Cross: trifluorothymidine.**								
Imidazolidinyl urea	$C_{11}H_{16}N_8O_8$	388.31	C,H	2.0% aq	39236-46-9		x	x
Preservative for lotions, creams, hair conditioners, shampoos, deodorants and topical drugs. Formaldehyde releaser (Germall 115, Imidurea NF, Sept 115, Unicide U-13, Tristat IU, Biopure 100).								
Isoeugenol	$C_{10}H_{12}O_2$	164.21	B,D,F	2.0%pet	97-54-1	5054	x	x
Fragrance in perfumery, over-the-counter medicines, dental materials, foods. In the production of vanillin flavor. Found in oils of nutmeg, ylang-ylang etc. **Cross: eugenol**								
Isophorone diamine	$C_{10}H_{22}N_2$	170.29	E,I	0.1%pet	2855-13-2		x	x
Common hardener for epoxy resins. Also a degradation product from Isophorone diisocyanate (IPD).								

Isophorone diisocyanate $C_{12}H_{18}N_2O_2$ 170.29   I,PG   1.0% pet   4098-71-9   x
Used in the manufacture of polyurethane plastics and lacquers (IPDI). **Cross: Isophorone diamine.**

4-Isopropyl-dibenzoyl-methane $C_{18}H_{18}O$ 266.34   C,SU   2.0% pet   63250-25-9   x   x
UV-A absorbing agent in sunscreen cosmetics of the type creams, lotions, lipsticks, sun oils, etc. (Eusolex 8020).

Isopropyl myristate $C_{17}H_{34}O_2$ 270.44   C,ME   20.0% pet   110-27-0   5103   x
Emollient in cosmetic and pharmaceutical bases. Has solvent properties.

N-Isopropyl-N-phenyl--4-phenylene-diamine $C_{15}H_{18}N_2$ 226.32   R,SH   0.1% pet   101-72-4   x   x
Antidegradant in natural rubber, styrene-butadiene, nitrile-butadiene, butadiene and chloroprene rubber (IPPD).

Jasmine   F   2.0% pet   x
Synthetic jasmine for use as fragrance in perfumery. **Cross: benzylsalicylate**

Jasmine absolute, Egyptian   F   2.0% pet   x
Natural jasmine for use as fragrance in perfumery. **Cross: benzylsalicylate. May produce hyperpigmentation.**

Juniper tar   F,ME,V   3.0% pet   5153   x
Tar obtained from distillation of <u>Juniperus oxycedrus</u> for use in, e.g., eczema and psoriatic medications and perfumes.

Kanamycin sulfate $C_{18}H_{36-37}N_{45}O_{10-11}.H_2SO_4$ ME   10.0% pet   25389-94-0   5161   x
Antibacterial agent similar to neomycin. **Cross: neomycin, streptomycin, gentamicin sulfate, dihydrostreptomycin.**

Lavender absolute   F   2.0% pet   5261   x
Fragrance for use in various perfumes. Flavor and carminative. **Cross: Geranial .**

TABLE A-3. (Continued)

Name/Information	Formula	FW	Exp.	RPC	CAS	MI	CT	H
Levobunolol-hydrochloride	$C_{17}H_{26}ClNO_3$	270.84	OP	1.0% aq	27912-14-7	5343		
Used as antiglaucoma agent in ophthalmic solutions.								
Lidocaine	$C_{14}H_{22}N_2O$	234.33	ME	5.0% pet	137-58-6	5359	x	x
Used as a local anesthetic and as antiarrhythmic agent.								
Lindane	$C_6H_6Cl_6$	290.85	PE	1.0% pet	58-89-9	5379		
Insecticide widely used in agriculture, horticulture, in the household, and as a scabicide.								
Malathion	$C_{10}H_{19}O_6PS_2$	330.36	PE	0.5% pet	121-75-5	5582		
Insecticide for fruits and other plants in household and greenhouses. Also used in veterinary medicine as ectoparasiticide for lice and fleas (Milon).								
Melamine formaldehyde	$C_6H_{12}N_6O_3$	216.20	TF	7.0% pet			x	x
Textile resin of formaldehyde releasing type for the treatment of draperies, collars, apparel, etc.								
Menthol	$C_{10}H_{20}O$	156.26	B,ME,V	2.0% pet	1490-04-6	5723	x	
In confectionery, perfumery, cough drops, cigarettes, liqueurs, etc. Topical antipruritic, local anesthetic, gastric sedative. ICU.								

2-Mercaptobenzo-thiazole $C_7H_5NS_2$ 167.25 O,R,SH,V 2.0% pet 149-30-4 5759 x x

Accelerator, retarder, and peptizer for natural and other rubber products such as shoes, gloves, rubber in undergarments and clothing, condoms and diaphragms, medical devices, toys, tires and tubes, renal dialysis equipment, swimwear. Fungicide. Corrosion inhibitor in soluble cutting oils and antifreeze mixtures. Also used in greases, adhesives, photographic film emulsions detergents, veterinary products such as tick and flea powders and sprays (MBT).

Mercuric chloride $HgCl_2$ 271.50 P,V 0.1% pet 7487-94-7 5770 x

In tanning leather. Intensifier in photography. Topical antiseptic and disinfectant. **Cross: other mercurials.**

Mercury Hg 200.59 D,V 0.5% pet 7439-97-6 5801 x

As chemical reagent. In thermometers and dental amalgams. In pharmaceuticals, antifouling paints, agricultural chemicals. **May cause airborne contact dermatitis.**

Mercury ammonium chloride $Cl_4H_8HgN_2$ 378.52 ME 1.0% pet 33445-15-7 5771 x x

Inorganic mercurial compound used in creams as a topical antiinfective agent (formerly used in the treatment of psoriasis and in skin-lightening formulations). **May cause pigmentation and depigmentation.**

2,2-bis(4-(2-Methacryl-oxyethoxy) phenyl) propane $C_{27}H_{32}O_6$ 452.55 D,MP 1.0% pet 24448-20-2 x

Methacrylic monomer based on bisphenol A. In dental restorative composite materials. As reactive monomer in adhesive products (BIS-EMA).

2,2-bis(4-Methacryloxy) phenyl) propane $C_{23}H_{24}O_4$ 364.44 D,MA 2.0% pet 3253-39-2 x

Methacrylic monomer based on bisphenol A. In dental restorative composite and adhesive materials (BIS-MA).

2-Methoxy-6-n-pentyl-4-benzoquinone $C_{12}H_{16}O_3$ 208.26 PL 0.01% pet x x

Primary allergen of the plant Primula Obconica found in glandular hairs on the leaves and the stem. (**Primin**). **May cause airborne contact dermatitis from contact with Primula.**

TABLE A-3. (Continued)

Name/Information	Formula	FW	Exp.	RPC	CAS	MI	CT	H
Metol	$C_{14}H_{20}N_2O_6S$	344.39	H,P	1.0% pet	55-55-0	5940	x	x
Black & white photographic developer and pigment in hair dyes (4-Methylaminophenol sulfate). May induce lichen planus. **Cross: Para group of compounds.**								
Metoprolol	$C_{15}H_{25}NO_3$	267.38	ME,OP	3.0% aq	37350-58-6	6072		
β-Adrenergic blocking antihypertensive and antianginal agent. Used in ophthalmic preparations and for the treatment of myocardial infarcts.								
3-(4-Methylbenzylidene) camphor	$C_{18}H_{22}O$	254.37	C,SU	2.0% pet	36861-47-9		x	x
UV-B absorbing agent in sunscreen cosmetics of the type creams, lotions, lipsticks, sun oils, etc. (Eusolex 6300).								
6-Methylcoumarin	$C_{10}H_8O_2$	160.17	C,PH	1.0% pet	92-48-8		x	x
Synthetic fragrance in cosmetics, toiletries and soaps. **Cross (photo): 7-methylcoumarin, coumarin, 7-methoxycoumarin. PA.**								
N,N-Methylene-bis-acrylamide	$C_7H_{10}N_2O_2$	154.17	MP	1.0% pet	110-26-9		x	
Acrylamide compound cross-reacting with unidentified primary sensitizers in NAPP and Nyloprint UV-cured printing plates.								
α-Methylene-γ-butyrolactone	$C_5H_6O_2$	98.10	PL	0.01% pet	547-65-9	5981	x	
Tulipaline A, allergen in the Liliaceae family of plants to which species such as Tulip, Alstromeria, Erythronium dens canis & americanum belong. **May cause airborne contact dermatitis from contact with Tulip and Alstroemeria.**								

Methylhydroquinone $C_7H_8O_2$ 24.14 D 1.0% pet 95-71-6 x
Stabilizer and antioxidant in acrylic monomers to prevent polymerization.

Methyl-4-hydroxy-benzoate $C_8H_8O_3$ 152.15 B,C,ME 3.0% pet 99-76-3 6021 x x
Preservative in foods (salad dressings, mayonnaise, spiced sauces, mustard, frozen dairy products, baked products), cosmetics and pharmaceutical preparations (Methylparaben, Nipagin).
Cross: other parabens, hydroquinone monobenzylether, para group of compounds. ICU. NICU.

2-Methyl-4-isothia-zoline-3-one C_4H_5NOS 115.15 C_3H_6OSH 0.01% aq* 2682-20-4 x x
Component in Kathon CG preservative for use in cosmetics, shampoos, cooling fluids, detergents etc. *) Mixed with 5-Chloro-2-methyl-4-isothiazolin-3-one (see this compound for further information).

Methyl methacrylate $C_5H_8O_2$ 100.12 D,MA,MP 2.0% pet 80-62-6 5849 x x
Methacrylic monomer in plastics for dentures, bone cement, artificial nails, hearing aids etc. (MMA).

N-Methylolchloro-acetamide $C_3H_6ClNO_2$ 123.54 C,O 0.2% pet x
Preservative in cooling fluids and cosmetics. (Grotan HD, Parmetol K 50). **May cause airborne contact dermatitis.**

Miconazole $C_{18}H_{14}Cl_4N_2O$ 416.12 ME 1.0% alc 22916-47-8 6101 x
Antifungal agent of the imidazole type which is used in topical and vaginal preparations to prevent growth of dermatophytes, yeast and molds. **Cross: econazole, enilconazole.**

2-Monomethylol phenol $C_7H_8O_2$ 124.14 ME,PG 1.0% pet x
Intermediate in the production of phenol formaldehyde resins which may remain after condensation of the resin. Sensitizer in phenol formaldehyde resins. Also in local anesthetic (Saligenin).

TABLE A-3. *(Continued)*

Name/Information	Formula	FW	Exp.	RPC	CAS	MI	CT	H
2-(4-Morpholinylmercapto) benzothiazol	$C_{11}H_{12}N_2OS$	252.47	R	1.0% pet			x	x
Accelerator for natural rubber, isoprene butadiene, styrene-butadiene, nitrilebutadiene rubber products (MOR).								
Musk ambrette	$C_{12}H_{16}N_2O_5$	268.41	B,F,PH,V	1.0% pet	123-69-3		x	x
Synthetic nitro musk compound for use as fragrance and fixative in after-shave lotions, perfumes, etc. Also permitted as food flavor. Cross (photo): **musk xylene**. **May cause hyperpigmentation. May cause airborne contact dermatitis. PA. PL.**								
Musk ketone	$C_{14}H_{18}N_2O_5$	294.30	C,F	1.0% pet	81-14-1		x	x
Synthetic nitro musk compound for use as fragrance and fixative in after-shave lotions, perfumes, etc.								
Musk moskene	$C_{14}H_{18}N_2O_4$	280.33	C,F	1.0% pet			x	
Synthetic nitro musk compound for use as fragrance and fixative in after-shave lotions, perfumes, etc.								
Musk tibetine	$C_{18}H_{18}N_2O_4$	266.29	C,F	1.0% pet			x	
Synthetic nitro musk compound for use as fragrance and fixative in after-shave lotions, perfumes, etc.								
Musk xylene	$C_{12}H_{15}N_3O_6$	297.45	C,F,PH	1.0% pet	81-15-2		x	x
Synthetic nitro musk compound for use as fragrance and fixative in after-shave lotions, perfumes etc. The musk compound of choice for soap and detergent fragrances. **Cross (photo): musk ambrette. PA.**								
Neomycin sulfate			ME	20.0% pet	1405-10-3	6369	x	x
Broad-spectrum antibiotic in topical creams, powders, ointments, eye and ear drops. Also as systemic antibiotic and growth promotor in veterinary use. **Cross: streptomycin, gentamycin, framycetin, dihydrostreptomycin, kanamycin, spectinomycin, tobramycin, paromomycin, butirosin, bacitracin. UCU.**								

Nickel sulfate-hexahydrate $NiO_4S.6H_2O$ 262.86   D,H,SH,V   5.0% pet   10101-97-0   6424   x   x

Nickel metal: a common allergen present in various alloys, electroplated metal, earrings, watches, buttons, zippers, rings, utensils, tools, instruments, batteries, machinery parts, working solutions of metal cutting fluids, nickel plating for alloys, coins, pigments, dentures, orthopedic plates, keys, scissors, razors, spectacle frames, kitchenware etc. May produce erythema-multiforme-like eruptions. **May cause airborne contact dermatitis. ICU.**

Nitrofurazone $C_6H_6N_4O_4$ 198.14   ME   1.0% pet   59-87-0   6521   x   x

Topical antibiotic for use in human and veterinary medicine and is sometimes also added to animal feeds (Furacin). **May cause airborne contact dermatitis.**

Nigrosin   V   1.0% pet   11099-03-9   x

Dye for use in carbon papers, inks, typewriter ribbons, shoe polishes, etc. (C.I. 50415).

4-(2-Nitrobutyl)morpholine $C_8H_{16}N_2O_3$ 188.23   O   0.5% pet*   2224-44-4   x

Preservative for use in cooling fluids, crude oil, diesel fuel, heating oil etc. (70% in Bioban P 1487). *) Concentration is valid for Bioban P 1487.

2-Nitro-4-phenylene-diamine $C_6H_7N_3O_2$ 153.14   H   1.0% pet   5307-14-2   x   x

Dye present in different hair dyeing preparations. These are of the semipermanent type and do not require the use of hydrogen peroxide.

Oakmoss absolute   F,PL   2.0% pet   x   x

Extract of oak moss for use as fragrance in many perfume mixtures, after-shave lotions etc. Extract made mainly from Evernia prunastri (oak moss) and Pseudevernia furfuracea (tree moss). Contains atranorin, evernic acid and usnic acid. **PA.**

TABLE A-3. (Continued)

Name/Information	Formula	FW	Exp.	RPC	CAS	MI	CT	H
Octyl gallate	$C_{15}H_{22}O_5$	282.34	B,C,ME	0.25% pet	1034-01-0		x	
Antioxidant for use in cosmetic and pharmaceutical products and in food products such as margarine and peanut butter. **May cause airborne contact dermatitis.**								
2-n-Octyl-4-isothiazolin-3-one	$C_{11}H_{19}NOS$	213.34	O,PG,SH	0.1% pet	26530-20-1	6677	x	
Fungicide for use in paints, cutting oils, wallpaper adhesives, etc. Also used for the preservation of leather (Skane M-8, Kathon 893).								
Olaquindox	$C_{12}H_{13}N_3O_4$	263.25	B,ME	0.5% pet	23696-28-8	6783		
Widespread growth promotor in pig breeding acting as a chemotherapeutic agent prophylactically used to lower the frequency of bacterial enteritis in pigs. N-(2-Hydroxyethyl)-3-methyl-2-quinoxalinecarboxamide-1,4-dioxide. **PA. PL.**								
Oleamidopropyl-dimethylamine	$C_{23}H_{46}N_2O$	366.25	C,H	0.1% aq			x	
Cationic emulsifier used in cosmetics such as body lotions, creams, shampoos, hair rinse preparations, etc.								
Oligotriacrylate		480	MP	0.1% pet			x	
Multifunctional acrylic monomer for use in lithographic inks, overprinting varnishes, coatings on wood, paper, etc. cured by UV-light (OTA 480).								
Olive oil			B,C,ME,V	100%	8001-25-0	6796	x	
Used as food in salads, with sardines, etc. Also used as emollient and for treatment of leg ulcers. In the manufacturing of soaps, textile lubricants, cosmetics, and pharmaceutical products.								

Palladium chloride   PdCl$_2$ 177.31   D,V   2% pet   7647-10-1   6941   x   x

Catalyst in jewelry. Present in dental alloys and electroplating parts of clocks and watches.

Pentaerythritol-triacrylate   C$_{14}$H$_{18}$O$_7$ 298.30   MP   0.1% pet   3524-68-3   x

Trifunctional cross-linking acrylic monomer for use in adhesives, coatings, inks, photoresists, castings, etc. cured by UV radiation.

Petrolatum   C,SH,V   100%   7138   x   x

White petrolatum which is a purified mixture of semisolid hydrocarbons. As ointment base in cosmetics. Leather grease and shoe polish component. **May cause hyperpigmentation.**

Phenidone   C$_9$H$_{10}$N$_2$O   162.19   P   1.0% pet   92-43-3   7281   x   x

Black & white developer in photography (1-Phenyl-3-pyrazolidinone).

Phenol formaldehyde resin   PG,V   1.0% pet   x

Resol based on phenol, resorcinol and formaldehyde. Contains methylol phenols. Used in binders, adhesives, laminates, impregnation products, surface coatings, casting sand, etc. (P-F-R-2). **May cause airborne contact dermatitis.**

2-Phenoxyethanol   C$_8$H$_{10}$O$_2$ 138.16   C,V   1.0% pet   122-99-6   7226   x

Fixative for perfumes, as bactericide in conjunction with 1,2-dibromo-2,4-dicyanobutane (Euxyl K 400) as well as quaternary ammonium compounds. Also used as insect repellent and topical antiseptic.

Phenylbenzimidazol-5-sulfonic acid   C$_{13}$H$_{10}$N$_2$O$_3$S   274.30   SU   2.0% pet   27503-81-7   x

Sun-screening agent for use in various sunscreen products. Trade names: Eusolex 232 and Novantisol.

TABLE A-3. (Continued)

Name/Information	Formula	FW	Exp.	RPC	CAS	MI	CT	H
4-Phenylenediamine	$C_6H_8N_2$	108.14	H,PG,R	1.0% pet	106-50-3	7256	x	x
Phenylephrine-hydrochloride	$C_9H_{13}NO_2xHCl$	203.67	OP	10.0% aq	61-76-7	7257			
2-Phenylglycidyl ether	$C_9H_{10}O_2$	150.18	E	0.25% pet	122-60-1			x	x
2-Phenylindole	$C_{14}H_{11}N$	193.25	PG	2.0% pet	948-65-2		x		
Phenylmercuric acetate	$C_8H_8HgO_2$	336.74	C,ME,OP,PE	0.01% aq	62-38-4	7271	x		x
N-Phenyl-2-naphtylamine	$C_{16}H_{13}N$	219.29	R	1.0% pet	135-88-6		x		

4-Phenylenediamine
Primary intermediate in permanent hair dyes and fur dyes (valid for 4-Phenylenediamine). Also used in photographic developers, lithography, photocopying, oils, greases, gasoline and as antioxidant/accelerator in the rubber and plastic industry. The hydrochloride is used as blood reagent. **Cross: parabens, PABA, para compounds. May produce erythema-multiforme-like eruptions. May cause airborne contact dermatitis. PA. UCU.**

Phenylephrine-hydrochloride
Mydriatic agent used in ophthalmic preparations.

2-Phenylglycidyl ether
Reactive diluent in epoxy resin systems. Forms chemical bonds with the resin during cure and accelerates the curing process.

2-Phenylindole
Stabilizer in PVC-plastic products (α-phenylindole).

Phenylmercuric acetate
Used as herbicide and fungicide. As preservative in antibiotic eye drops, eye cosmetics, shampoos, etc. (Advacide PMA 18, Cosan PMA, Mergal A25, Metasol 30, Nildew AC 30, Nuodex PMA 18, Nylmerate). **Cross: p-chloromercuriphenol. ICU.**

N-Phenyl-2-naphtylamine
Antidegradant for various rubber products such as natural rubber, styrene-butadiene, nitrile, butadiene and chloroprene (Phenyl-β-naphtylamine, PBN).

2-Phenylphenol $C_{12}H_{10}O$ 170.20 C,O,P,E,V 1.0%pet 90-43-7 7276 x
Preservative in cosmetics, cooling fluids, detergents and as agricultural fungicide for citrus fruits, etc. (Dowicide 1, o-Phenylphenol). **Photosensitizer. May cause depigmentation.**

Phenyl salicylate $C_{13}H_{10}O_3$ 214.22 C,P,G,S,U,V 1.0%pet 118-55-8 7282 x x
Used as UV-light adsorber in plastics, suntan oils, and creams. Also in waxes, adhesives, polishes etc. Analgesic, antipyretic, and anti-rheumatic agent. In veterinary use as external disinfectant and intestinal antiseptic agent (Salol).

Pilocarpine hydrochloride $C_{11}H_{16}N_2O_2xHCl$ 244.72 OP 1.0%aq 154-71-7 7395
Miotic and antiglaucoma agent used in ophthalmic preparations.

Pine tar ME 3.0%pet 7417 x
Product obtained by distillation of wood of pine. Consists of turpentine, various phenols, xylene, etc. Topical antieczematic and rubefacient.

Polymyxin B sulfate $C_{55-56}H_{96-98}N_{16-}O_{13-}\cdot 2H_2SO_4$ 1385.63 ME,OP 5.0%pet 1405-20-5 7550 x
Topical antibiotic agent widely used, often in combination with neomycin. Polymyxin B is an important allergen in leg ulcer dermatitis. Products include ointments, creams, eye and ear drops. **Cross: bacitracin.**

Polyoxyethylenesorbitan monooleate B,C,ME 5.0%pet 9005-65-6 7559 x x
Emulsifier and dispersing agent for medicinal products for internal use. Emulsifier in cosmetics, pharmaceuticals & food. Tween 80.

Potassium dichromate $Cr_2K_2O_7$ 294.21 D,P,SH,V 0.5%pet 7778-50-9 7608 x x
Hexavalent form of chromium. In cement, tanning of leather, textile dyes, wood preservatives, alloys in metallurgy, safety matches, photography, electroplating, anticorrosives, engraving and lithography, ceramics, automobile industry, TV manufacturing, photocopy paper, tattoos, mascara/eye shadow pigments (chromium oxide), milk testing, welding, floor waxes, shoe polishes, paints, glues, pigments, detergents, etc. **May cause airborne contact dermatitis.**

TABLE A-3. (*Continued*)

Name/Information	Formula	FW	Exp.	RPC	CAS	MI	CT	H
Potassium dicyanoaurate	C_2AuKN_2	288.13	V	0.1% aq	13967-50-5	7609	x	x

Gold salt used in the electroplating industry.

Name/Information	Formula	FW	Exp.	RPC	CAS	MI	CT	H
Procaine hydrochloride	$C_{13}H_{21}ClN_2O_2$	272.77	ME	1.0% pet	51-05-8	7763	x	x

Local anesthetic agent (Novocaine, Ethocaine, Allocaine, Topocaine, Neocaine, Syncaine, etc.). **Cross: para group of compounds, parabens, butethamine, PABA.**

Name/Information	Formula	FW	Exp.	RPC	CAS	MI	CT	H
Promethazine hydrochloride	$C_{17}H_{21}ClN_2S$	320.87	ME,PH	1.0% pet	58-33-3	7797	x	x

Antihistaminic, antiemetic, CNS depressant used in pills, syrup, injections and suppositories (Phenergan, Lergigan, Atosil, Fenazil etc.). **Cross: phenothiazines, ethylenediamine-HCl, para compounds, chlorpromazine HCl, tripelennamine. May produce erythema-multiforme-like eruptions. PA. UCU. PL.**

Name/Information	Formula	FW	Exp.	RPC	CAS	MI	CT	H
Propionic acid	$C_3H_6O_2$	74.08	B,F	3.0% pet	79-09-4	7837	x	

As food additive for the preservation against moulds in, e.g., cheese products. Also in the production of fruit flavors and perfume bases.

Name/Information	Formula	FW	Exp.	RPC	CAS	MI	CT	H
Propolis			C,PL,V	10.0% pet		7848	x	x

A resinous substance found in beehives (bee glue). Collected by bees from poplar buds. Found in biocosmetics, face creams, ointments, lotions, solutions, varnish, toothpaste, mouthwashes, tablets, chewing gum, etc. Also found in wax for violins. Contains flavonoid aglycones and the main allergen is 1,1-dimethylallyl caffeic acid ester (LB-1). **Cross: balsam of Peru. May cause airborne contact dermatitis.**

Propylene glycol $C_3H_8O_2$ 76.09 C,ME,O 5.0% pet 57-55-6 7868 x x
Vehicle in pharmaceutical and cosmetic bases. In food as solvent for colors and flavors and to prevent growth of moulds. As humectant. In cooling fluids. UCU.

Propyl gallate $C_{10}H_{12}O_5$ 212.20 B,C,ME 1.0% pet 121-79-9 7872 x
Antioxidant in cosmetic and pharmaceutic creams, emulsions, various fats, oils and waxes. Also in foods like margarine, peanut butter, etc.

Propyl-4-hydroxy-benzoate $C_{10}H_{12}O_3$ 180.20 B,C,ME 3.0% pet 94-13-3 7879 x x
Preservative in foods (salad dressings, mayonnaise, spiced sauces, mustard, frozen dairy products, baked products), cosmetics and pharmaceutical preparations (propylparaben). **Cross: hydroquinone monobenzyl ether, other parabens, para compounds.**

Quinine sulfate $(C_{20}H_{24}N_2O_2)_2 \cdot H_2SO_4 \cdot 2H_2O$ 746.93 B,ME 1.0% pet 6119-70-6 8089 x x
Antimalarial agent also used as antipyreticum and in liquids (tonic etc.). **PA.**

Resorcinol $C_6H_6O_2$ 110.11 C,H,ME,OP,P 1.0% pet 108-46-3 8158 x
Keratolytic agent in acne medications. In hair dyes, resins, tanning, cosmetics, Castellanis paint, eye drops, suppositories, photocopying and photographic solutions, explosives, etc. Topical antipruritic and antiseptic. **Cross: phenol. May cause orange-brown discoloration of lacquered nails and may darken fair hair.**

Resorcinol monobenzoate $C_{13}H_{10}O_3$ 214.22 PG,SU 1.0% pet 136-36-7 x x
UV-light absorber added mainly to out door plastics. Has caused dermatitis as additive in spectacle frames. **Cross: balsam of Peru.**

TABLE A-3. *(Continued)*

Name/Information	Formula	FW	Exp.	RPC	CAS	MI	CT	H
Rose oil								
Bulgarian			F,V	2.0% pet		6762	x	
Fragrance for use in various perfumes. For flavoring lozenges, ointments, toilet preparations, etc.								
Sandalwood oil (Indian)			C,F	2.0% pet		6765	x	
Fragrance for use in various perfumed products like soap, after-shave lotions, colognes and cosmetics. **PA. PT. PL.**								
Silver nitrate	$AgNO_3$	169.89	P,V	1.0% aq	7761-88-8	8464	x	
Used in photography, silver plating, coloring porcelain, manufacturing of mirrors, etching ivory, analytical reagent. Astringent and antiseptic agent. **May cause gray-brown discoloration of the conjunctivae and black discoloration of the fingernails.**								
Sodium benzoate	$C_7H_5NaO_2$	144.11	B,C,ME	5.0% pet	532-32-1	8527	x	
Preservative especially for food products (drinks, jams, jellies, pickles, syrups, etc.) Also common in cosmetic and pharmaceutical products. NICU.								
Sodium omadine	C_5H_4NOSNa	149.14	C,O,V	0.1% aq	3811-73-2		x	
Bactericide for use in cooling fluids and short term -in can- preservation of vinyl acetate latex, paints and synthetic fiber lubricants.(Sodium-2-pyridinethiol-1-oxide). Preservative for cosmetic rinse-off products.								
Sorbic acid	$C_6H_8O_2$	112.13	B,C,ME,O,V	2.0% pet	110-44-1	8677	x	x
Preservative (antifungal) in foods like cheese syrup etc. and in cosmetic and pharmaceutical products. Also in alkyd coatings and drying oils, adhesives, glues, inks, paints, varnishes, tanning agents, metalworking fluids. **Cross: potassium sorbate. ICU, NICU.**								

Sorbitan monooleate

C,ME   5.0% pet   1338-43-8   8689   x

Monoester of oleic acid and hexitol anhydrides derived from sorbitol. Emulsifier in cosmetic and pharmaceutical ointments and creams (Span 80). **Cross: sorbitan sesquioleate (Arlacel 83).**

Sorbitan sesquioleate

C,ME   20.0% pet   8007-43-0   x   x

Mixed ester of oleic acid and hexitol anhydrides derived from sorbitol. Emulsifier in cosmetic and pharmaceutical ointments and creams (Arlacel 83).

Stearyl alcohol

$C_{18}H_{38}O$ 270.48   C,ME,TF   30.0% pet   112-92-5   8762   x

Lubricant and antifoam agent in cosmetic and pharmaceutical creams and in textile oils and finishes. UCU.

Streptomycin sulfate

$C_{42}H_{84}O_{36}S_3$ 1457.38   PE,V   1.0% pet   3810-74-0   8786

As bactericide in combination with tetracycline to control fireblight in apples and pears and blight of ornaments like roses, begonias etc. Also used in veterinary medicine and in laboratory research applications to control microbial contamination in tissue culture. **Cross: dihydrostreptomycin, kanamycin, neomycin. May produce systemic contact dermatitis. May cause airborne contact dermatitis.** ICU.

Styrax

F,PL   2.0% pet   8046-19-3   8778   x   x

Balsam obtained from the trunk of trees. Contains cinnamates, styrene, etc. Used in perfumery. **Cross: balsam of Peru, tincture of benzoin, dieythylstilbestrol.**

Sulfanilamide

$C_6H_8N_2O_2S$ 172.21   ME   5.0% pet   63-74-1   8898   x   x

Topical and vaginal antibiotic of sulfonamide type. **Cross (photo): para group of compounds. May produce erythema-multiforme-like eruptions. PA, PL.**

Tanacetum vulgare (Tansy)

PL   1.0% pet*   x   x

A strongly aromatic weed growing in uncultivated areas, along roadsides, rivers etc. Grows all over Europe and in North America. Used as a herbal remedy, for seasoning and for making a tea. The oil is used as a vermifuge and in perfumery. Contains the sesquiterpene lactones arbusculin-A and tanacetin. *) Extract. **Cross: other plants within the Compositae family.**

TABLE A-3. *(Continued)*

Name/Information	Formula	FW	Exp.	RPC	CAS	MI	CT	H
Taraxacum officinale (dandelion)			ME,PL	2.5%pet*				x
Weed that grows in open fields, on prairies, in garbage dumps, etc. and spread all over the world. It is a popular folk medicine plant (laxative, diuretic, tonic, etc.). Allergenic substance is taraxin acid glucoside.*) Extract. **Cross: other plants within the Compositae family. May cause airborne contact dermatitis.**								
Tetracaine hydrochloride	$C_{15}H_{25}ClN_2O_2$	300.83	ME	5.0%pet	136-47-0	9123	x	x
Used as topical and local anesthetic. Amethocaine. **Cross: Amylocaine hydrochloride.**								
Tetrachloro-isophthalonitrile	$C_8Cl_4N_2$	265.89	PE,V	0.001%ac	1897-45-6	2167		
Fungicide used in agriculture to protect potatoes, seed etc. and horticulture and for wood preservation. Also used as fungicide in wet room paints. (Chlorothaloni). **May cause airborne contact dermatitis.**								
3,3′,4′,5-Tetrachloro-salicylanilide	$C_{13}H_7Cl_4NO_2$	351.02	O,PH,V	0.1%pet	1154-59-2	9127	x	x
Bacteriostat in shampoos, surgical and laundry soaps, polishes, rinses, deodorants etc. Also in cooling fluids, textile finishes (Irgasan BS 200, TCS). **Cross (photo): other halogenated salicylanilides, hexachlorophene. PA. PT. PL.**								
Tetraethyleneglycol dimethacrylate	$C_{16}H_{26}O_7$	330.00	MA	2.0%pet	109-17-1		x	
Methacrylate present in adhesives and constitutes the main component in polyethyleneglycol dimethacrylate in Loctite anaerobic sealants.								

Tetraethylthiuram disulfide $C_{10}H_{20}N_2S_4$ 296.54 PE,R,SH,V 1.0% pet 97-77-8 3370 x x
Accelerator, activator, stabilizer and vulcanizing agent for various rubber products. Also as fungicide, seed disinfectant, and alcohol deterrent (disulfiram, antabuse, TETD).

Tetrahydrofurfuryl-methacrylate $C_9H_{15}O_3$ 170.20 D,MN 2.0% pet 2455-24-5 x
Methacrylic component in dental materials such as crown and bridge products. Also a component in artificial nails.

Tetramethylol acetylene-diurea $C_8H_{14}N_4O_6$ 262.23 TF 5.0% aq x
Formaldehyde type of textile finish resin (Fixapret 140).

3,3,5,5-Tetramethyl-benzidine $C_{16}H_{20}N_2$ 240.35 V 0.1% pet 54827-17-7 x
Non carcinogenic substitute for benzidine as reagent for the detection of blood and determination of hemoglobin content.

Tetramethylthiuram disulfide $C_{16}H_{12}N_2S_4$ 240.44 PE,R,SH,V 1.0% pet 137-26-8 9304 x x
Rubber accelerator and vulcanizer. Fungicide, disinfectant for seed, bacteriostat in soap, animal repellent, etc. (Thiram, TMTD). **Cross: tetraethylthiuram monosulfide, tetraethylthiuram disulfide.**

Tetramethylthiuram monosulfide $C_6H_{12}N_2S_3$ 208.37 R,SH 1.0% pet 97-74-5 x
Accelerator and activator for natural rubber nitrile-butadiene and butyl rubber (TMTM).

Thimerosal $C_9H_9HgNaO_2S$ 404.84 C,ME,OP 0.1% pet 54-64-8 9244 x x
Preservative in vaccines, antitoxins, skin testing antigens, antiseptics, eye-drop solutions, contact lens solutions, and cosmetic products like eye makeup (Merthiolate, Thiomersal).

TABLE A-3. (Continued)

Name/Information	Formula	FW	Exp.	RPC	CAS	MI	CT	H
Thiourea	CH_4N_2S	76.12	P,R,V	0.1% pet	62-56-6	9299	x	x
Timolol	$C_{13}H_{24}N_4O_3S$	316.42	ME,OP	0.5% aq	26839-75-8	9374		
Tin	Sn	118.69	D,V	50.0% pet	7440-31-5	9376	x	
Tixocortol-21-pivalate	$C_{26}H_{38}O_5S$	462.35	CS,ME	1.0% pet	55560-96-8	9408	x	
Toluene-2,4-di-isocyanate	$C_9H_6N_2O_2$	174.15	L,PG	2.0% pet	584-84-9	9456	x	x
Toluenesulfonamide formaldehyde resin			C,PG	10.0% pet			x	x

Thiourea
Photographic fixing agent and stain remover. Rubber accelerator. In the manufacture of resins. Antioxidant in photocopy paper to prevent discoloration. **May cause airborne contact dermatitis. PA.**

Timolol
β-Adrenergic blocker used in antihypertensive, antiarrhythmic, antianginal, and antiglaucoma pharmaceuticals.

Tin
Metal used in tin plating, soldering and dental alloys, collapsible tubes. In the production of tin salts.

Tixocortol-21-pivalate
Topical corticosteroid belonging to the group A (hydrocortisone) type of steroids used in nasal sprays for the treatment of rhinitis. Good marker for group A corticosteroid contact allergy. **May cause airborne contact dermatitis.**

Toluene-2,4-di-isocyanate
Used in the production of polyurethane foams, elastomers, adhesives, printing plates, etc. (TDI). **May cause allergic asthma.**

Toluenesulfonamide formaldehyde resin
Modifier and adhesion promotor for film forming natural and synthetic resins. Occurs in vinyl lacquers, nitrocellulose compositions (e.g., nail lacquers), PVA adhesives, acrylics.

4-Tolyldiethanolamine C$_{11}$H$_{17}$NO$_2$ 195.26 D 2.0% pet x
Amine accelerator for the polymerization of e.g. dental acrylic composite restorative materials.

3,4´,5-Tribromo-salicylanilide C$_{13}$H$_8$Br$_3$NO$_2$ 449.96 PH,V 1.0% pet 87-10-5 9529 x x
Bacteriostatic agent in detergents and soaps, disinfectants, pet flea powders (Tribromsalan, TBS). Cross (photo): **bithionol and other halogenated salicylanilides, triclocarban, hexachlorophene, fentichlor. PA, PT.**

3,4,4´-Trichloro-carbanilide C$_{13}$H$_9$Cl$_3$N$_2$O 315.59 PH,V 1.0% pet 101-20-2 9568 x x
Bacteriostat and antiseptic agent in soaps and other cleansing compositions. Disinfectant (Triclocarban, TCC). Cross (photo): **bithionol and other halogenated salicylanilides. PA. PT. May cause pigmentation of the face.**

Triclosan C$_{12}$H$_7$Cl$_3$O$_2$ 289.53 C,PH,V 2.0% pet 3380-34-5 9573 x x
Preservative in cosmetic products, soaps, detergents, shampoos, bath additives, deodorants, foot powders and sprays, disposable paper products, antiodor insoles and hose, laundry products. Also in the treatment of textiles. As antifungal agent in PVC wet room carpets (Irgasan DP 300). **PA.**

Tricresyl phosphate C$_{21}$H$_{21}$O$_4$P 368.36 PG,V 5.0% pet 1330-78-5 9675 x x
Plasticizer in vinyl plastics, spectacle frames. As flame retardant and additive to extreme pressure lubricants. Solvent for nitrocellulose, etc.

Triethanolamine C$_6$H$_{15}$NO$_3$ 149.19 C,O 2.0% pet 102-71-6 9581 x x
Surface-active agent in soaps, shampoos, creams, waxes, cutting oils etc. In making emulsions with mineral and vegetable oils.

Triethyleneglycol-diacrylate C$_{12}$H$_{18}$O$_6$ 258.28 MN,MP 0.1% pet 1680-21-3 x
Cross-linking acrylate monomer for use in coatings, adhesives, and in printing plates of photoprepolymer type (TEGDA).

TABLE A-3. (*Continued*)

Name/Information	Formula	FW	Exp.	RPC	CAS	MI	CT	H
Triethyleneglycol-dimethacrylate	$C_{14}H_{22}O_6$	286.33	D,MA,MN	2.0% pet	109-16-0		x	x
Methacrylic monomer for use as cross-linking agent for adhesives and dental restorative materials (TREGDMA).								
Triethylenetetramine	$C_6H_{18}N_4$	146.23	E,V	0.5% pet	112-24-3	9579	x	x
As thermosetting resin, epoxy curing agent, lubricating oil additive, chelating and analytical agent (TETA).								
Trifluridine	$C_{10}H_{11}F_3N_2O_3$	296.21	OP	5.0% pet	70-00-8	9599		
Antiviral agent in ophthalmic preparations (Trifluorothymidine).								
Triglycidyl isocyanurate	$C_{13}H_{15}N_3O_6$	309.13	PG,V	0.5% pet			x	
Trifunctional epoxy compound used as cross-linker in heat-cured polyester paints such as laminated sheetings, printed circuits, tools, inks, adhesives, lining materials etc. (TGIC). **May cause airborne contact dermatitis.**								
Triamcinolone acetonide	$C_{24}H_{31}FO_6$	434.49	CS,ME	1.0% pet	76-25-5	9512	x	
Topical and systemic corticosteroid belonging to the group B (triamcinolone acetonide) type of steroids.								
2,2,4-Trimethyl-1,2-dihydro-quinoline	$(C_{12}H_{15}N)n$		PG,R,V	1.0% pet				
Antioxidant for use in rubber and plastic materials. Also used in hydraulic fluids and greases (Flectol H, Agerite resin D).								

Trimethylol propane-triacrylate

$C_{15}H_{20}O_6$ 296.31   MN,MP   0.1%pet   15624-89-5   x

Triacrylate for use in UV-curable lithographic inks, varnishes, artificial nails, wood finish solder, and etch resists in the electronics industry (TMPTA).

3,4-Trimethyl-oxazolidine

$C_6H_{15}NO$ 115.18   O,V   1.0%pet*   x

Component in Bioban CS 1135 preservative (2.5%) for use in latex paints, resin emulsions, and cooling fluids.
*) Concentration is valid for Bioban CS 1135.

Triphenyl phosphate

$C_{18}H_{15}O_4P$ 326.28   PG   5.0%pet   115-86-6   9656   x   x

Plasticizer in plastics (e.g., cellulose acetate) lacquers, varnishes, etc. Also in impregnating roofing paper.

Tripropyleneglycol-diacrylate

$C_{15}H_{24}O_6$ 300.36   MP   0.1%pet   42978-66-5   x

Diacrylate monomer for use in UV-curable flexographic and silk screen inks, wood-finish varnishes, coatings on plastics, etc. (TPGDA).

Tromantadine hydrochloride

$C_{16}H_{28}N_2O_2$ 280.41   ME   1.0%pet   53783-83-8   9683

Antiviral agent effective against herpes simplex infections. **Cross: amantadine.**

Turpentine peroxides

O,V   0.3%o.o.   x

Mixture of hydroperoxides of terpenes found in oil of turpentine. Main allergen is the hydroperoxide of delta-3-carene. In solvents or lacquers for printing, etching and art painting. In sealing wax, coolants, tapes, polish, metal cleaners, deodorizers, paints, cosmetics like soaps and bath oils. **Cross: <u>chrysanthemum</u>, pyrethrin. May cause airborne contact dermatitis.**

TABLE A-3. (*Continued*)

Name/Information	Formula	FW	Exp.	RPC	CAS	MI	CT	H
Tylosin tartrate	$C_{46}H_{77}NO_{17}$ x $C_4H_6O_6$	1066.20	ME	5.0% pet	74610-55-2		x	x
Urea formaldehyde	$C_3H_8N_2O_3$	120.11	TF	10.0% pet			x	x
Urethane diacrylate, aliphatic		1500	MP	0.1% pet			x	
Urethane diacrylate, aromatic		1000	MP	0.05% pet			x	
Urethane dimethacrylate	$C_{24}H_{40}N_2O_8$	484.60	DMA	2.0% pet			x	

Tylosin tartrate — Chemotherapeutic agent used to treat pigs with enteritis and household pets with respiratory infections as well as mastitis in cows. **May cause airborne contact dermatitis.**

Urea formaldehyde — Textile finish resin of formaldehyde type for treatment of, e.g., cotton and rayon materials. Also in wood glue industry.

Urethane diacrylate, aliphatic — UV-reactive prepolymer based on an acrylated aliphatic isocyanate. For use in curable coatings, inks, and varnishes (Ebecryl 270).

Urethane diacrylate, aromatic — UV-reactive prepolymer based on an acrylated aromatic isocyanate. For use in curable coatings, inks and varnishes. (Ebecryl 220).

Urethane dimethacrylate — Methacrylate based on a methacrylated aliphatic isocyanate. For use in dental bonding agents, resin veneering, and restorative materials (UEDMA).

(+)-Usnic acid $C_{18}H_{16}O_7$ 344.31   ME,PL   0.1%pet   7562-61-0   9806   x   x

Antibacterial substance found in many lichens. Occurs in oak moss absolute used as fragrance. Preservative in deodorants, antiacne formulations, and as antibiotic for topical application. **Cross: oak moss. May cause airborne contact dermatitis.**

Vanillin $C_8H_8O_3$ 152.14   B,F,ME   10.0%pet   121-33-5   9839   x   x

Flavoring agent in beverages, confectionery, foods, galenicals. In perfumery and pharmaceuticals. Also as chemical reagent. **Cross: coumarin, propolis. ICU.**

Vitamin E acetate $C_{31}H_{52}O_3$ 472.76   B,C,ME,V   10.0%pet   7695-91-2   9806   x

Vitamin E (α-tocopherol) occurs naturally in most vegetable oils. The highest concentrations are found in corn, soybean oils, sunflower seed, wheat germ, rapeseed, alfalfa, and lettuce. It occurs in a number of cosmetic products and is claimed to have age-retardant properties. Vitamin E creams are also used for scars, striae, and burns. Vitamin E is also used in pharmaceutical creams and deodorants and sometimes also as antioxidant in foods. Tocopheryl acetate.

Wool alcohols   C,ME   30.0%pet   x   x

Different types of alcohols (aliphatic, steroid, triterpenoid) present in wool fat (lanolin). As ointment base in cosmetic and pharmaceutical products. **Cross: eucerin, lanette wax.**

Ylang–Ylang oil   F   2.0%pet   10008   x

Fragrance for use in various perfumed products. **Cross: benzyl salicylate, geranial. May cause pigmentation of the face.**

Zinc   Zn   65.38   V   2.5%pet   7440-66-6   10025   x

Metal used for galvanizing sheet iron. Ingredient in alloys (bronze, brass, etc.), protective coatings for other metals, household utensils, etc.

Zinc dibutyldithio-carbamate $C_{18}H_{36}N_2S_4Zn$ 474.14   R   1.0%pet   136-23-2   x

Activator, antidegradant and accelerator for natural rubber, butadiene, styrene-butadiene, nitrile-butadiene, butyl rubber, and ethylene-propylene-diene terpolymers (ZBC).

TABLE A-3. (*Continued*)

Name/Information	Formula	FW	Exp.	RPC	CAS	MI	CT	H
Zinc diethyldithio-carbamate	$C_{10}H_{20}N_2S_4Zn$	361.91	R	1.0% pet	136-94-7		x	
Activator and accelerator for natural rubber, styrene-butadiene, nitrile-butadiene, and butyl rubber (ZDC). **ICU.**								
Zinc dimethyldithio-carbamate	$C_6H_{12}N_2S_4Zn$	305.82	PE,R,V	1.0% pet	137-30-4	10075	x	x
Activator and accelerator for natural rubber, styrene-butadiene, and butyl rubber. Agricultural fungicide for seeds, plants, and fruit (Ziram).								
Zinc ethylenebis-(dithiocarbamate)	$C_4H_6N_2S_4Zn$	275.75	O,PE	1.0% pet	12122-67-7	10071	x	x
Fungicide for use in cooling fluids and as pesticide for seeds, plants, and fruit (Zineb).								
Zinc pyrithione	$C_{10}H_8N_2S_2O_2Zn$	317.70	H	1.0% pet	13463-41-7	8004	x	
Antifungal, antibacterial and antiseborrheic agent used in many shampoos and hair creams (Zinc omadine). Reactions may lead to photosensitive eczema and actinic reticuloid syndrome.								

TABLE A-4. Synonyms and Trade Names in the Table of Contact Antigens

Name	Synonyms
Abitol	Hydroabietyl alcohol
Alantolactone	Helenin
Amethocaine	Tetracaine
Amylocaine HCl	1-dimethylamino-2-methyl-2-butanolbenzoate-hydrochloride: Stovaine
Anthemis nobilis	Chamaemelum nobile
Arlacel 83	Sorbitan sesquioleate
Benzylparaben	Benzyl-4-hydroxybenzoate
Bithionol	2,2-Thiobis(4,6-dichlorophenol)
Bronopol	2-Bromo-2-nitropropane-1,3-diol
Butylparaben	Butyl-4-hydroxybenzoate
Captan	N-(Trichloromethylthio)-4-cyclohexene-1,2-dicarboximide: Vancide 89
Captafol	Difolatan
Chloramine T	N-Chloro-(4-toluenesulfonamido)sodium
Chlorquinaldol	Sterosan: 5,7-Dichloro-2-methyl-8-quinolinol
Cinchocaine	Dibucaine, Percaine
Clioquinol	Chinoform: Vioform: 5-Chloro-7-iodoquinolinol
Cocamide-DEA	Coconut diethanolamide
Diaminodiphenylmethane	Methylenedianiline
Dibucaine-HCl	2-Butoxy-N-(2-(diethylamino)ethyl)-4-quinoline-carboxamide hydrochloride: Cinchocaine
Dioctylphthalate	Di(2-ethylhexyl)phthalate
Disulfiram	Antabuse (tetramethylthiuram disulfide)
Dandelion	Taraxacum officinale
Dowicil 200	1-(3-Chloroallyl)-3,5,7-triaza-1-azoniaadamantane chloride: Quaternium 15
Dodecyl gallate	Lauryl gallate
Ethoxyquin	6-Ethoxy-1,2-dihydroxy-2,2,4-trimethylquinoline
2-Ethylhexyl-4-dimethylaminobenzoate	Octyldimethyl-4-aminobenzoic acid

TABLE A-4. *(Continued)*

Name	Synonyms
Ethylparaben	Ethyl-4-hydroxybenzoate
Feverfew	Chrysanthemum parthenium, Tanacetum parthenium
Germall 115	Imidazolidinylurea, Biopure 100, Euxyl K 200
Germall II	Diazolidinylurea
Hexamin	Hexamethylenetetramine, Urotropin, Aminoform, Formin, Cystamin
Lidocaine	2-(Diethylamino)-N-(2,6-dimethyl-phenyl)acetamide: Lignocaine, Xylocaine
Limonene	Dipentene
Methylhydroquinone	Toluhydroquinone
Methylparaben	Methyl-4-hydroxybenzoate
Metol	4-Methylaminophenol sulfate
Mountain Tobacco	Arnica montana
Phenidone	1-Phenyl-3-pyrazolidone
Prilocaine	N-(2-Methylphenyl)-2(propylamino)propanamide: Propitocaine
Primin	2-Methoxy-6-n-pentyl-4-benzoquinone
Procaine-HCl	Novocaine, Ethocaine, Allocaine, Topocaine, Neocaine, Syncaine
Promethazine-HCl	Phenergan, Lergigan, Atosil, Fenazil
Propylparaben	Propyl-4-hydroxybenzoate
Pyrethrum	Chrysanthemum cinerariaefolium
Salol	Phenyl salicylate
Sodiumomadine	Sodium-2-pyridinethiol-1-oxide
Span 80	Sorbitan monooleate
Tansy	Tanacetum vulgare
Tetracaine HCl	4-(Butylamino)benzoic acid-2-(dimethylaminoethyl ester hydrochloride: Amethocaine HCl
Tetrachloroisophthalonitrile	Chlorothalonil
Thimerosal	Merthiolate: Thiomersal
Tribromsalan	3,4,5-Tribromsalicylanilide
Triclocarban	3,4,4-Trichlorcarbanilide
Triclosan	2,4,4-Trichloro-2-hydroxydiphenyl ether: Irgasan DP 300
Tween 80	Polyoxysorbitan monooleate
Yarrow	Achillea millefolium
Zineb	Zinc ethylenebis(dithiocarbamate)
Ziram	Zinc dimethyldithiocarbamate
Zinc pyrithione	Zinc omadine, Vancide

TABLE A-5.   Active Components and Trade Names in the Table of Contact Antigens

Active Component	Trade Names
1-Aza-3,7-dioxa-5-ethylbicyclo(3,3,0)octane	Bioban CS 1246
4-tert.Butyl-4'-methoxy-dibenzoylmethane	Parsol 1789
5-Chloro-2-methyl-4-isothiazolin-3-one +	
2-Methyl-4-isothiazolin-3-one	*Kathon CG*, Acticide, Algucid CH 50, Amerstat 250, Euxyl K 100, Fennosan IT 21, GR 856 Izolin, Grotan TK2, Kathon 886 MW, Kathon LX, Kathon WT, Mergal K7, Metatin GT, Mitco CC 31L, Mitco CC 32L, Special Mx 323, Parmetol DF 35, -DF 12, -A23, -K50, -K40, -DF18, -P3, Multan D, Piror P109.
Cocamidopropyl betaine	Tegobetaine L7
Cycloaliphatic epoxy resin	Araldit CY 184
Cyclohexanone resin, condensation product	Laropal K 80
Diazolidinylurea	Germall II
1,2-Dibromo-2,4-dicyanobutane	Tektamer 38
1,2-Dibromo-2,4-dicyanobutane +	
2-Phenoxyethanol	Euxyl K 400
Dicyclohexylmethane-4,4-diisocyanate	Desmodur W
Dimethylol dihydroxyethylene urea	Fixapret CPN
Dimethylol propylene urea	Fixapret PH
3,4-Dimethyloxazolidine +	
3,4,4-Trimethyloxazolidine	Bioban CS 1135
Ethyleneurea, melamineformaldehyde	Fixapret AC
2-Ethylhexyl-4-dimethylaminobenzoate	Eusolex 6007, Escalol 507
2-Ethylhexyl-4-methoxycinnamate	Parsol MCX, Escalol 557
Hexahydro-1,3,5-tris(2-hydroxyethyl)triazine	Grotan BK, Bacillat 35
2-Hydroxy-4-methoxybenzophenone	Eusolex 4360, Escalol 567, Oxybenzone
2-Hydroxy-4-methoxy-benzophenon-5-sulfonic acid	Sulizobenzone, Uvinyl MS 40, Benzophenone 4
2-Hydroxy-methoxymethylbenzophenone	Mexenone
2-Hydroxymethyl-2-nitro-1,3-propanediol	Tris nitro
2(2-Hydroxy-5-methylphenyl)benzotriazol	Tinuvin P
Imidazolidinyl urea	Germall 115, Imidurea NF, Sept 115, Unicide U-13, Tristat IU Biopure 100

TABLE A-5. *(Continued)*

Active Component	Trade Names
4-Isopropyl-dibenzoylmethane	Eusolex 8020
Lanolin alcohols	Amerchol L 101
Melamine formaldehyde	Kaurit M 70
3-(4-Methylbenzyliden)camphor	Eusolex 6300
N-Methylolchloroacetamide	Grotan HD, Parmetol K 50
N-Methylolchloroacetamide +	
5-Chloro-2-methyl-4-isothiazolin-3-one	Parmetol A 23
4-(2-Nitrobutyl)morpholine +	
4,4-(2-Ethyl-2-nitrotrimethylene)-	
dimorpholine	Bioban P 1487
2-n-Octyl-4-isothiazolin-3-one	Kathon 893, Skane M-8
Oligotriacrylate	OTA 480
Phenylbenzimidazol-5-sulfonic acid	Eusolex 232, Novantisol
Phenylmercuric acetate	Advacide PMA 18, Cosan PMA, Mergal A25, Metasol 30, Nildew
	AC 30, Nuodex PMA 18, Nylmerate, Troysan
2-Phenylphenol	Dowicide 1, Preventol O
3,3′,4′,5-Tetrachlorosalicylanilide	Irgasan BS 200
Tetramethylol acetylene diurea	Fixapret 140
2,2,4-Trimethyl-1,2-dihydroquinoline	Agerite resin D, Flectol H
Urea formaldehyde	Kaurit S
Urethanediacrylate (aromatic)	Ebecryl 220
Urethanediacrylate (aliphatic)	Ebecryl 270

REFERENCES

1. Marks JG, DeLeo VA: *Contact and Occupational Dermatology.* St. Louis, Mosby-Year Book, 1992.
2. Rycroft RJ, Menne'T, Frosch PJ, Benezra C: *Textbook of Contact Dermatitis.* Berlin, Springer-Verlag, 1992.
3. Budavari S, O'Neil MJ, Smith A, Heckelmann PE: *The Merck Index.* 11th ed. Rahway, NJ, Merck & Co., Inc., 1989.
4. Adams RM: *Occupational Skin Disease.* 2d ed. Philadelphia, Saunders, 1990.
5. Niklasson B: *Product Catalogue 1992/93.* Malmö, Sweden, Chemotechnique Diagnostics, 1992.
6. Nater P, de Groot AC: *Unwanted Effects of Cosmetics and Drugs Used in Dermatology.* 2d ed. Amsterdam, Elsevier, 1985.
7. de Groot AC: *Patch Testing.* Amsterdam, Elsevier, 1986.
8. Dooms-Goossens AE, Debusschere KM, Gevers DM: Contact dermatitis caused by airborne agents. *J Am Acad Dermatol* 15:1, 1986.
9. Dooms-Goossens AE, Deleu H: Airborne contact dermatitis: An update. *Contact Dermatitis* 25:211, 1991.
10. Kabara JJ: *Cosmetic and Drug Preservation.* New York, Dekker, 1984.
11. Benezra C, Ducombs G, Sell Y, Fousserau J: *Plant Contact Dermatitis.* Philadelphia, B.C. Decker Inc., 1985.
12. Fisher AA: *Contact Dermatitis,* 3d ed. Philadelphia, Lea & Febiger, 1986.
13. Herbst RA, Maibach HI: Contact dermatitis caused by allergy to ophthalmic drugs and contact lens solutions. *Contact Dermatitis* 25:305, 1991.

APPENDIX B

QUESTIONNAIRE FOR CONTACT DERMATITIS

Date _____ 19 _____

Name _____ Age _____ Sex _____

Address _____

City _____

State _____ Zip _____

Telephone: Home ( ) _____ Work ( ) _____

Occupation _____

Employer _____

_____

Referred by _____

Address _____

City _____

State _____ Zip _____

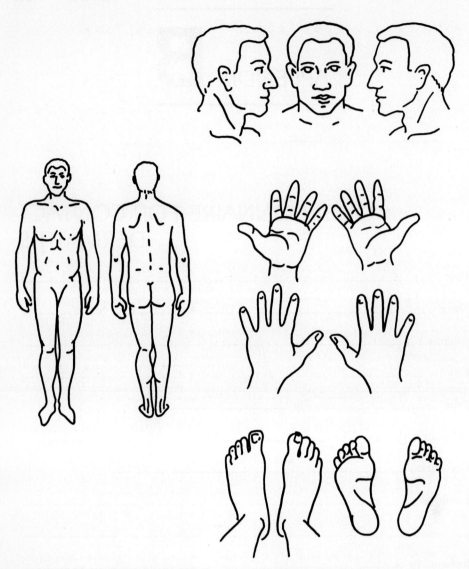

Please indicate the areas where you have broken out by shading them on the diagram (opposite page).

How long have you had the condition? _____

Does it get better: Away from work? _____

On weekends? _____

On vacations? _____

Away from home? _____

Have you ever been found to be allergic to anything? _____

What? _____

Jewelry, such as earrings, or watch band? _____

A cologne, perfume, deodorant, after-shave, cosmetic, or lotion? _____

Which? _____

Have you changed cosmetics? _____ What? _____ When? _____

Have you ever broken out to shoes? _____ Boots or sandals? _____

Gloves? _____ Clothing? _____ Hair dye? _____

Have you ever reacted to any medication you have applied? _____

Have you ever had patch-testing done? _____

If so, what, if anything, was positive? _____

_____

Did you ever have eczema (perhaps as a baby)? _____

Asthma? _____ Allergic runny nose? _____

Sinus problems? _____ Migraine? _____

Hives due to food? _____ Rubber? _____ Cosmetics? _____ Plants? _____

Have you (or a family member) ever had psoriasis? _____

Do you get worse in sunlight? _____ Outdoors? _____

Have you ever had a chronic unresponsive athlete's foot? _____

If so, was the diagnosis proved with a scraping or culture? _____

Have you been given a medication by a neighbor or relative?

What? _____
Please list all medications you have applied since the condition started:

1. _____   7. _____

2. _____   8. _____

3. _____   9. _____

4. _____   10. _____

5. _____   11. _____

6. _____   12. _____

Now circle those you have used in the last month.

Please list all cosmetics, after-shave lotions, colognes, sunscreens, hair dressings and shampoos, children's shampoo, and any other items applied in personal care:

1. _____   7. _____

2. _____   8. _____

3. _____   9. _____

4. _____   10. _____

5. _____   11. _____

6. _____   12. _____

Please note any recent outdoor activity:

Yard work _____ Camping _____ Pulling weeds _____ Picnics _____

Fishing _____ Cutting or gathering firewood _____ Mowing grass _____

Do you wear gloves? _____

Cloth? _____ Leather? _____

Rubber? _____ Plastic? _____

Have you applied a medication under your gloves? _____

What moisturizers (lotions and creams) have you used?

1. _____   5. _____

2. _____   6. _____

3. _____   7. _____

4. _____   8. _____

What detergent do you use to wash clothes? _____

How much do you use? _____ Do you measure? _____

What soap do you use to bathe or shower? _____

How often do you shampoo your own hair? _____ your children's hair? _____

What shampoo do you use? _____

How often do you bathe/shower? _____

Do you use a washcloth? _____

Do you bathe in hot/warm/tepid water? _____

What are your hobbies? Photography _____ Woodworking _____

Gardening _____ Automotive repair _____ Crafts _____ Cooking _____

Sewing _____ Furniture refinishing _____ Carpentry _____

Construction or masonry _____ Electronics _____

Others? Please list _____

Do you use any glues, paints, varnishes, or other such chemicals? _____

Do you do small engine repair? _____

What are your athletic activities?

Golf _____ Tennis _____ Swimming _____ Scuba diving _____ Running _____

Hiking _____ Softball _____ Football _____ Cycling _____ Skating _____

Bowling _____ Riding _____ Exercise _____ Aerobics _____ Ballet _____

Dancing _____ Others? Please name _____

Does the affected area contact any item of equipment you might wear or use? _____

If so, what? _____

OCCUPATIONAL HISTORY

Date _____ 19 _____

Name _____ Age _____ Sex _____

Address _____

City _____

State _____ Zip _____

Telephone: Home (   ) _____ Work (   ) _____

Occupation _____

Job Title _____

Place of Employment _____

Are you currently working? _____ If not, for how long have you been unemployed?

_____

Do you need approval at this visit to remain away from work? _____

Is this condition the result of a specific injury or accident? _____

If yes, what is the date? _____ Is this exact _____ or approximate? _____

Give details of this incident:

_____

_____

_____

_____

_____

_____

_____

_____

Is there an attorney involved who is to receive a report? _____

Name _____

Address _____

Do *you* associate your condition with your work? _____

Why? _____

_____

_____

_____

_____

_____

What do you do at work? _____

_____

Can you describe your daily tasks very simply, so that a child could understand? Use the back of the form if you do not have enough space.

_____

_____

_____

_____

_____

_____

_____

Is there any task you do or anything to which you are exposed that seems to be

causing or aggravating the problem? _____

Is anyone else in your area breaking out? _____

If yes, how many? _____ For how long? _____

Is the rash they have in the same location as yours? _____

Do you work with metals? _____ Ink? Ultraviolet-cured ink or resins? _____

Permanent-wave solutions? _____ Hair dye? _____ Bleach? _____

Cleansers? _____ Solvents? _____ Germicides? _____ Detergents? _____

Are you in contact with chemicals? _____ Medications? _____ Glues? _____

Do you work with coolants? _____ Solder? _____ Rosin? _____ Plastics? _____

Rubber? _____ Acids? _____ Alkalis? _____ Plants? _____ Foods? _____

Construction materials? _____ Formaldehyde? _____ Cement? _____

Do you work with trichloroethylene? _____ Methyl ethyl ketone (MEK)? _____

Solvents? _____

How do you clean your hands after work? _____

Name of soap or hand cleaner _____

How long does this take? _____

Do you wear protective gloves? _____ Clothing? _____ Salves? _____

Do you know the type of your special protective gloves? _____

If so please provide the type or name _____

What treatments have you received at work? _____

_____

Do you have Material Safety Data Sheets for the chemical and other materials in

your work area? _____ Did you bring them? _____

Insurance carrier for workmen's compensation claims

_____

_____

_____

Telephone number (if known) for contact (   ) _____

Summary of pertinent workup and history from referring physician:

_____

_____

_____

_____

_____

Summary of pertinent physical findings:

_____

_____

_____

_____

Photographs taken? Dates _____

Letter to referring physician, company, attorney dictated: Date _____

APPENDIX C

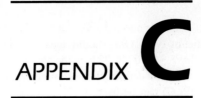

QUALITATIVE TESTS

METHOD OF TESTING FOR UNHARDENED BISPHENOL A TYPE OF EPOXY (TLC METHOD)[1,2]

The method of testing is as follows:

Chloroform/acetonitrile 90%:10% is solvent system.

1 *M* sulfuric acid is first spray reagent.

Anisaldehyde in methanol 2.5% in acetone (vol/vol) is second spray reagent.

A standard of 1% low-molecular-weight resin (weight/volume) is used as the positive control.

Ethanol extraction is made of solid samples. This may take from a few minutes to 24 h.

The extract is evaporated to a few milliliters.

2 to 5 μL of standard solution is applied a few millimeters from edge of the TLC silica plate.

2 to 5 μL of the sample to be tested is also applied next to the standard spot.

Dilutions of the unknown may be used for solids or when the concentration is unknown.

Allow the solvent of the samples to evaporate dry (a few minutes).

Develop in chloroform/acetonitrile in a glass tank.

Air dry.

Two methods are used for visualization:

1. Ultraviolet Light Method
   Examine by UV light, looking for darker spots as evidence of lower-molecular-weight oligomers. This is ten times as sensitive as detection with sprayed plates.[1]
2. Spray Method
   Spray with sulfuric acid until moist.
   Spray lightly with anisaldehyde.
   Dry 10 min at 110°C.
   Violet spots appear with smaller epoxy oligomers at the top.
   Weight corresponds to the standard(s).

A single dark spot in UV light or a violet spot is not sufficient to identify unhardened epoxy resin of the bisphenol type. One should look for spots corresponding to its different oligomers (e.g., MW 340, 624). This is the standard test for epoxy oligomers in uncured resins. In systems where certain plasticizers cause interference, high-pressure liquid chromatography (HPLC) can be used.[1]

METHOD OF TESTING FOR BISPHENOL A TYPE OF EPOXY (FILTER-PAPER METHOD)[1]

The method of testing is as follows:

Dissolve about 0.1 g of the sample in 2 mL of concentrated sulfuric acid by heating 40 to 50°C on a water bath.

Dilute as necessary to produce a color (orange) equivalent to that of 0.1 M potassium dichromate solution.

Using a glass rod, streak a drop of epoxy solution across a filter paper.

A positive test will turn purple in 1 min; ultimately, it turns blue.

A bisphenol A monomer should be used as a positive control.

Both cured and uncured epoxy resins should show a positive test. Certain oils (fish, tung, and linseed treated with cyclopentadiene), rosin, and certain phenolic resins also give positive tests, so this test is used at most for screening purposes.

While this method has appeal because of its ease and simplicity, it is less specific and Fregert considers it to be of limited value.

SPOT TEST FOR NICKEL

1. Two reagents are used in the test: 1% dimethylglyoxime in alcohol and 10% ammonia water.
2. A few drops of each reagent are placed on a cotton-tipped applicator so that it is moist. Two or three are usually enough.
3. The metal surface is rubbed with the applicator and observed for a red color.
4. The color change to red indicates the presence of free nickel.

A positive test is important, but a negative test is no guarantee. While this very simple test will detect relatively low levels of free nickel, some very sensitive persons may occasionally break out to metal objects that test negative. "Hypoallergenic" jewelry often does not have enough free nickel to cause a rash, but testing an object first is advised, as some articles that are said to be safe may not be.

Steel other than stainless steel is suspect, and even stainless can occasionally cause a problem. However, one can test jewelry and metal objects for free nickel with a "nickel spot test." Test kits for this purpose can easily be made up by a local pharmacist. Dimethylglyoxime is the only ingredient that must be ordered, as the others are standard items. If such kits are dispensed on prescription, written instructions should accompany them. A commercial product is marketed by Allerderm Laboratories. If your local pharmacy does not carry it, you can purchase one by mail from the Skin and Allergy Shop, 310 East Broadway, Louisville, KY 40202 or calling (800) 366-6483.

COBALT ANALYSIS[3]

The pH of a solution to be tested should be adjusted to 7 to 8. A 1% aqueous solution of 2-nitroso-1-naphthol-4-sulfonic acid is added to test for cobalt. This reagent supposedly detects cobalt by producing a red coloration.

According to Fregert,[2] no reliable spot test for cobalt is available. For cobalt in solution, he suggests the use of UV spectroscopy with alpha-nitroso-beta-naphthol as a reagent; but atomic absorption is probably the best method.

SPOT TEST FOR HEXAVALENT CHROMIUM*[2,4]

Reagents are as follows:

1. Concentrated sulfuric acid.
2. Diphenylcarbazide 0.5% to 1.0% dissolved in absolute alcohol which has been adjusted to <pH 2 by addition of a few drops of sulfuric acid. Dissolution may require ultrasonic mixing.[4]

For a solution containing suspected (hexavalent) chromium, add a few drops of concentrated sulfuric acid and then a few drops of 0.5% *sym*-diphenylcarbazide in ethanol. A red color indicates the presence of chromate or dichromate.

For a positive control, use a match head dipped in water to which a few drops of the reagents have been added. For solid objects, dip the object in water and test the dilute solution as above. Iron causes a false-positive reaction.

LUTIDINE (ACETYLACETONE) METHOD FOR DETECTION OF FORMALDEHYDE[5]

Formaldehyde can be detected by two methods that seem to complement each other. Fregert et al.[5] have reported a method using acetylacetone.

Reagents are as follows:

Ammonium acetate 15 g
Acetylacetone 0.2 mL
Glacial acetic acid 0.3 mL
Distilled water to 100 mL

All chemicals must be analytical grade.

Reagents should be made up at the time of the test for most purposes. Investigators who test regularly may make up reagents weekly.

Stock solutions can be made of formaldehyde 100 μg/mL, 2.5 μg/mL, 5 μg/mL, and 10 μg/mL. These also should be made up weekly and kept under refrigeration.

---

*Note: This test is usually done together with atomic absorption spectroscopy, used for quantitative readings.

QUALITATIVE METHOD

The sample to be tested (0.5g for solid samples; 1.0 mL for liquid samples) is placed in a glass jar (25-mL capacity, approximately) with a glass stopper.

Oily materials (e.g., ointments) should be emulsified using a formaldehyde-free emulsifier. Fregert uses Triton X-100 (Merck) as an example.

Solids are used as is.

Place 1 mL of each standard formaldehyde solution in a glass jar (as a positive control) and 1 mL distilled water in a glass jar (as a negative control). Add 2.5 mL of the reagent to each glass jar and agitate.

Warm to 60°C in a heated cabinet for 10 min.

A yellow color indicates the presence of formaldehyde (not used with yellow or green substances).

QUANTITATIVE METHOD

Estimate the reading by the qualitative method.

Use standard formaldehyde solutions of 2.5, 5.0, 10.0, and 20.0 μg/mL.

Make an aqueous solution of the sample calculated to approximate 10 μg/mL.

Place in 10-mL volumetric flasks 1 mL distilled water and 1 mL of the dissolved sample and stock solutions.

Add 1.5 mL of the reagent to each flask.

Heat at 60°C in a cabinet for 10 min, cool to room temperature, and add water to make 10 mL.

Measure the absorption of each sample in a spectrophotometer at 412 nm.

Plot a graph of readings for the standard reagents and locate the reading of the unknown on the graph. Read the amount of formaldehyde from the graph.

For colored products, butanol extraction is necessary.

Check the color extraction by adding N-butanol to confirm that the color is not extractable with N-butanol.

Place 2 mL of each solution, the control, and the sample in separate centrifugation tubes.

Add 4 mL of N-butanol to each tube.

Agitate for 30 s.

Centrifuge for 10 min.

Measure the N-butanol extract at 412 nm in a spectrophotometer.

Measure the N-butanol extract of the standard samples in the same manner and plot a graph.

Read the level detected by plotting the reading on the graph.

CHROMOTROPIC ACID TEST FOR FORMALDEHYDE[6]

The procedure is as follows below.

The reagent is made up with 40 mg of chromotrophic acid in 10 mL concentrated sulfuric acid.

Three or more glass jars (25 to 50 mL in volume) with ground glass stoppers are used to hold the test tubes used for analysis, one each for the positive and negative controls and one for each sample.

The positive control is 10 μg/mL formaldehyde in a 2- to 3-mL test tube to which 0.5 mL of the reagent is added. This is placed in a glass jar (as above) and labeled.

The negative control is 0.5 mL of the reagent in a 2- to 3-mL test tube. The jar is then marked or labeled.

The sample should be about 0.5 to 1.0 g or 3 to 5 cm² of textile material. Measure and add 0.5 mL of the reagent to the sample in a 2- to 3-mL test tube and place it in a clearly labeled separate glass jar.

The jars are kept in a dark place and observed at 1 to 2 days. A violet color is considered positive. Multiple standards allow rough quantitation.

Some precautions are in order in the chromotropic acid test. The glassware must be washed with detergent, rinsed with distilled water, and stored in a dust-free place.

Some samples of chromotropic acid turn color with time.

Acetone, methylethylketone, other ketones, proprionaldehyde, isopropanol, and propanol will cause discoloration.

Organic material causes a yellow color to appear.

Perfumes and substances causing discoloration may be a problem in many cosmetic products.

Polyethylene glycols form formaldehyde when heated.

The laboratory facilities should be equipped to handle concentrated sulfuric acid with all necessary safety precautions.

ANALYSIS FOR FORMALDEHYDE IN FABRICS[7]

Vapor extraction is used to extract formaldehyde from fabric. Fineman[7] calls the "sealed jar test" of the American Association of Textile Chemists and Colorists (AATCC Test Method 112-1982) one of the most severe extraction procedures for formaldehyde in textiles. The fabric is suspended in hot water vapor in a sealed jar, either at 49°C for 20 h or at 65°C for 4 h.

The sample is cooled to room temperature and the liquid is analyzed for formaldehyde spectrophotometrically, usually with acetylacetone. This method measures both free and cross-linked formaldehyde.

Results in AATCC Method 112-1982 depend upon the humidity in the jar, the length of extraction, and the oven temperature; higher formaldehyde levels are given when the length of extraction, the temperature used, or the humidity is increased.

Following extraction, analysis for formaldehyde can be done by any of several methods given, but usually it is done by the lutidine method described above using acetylacetone, which reacts with formaldehyde in the presence of ammonia to form a yellow compound, 3,5-diacetyl-1,4-dihydrolutidine.

Lutidines are dimethyl derivatives of pyridine. This method is relatively specific for formaldehyde. The chromotropic acid determination has been given previously. It is less specific than the lutidine or Nash test, as several agents produce interference. A more sensitive reagent is 3-methyl-2-benzothiazolinone hydrazone hydrochloride (MBTH), which forms a violet color with formaldehyde.

Pararosaniline combined with sulfite (Schiff's reagent) gives a rose-violet color and is specific for formaldehyde at 560 nm.

Table C-1, gives the relative sensitivity of analytical tests for extracted formaldehyde. Wall,[4] however, says that the limit of detection is 2.5 μg/mL for chromotropic acid test and 1 μg/mL for the Lutidine (acetylacetone) method.

TABLE C–1. Relative Sensitivity of Analytical Tests for Extracted Formaldehyde

Method	Minimum Conc., Detectable, μg/mL	Wavelength, Max., nm	Interferences
Chromotropic acid	0.25	580	Nitrogen dioxide, alkenes, phenol, acrolein, acetaldehyde
Pararosaniline	0.1	570	Sulfur dioxide, cyanide
	0.1	560	Specific
MBTH	0.05	628	Higher aldehydes
Lutidine	1.4	412	Specific

Source: From Feinman.[7] Used with permission.

WHAT FOLLOWS BELOW IS PRESENTED FOR COMPARISON RATHER THAN FOR PRACTICAL USE[7]

LIQUID EXTRACTION PROCEDURES

Cold Sulfite Analysis

This method measures free or unbound formaldehyde in textiles. The sample is incubated with sodium sulfite for 7 min at 0 to 10°C. This produces a bisulfite adduct and sodium hydroxide. The reaction product is then assayed by acid-base titration or by iodometry. The procedure is somewhat laborious but it is considered a good method to measure unbound formaldehyde.

Potassium Cyanide Measurement of Formaldehyde and Methylols

Cold extraction is used and formaldehyde and methylol groups are measured by their reaction with a known concentration of potassium cyanide to produce glyconitrile. The unreacted potassium cyanide is titrated with nickel sulfate to calculate the total free and released formaldehyde. Cold sulfite analysis can be performed simultaneously and the total formaldehyde subtracted to calculate N-methylol groups present.

Shirley Institute Method

This method is milder than the Nash method and was developed at the Shirley Institute to extract those fabric agents to which skin is normally exposed. Aqueous extraction procedure (10:1 liquid to fabric) is used at 20°C. The filtrate is subsequently measured spectrophotometrically with chromotropic acid and hot sulfuric acid. Problems with interference using chromotropic acid have been outlined above.

Japanese Test Method—Law 112-1973

A fabric sample is extracted by soaking for 1 h in water at 40°C (100:1 liquid-to-fabric ratio). This ostensibly simulates dissolution in sweat at body temperature. The Nash method is used with acetylacetone and spectroscopy.

Gas Chromatography

After weighing, a fabric sample is sealed in a glass vial and maintained at 65°C. For analysis, a needle is used to pierce the vial stopper and inject a portion of the head-space vapor onto the separation column of a specially modified gas chromatogram with a flame ionization detector.

Results are reproducible with levels between the Nash and Japanese method, which are higher, and the cold sulfite test, which is lower.

From a practical standpoint, many use the chromatropic acid test as a screening test. If it proves negative, the levels are probably relatively safe for most people. One must understand, however, that this method is less specific.

REFERENCES

1. Fregert S, Trulsson L: Simple methods for demonstration of epoxy resins of bisphenol A type. *Contact Dermatitis* 4:69–72, 1978.
2. Fregert S: Physicochemical methods for detection of contact allergens. *Dermatol Clin* 6:97–104, 1988.
3. Fisher AA: *Contact Dermatitis*. Philadelphia, Lea & Febiger, 1986, p. 723.
4. Wall LM: Spot tests and chemical analyses for allergen evaluation, in Rycroft RJG, Menne T, Frosch PJ, et al (eds): *Textbook of Contact Dermatitis*. Berlin, Springer-Verlag, 1992, pp. 277–285.
5. Fregert S, Dahlquist I, Gruvberger B: A simple method for the detection of formaldehyde. *Contact Dermatitis* 10:132–134, 1984.
6. Dahlquist I, Fregert S, Gruvberger B: Reliability of the chromotropic acid method for qualitative formaldehyde determination. *Contact Dermatitis* 6:357–358, 1980.
7. Feinman S: *Formaldehyde Sensitivity and Toxicity*. Boca Raton, FL, CRC Press, 1988.

INDEX

Note: Page numbers in italics indicate figures; page numbers followed by the letter "t" indicate tables.

AACAlc (alpha amylcinnamic alcohol), sensitivity to, 214
AACAld. *See* Alpha amylcinnamic aldehyde (AACAld)
Abietic acid, 708t
Abitol, 708t
Absolutes, in fragrances, 357
Accupatch test, 46
ACD. *See* Allergic contact dermatitis (ACD)
Achillea millefolium, 708t
Acid yellow 36, 708t
Acidic solutions, buffering of, 69
Acneiform irritant contact dermatitis, 9, 9t
Acrylates, epoxy, 443, 731t
Acrylic resin inhibitors, 409
Acrylic resin polymerization activators, 408–409
Acrylics, 447–457
  avoidance of exposure to, 457
  chain polymerization and, 447–449, *449*
  chemistry of, 447–450, *448, 449*
  cross-sensitivities and, 453–454
  dental. *See* Dental products
  irritation caused by, 456–457
  light-sensitive, 455–456
  nail complications caused by, 455
  patch testing with, 451, 452t–453t, 453–454
  recognition of sensitivity to, 450, *451*
  sources of contact with, 454–455
ACTH. *See* Adrenocorticotropic hormone (ACTH) gel
Acyclovir (Zovirax), 564t
Adhesives
  for patch testing, 52–53
  in shoes, 329–330
Adrenocorticotropic hormone (ACTH) gel, for allergic contact dermatitis, acute, 676
Age, irritant contact dermatitis and, 12
Agricultural chemicals, sensitivity to, 163–164
  morphology of reactions, 163–164
Airborne dermatitis, 55
  nickel causing, 274
  thiuram causing, 182
Alantolactone, 708t

Alclometasone-17,21-dipropionate, 708t
Alcohols
  benzyl, 714t
  cetyl, 718t
  cinnamic. *See* Cinnamic alcohol
  hydrocortisone, frequency of sensitivity to, 577, *577*
  lanolin (wool). *See* Lanolin (wool) alcohols
  stearyl, 753t
Alkaline solutions, buffering of, 69
Allergens, 97–293. *See also* Allergic contact dermatitis; Allergic contact dermatitis (ACD); *specific allergens*
  compound, 64
  concentration, 705
  contact, 3–4
    determinants of substances acting as, 3–4, *4*
    for patch testing. *See* Patch testing
  photocontact, 50
  sensitizing index of, 50
Allergic contact dermatitis (ACD), 31–39, 49–59, 50t. *See also specific allergens*
  acute, treatment of, 676t, 676–678
    compresses in, 677–678
    hyposensitization in, 677
    local corticosteroids in, 677
    recognizing and removing allergen and, 676
    systemic corticosteroids in, 676
  airborne, 55
  chromate causing, *662*
  chronic, treatment of, 678t, 678–680
    avoidance of cause and, 678
    environmental control and antigen substitution for, 679–680
    hazards of home and other treatment and, 679
    home treatment and, 680
    identification of specific allergens and, 678–679
  clothing causing. *See* Clothing dermatitis
  dermal, 51–52
  diagnosis of, 55, 58
  distribution in, 34
  education and, 58–59
  erythema multiforme in, 38
  formaldehyde causing, 199
  fragrances causing, *360,* 360–361, *361*
  of hands, 650–651

ISBN 0-07-025169-X

90000>

9 780070 251694